Textbook of Human Histology

with Color Atlas, 3D Illustrations and Flowcharts

As per CBME Guidelines | Competency Based Undergraduate Curriculum for the Indian Medical Graduate

Other book from the same author
Textbook of Human Embryology with Clinical Cases and 3D Illustrations

Textbook of Human Histology

with Color Atlas, 3D Illustrations and Flowcharts

As per CBME Guidelines | Competency Based Undergraduate Curriculum for the Indian Medical Graduate

Yogesh Ashok Sontakke MBBS MD

Additional Professor, Department of Anatomy
Jawaharlal Institute of Postgraduate Medical Education and Research (JIPMER)
(An Institute of National Importance under The Ministry of Health and Family Welfare, Government of India),
Puducherry, India

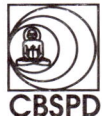

CBSPD

CBS Publishers & Distributors Pvt Ltd

New Delhi • Bengaluru • Chennai • Kochi • Kolkata • Lucknow • Mumbai
Hyderabad • Jharkhand • Nagpur • Patna • Pune • Uttarakhand

Disclaimer

Science and technology are constantly changing fields. New research and experience broaden the scope of information and knowledge. The author has tried his best in giving information available to him while preparing the material for this book. Although all efforts have been made to ensure optimum accuracy of the material, yet it is quite possible some errors might have been left uncorrected. The publisher, the printer and the author will not be held responsible for any inadvertent errors, omissions or inaccuracies.

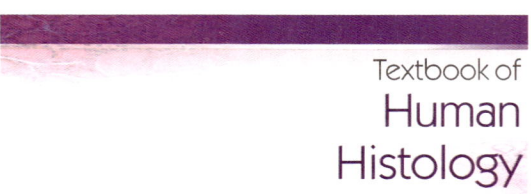

Textbook of **Human Histology**

with Color Atlas, 3D Illustrations and Flowcharts
As per CBME Guidelines | Competency Based Undergraduate Curriculum for the Indian Medical Graduate

ISBN: 978-81-94125-42-6

Copyright © Author and Publisher

Illustrations and Images © Yogesh Sontakke

First Edition: 2020
 Reprint: 2020
 Updated reprint: 2021, 2022

All rights reserved. No part of this book may be reproduced or transmitted in any form or by any means, electronic or mechanical, including photocopying, recording, or any information storage and retrieval system without permission, in writing, from the author and the publisher.

Published by Satish Kumar Jain and produced by Varun Jain for

CBS Publishers & Distributors Pvt Ltd
4819/XI Prahlad Street, 24 Ansari Road, Daryaganj, New Delhi 110 002, India.
Ph: 011-23289259, 23266861, 23266867 Fax: 011-23243014 Website: www.cbspd.com
 e-mail: delhi@cbspd.com; cbspubs@airtelmail.in

Corporate Office: 204 FIE, Industrial Area, Patparganj, Delhi 110 092
Ph: 011-4934 4934 Fax: 011-4934 4935 e-mail: publishing@cbspd.com; publicity@cbspd.com

Branches

- **Bengaluru:** Seema House 2975, 17th Cross, K.R. Road, Banasankari 2nd Stage, Bengaluru 560 070, Karnataka, India
  Ph: +91-80-26771678/79 Fax: +91-80-26771680 e-mail: bangalore@cbspd.com
- **Chennai:** 7, Subbaraya Street, Shenoy Nagar, Chennai 600 030, Tamil Nadu, India
  Ph: +91-44-26680620, 26681266 Fax: +91-44-42032115 e-mail: chennai@cbspd.com
- **Kochi:** 42/1325, 1326, Power House Road, Opp KSEB, Power House, Ernakulam 682 018, Kerala, India
  Ph: +91-484-4059061-65 Fax: +91-484-4059065 e-mail: kochi@cbspd.com
- **Kolkata:** 147, Hind Ceramics Compound, 1st Floor, Nilgunj Road, Belghoria, Kolkata-700056,
  West Bengal, India
  Ph: +91-33-25633055/56 e-mail: kolkata@cbspd.com
- **Lucknow:** Basement, Khushnuma Complex, 7-Meerabai Marg (Behind Jawahar Bhawan) Lucknow 226001, India
  Ph: +92-522-4000032 e-mail: tiwari.lucknow@cbspd.com
- **Mumbai:** PWD Shed. Gala no. 25/26, Ramchandra Bhatt Marg, Next to JJ Hospital Gate no. 2, Opp. Union Bank of India,
  Noorbaug Mumbai-400009, Maharashtra, India
  Ph: 022-66661880/89 e-mail: mumbai@cbspd.com

Representatives

• **Hyderabad**	0-9885175004	• **Jharkhand**	0-9811541605	• **Nagpur**	0-9421945513
• **Patna**	0-9334159340	• **Pune**	0-9623451994	• **Uttarakhand**	0-9716462459

Printed at HT Media Ltd., Greater Noida, UP, India

Preface

This *Textbook of Human Histology* has been written to fulfil the requirements of students and teachers as per *Competency Based Undergraduate Curriculum for Indian Medical Graduate*.[*]

As per new curriculum, histology learning involves
- Knowledge (K) and skill (S) learning domains
- Knows (K) and knows how (KH) levels of competencies as per Miller's pyramid[#]

Most of the histology topics are in the core level of competency (must know). Only few topics are in non-core levels of competency (nice to know/desirable to know) such as cardioesophageal junction, corpus luteum, olfactory epithelium, eyelid, lip, sclerocorneal junction, optic nerve, cochlea, organ of Corti, pineal gland, and ultrastructure of muscular tissue, nervous tissue, epithelium, and connective tissue. The histology-related competencies should be taught with lectures and practical classes. Assessment methods for histology competencies involve written examination and skill assessment to identify the given slide with interpretation. Various topics of histology need horizontal integration with physiology and vertical integration with pathology.

To fulfil above requirements, this textbook is provided with the following features:
- *Concise text with functional correlation* for quick recapitulation during examination *(horizontal integration)*.
- *117 Photomicrographs* help to identify the microscopic structures.
- *122 Flowcharts* help to revise and memorize the microanatomy.
- *106 Practice figures (H&E pencil drawings)* are easy to draw for *written assessments*.
- *175 Three-dimensional illustrations* provide a visual grasp and easier retention of difficult concepts.
- *Summary (examination guide)* to overcome the difficulty of summarizing the facts in *written assessments*.
- *Identification feature* markings focus readers on specific points (for knows, knows how levels of competencies).
- *Neet, MCQ, Viva voce, and Clinical fact* markings for preparation of various upcoming academic entrance examinations.
- *Tables* to summarize essential facts.
- *Boxes* to focus on important topics.
- *Some interesting facts* to isolate them from main text, so that these facts should not be missed.
- *Clinical correlation* orient toward pathogenesis of diseases *(vertical integration)*.

Students are suggested to read the book in the following sequence:

Text → Flowchart → Summary (examination guide) → draw practice figures in log book

Any suggestions from the reader for rectification and improvement are welcome.

Yogesh Ashok Sontakke
dryogeshas@rediffmail.com

---

[*]Medical Council of India, Competency Based Undergraduate Curriculum for the Indian Medical Graduate, 2018; Vol 1:pg 41–80.
[#]Miller GE. The assessment of clinical skills/competence/performance. Acad Med. 1990;65(9 Suppl):S63–7.

Acknowledgments

I am thankful to Professors Dr RP Swaminathan (Dean Academics), Dr Parkash Chand (former professor senior scale in Anatomy), Dr Ashok Badhe (Medical superintendent), Dr M Sivakumar (Professor, Anatomy and Dean, JIPMER, Karaikal), Jawaharlal Institute of Postgraduate Medical Education and Research (JIPMER), Puducherry for encouraging and inspiring me for writing the books. I am greatly indebted to Dr K Aravindhan (Professor and Head), Department of Anatomy, JIPMER for invaluable support and suggestions.

I am grateful for encouragement, support, and suggestions from Dr SD Joshi (Indore), Dr SS Joshi (Indore), Dr PS Bhuiyan (KEM, Mumbai), Dr GP Pal (Indore), Dr Sunetra Naidu (Nagpur), Dr SK Aggarwal (Dehradun), Dr Mehera Bhoir (Mumbai), Dr Vino Victor Jesudas (Madurai), Dr Manik Chaterjee (Raipur), Dr Brijendra Singh (AIIMS, Rishikesh), Dr Ashutosh Mangalgiri (Bhopal), Dr JP Patel (Ahmedabad), Dr Priya Ranganath (Bangalore), Dr K Chandra Kumari (Trivandrum), Dr Lalitha C (Bengaluru), Dr Aparna Veda Priya K (Hyderabad), Dr Deepti Shastri (Salem), Dr P Bapuji (Eluru), Dr Kurian P Palliadiyil (Kollam), Dr C Kishan Reddy (Karimnagar), Dr Narayana Govindraj (Wayanad), Dr Komala B (Bangalore), Dr RR Marathe (Akola), Dr Shailaja Shetty (Bangalore), Dr Manisha Rajanand Gaikwad (AIIMS, Bhubaneswar), Dr Ravi Kant (Amritsar), Dr SK Chatterjee (Kolkata), Dr Anjali Jain (Ludhiana), Dr Nusrat Jabeen (Jammu and Kashmir), Dr Gunapriya Raghunath (Chennai), Dr Anupama Mahajan (Amritsar), Dr L Hema (Nellore), Dr Hitant Vohra (Ludhiana), Dr Tallapaneni Sreekanth (Hyderabad), Dr Shema K Nair (Bhopal), Dr Vaishali V Inamdar (Nanded), Dr Nandita Datta (Kolkata), Dr Sujay Mistri (Rampurhat, WB), Dr Ramesh Chandra Jha (Dhanbad), Dr Sandhya Kurup (Kolencherry), Dr BS Lala (Indore), Dr Gayatri Muthiyan (AIIMS, Nagpur), Dr Prakash KG (Kollam), Dr V Dhanalakshmi (Tuticorin), Dr Satheesha KS (Mangalore), Dr Aloka Sharma (Bhagalpur), Dr PS Chithra (Trichi), Dr Kalpana Ramachandran (Chennai), Dr Haritha Kumari (Mumbai), Dr Shruthi BN (Bangalore), Dr P Sasikala (Madurai), Dr Tejaswi HL (Adichunchanagiri, Mandya), Dr T Suresh Kumar (Vellore), Dr Ravikumar (Shimoga), Dr S Sathish Kumar (Dharmapuri), Dr DH Gopalan (Chennai), Dr Lenin (Kanyakumari), Dr Prajakta Kishve (Hyderabad) and Dr Mani Kathapillai (Ammapettai).

I acknowledge the encouragements and continuous support from Dr Suma HY, Dr Sarasu J, Dr Raveendranath V, Dr Suman Verma, Dr Sulochana Sakthivel, Dr Rajasekhar SSSN (JIPMER, Puducherry), Dr Nagaraj S (JIPMER, Karaikal). I am especially thankful to Dr V Gladwin, Dr Dharmaraj Tamgire, Dr Dinesh Kumar V and Dr G Dhivya Lakshmi for their critical suggestions.

Special thanks to my colleagues and friends for exchanging their views, interesting ideas, and thoughts who made possible the completion of my books. I acknowledge the support from Dr Rashmoni Jana (Delhi), Dr J Pranu Chakravarthy (Chennai), Dr Mukesh Mittal (Shivpuri), Dr PS Mittal (Greater Noida), Dr Jagruti Agarwal (Raipur), Dr Natwar Agrawal (Jabalpur), Dr Jaideo Manohar Ughade (Raigarh, CG), Dr Prashant Chaware (AIIMS, Bhopal), Dr V Dharani (Villupuram), Dr Praveen Kurrey (Raipur), Dr Rupa Chhaparwal (Indore), Dr Amit Kumar (Bilaspur), Dr R Sarah (AIIMS, Mangalagiri), Dr Sushil Jivane (Bhopal), Dr Shrikant Verma (Raipur), Dr Garima Pardhi (Vidisha), Dr Harsh Kumar Chawre (Vidisha), Dr Aparna Muraleedharan (Puducherry), Dr M Siva Kumar (Thiruvannamalai), Dr Vishal Bhadkaria (Sagar), Dr Thuslima M (Thiruvannamalai), Dr Sujithaa N, Dr Kiran K (Palakkad), Dr Shanthini S (Pondicherry), Dr Rajeev Panwar (Kanchipuram), Dr Saleena N Ali (Palakkad) and Dr Tom J Nallikuzhy (Ernakulam).

I also acknowledge Drs Praveena R, Vani PC, Chandan Lal Gupta, Surraj S and Mrinmayee Deb Barma (Senior residents) for their support. I also acknowledge Drs Phoebe Johnson, Arun Prasad, Sabin Malik, Kavitha T, Sankaranarayanan G, Jahira Banu T, Lavanya R, CH Chaitanya Kumar, Raju Kumaran T, Srinivasan S, Sivasakthi M, Abbirami GR and Regina C (Junior residents) for their help. I am thankful to Mr S Kirubanandan for his help in the typing of this manuscript and Mr Sendhilvel for his technical support.

I am thankful for the acceptability of views and support of Mr SK Jain (CMD), CBS Publishers & Distributors Pvt Ltd. I am obliged for continuous support from Mr YN Arjuna (Senior Vice-President, Publishing, Editorial and Publicity), and his entire team, specially Mrs Ritu Chawla (GM), Production), Mrs Sunita Rautela, Mr Parmod Kumar (DTP operators), Mr Neeraj Prasad (Graphic Designer) and Mr Neeraj Sharma (Copyeditor). I appreciate the entire team of CBS Publishers & Distributors in shaping this book to its present form.

I thank my wife Dr Anindita for editing, proofreading and her continuous support. I appreciate my little girl Aripra for her unconditional love and support. My sincere regards to my family for moral support. I thank all my supporters who made this possible. I thank the Almighty for giving me the strength and patience to continue my work.

Yogesh Ashok Sontakke

Contents

Preface v

Section 1 INTRODUCTION TO HISTOLOGY

1. Microscope 3
2. Orientation to Histological Techniques 8
3. Cell 12

Section 2 GENERAL HISTOLOGY

4. Epithelial Tissue 27
5. Cell Surface Projections and Cell Junctions 38
6. Glands 45
7. General Connective Tissue 54
8. Cartilage 69
9. Bone 77
10. Muscle Tissue 92
11. Lymphoid Tissue 106
12. Nervous Tissue 122
13. Cardiovascular Tissue 136
14. Skin and its Appendages 150

Section 3 SYSTEMIC HISTOLOGY

15. Respiratory System 167
16. Digestive System I: Oral Cavity and Associated Structures 183
17. Digestive System II: Esophagus and Stomach 196
18. Digestive System III: Small and Large Intestine 209
19. Liver, Gallbladder and Pancreas 223
20. Urinary System 237
21. Male Reproductive System I: Testis, Epididymis, Ductus Deferens 249
22. Male Reproductive System II: Accessory Sex Glands and Penis 259
23. Female Reproductive System I: Ovary, Uterus and Vagina 266
24. Female Reproductive System II: Mammary Gland, Placenta and Umbilical Cord 279
25. Endocrine System 291
26. Nervous System 308
27. Special Senses I: Eye 316
28. Special Senses II: Ear 329

Index 325

Some Important Points

- Remember following units:
  - 1 mm = 1000 µm
  - 1 µm = 1000 nm
- Some spellings need to remember: 'Mucous cells secrete mucus'. Here, mucous is adjective and mucus is noun.
- Some commonly encountered singular and pleural words in histology are as follows:

Singular	Pleural
Alveolus	Alveoli
Bronchus	Bronchi
Canaliculus	Canaliculi
Cilium	Cilia
Cisterna	Cisternae
Crista	Cristae
Diaphysis	Diaphyses
Epiphysis	Epiphyses
Epithelium	Epithelia
Flagellum	Flagella
Foot	Feet
Ganglion	Ganglia
Lacuna	Lacunae
Metaphysis	Metaphyses
Microvillus	Microvilli
Mitochondrion	Mitochondria
Nucleolus	Nucleoli
Septum	Septa/septae
Stratum	Strata

Index of Competencies
Competency Based Undergraduate Curriculum for the Indian Medical Graduate

Code	Competency	Chapter	Page no[#]
AN25.1	Identify, draw and label a slide of trachea and lung	15	167
AN43.2	Identify, describe and draw the microanatomy of:		
	Pituitary gland, thyroid, parathyroid gland	25	291
	Tongue, salivary glands	16	183
	Tonsil	11	106
	Epiglottis	15	171
	Cornea, retina	27	316
AN52.1	Describe and identify the microanatomical features of gastrointestinal system:		
	Oesophagus, fundus of stomach, pylorus of stomach	17	196
	Duodenum, jejunum, ileum, large intestine, appendix	18	209
	Liver, gallbladder, pancreas	19	223
	Suprarenal gland	25	302
AN52.2	Describe and identify the microanatomical features of:		
	Urinary system: Kidney, ureter and urinary bladder	20	237
	Male reproductive system: Testis, epididymis, vas deferens	21	249
	Prostate and penis	22	259
	Female reproductive system: Ovary, uterus, uterine tube, cervix	23	266
	Placenta and umbilical cord	24	279
AN52.3	Describe and identify the microanatomical features of:		
	Cardiooesophageal junction	17	202
	Corpus luteum	23	271
AN64.1	Describe and identify the microanatomical features of:		
	Spinal cord, cerebellum and cerebrum	26	308
AN65.1	Identify epithelium under the microscope and describe the various types that correlate to its function	4	27
AN65.2	Describe the ultrastructure of epithelium	5	38
AN66.1	Describe and identify various types of connective tissue with functional correlation	7	54
AN66.2	Describe the ultrastructure of connective tissue	7	54
AN67.1	Describe and identify various types of muscle under the microscope	10	92
AN67.2	Classify muscle and describe the structure-function correlation of the same	10	92
AN67.3	Describe the ultrastructure of muscular tissue	10	92
AN68.1	Describe and identify multipolar and unipolar neuron, ganglia, peripheral nerve	12	122
AN68.2	Describe the structure-function correlation of neuron	12	122
AN68.3	Describe the ultrastructure of nervous tissue	12	122
AN69.1	Identify elastic and muscular blood vessels, capillaries under the microscope	13	136
AN69.2	Describe the various types and structure-function correlation of blood vessel	13	136
AN69.3	Describe the ultrastructure of blood vessels	13	136
AN70.1	Identify exocrine gland under the microscope and distinguish between serous, mucous and mixed acini	6	45
AN70.2	Identify the lymphoid tissue under the microscope and describe microanatomy of lymph node, spleen, thymus, tonsil and correlate the structure with function	11	106
AN71.1	Identify bone under the microscope; classify various types and describe the structure-function correlation of the same	9	77
AN71.2	Identify cartilage under the microscope and describe various types and structure-function correlation of the same	8	69
AN72.1	Identify the skin and its appendages under the microscope and correlate the structure with function	14	150

[#]Note: This is indicative page number for the topic. Please refer to the mentioned chapter for the details.

SECTION 1

Introduction to Histology

1. Microscope
2. Orientation to Histological Techniques
3. Cell

CHAPTER 1

Microscope[1]

Chapter Outline

- Introduction
- Compound light microscope
  - Optical parts
  - Nonoptical parts
- Objective lenses

INTRODUCTION

- Microscopy is an instrument used for magnification of objects.
- Zacharias Janssen and Hens Janssen (Dutch) developed the first microscope (1590). Giovanni Faber coined the term microscope (1625). *Antonie van Leeuwenhoek* (1675) invented a simple light microscope.
- Microscopes are classified into three groups as follows:
  1. Optical microscope that utilizes light (photons) for image formation.
  2. Electron microscope that utilizes electrons for image formation.
  3. Scanning probe microscope that utilizes physical probe for the formation of surface images.
- Optical microscopes are classified as follows:
  A. *Simple microscope:* It consists of a single convex lens or a single set of lenses for magnifying objects.
  B. *Compound light microscope:* It consists of two sets of lenses, one near the sample (objective lens) and the second lens near the eye (eyepiece). It is the most commonly used microscope.
- Compound light microscopes are of the following types:
  1. *Bright-field microscope:* In this microscope, the specimen is placed between the light source and the optical system. The specimen looks dark (colorful if stained) and background looks bright (white).
  2. *Dark-field microscope:* It has a special condenser that allows the light rays to hit the sample rather than a direct hit. Only the rays that hit specimen form the image. It is useful for observing unstained samples.
  3. *Phase-contrast microscope:* It is useful for visualization of live, unstained organism and living cells. This microscopy has phase annuls in condenser and phase plate in the objective. The object that changes phase of the light is observed (looks bright) against a dark background.
  4. *Fluorescence microscope:* It uses the fluorescence property of the stained specimen. A *fluorophore* is a chemical that changes the wavelength (color) of the light. This microscopy is useful for immuno-istochemistry (identification of specific antigen/protein), in situ hybridization, and so on.
  5. *Polarized light microscope:* It is useful for observing birefringent substances such as bone, teeth, striated muscles, and so on. Birefringent substance can produce double refraction of light.

COMPOUND LIGHT MICROSCOPE

- Compound light microscope is the most commonly used microscope.

- It consists of the following parts (Fig. 1.1):
  1. Optical parts: Sources of light, condenser, objective lenses, and eyepiece.
  2. Nonoptical parts: Arm, coarse and fine adjustment, nosepiece, stage, microscopic tube, and base.

Optical Parts

- The quality of image, resolution, and magnification mostly depend on the optical parts and the microscope.
- Optical parts include source of light, condenser, objective lenses, and eyepiece.

Source of Light

- Microscopes are provided with mirror for reflecting light or tungsten/halogen/LED light.
- Plane side of the mirror is useful in bright daylight, whereas concave mirror is useful for artificial light source.

Substage Condenser

- Substage condenser gathers light and focuses it to the sample to be viewed.
- Aperture/iris diaphragm controls the amount of light passing through the condenser.

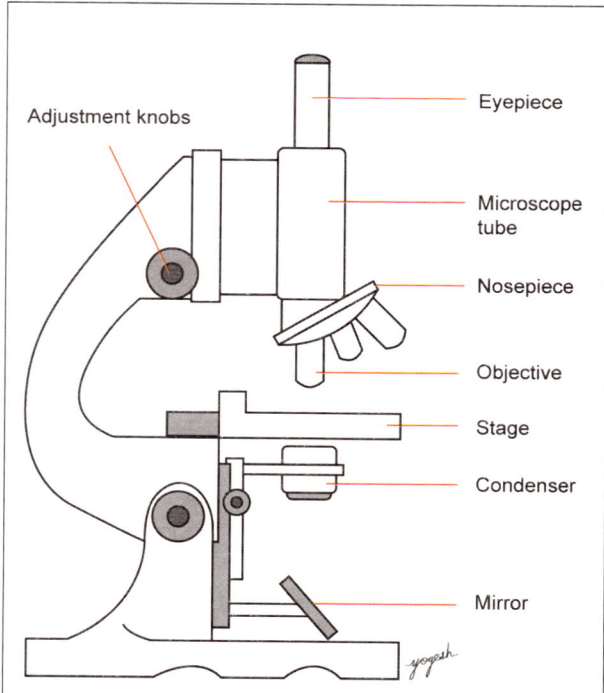

Fig. 1.1: Parts of microscope (practice figure).

- Position of condenser can be adjusted (up and down movements) to focus the light critically.

Objective Lens

- The lenses that receive light from the sample (lies near the sample) are called objective lenses.
- Objective lenses have different magnification powers, such as 4X (scanning objective), 10X (low power), 40X (high power), 100X (mostly called oil immersion). *Practical guide*
- Numerical aperture (NA) denotes light absorbing power and resolving power of objective.

Eyepiece (Ocular)

- The observer sees the image through the eyepiece.
- Eyepiece may be 10X (5X or 20X) and may be widefield.
- Monocular microscopes have only one eyepiece, whereas binocular microscopes have two eyepieces.
- Eyepiece produces a magnified virtual image.

Nonoptical Parts

- Each microscope consists of nonoptical parts that help in holding and moving the optical parts and specimen.
- Nonoptical parts include arm, fine and coarse adjustment, nosepiece, stage, and base/stand.

Base/Stand

It is a heavy metallic part that keeps the entire microscope steady.

Arm

- Arm connects base of the microscope with optical tube.
- Arm is usually used to hold the microscope during shifting of microscope from one place to another.

Adjustment Knobs

- Each microscope is filled with coarse and fine adjustment knobs.
- These knobs are useful for moving the sample upward and downward to bring it into focus.

Stage

- It is a platform for holding the sample.
- Stage is filled with
  - Clips to hold the glass slide

- Mechanical stage to move the specimen in X and Y axis. Mechanical stage is provided with Vernier graduation markings.

Microscope tube

- It is a tube that extends from objective lens to the eyepiece.
- Microscope tube is fitted with prism that changes the path of light.

Nosepiece

- Nosepiece links the objective lenses with the microscope tube and should be used for rotating the objective lenses.

Some Interesting Facts

Focal length
- It is a distance between the center of lens and its focus (Fig. 1.2).
- It is an indicator of capability of the lens to magnify or diverge parallel rays.

Magnification
- A lens magnifies the image. For a microscope, magnification is the multiplication of eyepiece magnification and objective magnification.
- For example, while using a microscope of 40X objective and 10X eyepiece, a sample is magnified 400 times (40 × 10).

Numerical aperture
- The numerical aperture denotes light gathering capacity of a lens (Fig. 1.2).
- NA = n sin θ
- Here, n = refractive index of the medium between objective lens and specimen.

Resolution
- Resolution is the ability of microscope to distinguish between closest two points as a separate entity.
- Resolution = 0.6λ/NA
  Here, λ = wavelength of light
  NA = Numerical aperture
- Higher NA of objective and condenser and shorter wavelength of light give better resolution.

Aberrations
- A defect in expected functioning of the lens or optical system is called an optical aberration.
- There are two types of axial aberrations: chromatic and spherical.

- *Chromatic aberration:* If a lens reflects the light according to wavelength (color), it is called chromatic aberration. Blue light gets refracted more than green and red. This phenomenon produces color halos around the magnified image (Fig. 1.3).
- *Spherical aberration*
  In spherical aberration, parallel rays passing from center of lens and that passing from peripheral part of lens are focused at different points (Fig. 1.4).
- Due to spherical aberration, blurred image is formed in the peripheral part.
- Other spherical aberrations include coma, astigmatism, field curvature, barrel distortion, pincushion distortion.

Kohler Illumination
- August Kohler (1893) described method for illumination in microscopy.
- It describes the steps (settings) by that source of light will not be visible in an image formed in microscopy and provide even illumination, high contrast, less specimen heating, and no glare.[2]

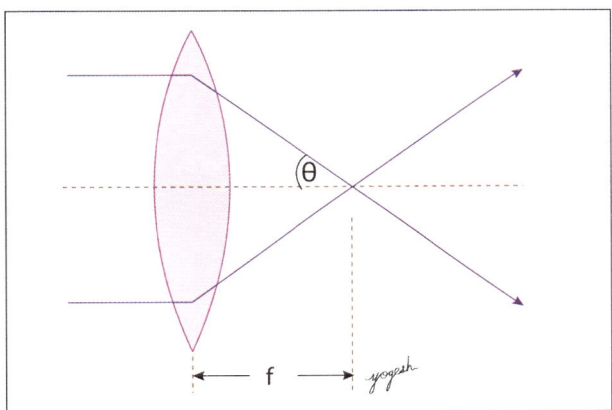

Fig. 1.2: Focal length (f) and numerical aperture (θ).

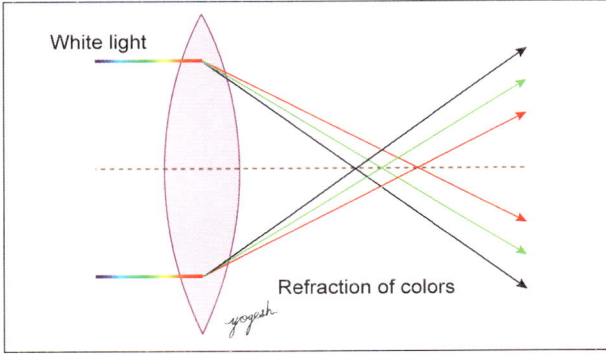

Fig. 1.3: Chromatic aberration.

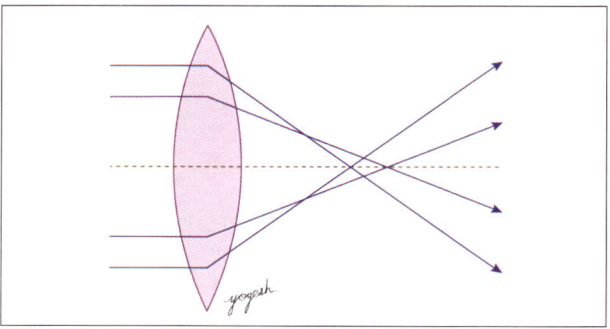

Fig. 1.4: Spherical aberration.

OBJECTIVE LENSES

- Objective lenses are of various types according to their correction for specific aberrations as follows:
  1. *Achromatic objectives:* These are corrected for axial chromatic aberration for colors (red and blue).
  2. Fluorites or *semi-apochromatic objectives:* These are constructed with fluorite and glass. They are corrected for 2–3 colors and field curvature aberrations. These are suitable for immune fluorescence microscopy, polarization, and differential interference contrast microscopy.
  3. *Apochromatic objectives:* These are corrected for all color aberrations and spherical aberration. These are suitable for confocal microscopy.
  4. *Plan objectives:* These are very costly lenses. These are corrected for curvature of field. For example, *plan-apochromatic objective* (corrected for maximum aberrations).^{MCQ}

Common markings on the objective lens are shown in Fig. 1.5.

Some Interesting Facts

Fluorescence microscopy
- Fluorescence microscopy utilizes the property of fluorescence. The sample is excited with high-energy light (shorter wavelength). The sample loses some energy and emits low energy light (higher wavelength).
- This microscope is fitted with mercury vapor lamp or high-power LEDs or LASER light and fluorescence filter cube.
- Fluorescence filter cube consists of excitation filter, dichroic filter and emission filter. The filter cube allows the specific wavelength of light (color) to pass through it (Fig. 1.6).

Confocal microscopy
- Confocal microscopy is modified fluorescence microscopy that forms an image of the sample from one focal plane. For this purpose, it is fitted with *spatial pinhole* that helps to collect images from different focal planes and forms three-dimensional images (Z stacking)
- It is useful for thick specimens that are stained with fluorescence dyes, for construction of *3-D images* of sample, live cell scanning, and colocalization of proteins.

Electron microscope
- Electron microscope utilizes the beam of electrons (instead of light) to illuminate the sample.

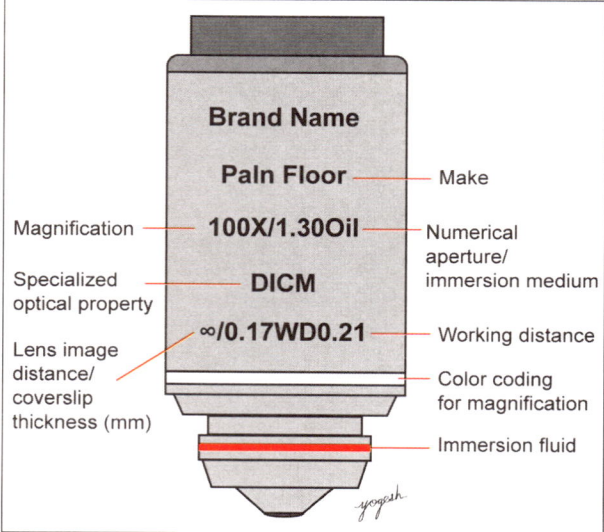

Fig. 1.5: Markings on objective lens.

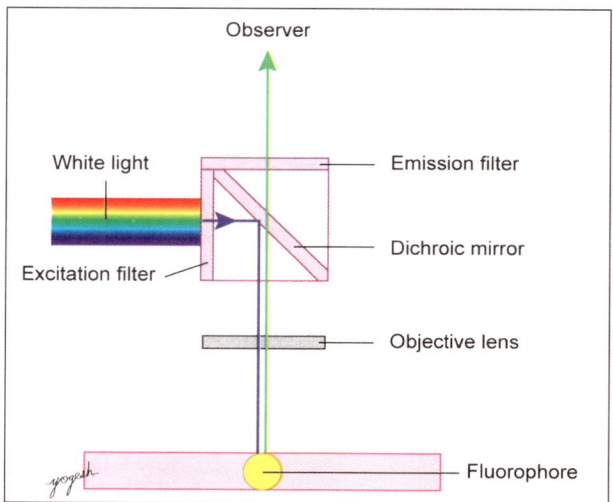

Fig. 1.6: Light path for fluorescence microscopy.

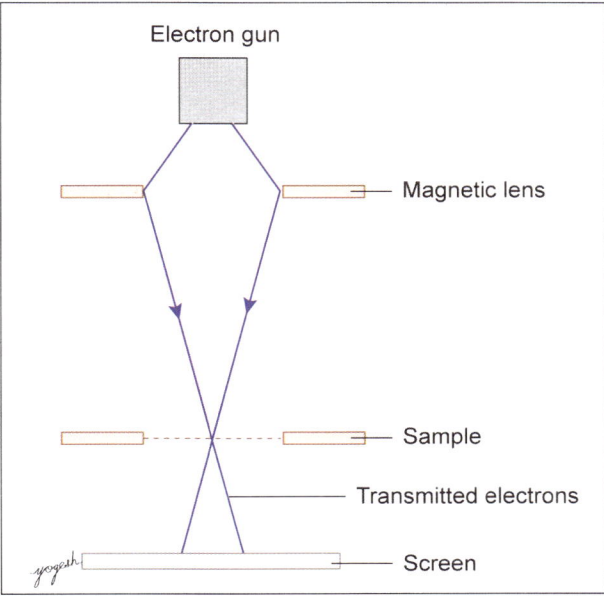

Fig. 1.7: Working principle of a transmission electron microscope.

- It can detect minute samples such as viruses, and atoms, but are not suitable for living tissue.
- There are various electron microscopes such as transmission electron microscope (TEM), scanning electron microscope (SEM), reflection electron microscope (REM), and so on.
- Electron microscopes utilize electromagnetic lenses, specimen (<100 nm thick) mounted on grid (Fig. 1.7).
- To cut such thin section, *ultra-microtome with glass knife* is required. The specimen is stained with uranyl acetate and lead citrate.

---

[1] This chapter is the zest of microscopy section of the book *Principles of Histological Techniques, Immunohistochemistry and Microscopy* by Yogesh Sontakke, Paras Medical Books, Hyderabad, India and reproduced with permission.

[2] For details, refer the book *Principles of Histological Techniques, Immunohistochemistry and Microscopy* by Yogesh Sontakke, 1st edn., Paras Medical Books Pvt. Ltd., Hyderabad, India.

CHAPTER 2

Orientation to Histological Techniques

Chapter Outline
- Tissue processing
- Special stains
  - Hematoxylin and eosin staining
  - Decalcification
- Orientation of sectional plane
  - Interpretation of Sections in Histology
    * Sections of solid structure
    * Sections of tubular structure

- Microscopic examination is based on thin sectioning of the tissue. AFJK Mayer (1819) coined the term *histology* (*histos* = tissue, *-logy* = science).
- This chapter provides brief overview of the histological techniques that are required for the section/slide preparation of tissue and orientation of sections (relationship of gross structure and microscopic section).

TISSUE PROCESSING

- In routine histology and histopathology, a specimen is sliced into 0.5 cm or so. These slices are processed and finally further sectioned into 5–7 µm thin sections. These sections are mounted and stained on glass slides to make them suitable for microscopic observation. This entire procedure is called *tissue processing.*
- Histological tissue processing involves the following major steps (Flowchart 2.1):

Tissue collection, grossing, tissue fixation, dehydration, cleaning, embedding, section cutting, staining, and mounting.

1. Tissue collection
- For histological studies, suitable tissue is collected from cadavers, forensic autopsies, surgical procedures, animals (goat, rat, dog, and so on) with

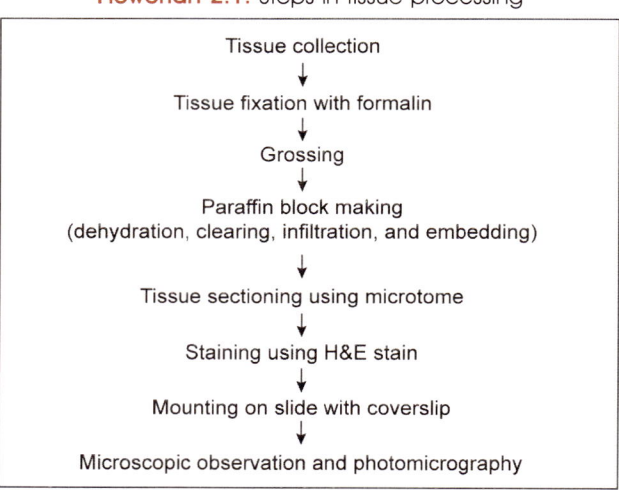

Flowchart 2.1: Steps in tissue processing

Tissue collection
↓
Tissue fixation with formalin
↓
Grossing
↓
Paraffin block making
(dehydration, clearing, infiltration, and embedding)
↓
Tissue sectioning using microtome
↓
Staining using H&E stain
↓
Mounting on slide with coverslip
↓
Microscopic observation and photomicrography

permission from authorities (ethics and research committees).

2. Tissue fixation
- Collected specimen is preserved for retaining their biological structure without any significant distortion or decomposition.
- 10% formalin is the most commonly used fixative.^{Viva}
- It cross-links proteins (enzymes and others) in the tissue. Other fixatives include glutaraldehyde, mercuric chloride, osmium tetroxide (highly toxic), and so on.

3. Grossing
- Grossing involves observing tissue for gross pathological changes and selecting a suitable part of the tissue for microscopic examination.
- The selected area is cut into ~5 mm thick slices.

4. Paraffin block making
- It is difficult to make thin sections of the tissue (5–7 μm) as most of the cells contain water (50–60%). Hence, the tissue is processed to replace water with firm material (paraffin wax) and to make the tissue suitable for cutting.
- It involves the following steps:
  - *Dehydration:* Tissue slice is treated with ascending grades of alcohols (50%, 70%, 90%, and absolute/100% alcohol) to gradually remove water from the tissue.
  - *Removal of alcohol/clearing:* Tissue slice is treated with xylene (clearing agent). Clearing agent makes the tissue clear by changing the refractive index of the tissue.
  - *Infiltration/removal of clearing agent:* Tissue slice is kept in melted paraffin that replaces xylene by infiltration in the tissue.
  - *Embedding/block making:* Tissue slice is kept fixed in the melted paraffin and allowed to form a solid block on cooling. This solid block makes the tissue suitable for sectioning.

5. Tissue sectioning
- Microtome is an instrument used for thin sectioning of tissue.
- Paraffin block is fitted on microtome and cut into thin sections (5–7 μm). These sections are transferred to glass slides.

6. Staining
- A section on a glass slide is stained with suitable staining.
- Hematoxylin and eosin (*H&E*) are commonly used stains.

7. Mounting
- Stained section is mounted with the help of a coverslip and DPX (glue) to make ready for observation under microscope and preserve.

SPECIAL STAINS
- Many structures or substances cannot be differentiated from each other with the help of routine hematoxylin and eosin staining.
- For the visualization and differentiation of specific structure, special stains are required.
- Some commonly used special stains and their uses are listed in Table 2.1.

Box 2.1: Hematoxylin and eosin staining
- Hematoxylin and eosin stain is most commonly used in routine histology and histopathology.
- Hematoxylin is a basic dye that is obtained from wood of *Hematoxylon campechianum* tree.
- Hematoxylin stains nuclei, calcium deposits, fibrin, muscle cross striations, matrix in cartilages, and so on. *Practical guide*
- Eosin is an acidic type that is derived from fluorescein.
- Eosin stains basic or eosinophilic compounds such as cytoplasm, connective tissue (collagen fibers), muscle fibers, red blood cells, and so on. *Practical guide*
- Steps involved in *H&E* staining.
  Deparaffinize the section using xylene, rehydrate the section with descending grades of alcohol (100% or absolute alcohol, 90% alcohol, 70% alcohol, and water), staining with hematoxylin, removal of excess hematoxylin (using acid-alcohol and water wash/bath), staining with eosin and dehydration. Dehydrated slide is preserved by fixing coverslip using DPX (transparent glue).

Box 2.2: Decalcification
- Calcified tissue (bones) cannot be sectioned properly using routine microtome.
- Decalcification is the technique useful for removing deposited minerals from the matrix of the tissue (bone) to facilitate microtome sectioning.
- The following agents are useful for decalcification strong mineral acids (nitric acid, hydrochloric acid), weak organic acids (formic acids), and calcium chelating agents (EDTA).

ORIENTATION OF SECTIONAL PLANE
- In histology, a two-dimensional view of a tissue section is observed under the microscope.
- The observer has to imagine a three-dimensional structure from a two-dimensional image.
  For example: If a circular structure is seen, the observer has to decide whether it is a sectional part of a tube or a sphere.
- *Microtome* is an instrument used for section cutting in histology. The knife/blade fitted to the microtome makes thin slices of the tissue.
- Tissue has various structures that have different size, shape, and orientations.
- Some structures are spherical, some are tubular, or solid. Some structures run parallel to the long axis of tissue, some run perpendicularly or obliquely. The resultant section of the tissue gives a two-dimensional image of these structures.

Table 2.1: Special stains and their uses

Structure	Stain	Color
Collagen fibers	Van Gieson technique	Red
	Masson's trichrome stain	Blue/green
Elastic fibers	Verhoeff–van Gieson method	Bluish black
	Weight's Resorcin–Fuchsin method	Blue-black
	Orcein stain	Dark-brown
Reticular Fibers	Gordon–Sweet's method	Black
	Gomori's silver impregnation method	Black
Basement membrane	Periodic acid–Schiff (PAS) method	Magenta
Carbohydrates (glycogen, amyloid, fungi, pancreatic zymogen granules, corpora amylacea in prostate, thyroid colloid)	PAS method	Magenta
Lipids/fat	Oil red-O	Brilliant red
Iron	Perl's Prussian blue reaction	Blue
Hemoglobin	Leuco patent blue V method	Dark blue-green
Bile pigment	Hall's method	Olive green
Melanin	Masson–Fontana method	Black
Lipofuscin	Pearse's staining method	Magenta
Calcium	Von Kossa method	Dark green-black
Uric acid	Hexamine–silver method	Black
Nissl substance in neuron	Cresyl Fast violet stain	Purple-dark blue
Myelin	Luxol fast blue method	Blue
	Osmium tetroxide method	Black
Astrocytes	Cajal's gold chloride method	Reddish-black

Interpretation of Sections in Histology

- To understand the histological section, the following examples are given:
  - Sections of solid structure
  - Sections of tubular structure

Sections of Solid Structure

- A boiled egg has an outer egg white and inner yellow/orange egg yolk.
- The nature of the section depends on orientation of the egg-like solid structure in the tissue (Fig. 2.1).
- For example: If an egg is oriented vertically, it will cut in longitudinal plane (*longitudinal section/LS*). If an egg is oriented horizontally, it will cut in transverse plane (*transverse section/TS*). If an egg is oriented obliquely, it will cut in oblique plane.
- In each plane, the egg is sectioned into various oval shapes depending on the depth of the section (from superficial to deep planes). In superficial or tangential planes egg yolk (similar to cell nucleus) may not be observed.*Practical guide*

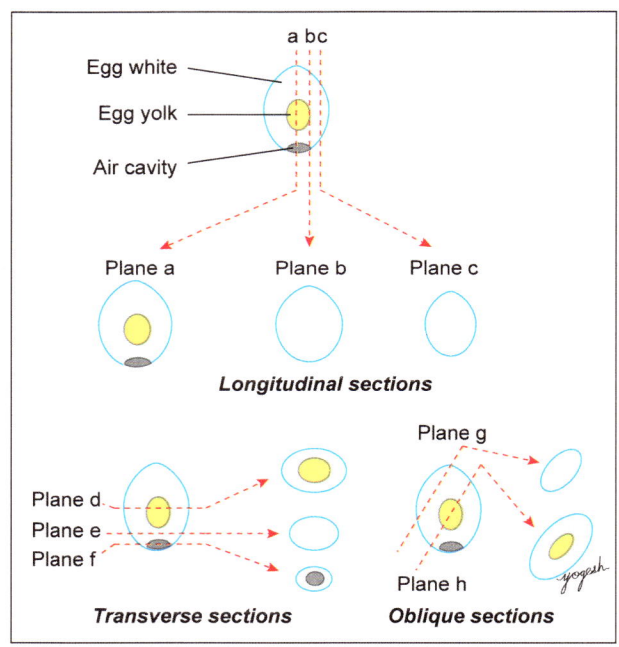

Fig. 2.1: Planes of sections of solid object.

Sections of Tubular Structure

- Many tissue structures are tubular, such as, blood vessels, intestine, renal tubules, seminiferous tubules, bronchi, and so on.
- The two-dimensional section of tubular structure depends on
  - Coiling of tubular structure
  - Orientation of the structure in the tissue
  - Plane of section
- If a tubular structure is straight, it produces only one appearance in a section. Based on the plane, it may be longitudinal, transverse or oblique section (Fig. 2.2).
- If a tubular structure is coiled, it may appear multiple time in the same section and its part may show various sections (longitudinal, transverse, oblique, and tangential) (Fig. 2.3).

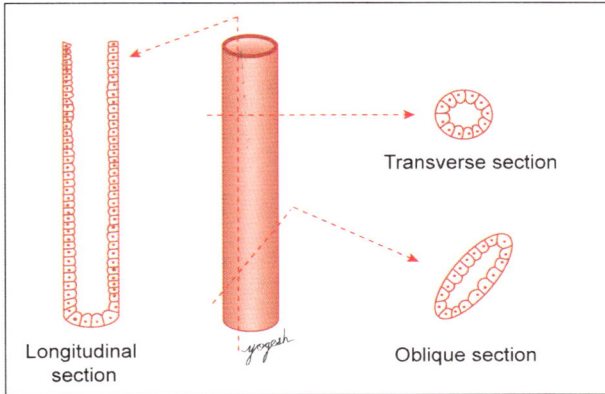

Fig. 2.2: Sections of straight tubular structure.

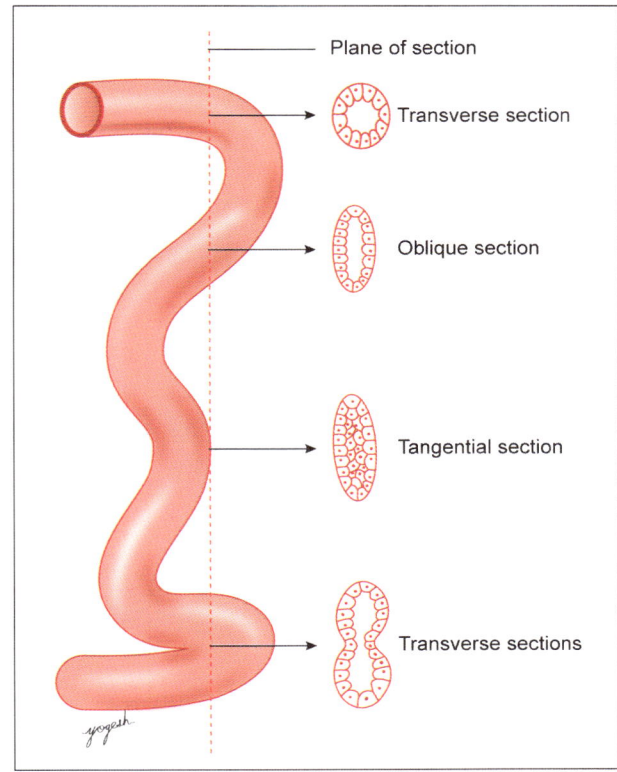

Fig. 2.3: Sections of coiled tubular structure.

Some Interesting Facts

Following points can be concluded with the understanding of plane of section:
- Sweat gland is a simple tubular gland having terminal coiled secretory portion. In a section, it may be seen as multiple oval (oblique) sections and round (transverse) sections. *Practical guide*
- In thyroid gland, some of the follicles may not show colloid, if the section does not pass through the colloid. In addition, it may show cluster of cells in tangential section. *Practical guide*
- In case of epithelium, some cells do not show nuclei, if the section does not pass through the nucleus of the **cell**.
- In smooth muscle, transverse section shows round central nucleus, whereas in longitudinal section, spindle-shaped nucleus is seen. *Practical guide*
- In a longitudinal section of a ground bone, parallel Haversian canals are present, whereas in transverse section round/oval-shaped Haversian canals are present.

Cell

Chapter Outline

- Plasma membrane
  - Modified fluid-mosaic model
  - Functions
- Transport across plasma membrane
- Endoplasmic reticulum (ER)
- Golgi complex
- Mitochondria
- Ribosomes
- Lysosomes
- Lysosomal storage diseases
- Peroxisomes
- Endosomes
- Cytoskeleton
  - Microtubules
  - Actin filaments/Microfilaments
  - Intermediate filaments
- Centrioles
- Nucleus
  - Nuclear envelope
  - Nucleoplasm
  - Chromatin
  - Nucleolus

INTRODUCTION

- Cell is basic structural and functional unit of all organisms.
- Human tissue consists of *eukaryotic cells* that have nucleus, cell organelles, and cytoplasm (Note: prokaryotic cells/unicellular organisms do not have membrane-bound nucleus and membrane-bound cell organelles).
- Each cell is bounded by a cell/plasma membrane that encloses *protoplasm.*
- Protoplasm consists of a nucleus and cytoplasm.
- Cytoplasm consists of gel-like matrix called *cytosol/hyaloplasm,* cell organelles, cytoskeleton, and inclusions. Cytoskeleton consists of microtubules, intermediate, and actin filaments.
- Cell organelles are grouped as membrane-bound and non-membrane-bound (Fig. 3.1).
- *Membrane-bound organelles* include plasma/cell membrane, rough endoplasmic reticulum (rER), smooth-surfaced endoplasmic reticulum (sER), Golgi apparatus, endosomes, lysosomes, pinocytic vesicles, endocytic vesicles, mitochondria, and peroxisomes.
- Membranes of intracellular organelles increase intracellular surface area and create intracellular microcompartments for proper physiological functions.
- *Nonmembrane-bound organelles* include microtubules, filaments (actin and intermediate filaments), centrioles, ribosomes, and proteasomes.
- Various cell organelles and their functions are listed in Table 3.1.

PLASMA MEMBRANE (CELL MEMBRANE)

- Plasma membrane is also called cell membrane or *plasmalemma.*
- It separates intracellular compartment from extracellular compartment of the tissue.
- Plasma membrane is a dynamic structure. It consists of an amphipathic lipid bilayer, integral membrane proteins, and peripheral proteins (Fig. 3.2).

Cell

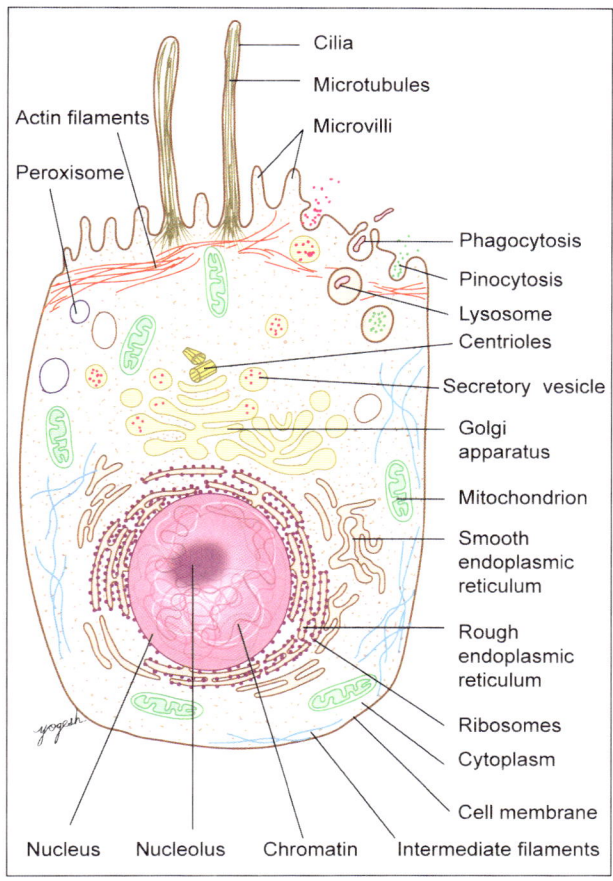

Fig. 3.1: The cell and cell organelles (practice figure).

Modified Fluid-Mosaic Model (Singer and Nicolson, 1972):

- Transmission electron microscopy (TEM): On TEM examination, plasma membrane consists of two electron-dense layers separated by middle electron lucent layer (Fig. 3.2).
- Thickness is 8–10 nm.

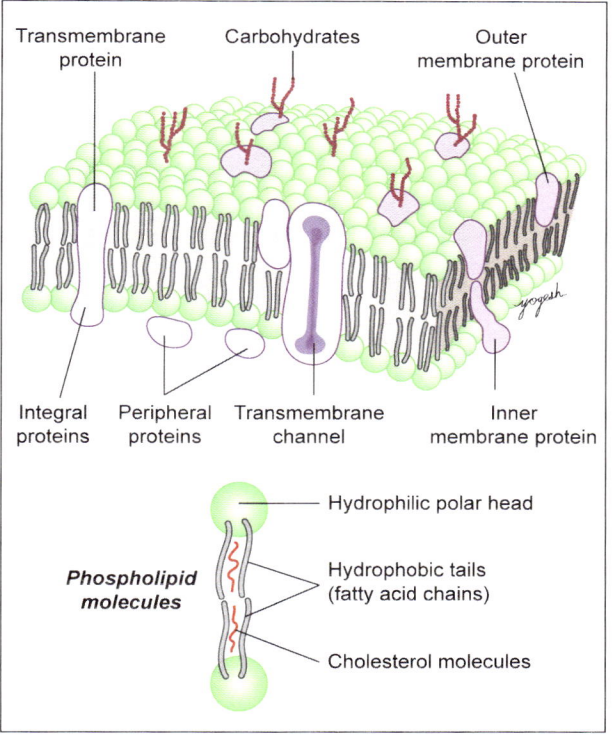

Fig. 3.2: Structure of cell membrane.

Lipids of Plasma Membrane

- Plasma membrane has three types of lipids: phospholipids, cholesterol, and glycolipids.
- *Phospholipid* molecules have polar hydrophilic end/head and nonpolar hydrophobic end/tail. The head consists of choline, phosphate, and glycerol. Nonpolar end consists of two fatty acid chains.
- Hydrophilic ends face toward extracellular and intracellular surfaces.
- *Lipid rafts* are microdomains of the plasma membrane. It consists of high concentration of cholesterol and glycolipids.

Table 3.1: Cell organelles and functions

Cell organelles	Functions	Remarks/characteristics
Plasma membrane	Selective barrier, cell adhesion	Bilipid layer
rER	Synthesis and transfer of proteins to Golgi complex	Flattened sheets with attached ribosomes
sER	Lipid and steroid metabolism	Flattened sheets without ribosomes
Golgi apparatus	Posttranslational modification of proteins	Flattened sheets
Secretory vesicles	Transport and storage of secretory proteins	Small membrane-bound vesicles
Mitochondria	Power house of cell	Outer and inner membranes
		Inner membrane shows cristae (folds)
Lysosomes	Disintegration of phagocytosed material	Membrane-bound vesicles
Peroxisomes	Oxidation of fatty acids, detoxification	Membrane-bound vesicles
Ribosomes	Protein synthesis	Have 40S and 60S subunits

- Lipid rafts also contain integral and peripheral membrane proteins that are involved in cell signaling.
- *Freeze fracture:* It is a method of tissue processing for electron microscopy. On freeze-fracture, cell membrane shows *E-face* (backed by extracellular compartment) and *P-face* (backed by protoplasm/cytoplasm). This method is useful for identification of integral proteins of cell membrane.

Proteins of Plasma Membrane

- Plasma membrane has two types of proteins: integral membrane proteins and peripheral membrane proteins.
- *Integral proteins* are confined within the plasma membrane and cross the entire or partial thickness of the cell membrane, whereas *peripheral proteins* are confined only on the surfaces of plasma membrane.
- Integral proteins form pumps (Na^+ pump), channels (gap junctions), receptor proteins, linker proteins (anchor cytoskeleton), enzymes (ATPase), and structural proteins.
- Integral proteins can move within the lipid bilayer.

Carbohydrates of Plasma Membrane

- Carbohydrates of plasma membrane form glycoproteins and glycolipids.
- They form *glycocalyx coat* on the outer surface of the plasma membrane.
- They help cell to interact with extracellular environment, cell recognition, cell adhesion, and metabolism.
- Glycocalyx also forms major histocompatibility complexes (MHC) and blood group antigens on RBCs. *Neet*

Functions of Plasma Membrane

1. *Selective barrier:* Plasma membrane limits the mobility of the substances across it.
2. *Protection:* Plasma membrane isolates the intracellular environment from extracellular environment.
3. *Cell shape/adhesion:* Plasma membrane anchors the cytoskeleton and provides attachment with adjacent cells and basement membrane to provide a particular shape to the cell.
4. *Polarity:* Plasma membrane maintains ionic polarization and respond to stimuli by depolarizing.
5. *Receptors:* Plasma membrane has receptors for specific molecules (hormones).
6. *Transport:* Plasma membrane help in transport across it by endocytosis, exocytosis, pinocytosis, and so on.

TRANSPORT ACROSS PLASMA MEMBRANE

Selective substances can enter or leave the cell through the plasma membrane. These substances follow one of the following modalities of transport (Fig. 3.3):
1. Passive transport
2. Active transport
3. Vesicular transport

Passive Transport

- For passive transport, energy is not required for transport of substances across plasma membrane. It can take place by simple diffusion or facilitated diffusion (Fig. 3.3).
- *Simple diffusion*
  By simple diffusion, lipid-soluble and uncharged molecules cross plasma membrane from higher to lower concentration.
- For example, oxygen, carbon dioxide, glycerol, and so on.

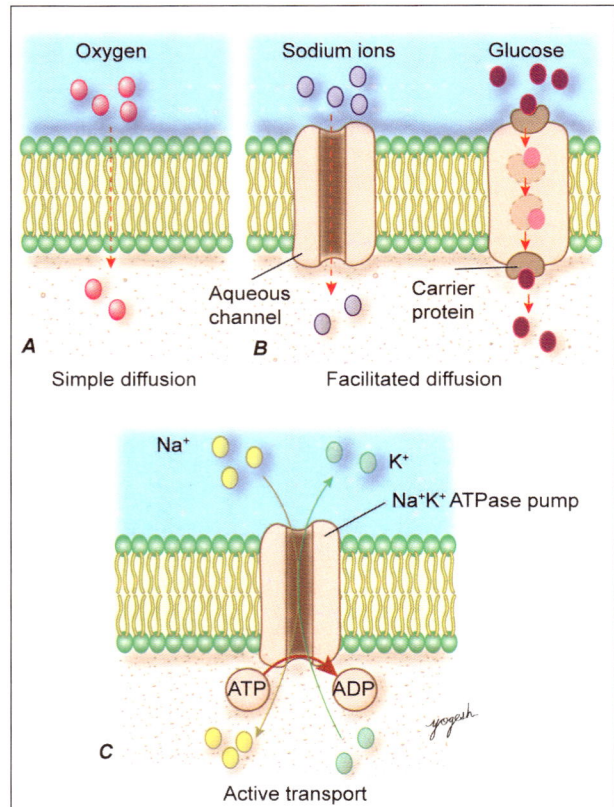

Fig. 3.3: Transport across the cell membrane. (A) Simple diffusion, (B) Facilitated diffusion, (C) Active transport.

- *Facilitated diffusion*
  In facilitated diffusion, *channel/carrier proteins* or channels of the plasma membrane help in transport of certain small, and water-soluble molecules.
- *Carrier proteins* move across the plasma membrane and help in the transport of small, water-soluble molecules.
- *Channel proteins* are transmembrane (integral) proteins. They have pore domain that regulates entry or exit of substances.

Channel proteins are:
- *Voltage-gated ion channels* regulated by membrane potentials
- *Ligand-gated ion channels* regulated by neuro-transmitters
- *Mechanical-gated ion channels* regulated by stress (hair cells in internal ear)

Active Transport

- The transport of molecules across the plasma membrane against the concentration gradient requires energy (ATPs). Such transport of molecules is called active transport.
  For example, sodium pump for Na^+ ion transport

Vesicular Transport

- Large molecules are transported with vesicular transport across the plasma membrane.
- It is of two types: Endocytosis and exocytosis.
- *Endocytosis*
  In endocytosis, the extracellular molecules are brought inside the cell as membrane-bound vesicles. Endocytosis may be pinocytosis, phagocytosis, or receptor-mediated endocytosis (Fig. 3.4).

Pinocytosis (*cell drinking*, in Greek): In pinocytosis, cell ingests liquid and form pinocytic vesicles.

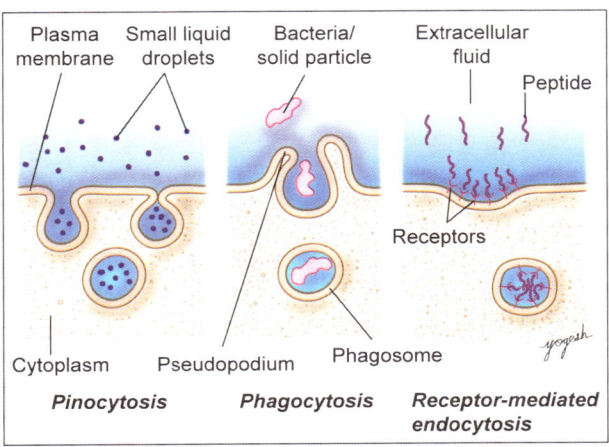

Fig. 3.4: Modalities of endocytosis.

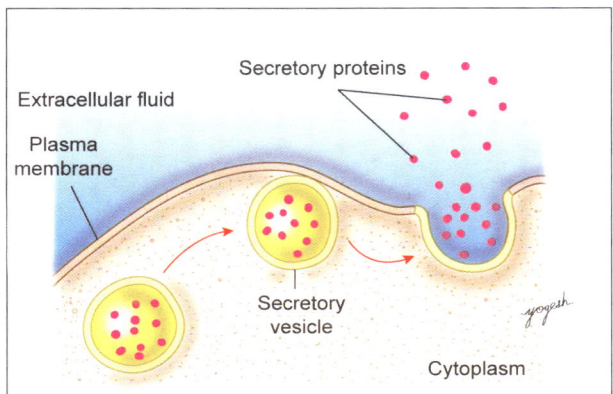

Fig. 3.5: Modalities of exocytosis.

Phagocytosis (*cell eating*, in Greek): In phagocytosis, cell ingests large substances such as cell debris, bacteria, and so on and forms large phagocytic vesicles (phagosomes).

Receptor-mediated endocytosis: Specific molecules (ligand) enter cell with the help of receptor-mediated endocytosis. For example, peptide hormones
- *Exocytosis*
  In exocytosis, molecules covered in a vesicle is expelled out of the cell through the plasma membrane (Fig. 3.5).

There are two types of exocytosis:
1. Constitutive pathway: In this process, substance is exocytosed immediately after its synthesis. For example, secretion of immunoglobulins.
2. Regulated pathway: In this process, substance is stored temporarily in vesicle after its synthesis in cytoplasm and exocytosed on extracellular signaling. For example, zymogen granules secretion.

CELL ORGANELLES

- Cytoplasm contains numerous structures that perform various functions. These are called cell organelles.
- Cell organelles are grouped as follows:
  1. Membrane-bound cell organelles: Endoplasmic reticulum, Golgi complex, mitochondria, phagosomes, lysosomes, peroxisomes, exocytic vesicles.
  2. Nonmembranous cell organelles: Cytoskeleton elements (microfilaments, microtubules, intermediate filaments).

Endoplasmic Reticulum (ER)

- Endoplasmic reticulum is a network of interconnecting membranes that form cistern, (Fig. 3.6).

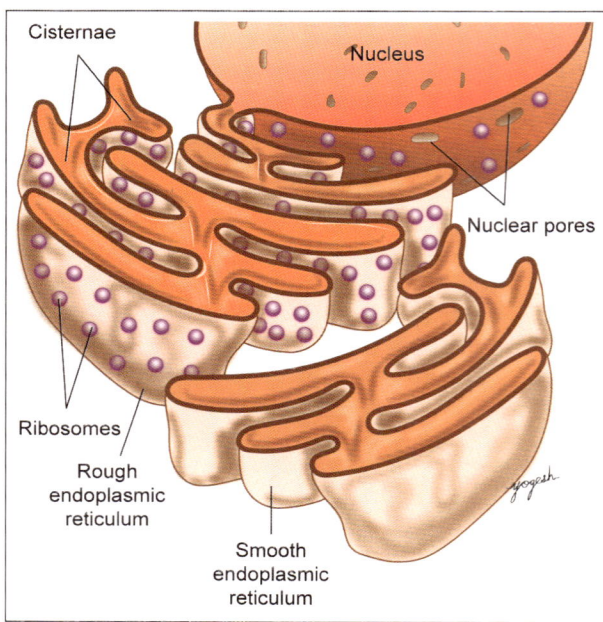

Fig. 3.6: Endoplasmic reticulum.

- The cytoplasm enclosed within the cisterns of endoplasmic reticulum is *vacuoplasm*, whereas the rest of the cytoplasm is hyaloplasm/cytosol.
- There are two varieties of ER: Rough-surfaced ER (having coating of ribosomes) and smooth-surfaced ER (without ribosomes).

Rough-Surfaced Endoplasmic Reticulum (rER)

- Ribosomes are present on the surface of rough endoplasmic reticulum (Fig. 3.6).
- As ribosomes contain RNA, they give basic (hematoxylin) staining to the cell.*Practical guide* *Ergastoplasm* is the portion of cytoplasm that stains with basic dyes.
- Ribosomes are attached on outer surface of rER by *ribosome docking proteins*.
- Mostly, rER is continuous with outer nuclear membrane.
- The mRNA binds with many ribosomes to form polyribosome complex or *polysome*.
- Newly synthesized proteins have signal sequences/peptides that direct the protein to get transferred to its destination site within the cell.
- Newly synthesized protein enters the lumen/cisternae of rER and undergoes posttransitional modifications such as glycosylation, folding, and so on. Later, modified proteins are delivered to the Golgi apparatus.
- Clinical fact: In *emphysema*, there is an inability of rER to deliver the synthesized enzyme α-1 antitrypsin to Golgi apparatus that results in *α-1 antitrypsin deficiency*.*Neet*

- rER is predominantly present in active protein secretory cells such as serous cells in the pancreas and salivary glands.
- Note: Free ribosomes synthesize cytoplasmic, structural and functional elements. For example, hemoglobin synthesis in precursor cells of RBCs, contractive protein synthesis in developing muscle.
- rER and free ribosomes produce Nissl bodies in neurons and cytoplasmic basophilia in other secretory cells.*Practical guide*

Functions

1. Protein synthesis: Site for translation (mRNA → proteins)
2. Checkpoint: rER destroys defective proteins.

Smooth-Surfaced Endoplasmic Reticulum (sER)

- Smooth-surfaced endoplasmic reticulum consists of short anastomosing tubules (Fig. 3.6).
- The sER lacks ribosome docking proteins, hence they do not have ribosomes.
- As sER is not associated with ribosomes, it gives eosinophilic (pink) color to cytoplasm.*Practical guide*

Functions

1. Lipid metabolism: sER is the main site for lipid synthesis. They are abundant in cells of liver, cells of adrenal cortex, and Leydig cells of testis.
2. *Sarcoplasmic reticulum:* In smooth and cardiac muscles, sER forms sarcoplasmic reticulum that acts as Ca^{++} ion reservoir.
3. Detoxification: sER is involved in detoxification of drugs and other chemicals.
4. Glycogen metabolism.
5. Membrane formation and recycling.

Golgi Complex [Camillo Golgi, 1843–1926]

- It is made up of 3–20 flattened curved membranous cisternae (sacs) that forms a shallow cup-like structure.
- It has convex/forming face (*cis-face*) and concave/maturing face (*trans-face*) (Fig. 3.7).
- Its *cis-face* faces toward rER and nucleus, whereas *trans-face* faces toward cell membrane.
- Middle part of Golgi apparatus is called media-*Golgi network*.
- Functions
  1. Posttranslational modification of proteins: Freshly synthesized proteins are transferred from rER to the Golgi apparatus. These proteins are modified by the Golgi apparatus.
  2. Formation of secretory vesicles: Modified proteins are wrapped around by the membrane of Golgi

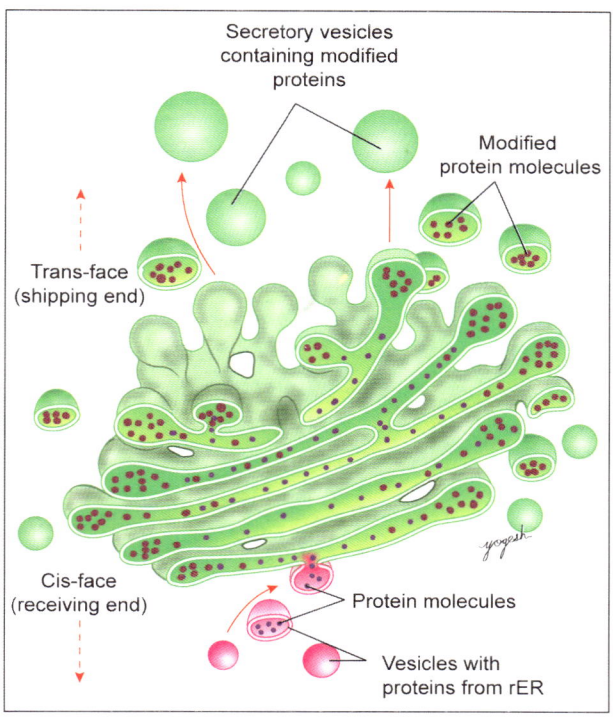

Fig. 3.7: Golgi apparatus.

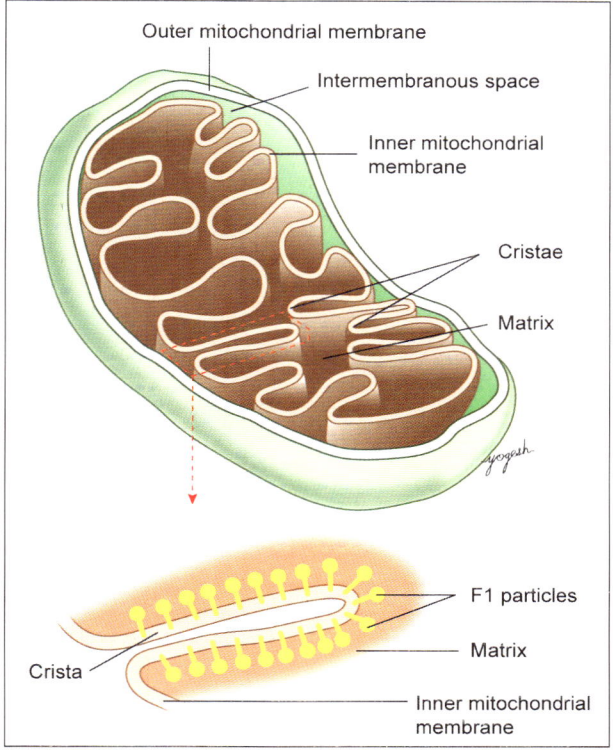

Fig. 3.8: Mitochondrion.

apparatus and get separated to form membrane-bound secretory vesicles or endosomes or lysosomes.
- Location: Usually, Golgi apparatus is located toward secretory portion (apical portion) of the cell membrane.

Mitochondria

- Mitochondria are *power houses* that generates energy (ATPs).
- Mitochondria are absent in RBCs and terminal keratinocytes of skin.^{MCQ}
- Size: 0.5–2 µm, elliptical-shaped.
- It is bounded by bilaminar membrane (similar to plasma membrane) with intermembranous space and matrix (Fig. 3.8).
- *Outer mitochondrial membrane* is smooth and has voltage-dependent anion channels called *mitochondrial porins*.
- Inner mitochondrial membrane shows folding called *cristae* (for increasing surface area).
- Inner mitochondrial membrane is impermeable to ions due to its cardiolipin phospholipids. It is a site for oxidation reactions, respiratory electron transport chain, and ATP synthesis.
- *Mitochondrial matrix* contains enzymes of Krebs cycle and fatty acid β-oxidation, Ca^{++} storing matrix granules, mitochondrial DNA, and so on.

- *Mitochondrial DNA* is a small circular double helix DNA that contains 37 genes.^{MCQ}
- Mitochondrial DNA is inherited from mother (ooplasm of ovum), as cytoplasm of sperm do not contribute to zygote.^{Neet}
- Due to mitochondrial DNA, mitochondria are self-replicating.
- Life span: ~10 days.
- Functions
  1. Powerhouse of cell: Mitochondria produces ATP by aerobic respiration.
  2. Self-replication: Mitochondrial DNA helps in certain protein synthesis and replication of mitochondria.
  3. Apoptosis (programmed cell death): Mitochondria sense cellular stress and release cytochrome C from intermembranous space into the cytoplasm. This cytochrome C initiates programmed cell death (apoptosis).
- *Mitochondrial cytopathy syndrome:* It is produced by defective mitochondrial DNA. It produces muscle weakness, neurological degenerative lesions, and lactic acidosis.^{Neet}
- *Myoclonic epilepsy with ragged red fibers* (MERRF) is produced because of defective enzymes of ATP synthesis. It produces muscle weakness, ataxia, seizures, and cardiac and respiratory failure. Red

muscle fibers show accumulation of abnormal mitochondria giving ragged-appearance on microscopic examination.

Ribosomes

[Discovered by *George Emil Palade, 1955*]
- Ribosomes are small cytoplasmic particles (15–20 nm)
- Ribosome consists of two subunits: Small (40S) and large (60S) (Fig. 3.9).
- Ribosomes lie in association with rER or in freeform in the cytoplasm.
- Polyribosome: It is a cluster of ribosomes bound to a single strand of messenger RNA.
- Ribosome synthesis is controlled by nucleolus (site of rRNA synthesis).
- Functions

Ribosomes synthesize protein as follows:
1. Free ribosomes produce structural proteins of a cell
2. Membrane-bound ribosomes (rER) produce secretory proteins

Lysosomes

- *Christian de Duve, 1955* discovered lysosomes (He termed them as suicide bags).
- Lysosomes are membrane-bound spherical cytoplasmic vesicles (0.2–0.8 μm in diameter).
- Electron microscopy: Lysosomes are electron-dense bodies.
- Formation: Lysosomes are derived from Golgi apparatus as primary lysosomes (Fig. 3.10).
- Primary lysosomes fuse with endocytic vesicle that contains material for digestion/destruction and forms secondary lysosome.
- Content: Lysosomes contain hydrolytic enzymes such as proteases, nucleases, glycosidases, lipases, and phospholipases.
- *New concept:* Endosomes receive hydrolytic enzymes from Golgi apparatus to form lysosomes.^{Neet}

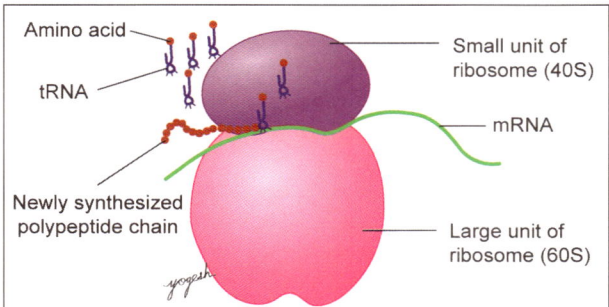

Fig. 3.9: Ribosome.

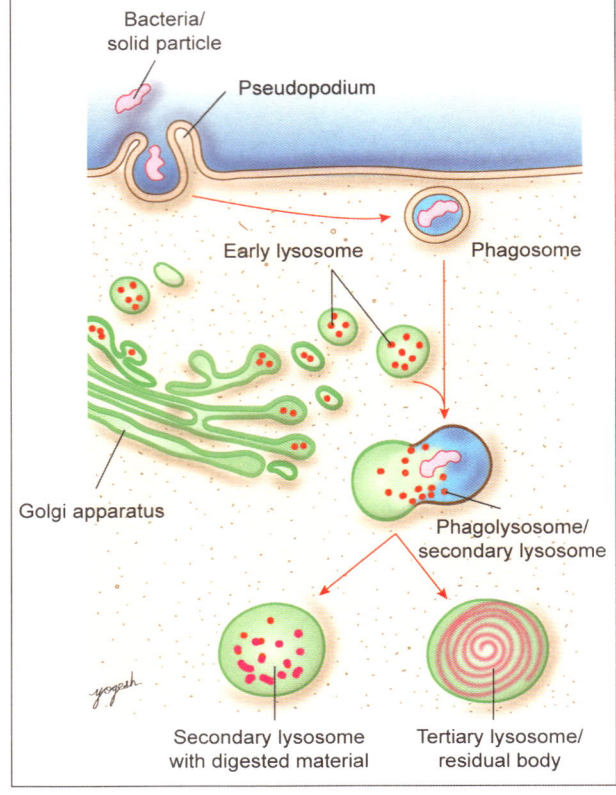

Fig. 3.10: Role of lysosome.

- Note: Proton (H^+ ion) pumps in lysosomal membrane make the content of lysosome highly acidic (<5 pH).
- Lysosomal membrane has unique lipid lysophosphatidic acid and other proteins. The inner surface of these lipids and proteins are covered by sugar molecules that protect lysosome from its own digestion by lysosomal enzymes.^{Viva}
- Functions
  1. Digestion of foreign material (*Heterophagy*): Lysosomes digest material (bacteria) that entered in to the cell by endocytosis.
  2. *Autophagy* (removal of old cell organelles): Lysosome removes worn-out organelles of cytosol.
  3. *Autolysis:* In case of diseases/lack of oxygen supply to the cell, lysosomal enzymes destroy own cells (autolysis).
  4. Inflammation: Neutrophil releases lysosomal enzymes in extracellular space that digest extracellular matrix and initiates acute inflammation.
- Recognizable lysosomes in histology^{Neet}
  1. Azurophilic granules in neutrophils.
  2. Lipofuscin granules (age pigment) are residual bodies in old cells. They are brown-pigmented granules developed due to lysosomal degradation.^{Viva}

Cell

> **Box 3.1: Lysosomal storage diseases**
> - Many genetic disorders cause lysosomal storage disease because of deficiency of certain lysosomal enzymes.
> - Table 3.2 includes some lysosomal storage diseases and responsible enzymes.
> - *Tay-Sachs disease* is an inherited lysosomal disorder due to deficiency of *β-hexosaminidase*. It results in accumulation of gangliosides in neurons that cause seizures, muscle rigidity, and death (before 5 years of age).^Neet

Table 3.2: Lysosomal storage diseases^Neet

Disease	Deficient enzyme
Gaucher disease	Glucocerebrosidase
Tay–Sachs disease	β-hexosaminidase
Krabbe disease	Galactosyl ceramidase
Niemann–Pick disease	Sphingomyelinase
Hurler syndrome	α-L-iduronidase
Hunter syndrome	L-iduronate sulfatase
Maroteaux–Lamy syndrome	Arylsulfatase B
Pompe disease	α-1, 4-glucosidase

Peroxisomes

- Peroxisomes are membrane-bound organelles.
- Peroxisomes contain oxidative enzymes that are required for the following:
  1. Amino acid oxidation
  2. β-oxidation of fatty acids
- Oxidation of these compounds generate hydrogen peroxide (H_2O_2) that is toxic for cell.
- H_2O_2 is broken down by enzyme *catalase* of peroxisomes.^MCQ
- Peroxisomes help for detoxification in liver and kidney.
- *Zellweger syndrome/cerebrohepatorenal syndrome:* It is an inherited nonfunctioning peroxisomal disorder. [Hans Ulrich Zellweger, 1909–1990, Swiss-American pediatrician].

Endosomes

- Endosomes are derived from *endocytosis*.
- *Early endosomes:* On endocytosis, the membrane-bound organelle called early endosome is formed.
- *Late endosomes/lysosomes:* Golgi apparatus transfers hydrolytic enzymes and convert early endosomes to late endosomes or lysosomes.
- Transfer of prohydrolase to endosome takes place with the help of mannose-6-phosphate (M-6-P) receptors that are present on endosome surface.
- Mannose-6-phosphate gets separated from prohydrolases by acidic environment to form active hydrolases.

CYTOSKELETON

- Cytoskeleton is a supporting network of protein filaments in cytoplasm.
- Cytoskeleton helps in the following:
  1. Maintaining cellular architecture
  2. Cellular mobility and migration
  3. Movement of cilia, microvilli, tail of sperms
  4. Anchoring the cell on basal lamina
  5. Form cell junctions
  6. Intracellular vesicular transport
- Components of cytoskeleton:
  1. Microtubules
  2. Microfilaments
  3. Intermediate filaments

Microtubules

- Microtubules are nonbranching hollow tubules made up of tubulin proteins (α and β tubulin) (Fig. 3.11).
- Locations: Cilia, flagella, centrioles, mitotic spindle, elongating cell processes, and growing axons.
- **Structure**
  - Microtubules are 20–25 nm in diameter with 5 nm thick wall.
  - It consists of 13 protofilaments of dimeric tubulin molecules that have α-tubulin and β-tubulin subunits.

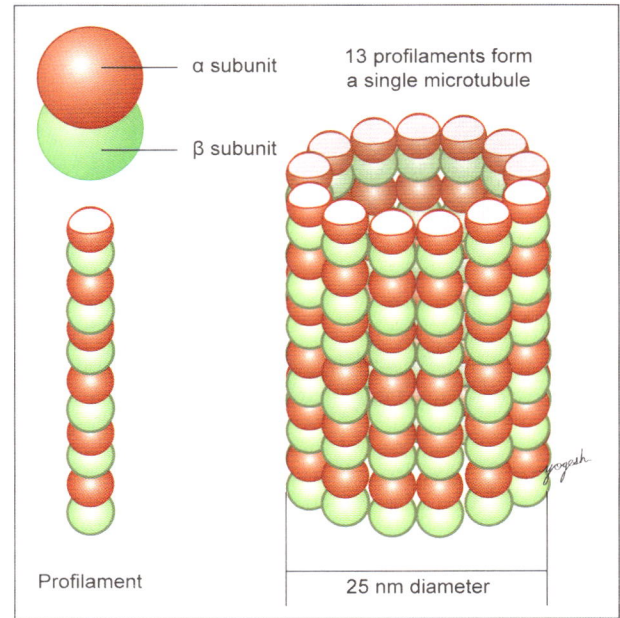

Fig. 3.11: Structure of microtubules.

- Centriole has *microtubule organizing center* that gives rise to microtubules.
- Formation of microtubules requires guanosine triphosphate (GTP) and Mg^{++}.
- Microtubule-associated proteins stabilize the microtubules.
- Functions
    1. Movement of cilia, flagella (tail of sperm)
    2. Intracellular transport of vesicles
    3. In cell division, formation of mitotic spindle
    4. Maintenance of cell shape.
- Molecular motor proteins help in the movement of cell organelles along the microtubules. For example, dynein (present in cilia and flagella), and kinesins.
- Dynein moves organelles toward the center of cell, whereas kinesins move organelles toward the periphery.

Actin Filaments/Microfilaments

- G-actin molecule assembles to form F-actin (filamentous actin) or microfilaments (Fig. 3.12).
- Microfilament is 6-8 nm in diameter.

- *Actin-binding proteins* (ABPs): They controls polymerization of G-actin, thus determining the length of actin filaments. They cross-link actin filaments to form bundles. For example, fascin, fimbrin in microvilli.
- Actin capping proteins (for example, tropomodulin) block further addition of actin molecules.
- Functions
    1. Anchor the cell membrane by forming cell junctions
    2. Forms core of microvilli (Chapter 5)
    3. Forms terminal web (Chapter 5)
    4. Cell movement by forming extension of plasma membrane called *lamellipodia*.
    5. *Filopodia* are small spikes/processes on the surface of cell processes (lamellipodia). Filopodia contain actin filaments.

Intermediate Filaments

- The diameter of intermediate filament (8–10 nm) is intermediate between that of microtubules (20–25 nm) and actin filaments (6–8 nm). Hence, these are called intermediate filaments.
- Intermediate filaments are grouped into six major classes based on their protein composition and cellular distribution (Table 3.3).
- Functions
    1. To link cells together with basal lamina.
    2. Keratins form superficial layers of stratified epithelium, core of hair and nails.
    3. Neurofilaments help to maintain shape of nerve processes.
    4. Lamins maintains shape of nucleus, whereas beaded filaments maintain eye lens integrity.
    5. Intermediate filament-associated proteins: These include desmoplakins, desmoplakin-like proteins, and plakoglobins. These molecules help in cell to cell and cell to extracellular matrix junctions.

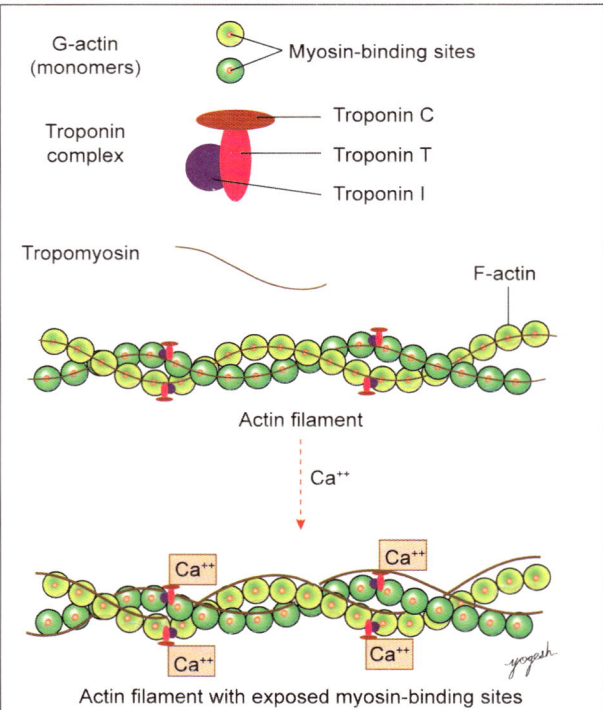

Fig. 3.12: Structure of thin filament. Actin consists of polypeptide chain of G actin monomers. In relaxed stage, tropomyosin covers the active binding sites of F-actin for myosin. Ca^{++} ions bind with troponin C and results in release of tropomyosin from F-actin. Thus, Ca^{++} exposes myosin-binding sites of actin.

Table 3.3: Types of intermediate filaments

Type of protein	Examples	Location
Class 1 and 2	Keratins	All epithelial cells
	Vimentin	Mesenchymal cells
Class 3	Desmin	Muscles
	Glial fibrillary acidic protein	Neuroglial cells, Schawnn cells
Class 4	Peripherin	Peripheral neurons
Class 5	Neurofilaments	Neurons
Class 6	Lamins	Nucleus

Centrioles

- Centrioles are small spherical area of cytoplasm situated near the nucleus.
- Centrioles are hollow cylindrical structures that are made up of nine microtubule triplets arranged in cylindrical pattern (Fig. 3.13).
- There are two centrioles in a cell. They are arranged at right angle to each other.
- Centrioles are surrounded by *pericentriolar area.*
- Centrioles and pericentriolar area together called as *centrosome or microtubule organizing region.*
- Centrioles are self-replicating organelles.
- Functions
  1. Centrosome initiate formation of microtubules.
  2. Centrosome forms mitotic spindle.
  3. Centrosome provides basal bodies for cilia and flagella.
  4. Centrioles self-replicate just before cell division.

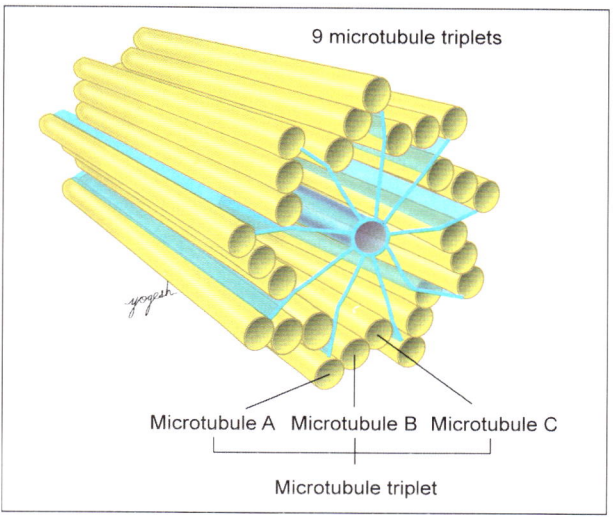

Fig. 3.13: Structure of centriole.

Clinical Correlation

- *Kartagener syndrome:* It is a defect in the organization of microtubules that results in *defective ciliary movement* in the respiratory tract, defective sperm movement, and defective ciliary movement of fallopian tubes. It results in repeated respiratory infections, and male and female infertility.[Neet]
- Colchicine and vinblastine prevent mitotic spindle formation and arrest cell division in mitosis. Colchicine is useful for chromosomal studies in cytogenetics.[Neet]
- *Alzheimer's disease:* Defective formation of neurofilaments (intermediate filaments) causes Alzheimer's disease. It results in accumulation of neurofibrillary tangles in neurons.
- In alcoholic liver cirrhosis, keratin filaments get accumulated in hepatocytes and form *Mallory bodies* (inclusions).
- *Duchenne muscular dystrophy* [Duchenne de Boulogne, 1806–1875, French Neurologist]: It is a X-linked recessive disorder that affects only boys. It involves a defective gene for dystrophin protein. Dystrophin is essential in binding contractile assembly to sarcolemma in skeletal muscles.[Neet]

NUCLEUS

- Nucleus is an oval or spherical membrane-bound structure.
- Most of the cell contain single nucleus except[MCQ]
  - RBCs and platelets do not have nuclei
  - Striated muscle cells are multinucleated
  - Few hepatocytes and transitional epithelial cells are binucleated

Box 3.2: Inclusions

- Inclusions are cytoplasmic or nuclear structures that are products of metabolic activity of cell.
- Inclusions have characteristic staining property.
- Examples: lipofuscin, hemosiderin, glycogen, lipid inclusions, and so on.

Lipofuscin[Viva]
- These are brownish-gold pigments.
- It is visible on *H&E* staining.
- Locations: Neurons, skeletal, and cardiac muscles, macrophages.
- It is a wear and tear pigment.
- Mechanism of formation: Digested bacteria in macrophages, accumulated oxidized lipids in other cells.

Hemosiderin
- These are iron complexes formed by indigestible residues of hemoglobin in phagocytic cells.

Glycogen
- It is a glucose polymer found mostly in hepatocytes and muscle cells.
- Toluidine blue or periodic acid–Schiff staining is useful for detecting glycogen.

Lipid inclusions
- These are fat droplets found in intestinal absorptive cells and adipocytes. They are also found in hepatocytes in lipid storage disease.

- Nucleus is present during interphase of the cell.
- It consists of the following components: chromatin, nucleolus, nuclear membrane, and nucleoplasm (Fig. 3.14).

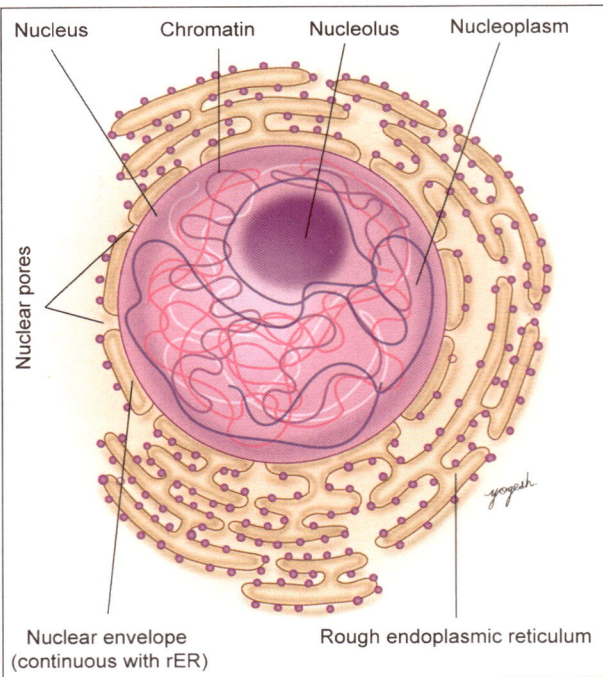

Fig. 3.14: Structure of nucleus.

Nuclear Envelope

- Nuclear envelope is bilaminar membrane that separates nucleoplasm from the cytoplasm.
- *Perinuclear cisternal* space lies between two layers of nuclear envelope.
- *Nuclear pores* are intervals in nuclear membrane that transport RNAs and proteins between the nucleus and the cytoplasm.
- Outer membrane of nuclear envelope is continuous with rough endoplasmic reticulum.
- Inner nuclear membrane is supported by intermediate filaments (lamin).
- Abnormal lamin proteins are detected in Emery-Dreifuss muscular dystrophy (progressive muscle weakness, *contractures* of tendons and weakening of heart muscle).*Neet*
- During cell division, nuclear envelope disappears to allow chromosomal separation. After cell division, nuclear envelope is reassembled.

Nucleoplasm

- Nucleoplasm is a material enclosed by nuclear envelope besides chromatin and nucleoli. It contains various proteins, ions, and inclusions.

Chromatin

- Genetic material of the cell located in the nucleus is in the form of a long thread called *chromatin*.

- Chromatin consists of (Human genome project-2003):
  – 1.8 m long DNA
  – 1000 times longer than the nucleus diameter
  – 46 chromosomes
  – 2.85 billion base pairs of nucleotides
  – 23,000 protein-coding genes
- Chromatin consists of DNA coiled around histone and nonhistone proteins (structural proteins). Presence of DNA and RNA (acids/negative charges) makes the chromatin basophilic (stained with hematoxylin).*Viva*
- Definition of gene: *"Gene is a union of genomic sequences encoding a coherent set of potentially overlapping functional products"* [Histology: A Text and Atlas, Pawlina W, 7th Ed].

Forms of Chromatin

- According to the functional activity, chromatin has coiled DNA and it produces two forms of chromatin as follows (Fig. 3.15):
- *Euchromatin**Viva*
  It is a partially condensed chromatin
  It is more active and lightly stained
  It is expressed during interphase
- *Heterochromatin**Viva*
  It is a condensed chromatin
  It is inactive and darkly stained
  It does not express during interphase
  – *Constitutive heterochromatin* remains inactive throughout the cell cycle. For example, around centromere, telomeres, and C-band of chromosomes.
  – *Facultative heterochromatin* remains active in certain phase of the cell cycle. For example, both the X chromosomes remain active during embryogenesis and later one X chromosome becomes inactive. Inactive X chromosome in females form *Barr body* or *drumstick body* in neutrophils.*MCQ*

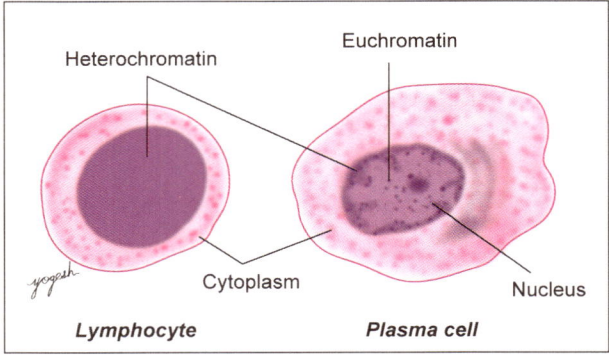

Fig. 3.15: Heterochromatic nucleus and euchromatic nucleus.

- Nucleosomes are the smallest units of chromatin. It consists of macromolecular complexes of DNA and histones.

Histone Proteins

- Histone proteins form an octamer having eight molecules of histone proteins. DNA wrapping around histone proteins produce *beads on a string* appearance.
- During cell division, chromatin condenses to form *chromosomes* (*color bodies* in Greek).

Nucleolus

- Nucleolus is a spherical mass of heterochromatin.
- It is a dark staining body, 1–3 µm in diameter.
- Each nucleus shows 1–2 nucleoli (maximum 5–6).^{Viva}
- It contains a protein nucleostemin that binds p53 protein and regulates cell cycle and cell differentiation.

- *Electron microscopy:* There are three regions of nucleolus inside outward as follows:
  - Fibrillar center
  - Fibrillar material
  - Granular material
- Function: Ribosomal RNA synthesis.

Some Interesting Facts

- In degenerative process, the nucleus loses its details and becomes shrunken, and darkly stained. Such nuclei are called *pyknotic nuclei.*^{Viva}
- Apoptosis is programmed cell death. It is an active gene-directed process that requires energy.^{Viva}
- Necrosis is not a programmed cell death. It may result from various factors such as mechanical chemical injury, infectious agents, toxins, and so on.^{Viva}

SECTION 2

General Histology

4. Epithelial Tissue
5. Cell Surface Projections and Cell Junctions
6. Glands
7. General Connective Tissue
8. Cartilage
9. Bone
10. Muscle Tissue
11. Lymphoid Tissue
12. Nervous Tissue
13. Cardiovascular Tissue
14. Skin and its Appendages

CHAPTER 4

Epithelial Tissue

Chapter Outline

- Classification of epithelia
- Simple epithelium
  - Simple squamous epithelium
  - Simple cuboidal epithelium
  - Simple columnar epithelium
- Pseudostratified epithelium
- Goblet cells
- Stratified epithelium
  - Stratified squamous epithelium
  - Stratified cuboidal epithelium
  - Stratified columnar epithelium
- Transitional epithelium/urothelium
- Basement membrane

Competency achievement: The student should be able to:

AN65.1 Identify epithelium under the microscope and describe the various types that correlate to its function

INTRODUCTION

- Human body consists of four basic tissue: Epithelium, nervous tissue, muscular tissue, and connective tissue.*Viva*
- Epithelium
  Definition: The surface of the body (inner and outer) and inner surfaces of tubular structures within the body are covered by a layer of cells that rests on the basement membrane. Such a covering layer is called *epithelium*.
- Epithelium is a basic tissue of body that consists of tightly adhered cells called epithelial cells.

Features of Epithelium

Epithelium has the following features:*Viva*

1. Epithelium consists of layers of cells that cover body surfaces.
2. Epithelium is an *avascular* structure. It receives nutrition by diffusion.*Viva*
3. Epithelial cells rest on basement membrane.
4. Epithelial cells show various types of junctions with adjacent cells and basement membrane.
5. Epithelial cells isolate deeper structures from surface environment.
6. Epithelial cells show surface modifications as per functional need. For example, microvilli in intestine increase absorptive surface area.
7. Epithelial cells undergo mitosis and can regenerate damaged portion.

Functions of Epithelium*Viva*

Q. List the functions of epithelium.

- Epithelial cells perform various functions based on their location. Some of their basic functions are listed as follows:
  1. Protection: Epithelium protects deeper structures. For example, in the skin, epithelium (called epidermis) protect deeper structures from external environment.
  2. Barrier: Epithelium acts as a mechanical barrier and may permit selective substances to cross it. For example, epidermis prevents entry of viruses but allows entry of some lipid soluble drugs (ointments).
  3. Absorption: Epithelium is involved in the absorption of substances. For example, in the intestine, epithelium absorbs nutrients from digested food.

4. Secretion/excretion: Epithelium can synthesize and secrete some products. For example, in salivary gland, epithelium is involved in saliva secretion.
5. Sensory perception: Epithelium is involved in receiving sensory signals from external environment. For example, epithelium of tongue (taste buds) are involved in perception of taste sensation.

Epithelial Cells

- Epithelial cells have different size and shape according to their locations and need for their functions. Epithelial cells have three basic shapes: squamous (flat), cuboidal, and columnar.

Surfaces of the Epithelial Cells

- Each epithelial cell has basal surface, apical surface, and lateral surfaces (Fig. 4.1).
  1. Basal surface remains in contact with basal lamina or deeper cells of epithelium.
  2. Apical surface of epithelial cells faces external environment in skin or luminal content in the tubular structures or may be attached with superficial epithelial cells.
  3. Lateral surfaces of epithelial cell form junctional complexes with adjacent epithelial cells.

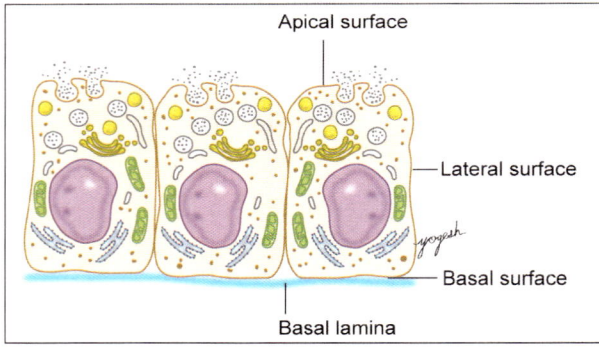

Fig. 4.1: Surfaces of epithelium.

> **Box 4.1: Histological practical aspects**
> - Always use special violet and lilac color professional pencils for drawing hematoxylin and eosin stained structures (Apsara, Faber-Castell, Staedtler or any other suitable brand).
> - Do not use routine pink and violet color pencils.
> - Use HB pencil or black pen for labeling.

- In a section, epithelial cells may be squamous, cuboidal, or columnar.
- However, on surface view, these cells are seen as polygonal or irregular in shape. Some cells show bulging on the surface at the site of underlying nucleus.

Note: Epithelioid cells or epithelioid histiocytes are activated macrophages that resemble epithelial cells. They have pale cytoplasm and central ovoid nucleus. These cells may merge to form giant multinucleated cells. Epithelioid cells are an essential feature of granuloma (an organized collection of epithelioid macrophages).*Neet*

CLASSIFICATION OF EPITHELIA

- Epithelia are classified according to two features (Flowchart 4.1):
  1. Layers of epithelial cells
  2. Shape of cells facing toward free surface of epithelium
- *Simple epithelium* has only one layer of cells.
- *Stratified epithelium* has two or more layers of cells.
- *Pseudostratified epithelium* has one layer of cells resting on basal lamina, but some of these cells do not extend up to free surface of epithelium.

Simple Epithelium

- Simple epithelium is a single layer of cells resting on basal lamina.

Flowchart 4.1: Classification of epithelium

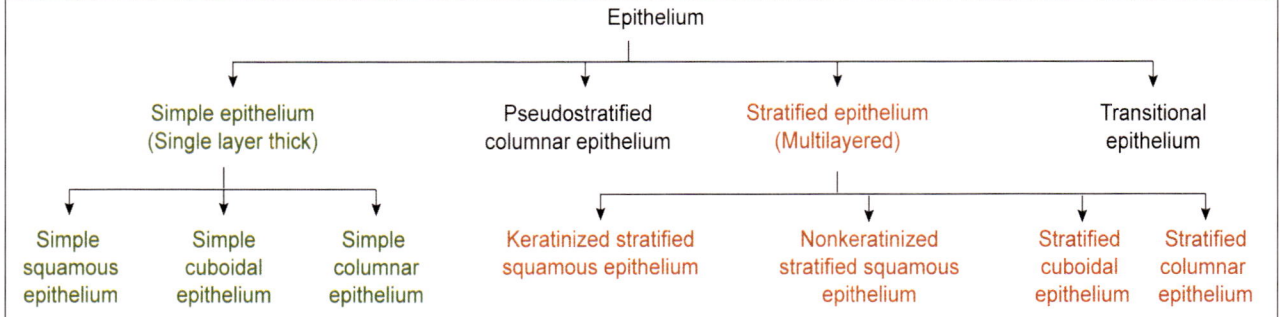

- Simple epithelium is classified into three groups based on shape of cells as follows (Flowchart 4.2):
  1. Simple squamous epithelium: Composed of flat cells
  2. Simple cuboidal epithelium: Composed of cells with equal height and width
  3. Simple columnar epithelium: Composed of cells with more height than width

Simple Squamous Epithelium

Features
- Simple squamous epithelium is composed of a single layer of flattened (*squamous* = flat) polygonal cells (Figs 4.2, 4.3 and Flowchart 4.2).
- These cells have thin layer of cytoplasm stained with eosin (pink).

Flowchart 4.2: Simple epithelium

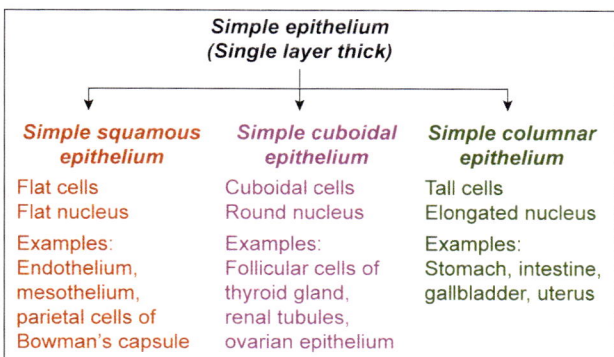

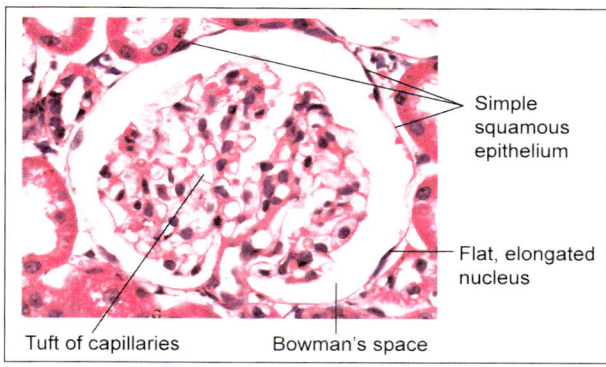

Fig. 4.3: Photomicrograph. Simple squamous epithelium (glomerulus in kidney, H&E stain, high magnification).

- Nuclei of these cells are elongated, flat, and produce bulging on cell surface. (Nuclei are stained dark with hematoxylin (violet).*Identification feature*
- *Top view:* Free surface (apical surface) of simple squamous epithelial cell is irregular or polygonal.
- *Section of cell:* It looks similar to a half-fried egg (consider nucleus as yolk and cytoplasm as egg white).

Locations*High yielding facts*
1. Lining epithelium of lung alveoli[Neet]
2. *Endothelium* (lining epithelium of blood and lymphatic vessels)
3. *Endocardium* (lining epithelium of heart)
4. *Mesothelium* (lining epithelium of serous cavities of body [pericardium, peritoneum, pleura])[Neet]
5. Parietal cells of Bowman's capsule and certain parts of nephron in kidney (ansa nephroni/loop of Henle)[Neet]

Functions
- As cells are very thin in simple squamous epithelium, small molecules can easily cross the epithelium. Thus, it helps in rapid transport of substances, diffusion of gases, and filtration of fluids.

Simple Cuboidal Epithelium

Features
- Simple cuboidal epithelium is composed of a single layer of cuboidal cells having equal width and height.
- Nuclei of cuboidal cells are rounded, placed centrally in cells. As width of cells is equal, their nuclei are seen to be equally placed in a single row (Figs 4.4 and 4.5).*Identification feature*
- Surface view: Cells are polygonal or hexagonal when seen from free surface.
- Cytoplasm: Cuboidal cells contain eosinophilic cytoplasm.

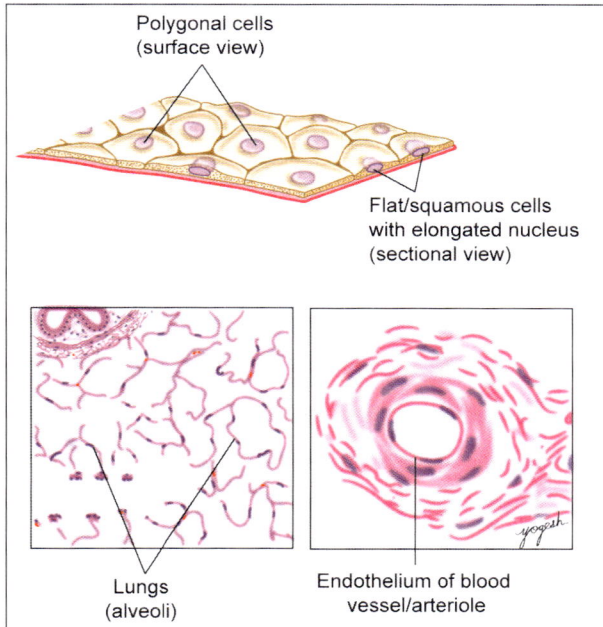

Fig. 4.2: Simple squamous epithelium (with practice figure).

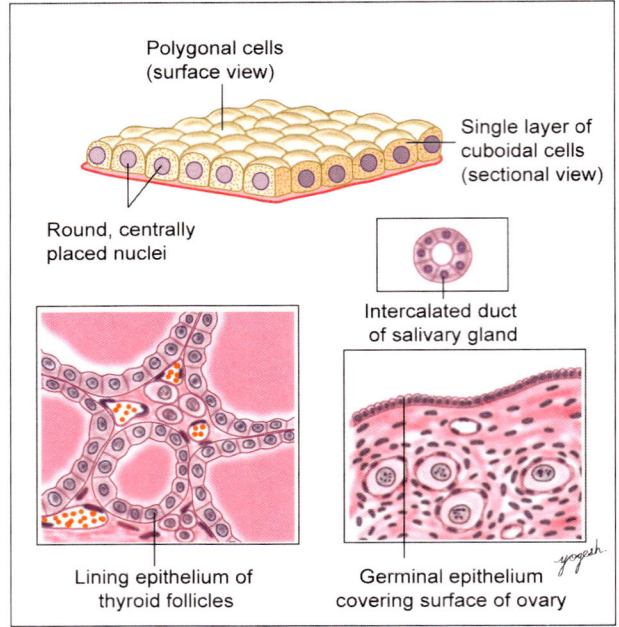

Fig. 4.4: Simple cuboidal epithelium (with practice figure).

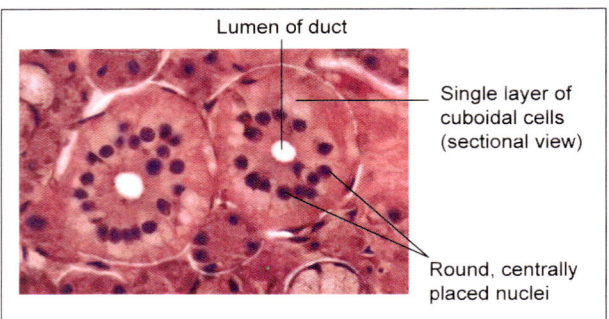

Fig. 4.5: Photomicrograph. Simple cuboidal epithelium (ducts in salivary gland, *H&E* stain, high magnification).

Locations
1. Lining epithelium of thyroid follicles[Neet]
2. Smaller ducts of exocrine glands
3. Epithelium covering the ovary (called germinal epithelium)
4. Choroid plexuses (produces cerebrospinal fluid)
5. Inner surface of lens of eyeball
6. Pigmented cell layer of retina
7. Duct of Bartholin gland[Neet]
8. Some part of tubules in kidney (distal convoluted tubule)[Neet]

Functions
- Cells of simple cuboidal epithelium have cytoplasm that contains required machinery for protein synthesis but does not have well-developed Golgi apparatus for storage of synthesized proteins and their substances. Hence, cuboidal epithelium is mainly involved in transport (absorption and excretion), synthesis, and secretion of substances.

Simple Columnar Epithelium

Features
- Simple columnar epithelium is composed of a single layer of columnar cells having more height than their width (Figs 4.6 and 4.7).*Identification feature*

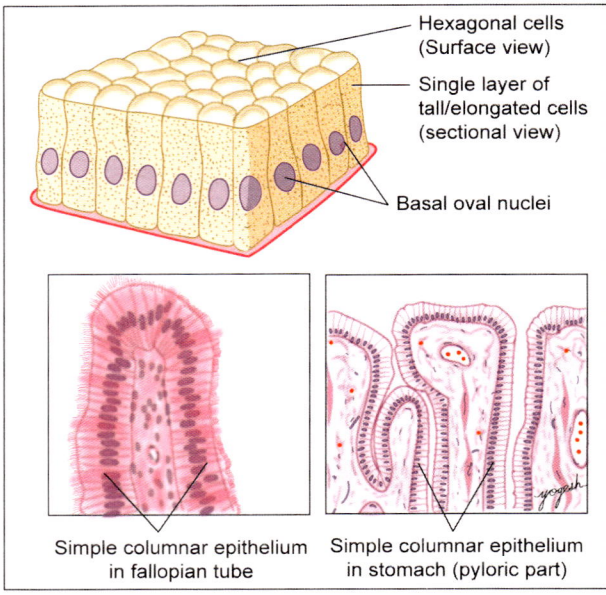

Fig. 4.6: Simple columnar epithelium (with practice figures).

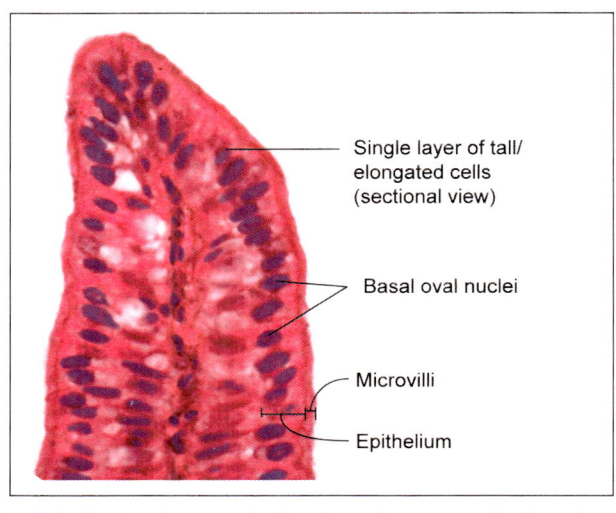

Fig. 4.7: Photomicrograph. Simple columnar epithelium (small intestine, high magnification).

- *Cytoplasm:* Columnar cells have abundant cytoplasm as these cells are involved in synthesis and storage of metabolites.
- *Staining:* Columnar cells take stain according to the presence of cell organelles.
  - *Apical eosinophilia:* Cells having well-developed Golgi apparatus and the presence of secretory granules show apical region stained with eosin (pink). It is known as apical eosinophilia.
  - *Basal basophilia:* Cells having well-developed rough endoplasmic reticulum in basal portion of cells show basal region stained with hematoxylin (violet). It is known as basal basophilia.
  - *Foamy appearance/empty appearance:* Some cells (mucous cells) contain carbohydrates (mucus or glycogen) or lipids in their cytoplasm. These substances are lost in the process of slide preparation. Such cells may show foamy appearance or empty cytoplasm.
- *Nuclei:* Nuclei of columnar cells are oval (elongated) and usually placed in basal region of cells.*Identification feature*
- Nuclei are lightly stained and show presence of one or two nucleoli. It indicates active involvement of nucleus in protein synthesis. All nuclei are placed at the same level.
- Surface modifications:
  Simple columnar epithelium at some locations shows certain surface modifications as follows:
  - *Cilia*: In fallopian tube, lining epithelium shows presence of cilia; hence, such epithelium is known as ***simple ciliated columnar epithelium***.
  - *Microvilli:* In gastrointestinal tract, bile duct, and gallbladder, lining epithelium shows microvilli. If villi are arranged in regular manner, it gives striated border appearance and if the villi are irregularly arranged, it gives brush border appearance on light microscopic examination.*Neet*

Locations
1. Lining epithelium of stomach, intestine, and gallbladder
2. Lining epithelium of uterus
3. *Simple ciliated columnar epithelium:* Fallopian tube, central canal of spinal cord, ventricles of brain, some part of respiratory tract, efferent ductules of testis, part of middle ear, Eustachian/auditory tube, ventricles of the brain [Bartolomeo Eustachi, 1500–1574, Anatomist].*Neet*

Functions
1. Secretory function: Secretion of enzymes, mucus and so on.
2. Absorptive function: Absorption of nutrients in intestine.
3. Ciliary beats: Propulsion of mucus in respiratory tract and ova in fallopian tube.
4. Microvilli: Help to increase absorptive surface area of cells in gall bladder and intestine.

Pseudostratified Epithelium

Features
- Pseudostratified epithelium consists of cells that rest on basal lamina and only some of these cells reach up to the free surface of epithelium (Figs 4.8 and 4.9).*Viva*

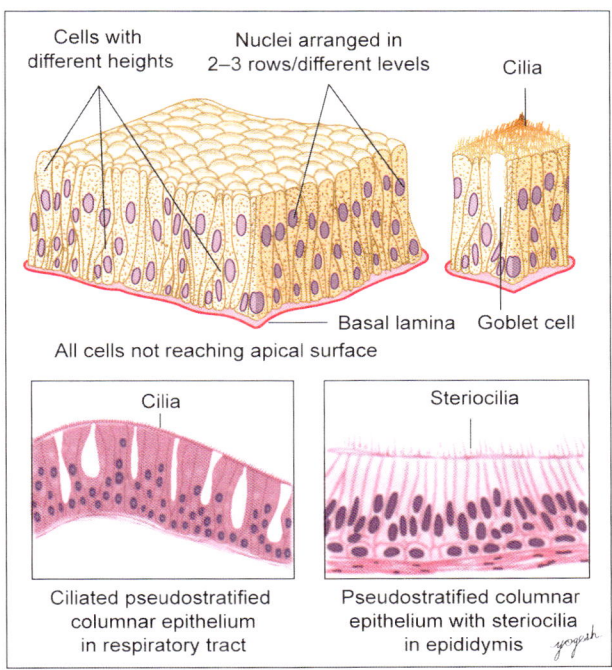

Fig. 4.8: Pseudostratified columnar epithelium (with practice figures).

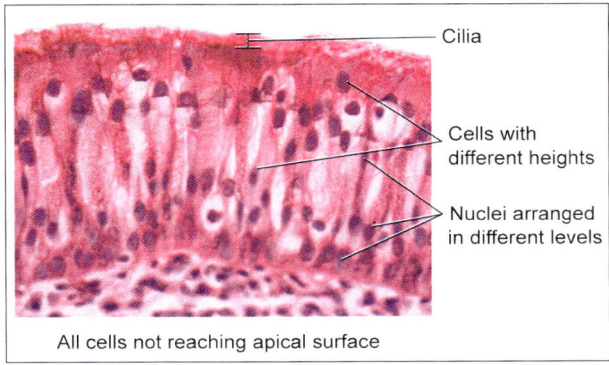

Fig. 4.9: Photomicrograph. Ciliated pseudostratified columnar epithelium (respiratory epithelium, high magnification).

- This epithelium *is not a true stratified* epithelium. It appears to be stratified.
- Because of differential height of cells, their nuclei lie at different levels and form two to three rows of nuclei.*Identification feature*
- Epithelium has small cuboidal basal cells that divide mitotically and replace other cells of epithelium.
- Fully matured cells are columnar and reach up to the free surface. Hence, this is called pseudostratified columnar epithelium.

Locations

1. Respiratory tract: In respiratory tract, tallest cells of epithelium show cilia on the free surface. Hence, it is called *ciliated pseudostratified columnar epithelium*. Cilia help in the removal of mucus.*Neet*
2. *In male reproductive tract:* In some part male reproductive tract (epididymis), pseudostratified columnar epithelium with stereocilia (long microvillus) is present. It helps in absorption of fluid.
3. Pseudostratified columnar epithelium (nonciliated) is present in the auditory tube, ductus deference, and membranous and penile urethra.*Neet*

Functions

1. Protection of underlying structures
2. Ciliary movements remove the mucus
3. Stereocilia help in absorption of fluid
4. Goblet cells secrete mucus
5. Basal cells act as stem cells for remaining cells of the epithelium

---

Box 4.2: Goblet cells

- These are mucus-secreting cells.
- Respiratory epithelium, epithelium of terminal part of small intestine, and large intestine show goblet cells.
- *Goblet* means cup with narrow beak in Greek.*Viva*
- Shape of goblet cell: Apical cup-shaped portion connected with basal stem-like part.
- Goblet cells show secretory granules (mucus) in upper part of cell and nucleus and other cell organelles in basal part of cell.
- H&E staining: Apical portion gives empty or *foamy appearance* as mucus is removed during tissue processing.*Neet, Identification feature*
- Basal portion shows flat, elongated nucleus.*Identification feature*
- PAS staining and fresh frozen section: Fresh frozen sections stained with periodic acid–Schiff's reagent gives dark magenta color to mucus.*Viva*
- Mucicarmine stain: It gives deep red color to goblet cells.

Functions
- Secretion of mucus
- Mucus protects underlying epithelium by forming gel-like coating. Mucus consists of large glycoprotein that can hold number of water molecules to form gel.

Locations
1. Respiratory epithelium
2. Gastrointestinal tract
3. Conjunctiva of upper eyelid

Clinical correlation
1. *Allergic asthm*a may result in excess production of mucus.
2. *Goblet cell carcinoid* is tumor formed by proliferation of goblet cells and neuroendocrine cells in gut.

Stratified Epithelium

- Stratified epithelium is a multilayered epithelium.
- In stratified epithelium, only the basal cell layer rest on basal lamina.
- Stratified epithelium is classified further based on shape of cells in superficial layer of epithelium as follows (Flowchart 4.3):
  1. Stratified squamous epithelium
  2. Stratified cuboidal epithelium
  3. Stratified columnar epithelium

Stratified Squamous Epithelium

Features

- Stratified squamous epithelium consists of several layers of cells (Figs 4.10 and 4.11).*Identification feature*
- Basal cell layer consists of cuboidal or columnar cells that rest on basal lamina. Nuclei of these cells are large, rounded, or oval.*Neet, Identification feature*
- Basal cells act as stem cells; they divide mitotically and migrate to superficial cell layers.
- Cells above basal layer gradually decrease in size and become flat (squamous). Nuclei of the superficial layer are elongated and flat.*Identification feature*
- Based on keratinization (dead cell layer), stratified squamous epithelium is further classified as follows:
  1. Keratinized stratified squamous epithelium
  2. Nonkeratinized stratified squamous epithelium

Keratinized stratified squamous epithelium

- Superficial cells show *keratohyalin granules* in their cytoplasm.
- The most superficial cells are dead. They do not have nuclei. Such dead cell layer is called *stratum corneum* (Figs 4.10 and 4.11).*Identification feature*
- Keratinization indicates dryness or friction exposed surface.
- Location: Epidermis of skin.

Flowchart 4.3: Stratified epithelium

Stratified epithelium (multiple layers)

Keratinized stratified squamous epithelium
- Multiple layers
- Basal cells - cuboidal
- Superficial cells - flat
- Stratified corneum: nonnucleated dead cell layer
- Examples: Skin

Nonkeratinized stratified squamous epithelium
- Multiple layers
- Basal cells - cuboidal
- Superficial cells - flat, nucleated
- Examples: Oral cavity, esophagus, vagina, anal canal, vocal folds, cornea

Stratified cuboidal epithelium
- Two cell layer thick
- Superficial cells - cuboidal
- Examples: Ducts of sweat and salivary glands

Stratified columnar epithelium
- Two cell layer thick
- Superficial cells - columnar
- Examples: Ducts of some glands, fornix of conjunctiva, cavernous urethra

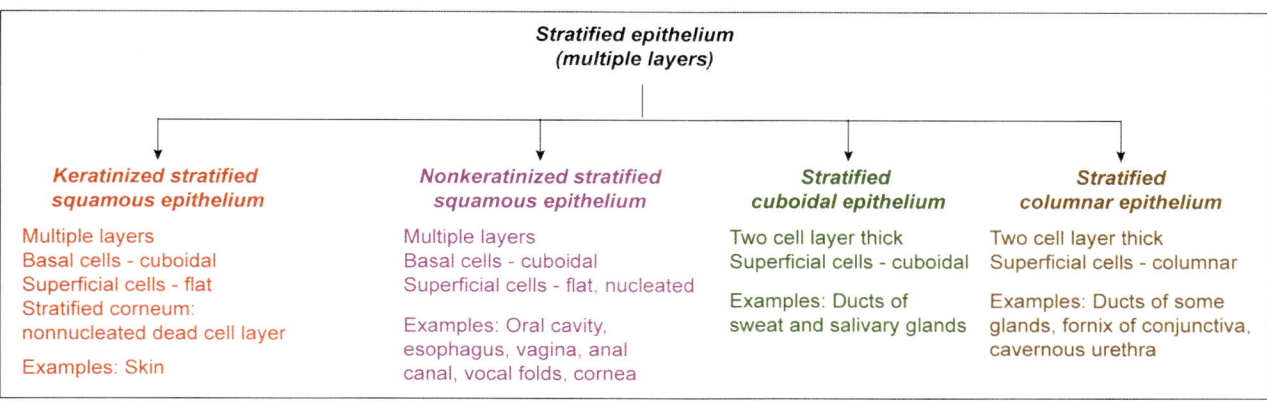

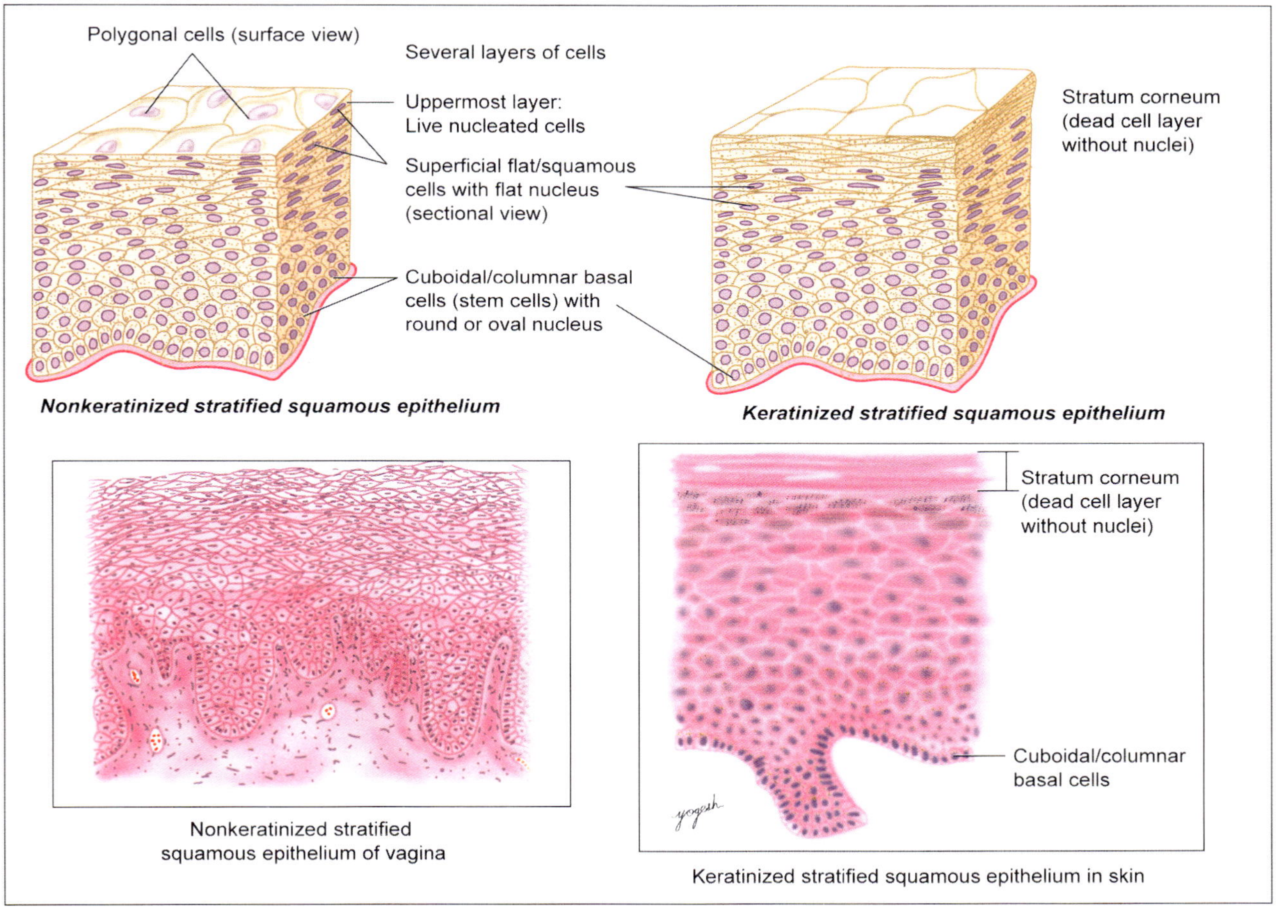

Fig. 4.10: Keratinized and nonkeratinized stratified squamous epithelium (with practice figures).

- *Functions*
  - It protects the deeper structures from mechanical injuries.
  - It acts as a barrier against infection.
  - It prevents water loss.

Nonkeratinized stratified squamous epithelium

- There is no stratum corneum. *Identification feature*
- Cells in the uppermost layer are live and nucleated (Figs 4.10 and 4.11). *Identification feature*
- Cells become increasing flattened as one move toward the superficial layer. *Identification feature*
- This epithelium remains always moist.
- Such moist epithelium with underlying thin connective tissue layer (lamina propria) is called mucosa.

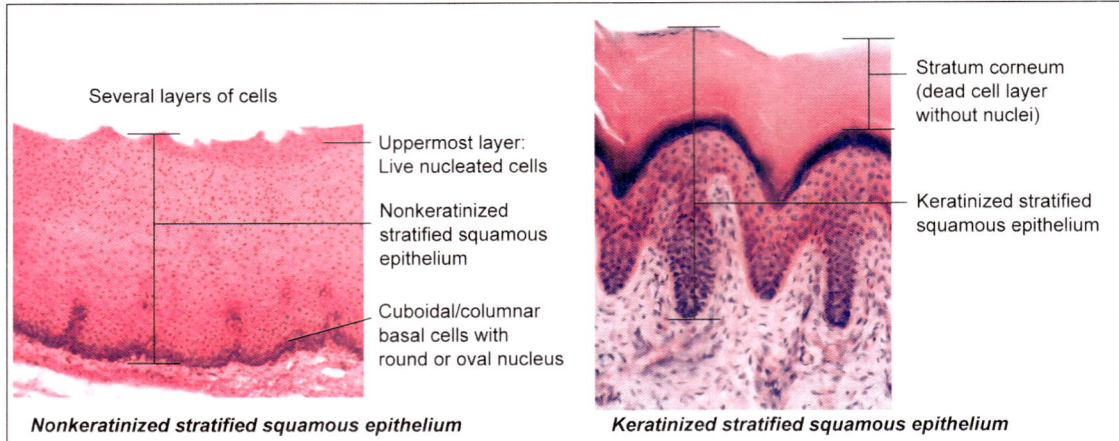

Fig. 4.11: Photomicrograph. Stratified squamous epithelium (nonkeratinized variety from esophagus and keratinized variety from thick skin, high magnification).

- Locations: Epithelial lining of oral cavity, oropharynx, laryngopharynx, esophagus, vagina, tonsil, vocal folds, and cornea.[Neet]
- *Functions*
  - It protects underlying structures.
  - It acts as a barrier against pathogenic organisms.
- Note: Epithelium covering the tongue remains moist, but it is exposed to continuous friction. Hence, the tongue is covered partly by keratinized and partly by nonkeratinized stratified squamous epithelium.

- *Parakeratinized epithelium* is similar to keratinized epithelium, except that in parakeratinized epithelium cell nuclei are present in stratum corneum. Example: masticatory mucosa located on hard palate and gingiva.
- Vitamin A deficiency may lead to keratinization of nonkeratinized stratified squamous epithelium.[Neet]

Stratified Cuboidal Epithelium

- Stratified cuboidal epithelium consists of two or more layers of cells (Figs 4.12 and 4.13).

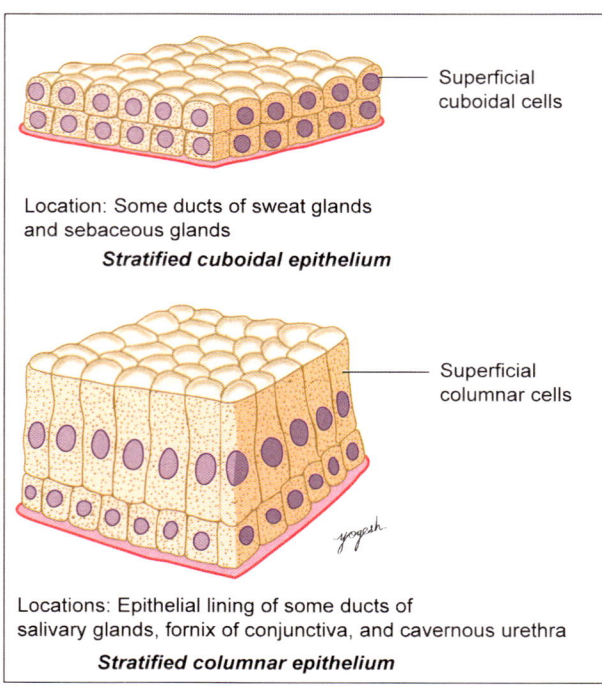

Fig. 4.12: Stratified cuboidal and columnar epithelium.

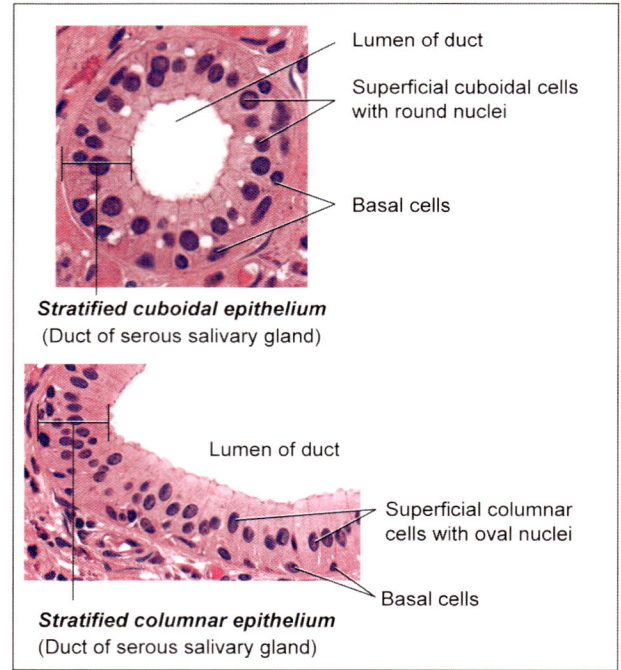

Fig. 4.13: Photomicrograph. Stratified cuboidal and columnar epithelium.

- Cells of superficial layer are cuboidal in shape.
- Location: Some ducts of sweat glands, salivary glands and sebaceous glands.
- *Function:* It acts as a barrier and provides passage for secretions.

Stratified Columnar Epithelium

- It is a two-layered thick epithelium.
- Superficial layer cells are columnar (Figs 4.12 and 4.13).
- Basal cells are cuboidal and rest on basal lamina.
- Locations: Epithelial lining of some ducts of salivary glands, fornix of conjunctiva, and cavernous urethra.
- Functions: It provides passage for secretions and acts as a barrier.

Transitional Epithelium/Urothelium

Q. Write a short note on transitional epithelium.

- Some authors consider transitional epithelium as a type of striated epithelium and some as a separate entity.

Features

- Transitional epithelium lines the major part of urinary passage; hence, it is also called **urothelium**.*Viva*
- Appearance (cell thickness) of transitional epithelium depends on stretching. In full (distended) bladder, transitional epithelium looks *only* 2–3 cell layer thick, whereas in empty bladder it looks 5–6 layer thick (Figs 4.14, 4.15 and Flowchart 4.4).*Viva* Thus, transitional epithelium has extra reserve of cell layer (number of cell layers decreases on stretching).*Neet*
- Cells become flattened on stretching due to distension of bladder. On relaxation in empty bladder, cells become cuboidal or polygonal.*Identification feature*
- Hence, this epithelium is called transitional epithelium.*Viva*
- Basal cells are cuboidal and rest on basal lamina.
- Cells of upper layer are polygonal.
- Cells of the most superficial layer are dome-shaped/ *umbrella-shaped* and more eosinophilic due to presence of plaque.*Identification feature*
- Plaque consists of intramembranous glycoproteins.
- Surface cells may show mitotic activity (two nuclei in single cell).*MCQ*

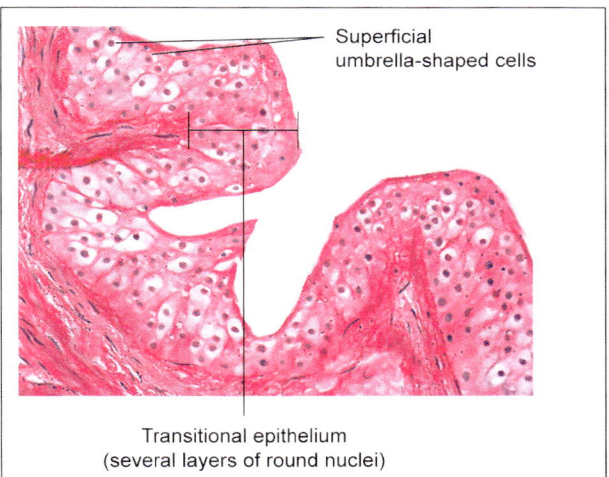

Fig. 4.15: Photomicrograph. Transitional epithelium/urothelium from ureter (ureter, high magnification).

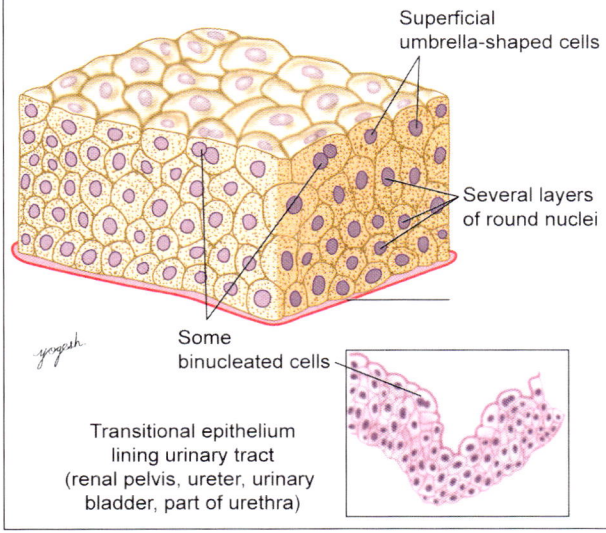

Fig. 4.14: Transitional epithelium (with practice figures).

Flowchart 4.4: Transitional epithelium

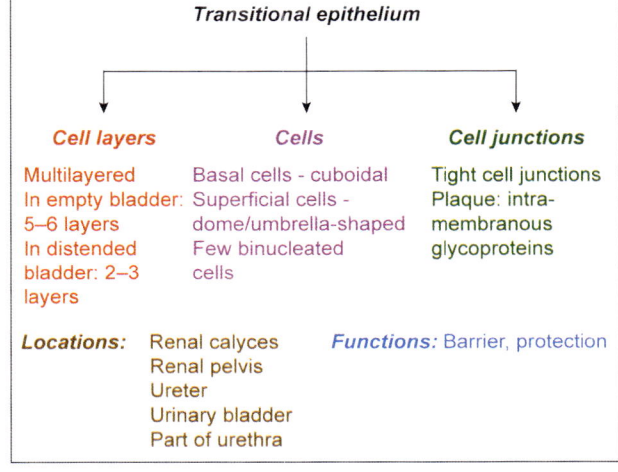

Location[Neet]
1. Renal pelvis and calyces of kidney
2. Ureter
3. Urinary bladder
4. Part of urethra

Functions
1. It provides ability of distension to urinary bladder.
2. It acts as a barrier because of presence of occluding junctions and intramembranous plaques.

- *Note:* Some workers consider that all cells of transitional epithelium are attached with basal lamina through thin processes.

BASEMENT MEMBRANE

Q. Write a short note on basement membrane.

- Basement membrane is a thin layer of extracellular matrix that supports the overlying epithelium

Staining
- *H&E staining:* Basement membrane is not clearly visible on H&E staining.
- *PAS staining:* Carbohydrates of basement membrane make it visible (magenta color) using periodic acid–Schiff staining method.[MCQ, Viva]

Structure
- Electron microscopically, basement membrane shows two layers: superficial basal lamina and deep reticular layer (Fig. 4.16, Flowchart 4.5).[Viva]
- **Basal lamina**
  – It lies just deep to the basal cell layer of epithelium
  – Basal lamina has two layers: lamina lucida and lamina densa.[Viva]
    * *Lamina lucida:* It lies immediately beneath the epithelium. It contains a network of type IV collagen fibers and amorphous matrix.
    * *Lamina densa:* It is deeper layer that contains numerous type IV collagen fibrils.
  – *New concept:* Electron microscopy revealed that basal lamina has only one layer. Lamina lucida is preparation artifact that is produced because of cell shrinkage.[Viva]
  – Basal lamina is a now commonly used terminology instead of basement membrane.
  – Collagen fibers and matrix of basal lamina are produced by epithelial cells.

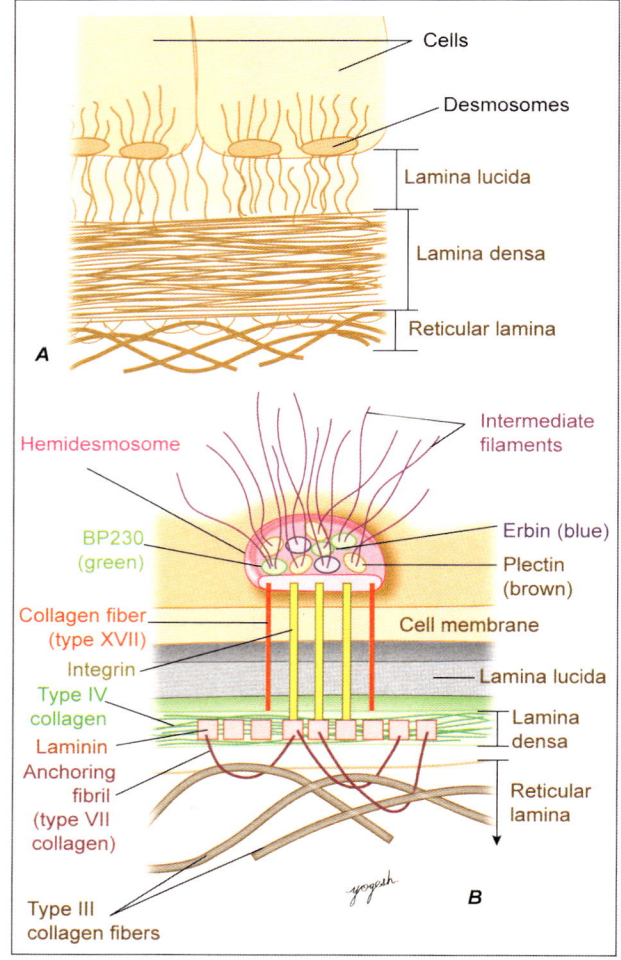

Fig. 4.16: Basement membrane (A) Practice figure, (B) Detailed ultrastructure of basement membrane.

Flowchart 4.5: Basement membrane

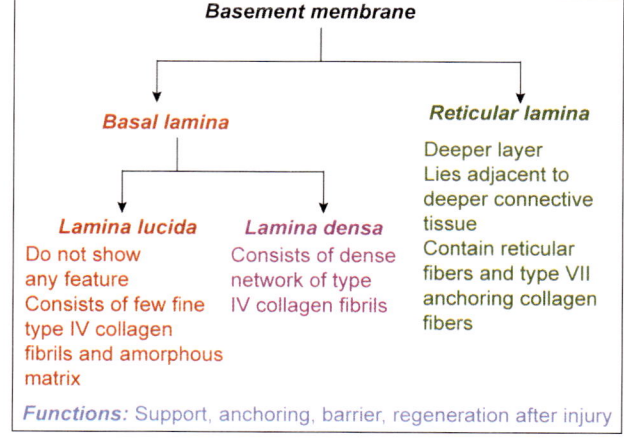

- *Reticular lamina*
  - It lies away from the epithelium, just adjacent to deeper connective tissue.
  - It contains reticular fibers that are produced by fibroblasts.
  - Type VII collagen fibrils anchor lamina densa and lamina reticularis.

Functions

1. It provides support to overlying epithelium.
2. It anchors overlying epithelium with underlying connective tissue.
3. It acts as a selective barrier that allows and restricts transport of many substances.
4. It helps in regeneration of epithelium after injury.

Some Interesting Facts

- Epithelium receives its nourishment by simple *diffusion* of substances from vessels that lie deep into the epithelium. *Viva*
- *Exfoliative cytology:* In exfoliative cytology, cells from the superficial layer of epithelium are scrapped and stained with a suitable stain. It is useful for detection of epithelial pathological changes. *Viva*
- *Metaplasia* is the abnormal conversion of one type of normal epithelium to another type of epithelium on exposure to certain factors. For example, loss of cilia from ciliated pseudostratified columnar epithelium of trachea on exposure to cigarette smoke. *Viva*

CHAPTER 5

Cell Surface Projections and Cell Junctions

Chapter Outline
- Cell junctions
  - Types of junctional complexes
  - Desmosomes
  - Zonula adherens
  - Fascia adherens
  - Hemidesmosomes
  - Zona occludens
  - Gap junctions
- Apical domain of cell and its modifications
  - Microvilli
  - Stereocilia
  - Cilia

Competency achievement: The student should be able to:
AN65.2 Describe the ultrastructure of epithelium

CELL JUNCTIONS

Q. List the various types of cell junctions.
- Cells in tissue are arranged in a specific manner and to perform their specific functions.
  - Cells in organ are closely packed and cell membranes of adjoining cells make contact with each other. At the point of contact, cell membranes are separated by an *intercellular space* (15–20 nm gap).
  - To avoid separation by mechanical forces, cells are connected by specialized junctional complexes with each other.

Types of Junctional Complexes (Fig. 5.1)
A. Adhesive/anchoring junctions
   - These junctions tie adjacent cells mechanically with each other.
   - There are four types of adhesive cell junctions:
     1. Desmosomes/maculae adherens/adhesive spot
     2. Adhesive belt/zonula adherens
     3. Fascia adherens/adhesive strips
     4. Hemidesmosomes
B. Occluding/tight junctions/zonula occludens
   - These junctions seal adjacent cell membranes with each other to create barrier for movement of material through interval between the cells.
C. Gap junctions/communicating junctions
   - These junctions permit transport of substances across cells.

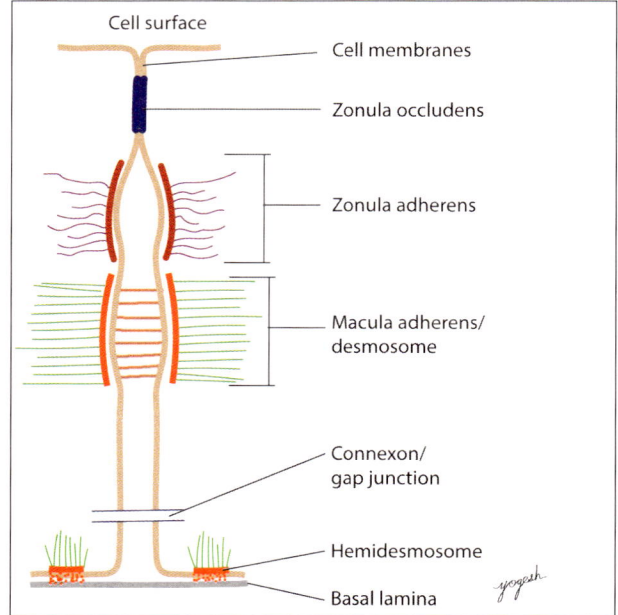

Fig. 5.1: Cell junctional complexes (practice figure).

38

Desmosomes/Macula Adherens/Adhesion Spots (Macula=Spot in *Latin*)

- They are also called *spot-welding*.^{Neet}
- Desmosome provides strong adhesion between cells.
- Electron microscopy: Desmosomes connect the lateral surfaces of the cells. Cell membranes are separated by 30 nm distance from each other.
- Desmosome consists of (Fig. 5.2) the following:
  1. Dense thick disc (made up of desmoplakin protein) on inner side of plasma membrane.
  2. Transmembrane linker proteins (cadherin) that extend across intercellular spaces and connect dense discs of two adjacent cells. *Autoantibodies* against *cadherin* produce intercellular separation and this condition is called *pemphigus vulgaris*.^{Neet}
  3. Intracytoplasmic fine intermediate filaments that run in cytoplasm and get attached with the dense disc.
- *Locations:* Epithelial cells exposed to mechanical stress, especially in epidermis of skin (*desmo* = bond and *soma* = body in Greek).
- *Functions*
  - Provides stability to epithelium.
  - Provides strong adhesion and helps to withstand physical and mechanical stress.

Zonula Adherens/Adhesive Belts

- Zonula adherens provides lateral adhesion to cell wall with adjacent cells.
- It completely encircles the cell.
- It permits gap of 15–20 nm between adjacent cell membrane (Fig. 5.3).^{Neet}
- Cell membranes show thickening due to deposited proteins on its inner (cytoplasmic) side.

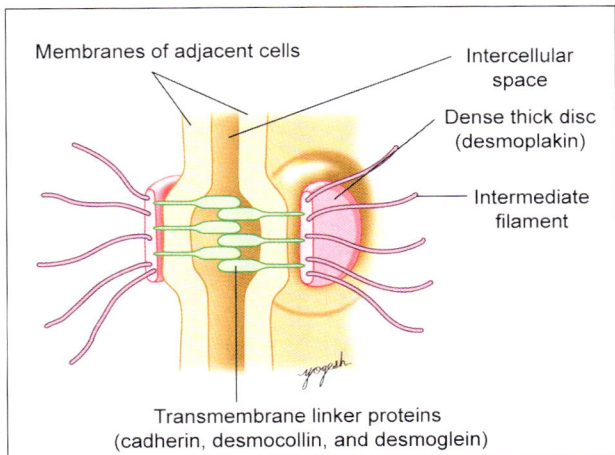

Fig. 5.2: Desmosome.

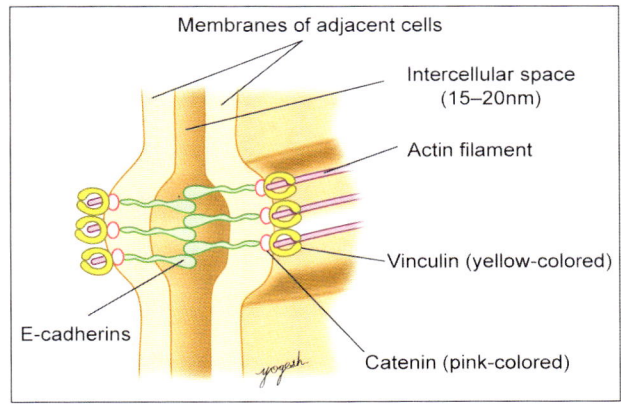

Fig. 5.3: Zonula adherens.

- These proteins provide attachment to cytoplasmic actin filaments from cytoskeleton.
- Transmembrane proteins (cadherin) attach with actin filaments.
- Apical part of cell has a network of actin filaments that runs horizontally and froms zonula adherens. These fibers form a **terminal web** (network). Contraction of actin filaments of terminal web spread out microvilli and increases the area for the absorption.
- *Functions*
  - Provides strong adhesion between adjacent cells.
  - Gives stability to terminal web of cells.

Fascia Adherens/Adhesive Strips

- Fascia adherens is similar to zonula adherens but it does not encircle entire circumference of cell.
- *Locations:* Intercalated discs of cardiac muscles, smooth muscles.

Hemidesmosomes

- These are similar to the half of the desmosome (*hemi = half*)
- Hemidesmosome anchors the cell to the basal lamina.
- Basal lamina shows thickening (intracellular attachment plaque) on inner surface of cell that gives attachment to cytoplasmic intermediate filaments.
- *Locations:* Cornea, skin, mucosa of oral cavity, esophagus, vagina.
- *Intercellular attachment plaque* consists of three proteins of desmoplakin family (Fig. 5.4):
  1. Plectin
  2. BP230
  3. Erbin
- Note: Absence of BP230 proteins or autoantibodies against BP230 proteins produces bullous

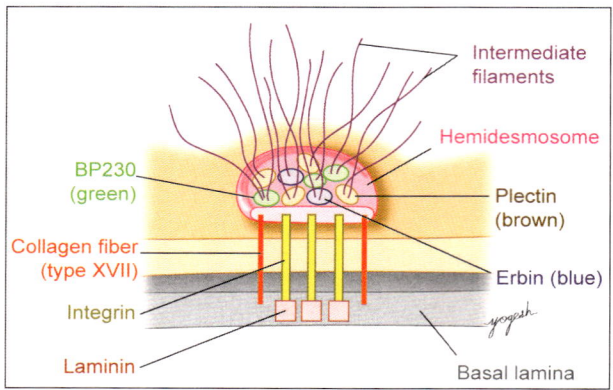

Fig. 5.4: Ultrastructure of hemidesmosome.

pemphigoid disease. This disease shows large fluid-filled blisters.*Neet*

- Hemidesmosome has integrin class of transmembrane proteins, such as α4β6 integrin, type XVII collagen, CD151. These molecules help to to anchor cell with the basal lamina.
- For example: α4β6 integrin binds with laminin-332 molecule of basal lamina. Note: Mutation of *laminin-332* gene results in blister forming skin disease called *junctional epidermolysis bullosa.*^{Neet}

Zona Occludens/Tight Junction

- *Zona occludens* are present near the apical surface of cells.
- It seals intercellular space along the entire circumference of cell.
- Several proteins are involved in formation of tight junction. They are occuldin, claudins, junctional adhesion molecule (JAM). These are transmembrane proteins. They join in intercellular space and provide attachment to intracellular actin filaments through zonula occludens (ZO) proteins (Fig. 5.5).
- *Locations:* Epithelium of intestine, renal tubules, and urinary bladder.
- *Functions*
  1. Provides firm cellular adhesion.
  2. Seals intercellular space.
  3. Provides barrier and prevents entry of content of organ into blood. For example, urinary bladder.

Gap Junctions/Nexus

- Gap junctions are cell-to-cell communication channels that have cytoplasmic connectivity between adjacent cells through a small canaliculus.*Neet*
- Adjacent plasma membranes lie very close to each other (<3 nm) (Fig. 5.6).

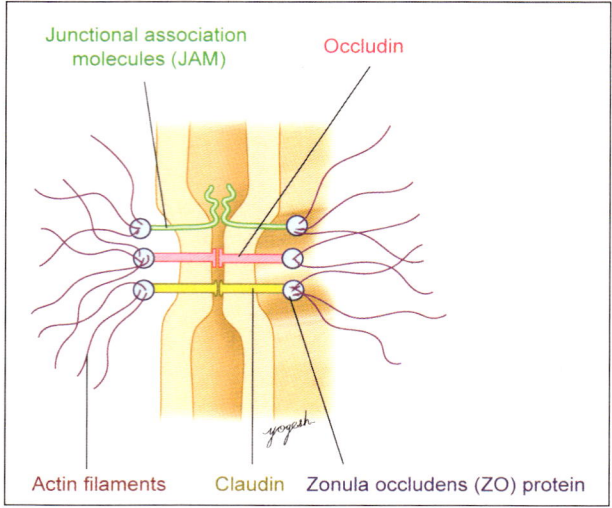

Fig. 5.5: Ultrastructure of zonula occludens/tight junction.

- Gap junction is formed by a protein called **connexons**.
- Six connexons molecules run across cell membranes and traverse through intercellular space. They create small canaliculus that has pores (openings in both cells).
- Opening and closing of gap junctions can regulate the transport of Ca^{++} ions and maintenance of pH

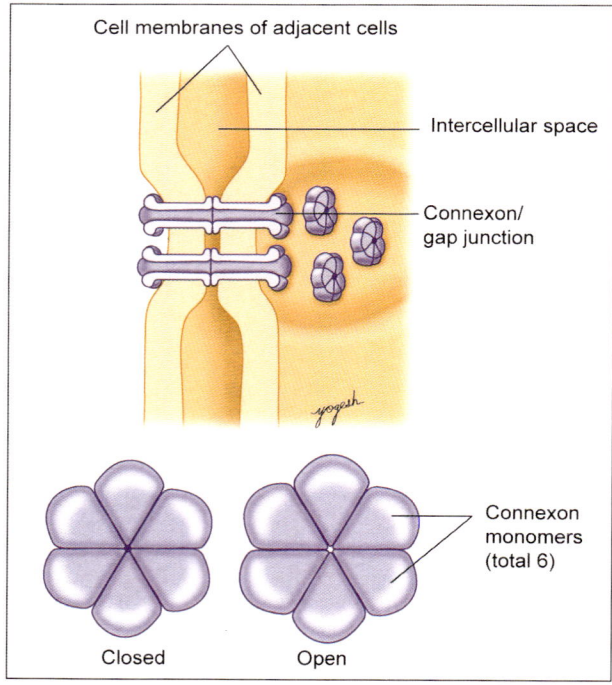

Fig. 5.6: Ultrastructure of connexon/gap junction.

among adjacent cells easily.
- *Locations*
  - Smooth muscle cells
  - Cardiac muscles
- *Functions*
  - Maintains cytoplasmic continuity of cells and make them *physiological syncytium* (single cell with multiple nuclei). It helps to pass substances between cells without entering extracellular fluid.[Neet]
  - Helps to excite and contract entire muscle together (smooth muscles, cardiac muscles).
  - Reduces need of neuromuscular signal transmission by exciting adjacent cells.

Summary of various types of cell junctions is given in Flowchart 5.1 and Fig. 5.7.

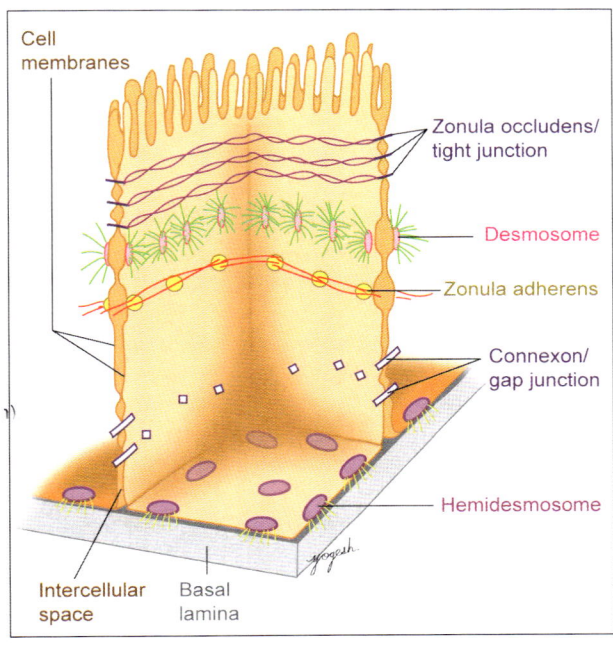

Fig. 5.7: Types of cell junctions.

APICAL DOMAIN OF CELL AND ITS MODIFICATIONS

- As per functional need, apical surface (luminal surface) of epithelial cells show surface modifications.
- Structural modifications are microvilli, stereocilia, and cilia (Fig. 5.8).[Viva]

Microvilli (Finger-like Projections)

Q. Write a short note on microvilli.

- Microvilli are *apical cell surface modifications*. The main function of microvilli is to increase cell surface area for absorption or secretion (Figs 5.9 and 5.10).

Locations
- Apical surface of epithelial cells in small intestine, gall bladder, and bile duct.[Neet]
- Few microvilli are seen on the surface of white blood cells, where microvilli help in WBC migration.
- Proximal convoluted tubules of kidney.

Dimensions
Length: 1–2 mm and diameter: 1–2 mm.

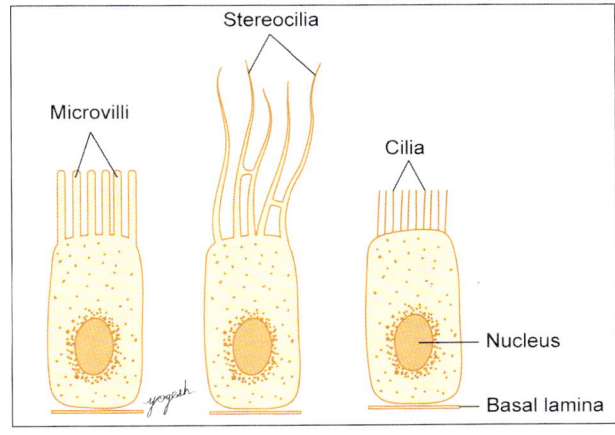

Fig. 5.8: Microvilli, stereocilia, and cilia (practice figure).

Flowchart 5.1: Cell junctions

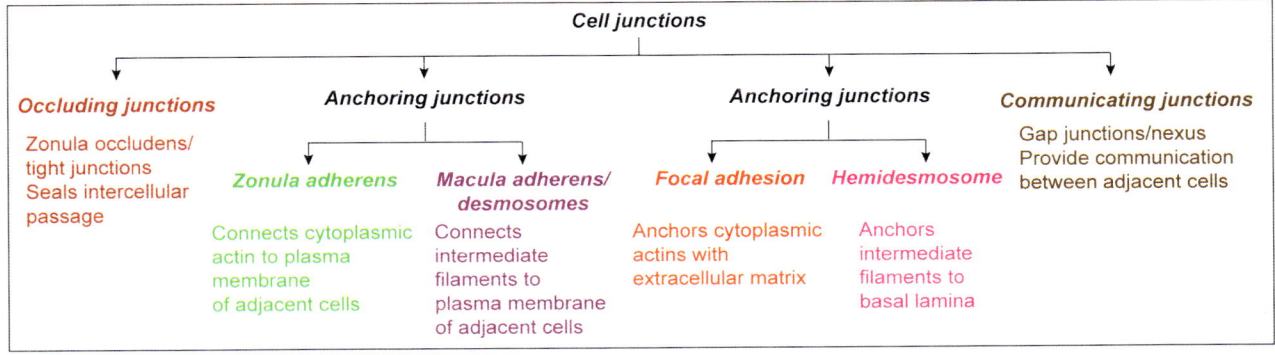

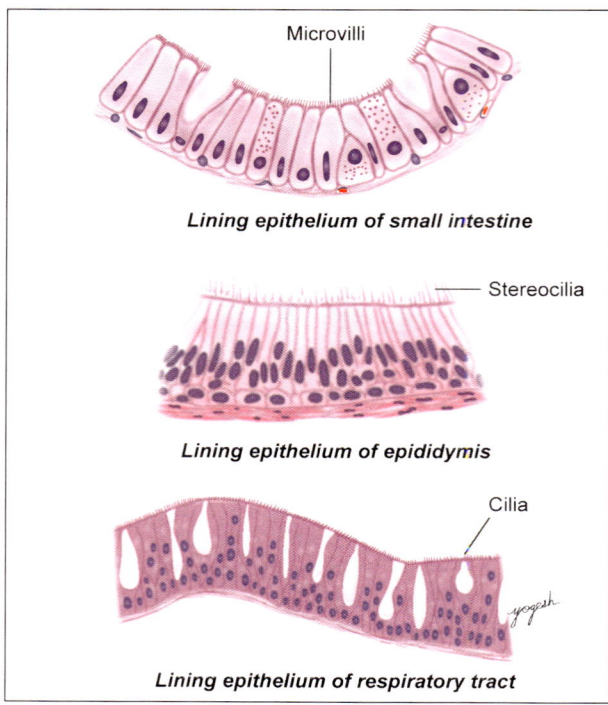

Fig. 5.9: Microvilli, stereocilia, and cilia on *H&E* staining.

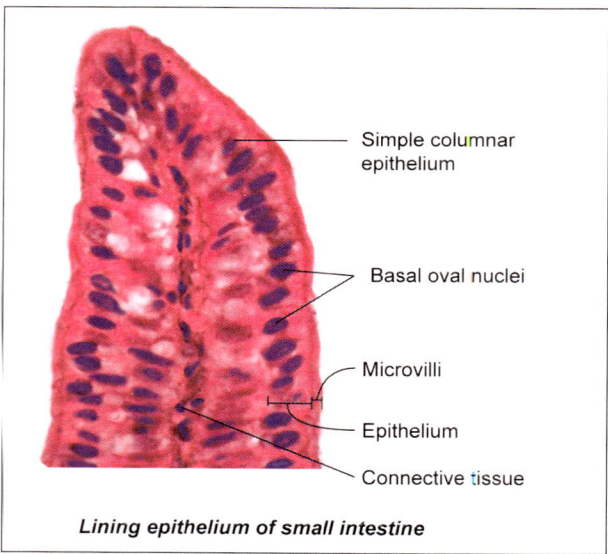

Fig. 5.10: Photomicrograph. Microvilli (simple columnar epithelium of small intestine, *H&E* stain, high magnification)

Structure
- Each microvillus has an outer covering of plasma membrane and a cytoplasmic core (Fig. 5.11).
- Cytoplasmic core contains core of 20–30 actin filaments that run from tip of microvillus to terminal web.
- Actin filaments are connected to the plasma membrane with the help of actin-binding proteins (fascin, epsin, fimbrin).

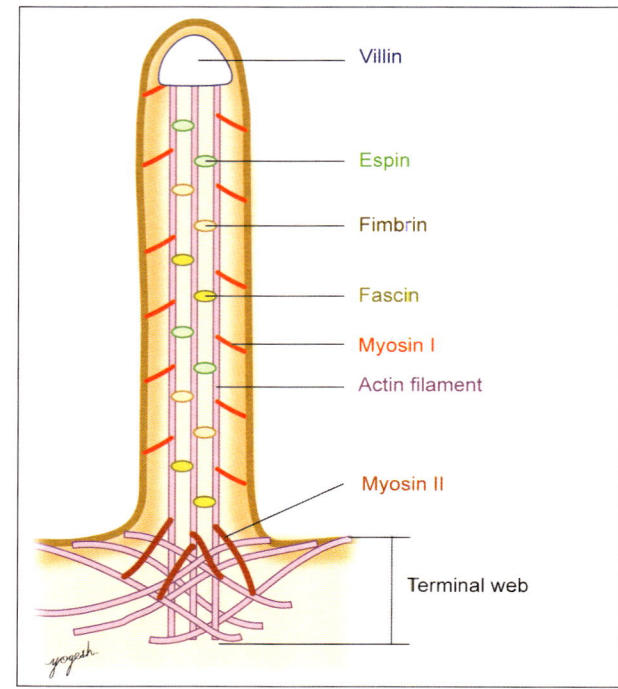

Fig. 5.11: Ultrastructure of microvillus.

- Myosin I molecules extend from plasma membrane to actin core filaments.
- Terminal web consists of horizontal network of actin filaments.
- Myosin II molecules are present at terminal web.
- These actin and myosin molecules help for mobility of microvilli.
- Surface of microvilli is covered by glycocalyx coat.

Functions
1. Increases surface area by 15–30 folds for absorption or secretion.
2. Slight motility of microvilli helps them to come in contact with newer food molecules in gut.
- Regularly arranged microvilli produce *striated border* over apical surface of absorptive cells of intestinal epithelium, whereas irregularly arranged long microvilli produce *brush border* (gall bladder and proximal convoluted tubule).[Neet]

Stereocilia
- Stereocilia is a *long, thick microvillus* (5–10 μm).
- Stereocilia are present on epithelium of receptor (hair) cells in internal ear and epithelial cells of epididymis.
- Stereocilia are nonmotile.
- Stereocilia increase cell surface area.

Structure
- Stereocilium is covered by plasma membrane and have a core of cytoplasm (Figs 5.12 and 5.13).

Cell Surface Projections and Cell Junctions

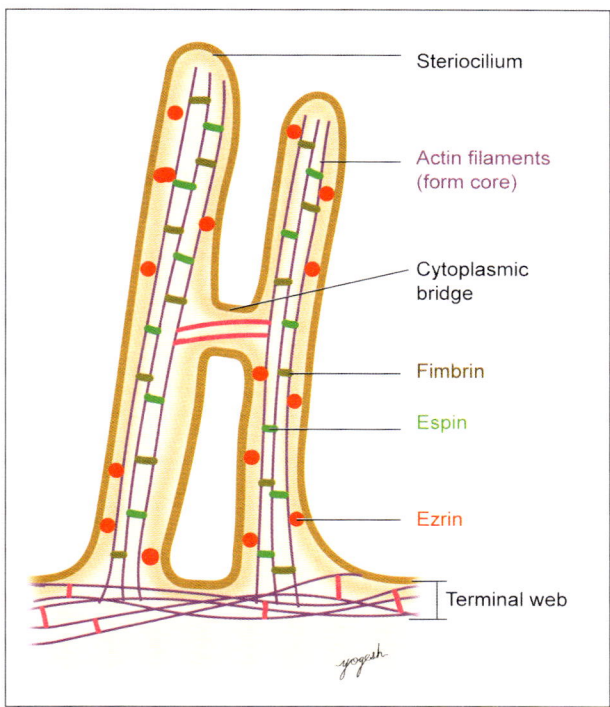

Fig. 5.12: Ultrastructure of stereocilia.

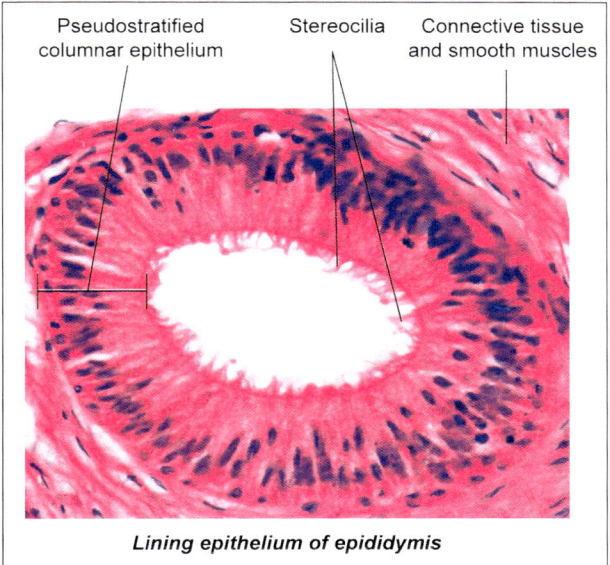

Fig. 5.13: Photomicrograph. Stereocilia (pseudostratified columnar epithelium of epididymis, H&E stain, high magnification).

- This cytoplasmic core contains bundles of actin filaments connected with plasma membrane by fimbrin.

Functions

1. In hair cells of internal ear: Here, stereocilia serve as a sensory mechanoreceptor. Vibration induces movement of stereocilia that generates signal.

2. In epididymis: Here, stereocilia increase the surface area for absorption of fluid.

Cilia

- Cilia are apical cell membranous hair-like projections.
- Cilia are *motile*.

Structure

- Cilia are covered by plasma membrane and have core of filaments (Figs 5.14 and 5.15).

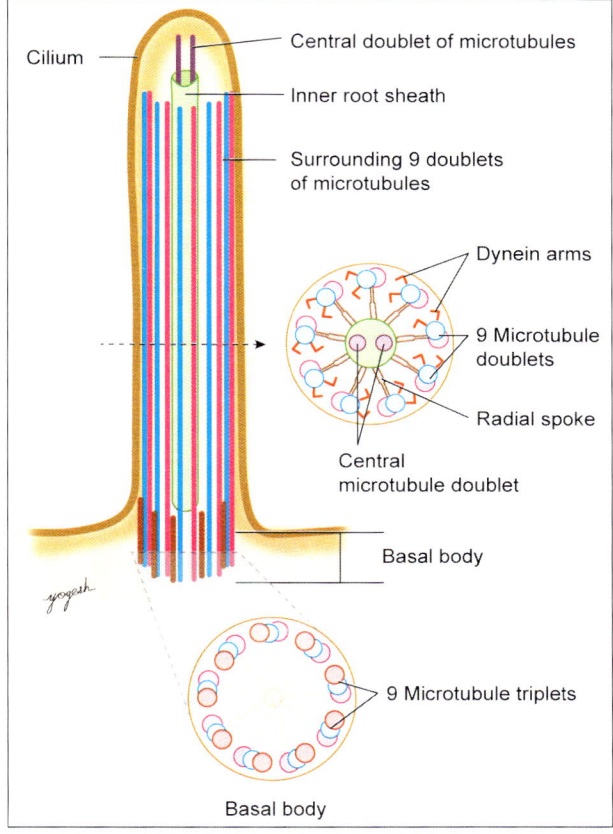

Fig. 5.14: Ultrastructure of cilium.

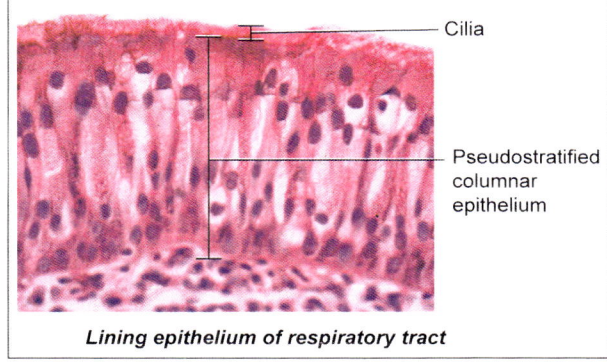

Fig. 5.15: Photomicrograph. Cilia (ciliated pseudostratified columnar epithelium of respiratory tract, H&E stain, high magnification).

- Each cilium has a free *shaft* and a basal *body*.
- Basal body of the cilium is attached with apical cell membrane.

■ *Dimensions*

10 μm length, 0.25 μm diameter
- Core or microtubule cytoskeleton of cilium (*axoneme*) is formed by microtubules arranged in specific manner.*Viva*
  - Centrally placed 2 microtubules (doublet)
  - Surrounding 9 pairs of microtubules (doublets)
- Surrounding microtubules have dynein arms. Dynein molecules help in bending of microtubules and movement of cilia.*Viva*
- All 9 pairs of surrounding microtubules are connected with the central microtubules by nexin.

Locations
- Respiratory tract (pseudostratified ciliated columnar) epithelium
- Sperms: Tail of sperm is flagellum (long cilium)*MCQ*
- Fallopian tube

Functions
1. In respiratory tract, ciliary movements help to remove the mucus from the epithelial surface.
2. For sperm, tail (flagellum/long cilium) helps in motility.
3. In fallopian tube, cilia help to bring gametes (ova/sperms) at site of fertilization and move fertilized egg toward the uterus.

Types of cilia

Cilia are classified into two groups as primary nonmotile cilia and motile cilia.

1. *Primary nonmotile cilia* are present at least one per cell on all cells.

   Examples, photoreceptor cells (rod and cones) of eye, dendritic knot of olfactory neurons.

   They help in chemical sensation, signal transduction, and so on.
2. *Motile cilia* include cilia of respiratory epithelium and fallopian tube.

Clinical Correlation

Immotile cilia syndrome
- It is also known as primary ciliary dyskinesia (PCD).
- It affects respiratory tract, sperms, and fallopian tube and collectively produce *Kartagener syndrome*.
- Cause: Deficient production of microtubule proteins such as dynein.*Neet*
- In respiratory tract, defective mucociliary movements cause repeated respiratory tract infections.
- In sperms and fallopian tube, it causes *infertility*
- If immotile cilia syndrome affects primitive node of the embryo, it may result in *situs invertus*. These cilia are called *nodal cilia*.

The summary of various types of apical cell surface modifications is given in Flowchart 5.2.

Flowchart 5.2: Cell surface modifications

Q. Enlist the differences between microvilli, stereocilia, and cilia.

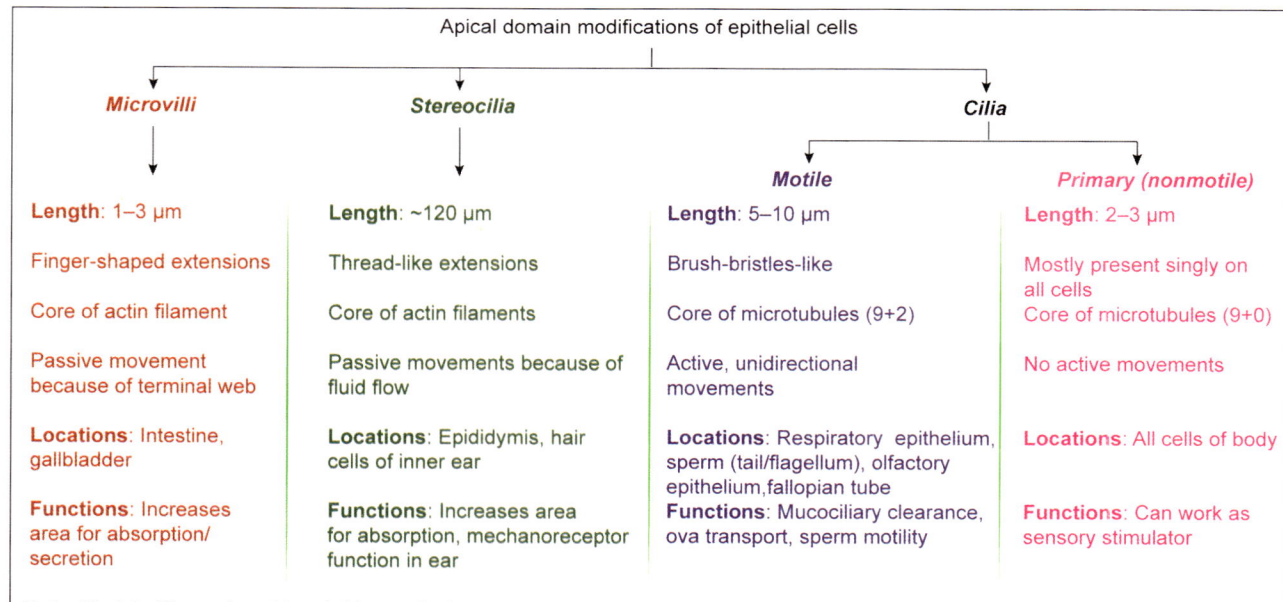

		Cilia	
Microvilli	**Stereocilia**	**Motile**	**Primary (nonmotile)**
Length: 1–3 μm	**Length:** ~120 μm	**Length:** 5–10 μm	**Length:** 2–3 μm
Finger-shaped extensions	Thread-like extensions	Brush-bristles-like	Mostly present singly on all cells
Core of actin filament	Core of actin filaments	Core of microtubules (9+2)	Core of microtubules (9+0)
Passive movement because of terminal web	Passive movements because of fluid flow	Active, unidirectional movements	No active movements
Locations: Intestine, gallbladder	**Locations:** Epididymis, hair cells of inner ear	**Locations:** Respiratory epithelium, sperm (tail/flagellum), olfactory epithelium, fallopian tube	**Locations:** All cells of body
Functions: Increases area for absorption/secretion	**Functions:** Increases area for absorption, mechanoreceptor function in ear	**Functions:** Mucociliary clearance, ova transport, sperm motility	**Functions:** Can work as sensory stimulator

Note: **Nodal cilia** are found in primitive node, have core of 9+0 microtubules, and determine right–left asymmetry of internal organs.

CHAPTER 6

Glands

Chapter Outline

- Classification of glands
- Exocrine glands
- Classification based on branching pattern of duct
- Classification based on nature of secretions
  - Serous glands
  - Mucous glands
  - Mixed gland
- Classification based on mode of secretion
  - Merocrine glands
  - Apocrine glands
  - Holocrine glands
  - Paracrine and autocrine glands
- Goblet cell

Competency achievement: The student should be able to:

AN70.1 Identify exocrine gland under the microscope and distinguish between serous, mucous and mixed acini

INTRODUCTION

- Gland is a specialized group of cells that synthesizes and secretes substances/hormones.
- Glands are derived from epithelium (Figs 6.1 and 6.2).
- Note: Mucus is a noun and mucous is an adjective. For example, mucous cells secrete mucus.

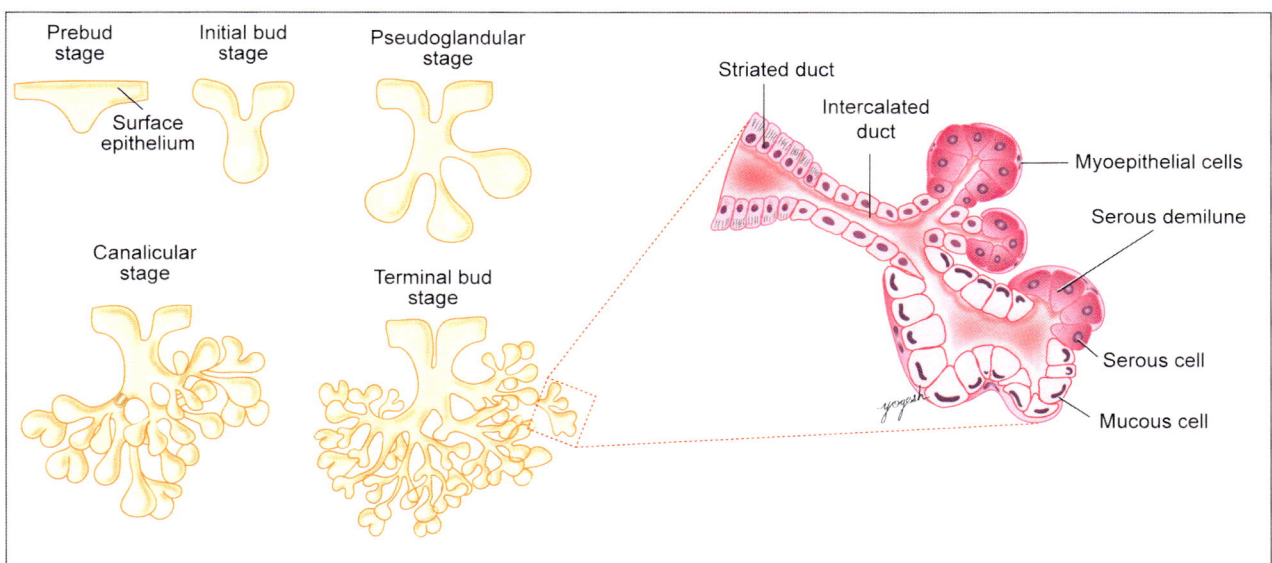

Fig. 6.1: Development of exocrine gland (salivary gland) (*Source:* Textbook of Human Embryology, Yogesh Sontakke, 1st edn., CBS Publishers).

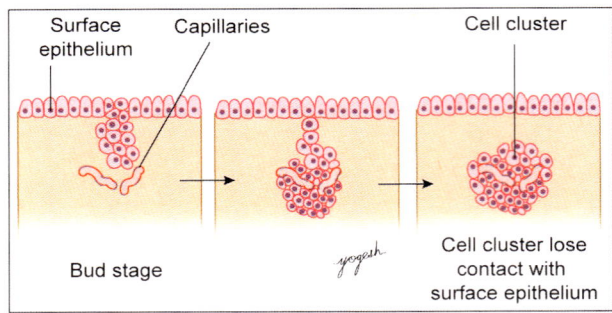

Fig. 6.2: Development of endocrine gland.

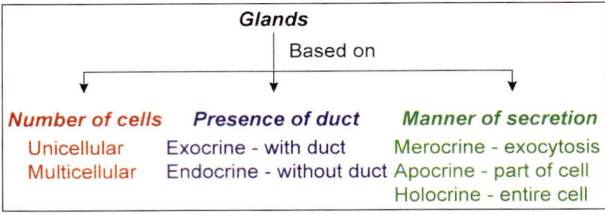

Flowchart 6.1: Classification of glands

CLASSIFICATION OF GLANDS

- Glands are classified in various ways as follows (Flowchart 6.1):*Viva*
  1. Based on number of cells
     - *Unicellular glands:* They have single cell that performs secretory function.
     - *Multicellular glands:* They have group of cells.
  2. Based on presence of duct
     - *Exocrine glands:* They use duct to convey their secretions
     - *Endocrine glands:* They do not have ducts and secrete secretions directly into the blood. For details on endocrine glands, *refer* Chapter 23.
  3. Based on the manner of secretion:
     - *Merocrine glands:* They secrete by exocytosis.
     - *Apocrine glands:* They secrete by shedding of apical portion of glands.
     - *Holocrine glands:* They secrete by disintegration of entire cell.

EXOCRINE GLANDS

- Exocrine glands convey their secretions with the help of duct.
- Exocrine glands are further classified as follows (Figs 6.3 to 6.12 and Flowchart 6.2):

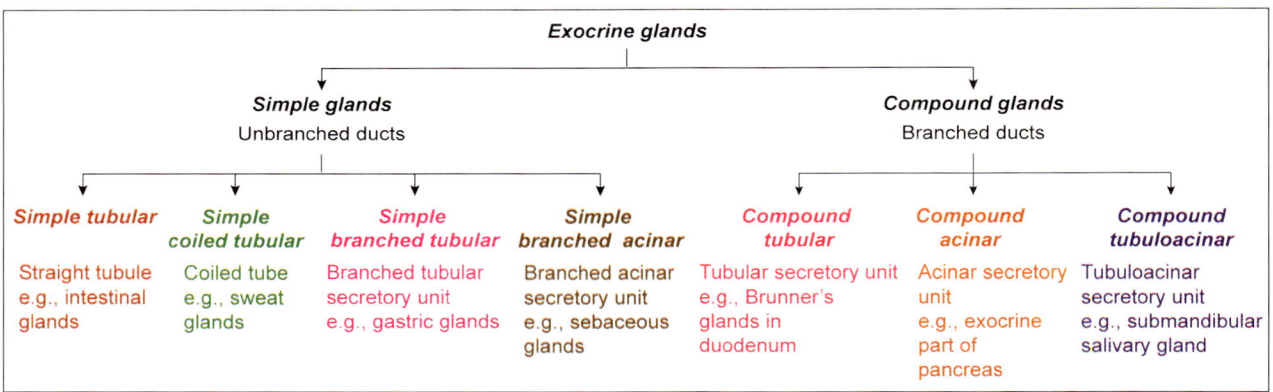

Flowchart 6.2: Classification of exocrine glands based on duct branching and shape of secretory unit

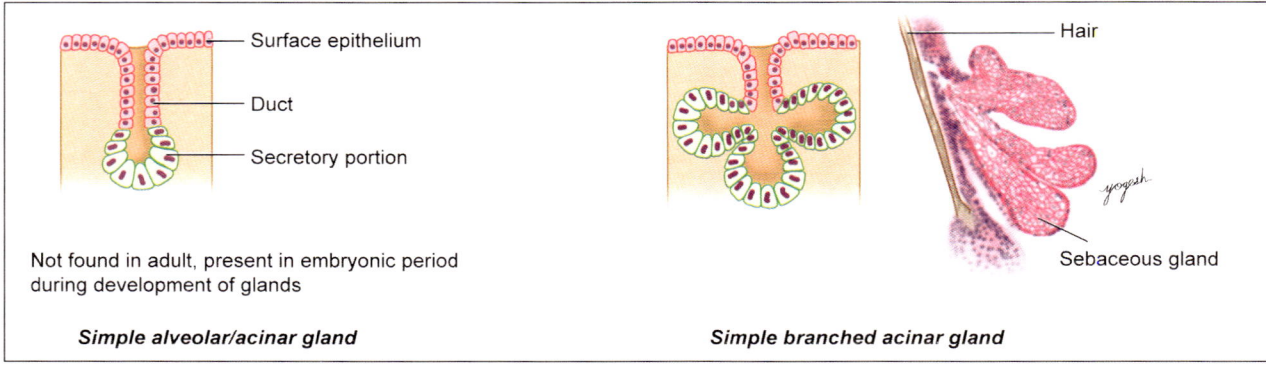

Fig. 6.3: Types of simple acinar glands.

Glands

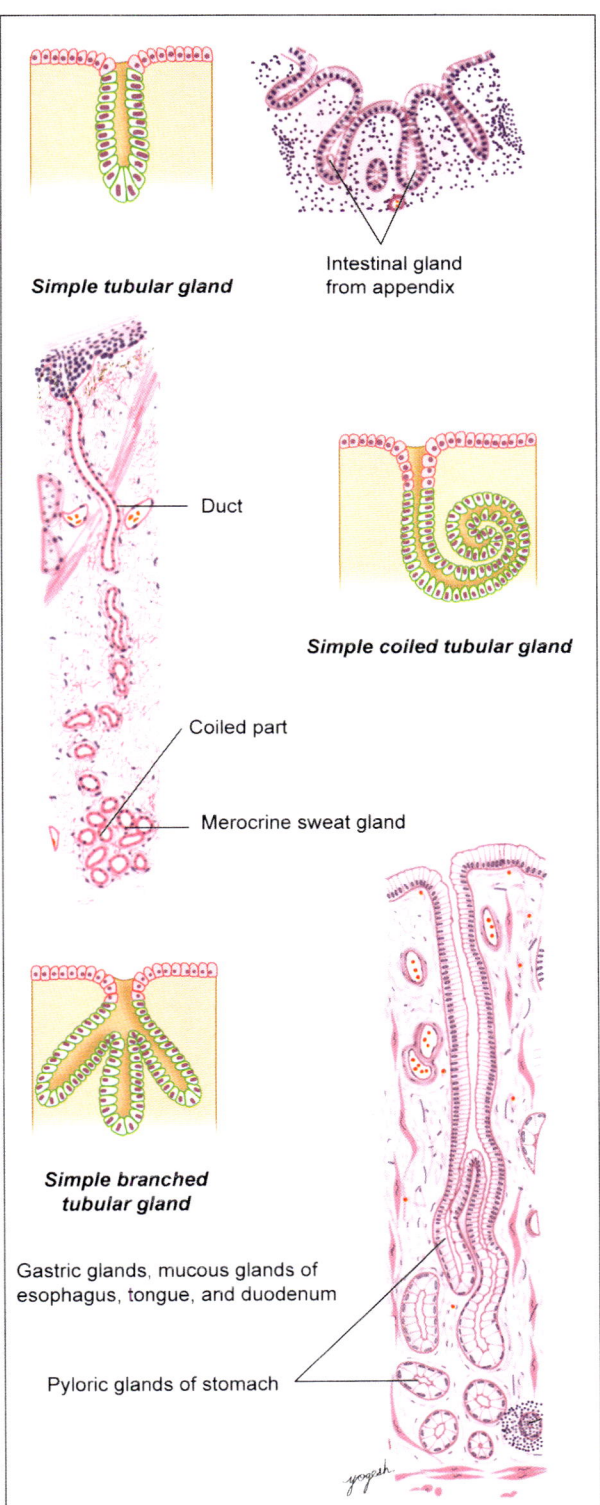

Fig. 6.4: Simple tubular glands.

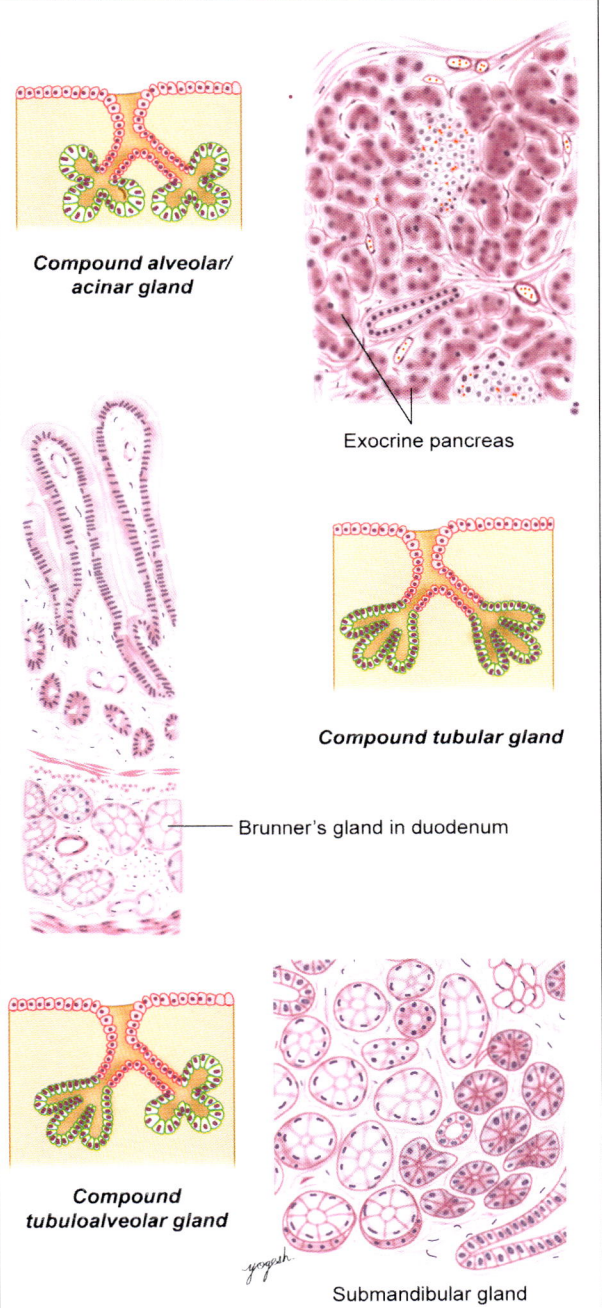

Fig. 6.5: Compound exocrine glands.

1. Number of branches of duct (simple, compound)
2. Shape of secretory unit (tubular, acinar, alveolar)
3. Nature of secretory product (serous, mucus, and mixed).
4. Some author includes classification based on the mechanism of secretion (merocrine, apocrine and holocrine) as fourth type of classification.

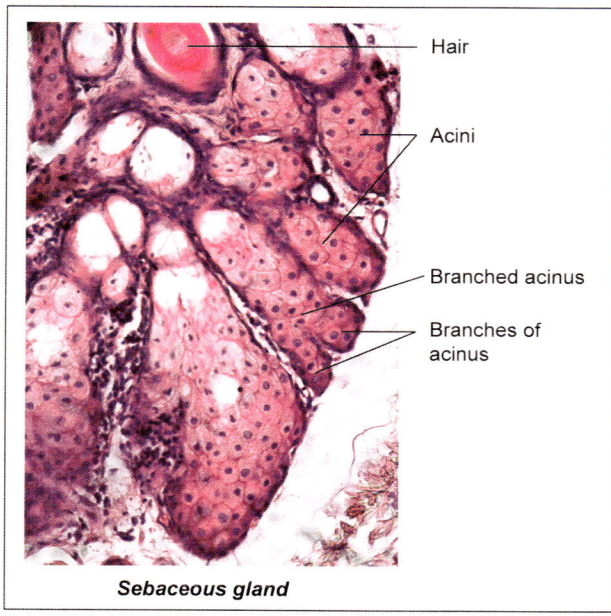

Fig. 6.6: Photomicrograph. Simple branched acinar gland.

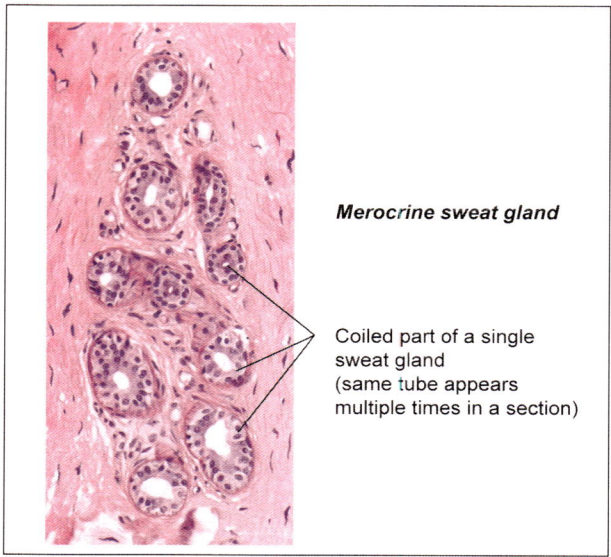

Fig. 6.8: Photomicrograph. Simple coiled tubular gland.

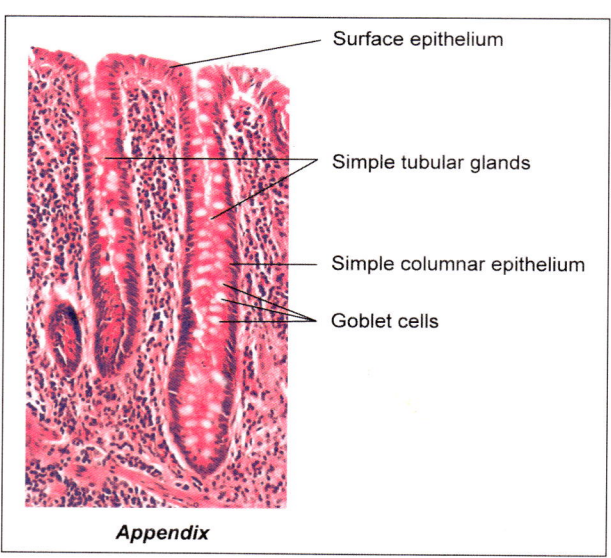

Fig. 6.7: Photomicrograph. Simple tubular gland.

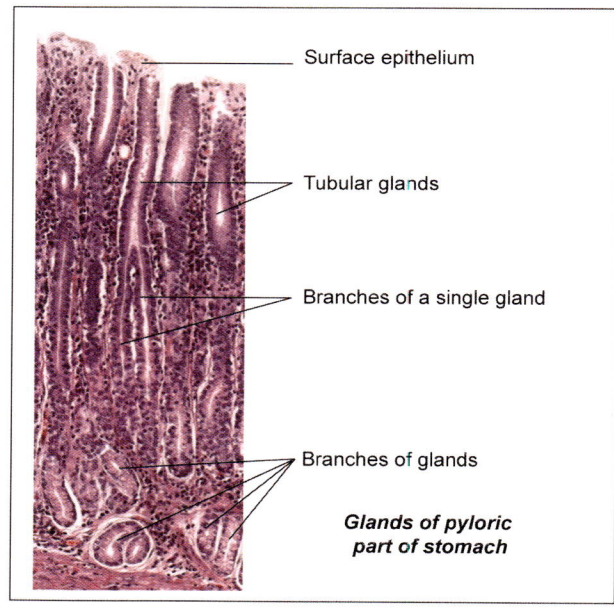

Fig. 6.9: Photomicrograph. Simple branched tubular gland.

Classification Based on Branching Pattern of Duct

- Exocrine glands can be grouped into two classes based on branching of the ducts as follows:
    1. *Simple glands:* These are exocrine glands that have only one unbranched duct (no branching).
       Examples, crypts of Lieberkühn, sweat glands, fundic glands of stomach, mucous glands of urethra, and Meibomian glands.
    2. *Compound glands:* These glands have branching of secretory duct.
       Examples, Brunner's glands, mammary gland, submandibular glands.

Classification Based on Shape of Secretory Unit

- Exocrine glands can be grouped into three groups based on the shape of secretory unit as follows:
    1. *Tubular glands:* The secretory unit is tube-shaped. The tube may be straight, coiled, or branched.
       Examples, intestinal glands, sweat glands (simple coiled tubular gland), gastric glands, Brunner's glands.

Glands

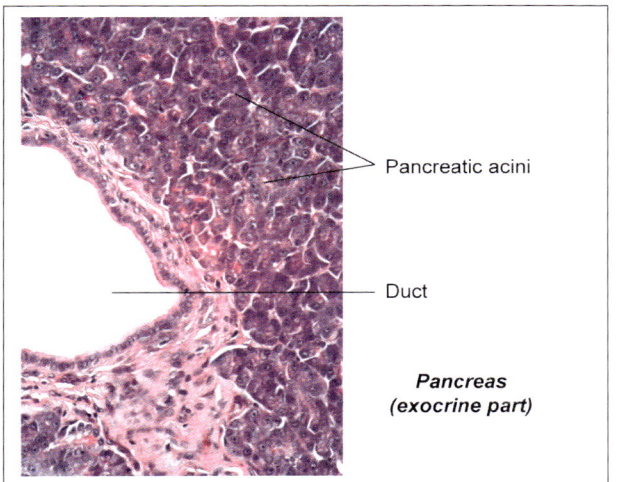

Fig. 6.10: Photomicrograph. Compound alveolar/acinar gland.

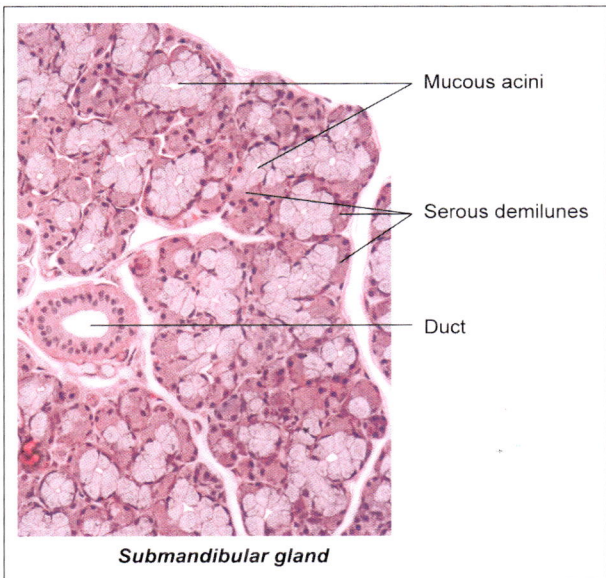

Fig. 6.12: Photomicrograph. Compound tubuloalveolar gland.

Classification Based on Nature of Secretions

- Based on the nature of secretions, exocrine glands are classified as serous, mucous, and mixed glands.

Serous Glands

Q. Draw a well-labelled diagram of serous gland.

- Serous glands secrete protein-rich watery secretions.*Viva*
- Serous gland has *serous acini* as secretory unit (Fig. 6.13).
- Serous acini are lined by pyramidal-shaped *simple columnar epithelium*.
- Serous cells have *Identification feature*
  - Rounded basal nucleus (located near basal lamina).
  - Large amount of rough endoplasmic reticulum for protein synthesis lie in basal region of cells. It gives *basal basophilia* (stained with hematoxylin).
  - Well-developed Golgi complex and many secretory vesicles (zymogen granules) lie in apical region of cells. It gives *apical eosinophilia* (stained with eosin).
- Serous acinus has *smaller lumen* than mucous acini.
- Examples, parotid gland, exocrine part of pancreas, lacrimal gland, von Ebner's glands in tongue.*Neet*

Mucous Glands

Q. Draw a well-labeled diagram of mucous gland.

- Mucous glands secrete thick mucoid secretions.
- Mucous gland has mucous acini as secretory unit.

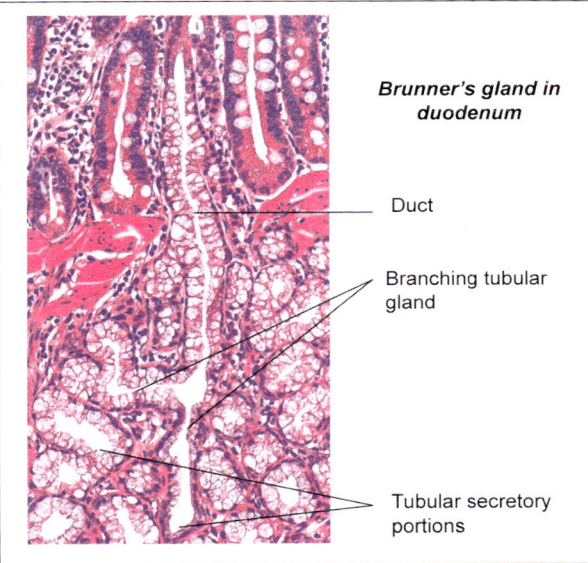

Fig. 6.11: Photomicrograph. Compound tubular gland.

2. ***Acinar glands:*** The secretory unit is spherical (round in cross-section).*Viva*
   Examples, exocrine part of pancreas, salivary glands.
3. ***Alveolar glands:*** The secretory unit is flask-shaped. The glands with distended secretory units are also called saccular glands.
   When the acinar glands become fully active or overactive, their secretory portions become flask-shaped or even saccular (alveolar in shape). For example, mammary gland, and exocrine pancreas.
4. ***Combination*** of secretory unit and branching of duct is commonly used in the classification of glands (Flowchart 6.2).

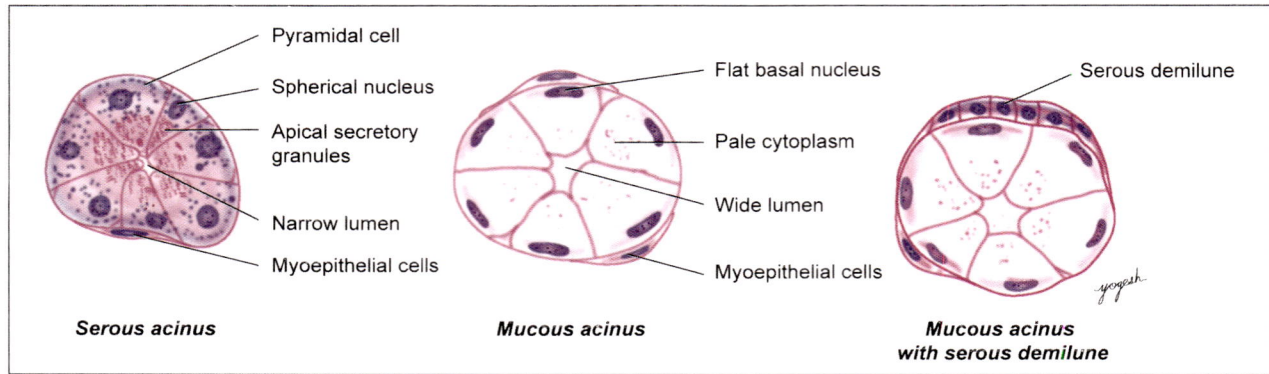

Fig. 6.13: Types of acini.

- Mucous acini are lined by pyramidal-shaped simple columnar epithelium (Figs 6.13 and 6.14).
- The mucous cell has^{Identification feature}
  - Flat, elongated basally-placed nucleus.^{Viva}
  - *Empty cytoplasm* on *H&E staining. Reason*:^{Viva} Mucous cells synthesize and store the mucous in the form of mucinogen granules. These granules are lost during tissue processing for slide preparation for *H&E staining*. Hence, mucous cells give an empty appearance on *H&E staining*.^{Viva}
- Mucous acinus has wider lumen than serous acinus.
- Mucous cells show positive staining with periodic acid–Schiff (PAS) staining. Mucus takes dark magenta stain.^{Viva}
- Example, sublingual salivary gland.

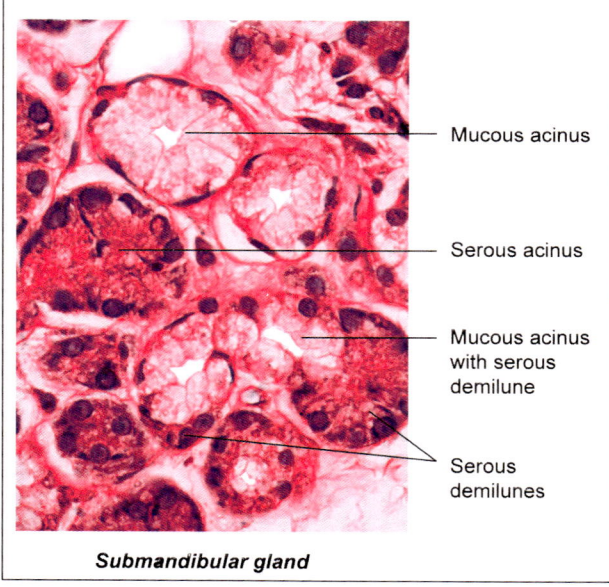

Fig. 6.14: Photomicrograph. Types of acini.

Mixed Gland

- Mixed gland secretes both mucus and enzyme-rich watery secretions.
- Mixed gland has *mucous acini with serous demilunes* as secretory unit (Fig. 6.13).
- Mucous acinus with serous demilunes^{Viva, Identification feature}
  - Mucous acinus is capped with serous cells that form serous demilunes.
  - Serous demilune is a half-moon shaped cap over mucous acinus that consists of serous cells.
  - All the serous cells of serous demilunes pore their secretions in the lumen of mucous acinus through fine canaliculi.
- *New concept:* Serous demilunes are preparation artifact that gets created due to swelling of mucous cells; during tissue processing. These swollen cells push serous cells to produce serous demilune. It is proved by rapid freezing method. It is observed that same acinus is lined by few serous and few mucous cells.
- Example: Submandibular salivary gland.

Differences between serous and mucous cells and acini are listed in Table 6.1 and 6.2.

Classification Based on Mode of Secretion

- Glands are classified based on the mode of secretion as merocrine, apocrine, and holocrine (Fig. 6.15 and Flowchart 6.3).^{Viva}

Merocrine/eccrine Glands

- Merocrine glands synthesize secretory product and seal, it into vesicles. These membrane-bound vesicles fuse with apical surface of cell and get secreted out by *exocytosis*. This mode of secretion is called *merocrine*.^{Viva}
- Most of the exocrine glands use merocrine mode of secretion.

Glands

Q. List the differences between serous and mucous cells.

Table 6.1: Differences between serous and mucous cells[Viva]

Feature	Serous cells	Mucous cells
Shape and size	Small pyramidal cells	Large pyramidal cells
H&E staining	Show basal basophilia and apical eosinophilia	Empty cytoplasm (mucus removed by tissue processing)
Nuclei	Rounded, placed in basal part of cell	Flat, placed toward basement membrane
Secretory granules	Zymogen granules	Mucinogen granules

Q. List the differences between serous and mucous acini.

Table 6.2: Differences between serous and mucous acini.

Feature	Serous acini	Mucous acini
Size	Smaller than mucous acini	Larger than serous acini
Acini type	Compound alveolar	Compound tubular or tubulo-alveolar
Lumen	Smaller than mucous acini	Wider lumen than serous acini
Cells	Serous cells	Mucous cells
Secretion	Thin, watery, enzyme-rich	Thick, mucoid secretions
Example	Parotid gland	Sublingual gland

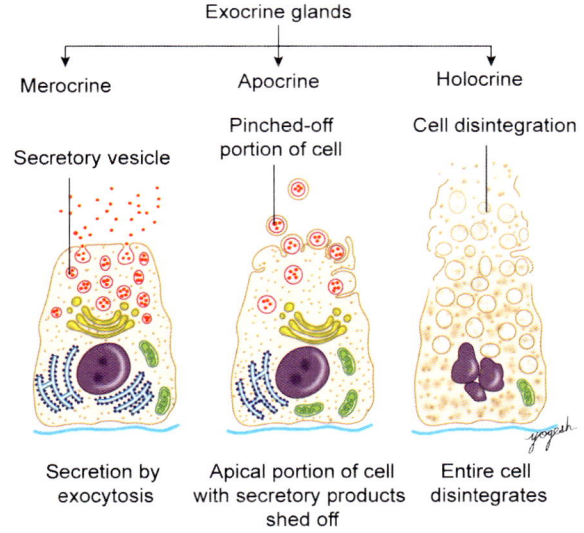

Fig. 6.15: Mode of secretion of exocrine glands.

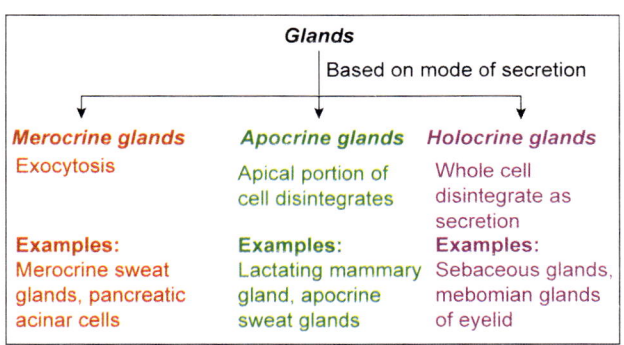

Flowchart 6.3: Classification of glands based on mode of secretion

- For example, pancreatic acinar cells, merocrine sweat glands.

Apocrine Glands

- Apocrine glands synthesize secretory product and accumulate it in apical portion. This apical portion of cell along with secretory products are shed off. This mode of secretion is called *apocrine*.[Viva]

- For example, lactating mammary gland, apocrine sweat glands, ceruminous glands of external ear.[Neet]

Holocrine Glands

- Holocrine glands synthesize and accumulate the secretory product. While discharging secretions, entire cell disintegrates and undergo programmed cell death on maturation. This mode of secretion is called *holocrine*.[Viva]

- For example, sebaceous glands, Meibomian (tarsal) glands of eyelids.[Neet]

Note: Endocrine glands secrete hormones directly into the bloodstream (Fig. 6.16).

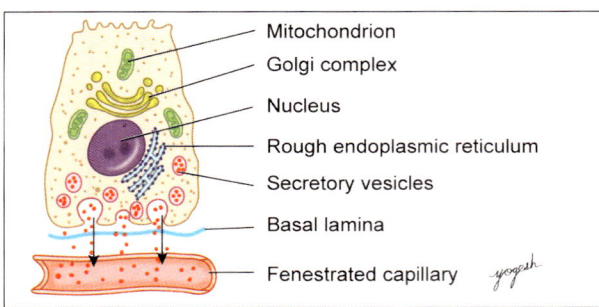

Fig. 6.16: Mode of endocrine gland secretion.

Paracrine and Autocrine Glands

Q. What are paracrine and autocrine glands?

- Some cells in epithelia (unicellular glands) function as paracrine or autocrine signaling mechanism (Fig. 6.17).

Paracrine Signaling

- Cells secrete substances that affect other nearby cells (secretions do not enter the bloodstream). This mechanism of glandular function is called paracrine signaling.
- Cells secrete paracrine substances into extracellular matrix and these substances reach the target cells by diffusion. For example, vasodilators released by endothelial cells act on vascular smooth muscles to produce relaxation of vascular wall.

Autocrine Signaling

- Cells secrete a molecule that acts on the same cell by binding with receptors. This mechanism of glandular function is called autocrine signaling.
- Autocrine signaling may activate (positive feedback) or inhibit (negative feedback) activity of the cell.
- For example, activation of cells of immune system by interleukins.

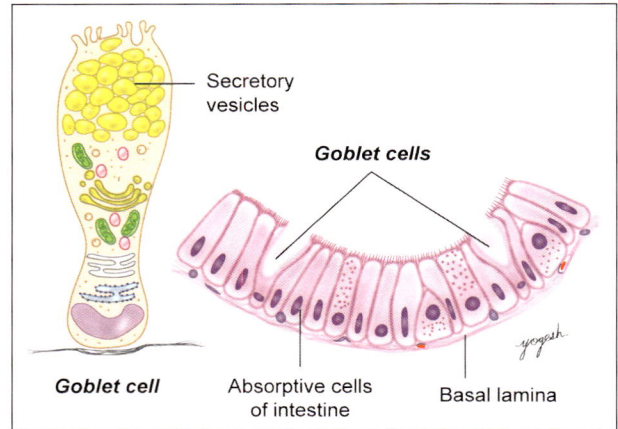

Fig. 6.18: Unicellular gland. For example, goblet cell.

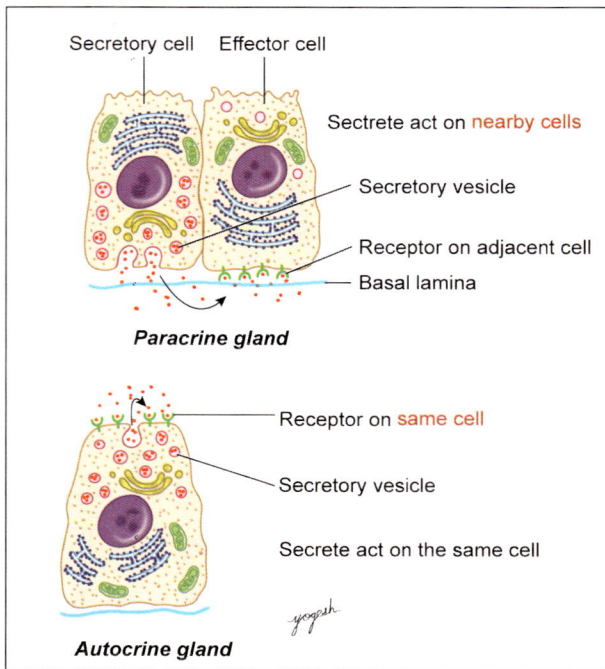

Fig. 6.17: Paracrine and autocrine mode of signaling.

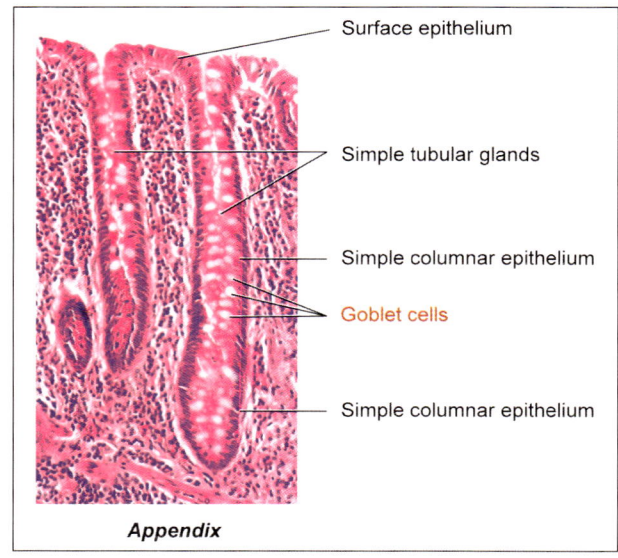

Fig. 6.19: Photomicrograph. Unicellular gland/goblet cell.

> **Box 6.1:** Goblet cell – as a gland

Q. Write a short note on goblet cell.

- Goblet cells are simple columnar cells that work as **unicellular glands.** *Viva*
- They lie among the lining epithelium singly or in other glands.
- Mode of secretion: *merocrine*, sometime apocrine.
- Shape: Goblet-shape = apical cup-shaped portion and base as narrow stem.
- Structure (Figs 6.18 and 6.19)
  In the apical portion, cytoplasm of goblet cell has numerous secretory vesicles filled with mucus.
- *H&E staining:* Apical portion gives an empty appearance as carbohydrate-rich proteins (mucin) are washed out during tissue processing for slide preparation. Nucleus is peripherally placed, flat and rests in basal portion of cell just adjacent to the basal lamina. *Viva*
- Special stains: Periodic acid–Schiff (PAS) staining imparts magenta color to mucin. Mucicarmine staining gives deep red color to goblet cells.

Functions
- Secretion of mucus.

Locations
- Epithelial lining of small and large intestine, respiratory tract, and conjunctiva.

CHAPTER 7

General Connective Tissue

Chapter Outline

- General connective tissue
- Components of connective tissue
- Fibers of connective tissue
  - Collagen fibers
  - Reticular fibers
  - Elastic fibers
- Marfan's syndrome
- Ground substance
- Cells of connective tissue
  - Fibroblasts
  - Myofibroblasts
  - Pericytes
  - Adipocytes
  - Macrophages
  - Mast cells
  - Lymphocytes
  - Plasma cells
  - Pigment cells
- Mononuclear phagocytic system
- Embryonic connective tissue
  - Mesenchyme
  - Mucous connective tissue
- Loose connective tissue
- Dense connective tissue
  - Dense irregular connective tissue
  - Dense regular connective tissue
- Adipose tissue
  - Yellow adipose tissue
  - Brown adipose tissue

Competency achievement: The student should be able to:

AN66.1 Describe and identify various types of connective tissue with functional correlation

AN66.2 Describe the ultrastructure of connective tissue

INTRODUCTION

- Tissue [*tissue* = woven in French, *texo* = weave in Latin] is a group of cells that are organized in a specific manner to perform a specific function.
- Tissue consists of cells and extracellular components.
- Human organ consists of *four basic tissue* types: Epithelial tissue, connective tissue, muscle tissue, and nerve tissue.^{Neet, Viva}

Epithelial tissue

- Epithelia/epithelial tissues covers surfaces of body, inner surfaces of body cavities and lining glandular tissue.
- Epithelial cells may be arranged in a single layer or in multiple layers.
- Cells of epithelium are connected with each other and with basal lamina by cell junctions.
- Adjacent cells are separated by intercellular spaces.

Connective tissue

- Connective tissue supports other three basic tissues of the body.
- Connective tissue consists of cells, connective tissue fibers, and intercellular matrix.
- There are some *specialized connective tissues* that include bone (with mineralized matrix), cartilage (with hydrated matrix), and blood (flowing connective tissue).^{Neet}

Muscle tissue

- Muscle tissue is a basic body tissue that has the property of contractility.
- Muscle tissue is further classified as skeletal, cardiac, and smooth muscles.

Nerve tissue

- Nerve tissue is a basic body tissue that has property of excitability and conduction.

- Nervous tissue receives information from external and internal environment, interpret the information, and convey it to other organs to control their functions.
- Nervous tissue is made up of nerve cells and supporting neurological cells.

GENERAL CONNECTIVE TISSUE

- Connective tissue is characterized by presence of *three components:*^{Viva}
  1. Cells
  2. Fibers
  3. Extracellular matrix
- Connective tissue gives definite shape to organ and body, supports other tissues, and performs various other functions.
- Connective tissues are classified into three groups (Flowchart 7.1):
  1. Embryonic connective tissue
     These are present only during embryonic life.
     They are mesenchymal and mucoid connective tissue.
  2. General connective tissue or connective tissue proper
     These are present in all organs of body and classified as loose and dense connective tissue.
  3. Specialized connective tissue
     These are characterized by specialized nature of their extracellular matrix.
     It includes bone, cartilage, blood, adipose tissue, and lymphatic tissue.
- This chapter includes description of embryonic connective tissue, general connective tissue, and adipose tissue.

Flowchart 7.1: Classification of connective tissue

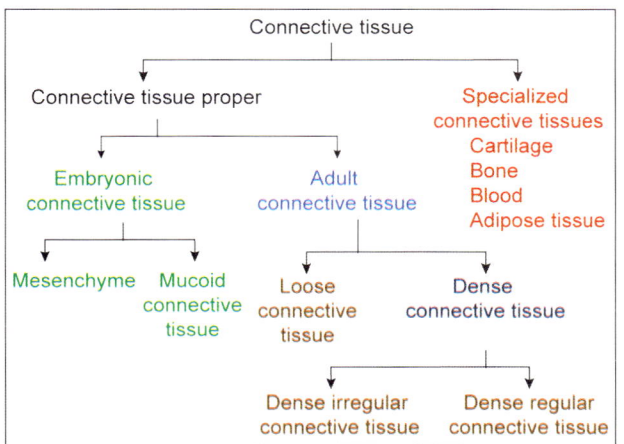

COMPONENTS OF CONNECTIVE TISSUE

Q. List the components of connective tissue.

- Connective tissue consists of the following three basic components (Fig. 7.1 and Flowchart 7.2):

A. Cells

- Cells of connective tissue are grouped as follows:
  1. *Resident cells:* Fibroblasts, adipocytes, macrophages, mast cells, adult stem cells, pigment cells.
  2. *Wandering/transient cells:* Lymphocytes, plasma cells, neutrophils, eosinophils, basophils, and monocytes.

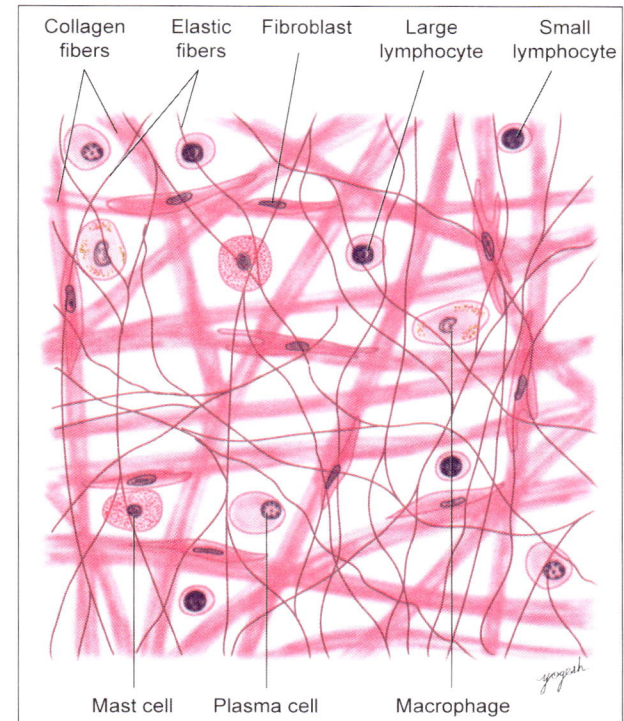

Fig. 7.1: Loose connective tissue (mesentery, high magnification, practice figure). Reticular fibers and blood vessels are not shown in this figure.

Flowchart: 7.2: Components of connective tissue

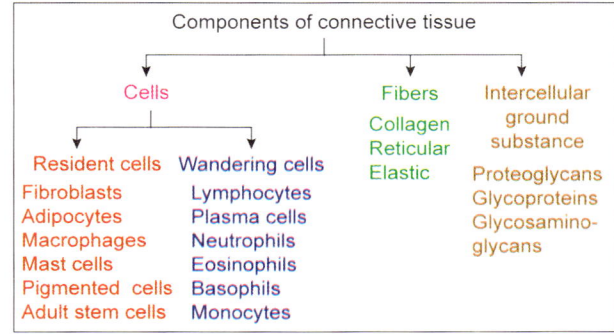

B. Fibers
- Connective tissue consists of collagen, elastic, and reticular fibers.

C. Intercellular ground substance
- It is a supportive amorphous substance that fills space between cells and fibers.
- It consists of proteoglycans, glycoproteins, and glycosaminoglycans.

FIBERS OF CONNECTIVE TISSUE
- Connective tissue has three different types of fibers in matrix: Collagen fibers, reticular fibers and elastic fibers (Fig. 7.1).
- Collagen fibers are found almost in all connective tissues.
- Reticular fibers are present in basement membrane, lymph nodes, and liver.
- Elastic fibers are present in blood vessels, lung, and ligamentum nuchae.

COLLAGEN FIBERS
- Collagen fibers are the most numerous connective tissue fibers.
- *Location:* Tendon, ligament, bone, cartilage, and most of the connective tissues of all organs.
- *Properties:* Collagen fibers are strong, flexible, inelastic and have high tensile strength.
- *Staining:* Collagen fibers are stained with eosin, fast green, methylene blue, aniline blue, and other acidic dyes. Special staining methods include Masson's trichrome stain and van Giesons stain.
- *Light microscopy:* Collagen fibers usually lie in *bundles*. Bundles show wavy appearance. *Bundles branch* and few fibers from bundles may join adjacent bundles. Thickness and length of collagen fibers vary from location to location. In tendon, they are very long and in skin (dermis) they are very short.*Identification feature*
- The 29 different types of collagen fibers have 42 different types of α-chains.*MCQ*
- For example (Fig. 7.2)
  - Type I collagen fiber has two identical α-1 chains and one α-2 chain
  - Type II collagen fiber has three identical α-1 chains.
  - Each third amino acid of the α-chain is glycine.
  - Alpha chain also has proline and hydroxyproline predominantly.

Types of Collagen Fibers
- Collagen fibers are of *29 different types*. They are classified using Roman numerals from I to XXIX.

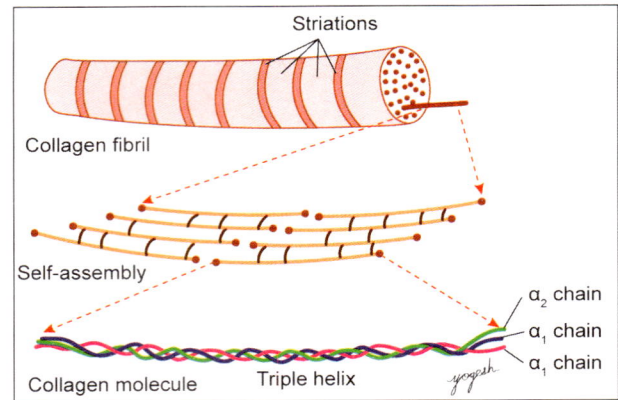

Fig. 7.2: Structure of collagen. On electron microscopic observation, collagen fiber shows striations. Each collagen molecule consists of three chains (triple helix).

- Some important collagen fibers are described below.

Type I Collagen
- They are found in connective tissue, tendons, fascia, ligaments, bones, skin, sclera, and organ capsules.*Viva*
- They are the commonest type of collagen (90%).*MCQ*
- They provide protection, resistance to stretch and tension.
- Disease: *Osteogenesis imperfecta* or *brittle bone disease* occurs because of lack of type I collagen fibers.

Type II Collagen
- It provides resistance to intermittent pressures.
- It is located in hyaline cartilage, elastic cartilage, vitreous of eye, nucleus pulposus of intervertebral disc, and notochord.*Neet, Viva*
- Disease: Deficiency of type II collagen fibers produces *Kniest dysplasia.*

Type III Collagen/Reticular Fibers
- They are also called *reticular fibers.*
- Location: Reticular lamina of basement membrane, loose connective tissues in livers, spleen, lung, kidney, and uterus, endoneurium, blood vessels, and skin.*Viva*
- They provide supportive meshwork in various organs.
- Diseases: Deficiency of reticular fibers produces *Ehlers-Danlos syndrome.*

Type IV Collagen
- These are present in the form of sheets of short filaments and they do not form bundles.
- Location: *Basal lamina* of all epithelia, glomeruli of kidney, and *lens capsule*.*Neet, Viva*

Flowchart 7.3: Collagen synthesis

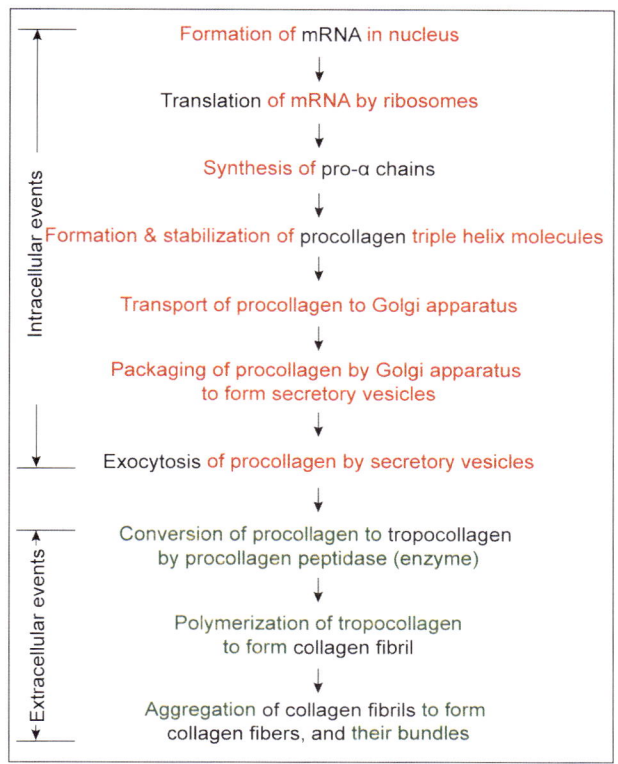

- These fibers provide support to overlying epithelia and form filtration barrier in kidney.
- Deficiency of type IV collagen fibers produces *Alport syndrome* [Cecil A Alport, 1927]. It is characterized by hematuria, progressive hearing loss, and ocular lesions.[Neet]

Synthesis of Collagen

- Synthesis of collagen by fibroblasts involves events that are grouped as intracellular events and extracellular events (Flowchart 7.3).

Some Interesting Facts

- Pro-α chain undergoes posttranslational modifications. It involves vitamin C dependent hydroxylation of proline and lysine residues. Hence, in *vitamin C deficiency (Scurvy)*, there is delayed wound healing due to lack of collagen synthesis.
- Collagen fibers are synthesized by fibroblasts, chondrocytes, pericytes of blood vessels, and epithelial cells.[Neet]
- Collagen can be degraded by mechanical injuries and various proteinases such as collagenases, gelatinases, matrix metalloproteinases (MMPs), and lysosomal enzymes.
- *Edema* is an excessive accumulation of extracellular fluid in the connective tissue.[Viva]
- Differences between collagen, elastic, and reticular fibers are listed in Table 7.1.

RETICULAR FIBERS

- Reticular fibers are fine fibers (~20 nm diameter).
- Reticular fibers are composed of *type III collagen*.[Neet]
- Locations: Reticular fibers form a supportive network of many organs such as liver, lymphatic tissue (*absent in thymus*), intestine, gland, nerves, bone marrow, and muscles.[Neet]
- Reticular fibers do not form bundles.
- Reticular fibers are produced by reticulocytes or fibroblasts.
- *Staining*
  - *Silver staining:* On silver impregnation, reticular fibers appear black because of their affinity for silver (*argyrophilic fibers*) (Figs 7.3 and 7.4).
  - *PAS staining:* Reticular fibers are positive for periodic acid–Schiff (PAS) reaction.

Table 7.1: Differences between collagen, elastic, and reticular fibers

Nature	Collagen fibers	Elastic fibers	Reticular fibers
Location	Tendons, ligaments, organ capsules	Large vessels, lungs, ligamentum nuchae	Basal lamina, dentine, pulp, liver spleen, lymph nodes
Course	Runs in bundles, Bundles are branching	Runs singly and branch	Form mesh-like network
Striations of TEM	Present	Absent	Present
Physical properties	Have high tensile strength and flexible but inelastic	Have highly elastic and little tensile strength	Have little elasticity and tensile strength
Special staining	van Giesons's method, Masson's trichrome chain	Orcein method, Verhoeff's method	Silver impregnation method
Another name	White fibers	Yellow fibers	Argyrophilic fibers

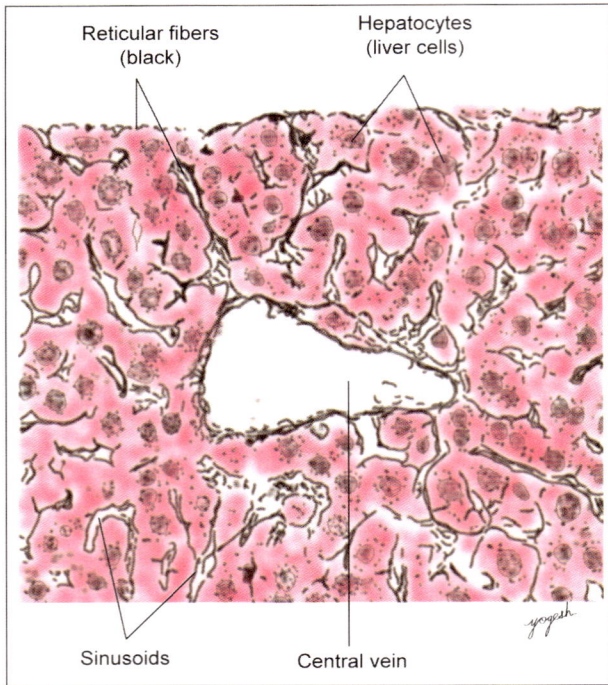

Fig. 7.3: Reticular fiber stained by Gorden and Sweet silver staining method (liver, high magnification, practice figure).

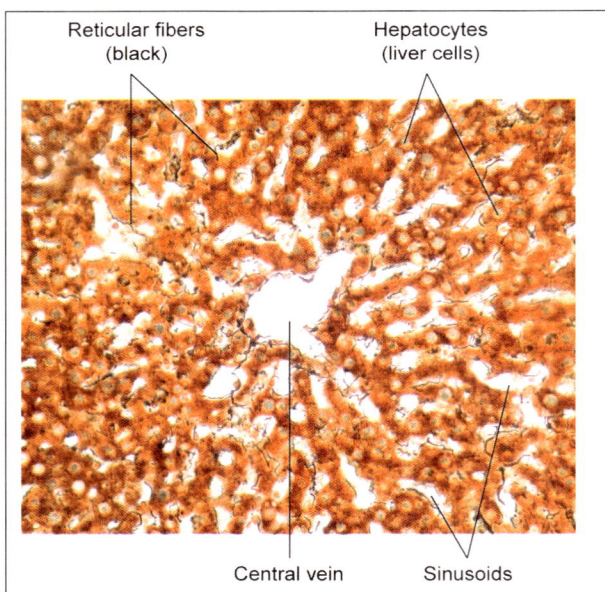

Fig. 7.4: Photomicrograph. Reticular fiber stained by Gomori's silver impregnation staining technique (Liver, high magnification).

- *Function:* Reticular fibers form supportive network around cells of many organs. They help to form basement membrane.

- Electron microscopically, reticular fibers also show striations.

ELASTIC FIBERS

- Elastic fibers are fine fibers (0.1–0.2 µm diameter).
- They *run single* (do not form bundles) and *branch* to form a network.^{Identification feature}
- *Locations:* Skin, blood vessels, in matrix of elastic cartilages, ligamentum nuchae, ligamentum flava, periodontal ligament, elastic ligaments of vocal folds of larynx, and lung.^{Neet, Viva}
- *Transmission electron microscopy:* Each elastic fiber has a central core of amorphous material. Surrounded by an outer layer of fibrils. Elastic fibers do not show striations (Fig. 7.5).
- *Chemical structure:* Elastin (protein) forms a central core of elastic fibers. Elastin has randomly distributed glycine that allows coiling and stretching of elastic fibers. Desmosine and isodesmosine are the amino acids that are present only in elastin (Fig. 7.6).^{Neet}
- Elastin is surrounded by fibrillin-1 (glycoprotein).
- *Synthesis:* Elastic fibers are synthesized by fibroblasts, smooth muscle cells, endothelium in vessels, and chondrocytes in cartilages.
- Absence of fibrillin-1 in vessels converts fine elastic fibers into elastic sheets or lamellae.^{Viva}
- *Staining:*
  – Elastic fibers cannot be well differentiated on *H&E* staining (*Previous concept:* Elastic fibers are not stained by *H&E* staining) (Fig. 7.7).

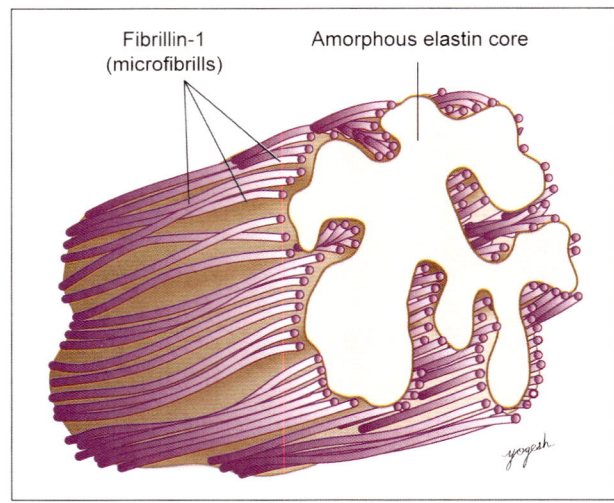

Fig. 7.5: Structure of an elastic fiber.

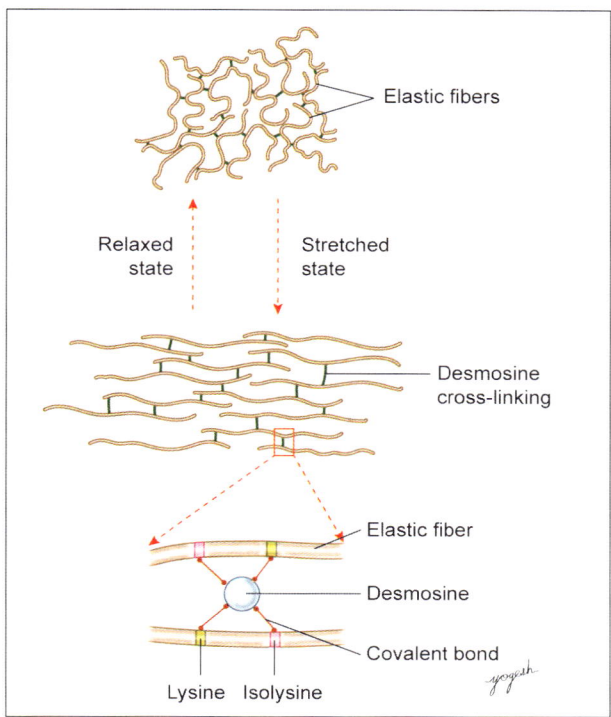

Fig. 7.6: Relaxed and stretched state of elastic fibers and role of desmosine in linking elastic fibers.

- Special stains such as *orcein* (gives dark brown color) and *Verhoeff's method* (gives black color) are useful for differentiation of elastic fibers (Fig. 7.8).

Box 7.1: Marfan syndrome

- Marfan syndrome is a genetic disorder due to abnormal development of elastic fibers.
- It was first described by **Antoine Marfan (French Pediatrician, 1858–1942)**.

Cause
- Abnormal FBN1 (fibrillin gene) located on chromosome 15 that encodes fibrillin-1 protein.^{MCQ}
- Mode of inheritance: Autosomal dominant.
- Fibrillin-1 is essential for formation of elastic fiber assembly during elastogenesis.

Signs and symptoms
- People with Marfan syndrome are tall and thin with long arms, legs, finger, and toes.^{MCQ}
- They may have highly flexible joints, eye lens dislocation causing blurring of vision, and aortic aneurysm/dilatation.^{MCQ}
- Incidence: 1 in 5,000–10,000 individuals.
- There is no cure for Marfan syndrome.
- Symptomatic treatment can be given.

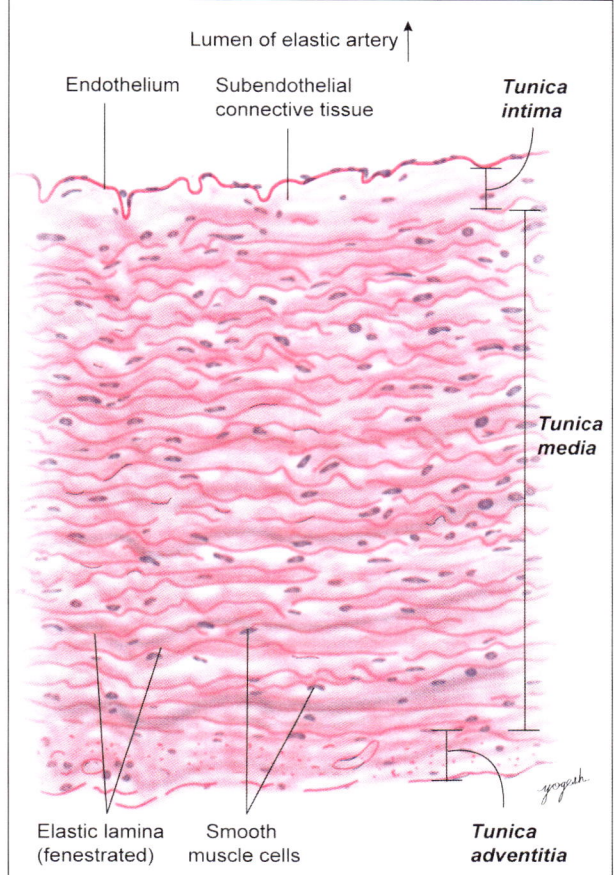

Fig. 7.7: Elastic fibers are seen in the form of lamina (section of elastic artery, *H&E* stain, high magnification).

GROUND SUBSTANCE/EXTRACELLULAR MATRIX

- Interfibrillar and intercellular spaces in the connective tissue are occupied by transparent, homogenous, extracellular matrix, or ground substance.^{Viva}
- Ground substance allows diffusion of metabolites and provides barrier for spread of microorganisms.^{Viva}

Staining

- On routine slide/section preparation, chemicals remove extracellular matrix. Hence, it gives *empty appearance* and only two components of loose connective tissue are observed that are cells and fibers.^{Practical guide}
- Freeze-drying method: Extracellular matrix stains metachromatically with toluidine blue.
- PAS method: Proteoglycans of ground substance make it PAS positive.

Composition

- Ground substance is made up of three groups of substances as follows (Fig. 7.9):^{Viva}

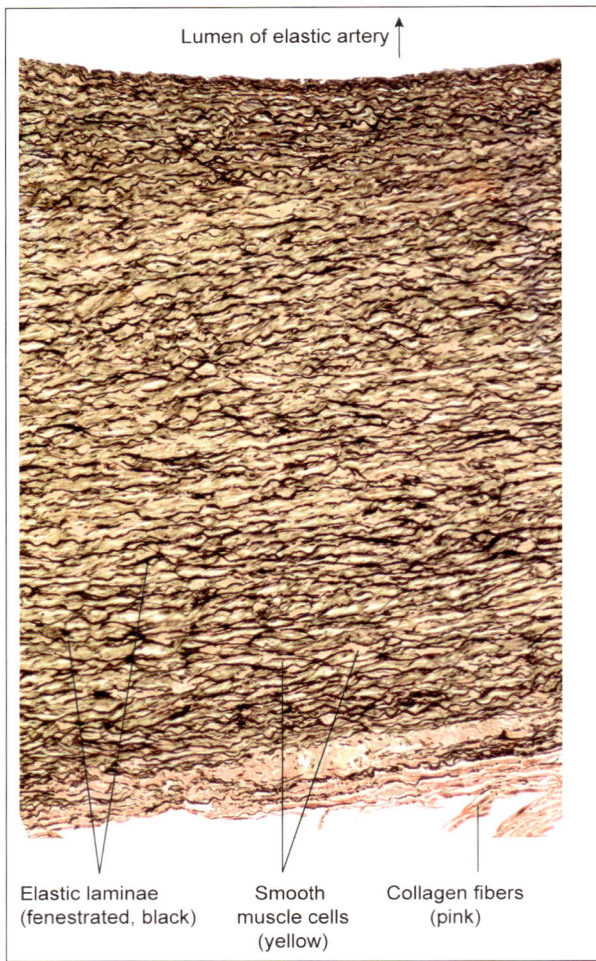

Fig. 7.8: Photomicrograph. Elastic fibers are seen in the form of lamina (section of elastic artery, Verhoeff–van Gieson stain, low magnification).

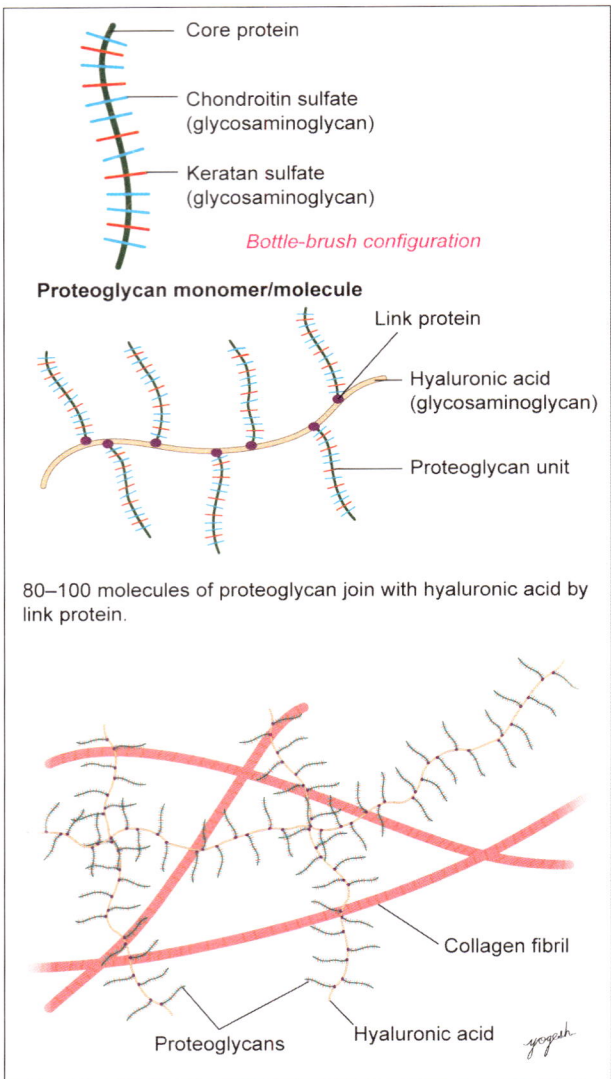

Fig. 7.9: Molecular organization of ground substance of the hyaline cartilage.

1. Glycosaminoglycans: dermatan sulfate, keratan sulfate, hyaluronan.
2. Proteoglycans: aggrecan, syndecan.
3. Glycoproteins: fibronectin, laminin.

Glycosaminoglycans (GAGs)
- GAGs are long chain, unbranched polysaccharides (Fig. 7.9).
- GAGs are highly negatively charged because of surface and carboxyl groups. Hence,
  i. GAGs attract water and form hydrated gel.
  ii. GAGs get stained with basic dyes (hematoxylin)
- GAGs are responsible for physical properties of ground substance.
- For example, hyaluronic acid (hyaluronan), chondroitin sulfate, dermatan sulfate, keratan sulfate, heparan sulfate.

- Hyaluronic acid form long rigid molecule that provides attachment to proteoglycan molecules with the help of link proteins.
- Hyaluronic acid binds with water molecules and converts extracellular matrix into gel-like substance.*Viva*

Proteoglycans
- Proteoglycans consist of a core protein that provides attachment to numerous glycosaminoglycans and forms *bottle-brush structure* (Fig. 7.9).
- Note: Hyaluronic acid does not bound to the core protein and hence, it does not form proteoglycans. However, proteoglycans bind with hyaluronic acid with the help of link proteins.

- Examples: Aggrecan (present in ground substance) and syndecan (present as transmembrane proteoglycan that connects cell to extracellular matrix).

Glycoproteins
- Glycoproteins stabilize extracellular matrix and bind the cells with extracellular matrix (Fig. 7.9).
- Examples:
  - Fibronectin: It is the most abundant multiadhesive glycoprotein. It binds cells with the extracellular matrix.
  - Laminin: It adheres epithelial cells with basal lamina (refer Fig. 4.16).
  - Entactin: It links laminin and type IV collagen in basal lamina.
  - Tenascin: It helps to bind cells of embryonic mesenchyme, perichondrium, periosteum and musculotendinous junctions with extracellular matrix.
  - Osteonectin: It helps in bone mineralization.
  - Chondronectin: It binds chondrocytes with extracellular matrix.

CELLS OF CONNECTIVE TISSUE

Q. List the cells of connective tissue and their functions.

- Cells of connective tissue are classified as resident/fixed cells and wandering cells (Table 7.2 and Fig. 7.10).

Fibroblasts
- These are the most numerous connective tissue cells (Fig. 7.10).

Table 7.2: Connective tissue cells

Fixed/resident cells	Wandering cells
– Fibroblasts	– Lymphocytes
– Adipose cells	– Plasma cells
– Macrophages	– Neutrophils
– Mast cells	– Eosinophils
– Pericytes	– Basophils
	– Monocytes

Cell description
- *Fibroblasts* are active cells that form collagen, elastic or reticular fibers, and extracellular matrix.
- Fibroblasts have abundant cytoplasm, oval or elongated nucleus, and branched cytoplasmic processes.
- *Fibrocyte* is a mature cell that is smaller cell, have less cytoplasm and flat elongated nucleus.
- *H&E staining:* Fibroblasts lie in close proximity of collagen fibers; hence, difficult to identify. Nuclei are clearly visible. Thin, pale-staining, flattened processes may also be visible. *Practical guide, Identification feature*
- The size and amount of cell organelles depend on activity of the cells. Fibroblasts are most active during wound healing.
- Fibroblast lie parallel to the long axis of adjacent collagen fibers.

Myofibroblast
- Myofibroblast has features of both smooth muscle cell and fibroblast.
- It is an elongated, spindle-shaped cell.
- On *H&E staining*, it cannot be differentiated.

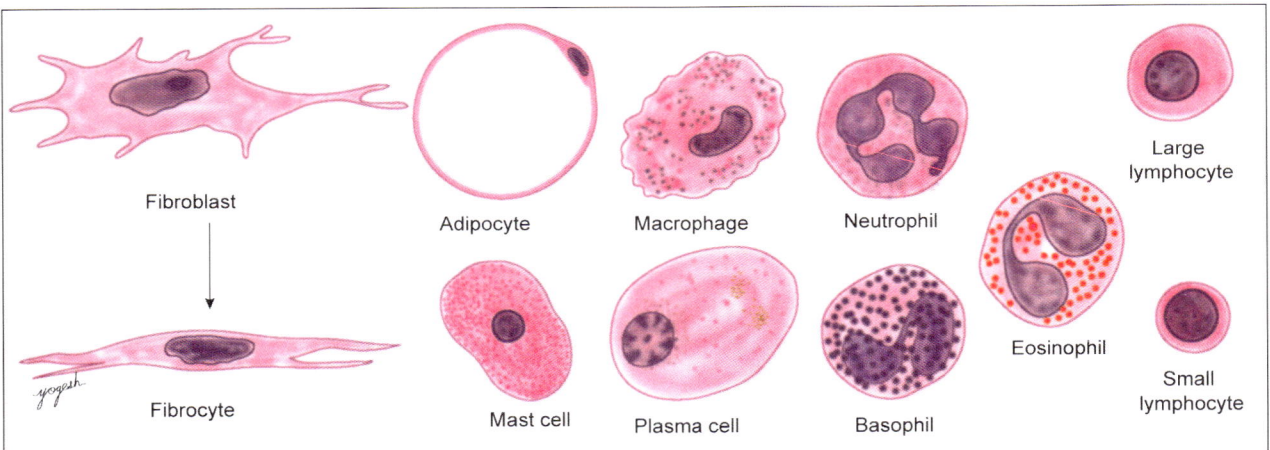

Fig. 7.10: Cells of connective tissue.

- It contains actin and myosin filaments; hence, have contractile property.
- In contrast to smooth muscle, myofibroblast is not covered by basal lamina.
- Functions: Myofibroblast plays a major role in wound healing and also plays a role in eruption of tooth (present in periodontal ligament).^{MCQ}

Pericytes

- These are present surrounding the endothelium of capillaries and venules.
- Pericytes lie embedded in the basal lamina of endothelium.
- Pericytes have a long oval euchromatic nucleus and several cytoplasmic processes that clasp capillary.
- Pericytes show features of both fibroblasts as well as smooth muscle cells.

Adipocytes (Fat Cells)

- Adipocytes synthesize and store large quantities of lipids in their cytoplasm (Fig. 7.10).^{Viva}
- There are two types of adipocytes: unilocular, and multilocular.^{Viva}

Unilocular Adipocytes

- Unilocular adipocytes are found in white/yellow adipose tissue. It mostly performs function of insulation and shock absorption.
- Structure: Unilocular adipocytes are large, spherical or polyhedral cells (ring-like). Cytoplasm contains large quantity of lipid mass that pushes nucleus toward one side. Cytoplasm forms a thin rim of cytoplasm surrounding a large lipid mass (Fig. 7.10).^{Identification feature}
- *H&E staining:* Because of routine histological processing of tissue for slide/section preparation, lipid is lost. Hence, on *H&E* staining, adipocytes show an empty appearance, a thin rim of cytoplasm, and peripheral, flat/elongated nucleus (Fig. 7.10).^{Viva, Practical guide}
- Special stains: For visualization of lipids/adipocytes, fresh frozen sections are suitable. In these sections, lipid can be stained using oil red O method, Sudan black B method, and Nile blue sulfate method.^{MCQ}
- Locations: Cushions around vital organs, *subcutaneous fat/panniculus adiposus*, mammary pad of fat, yellow bone marrow, *orbit*, retroperitoneal space, greater omentum.^{Neet}

Multilocular Adipocytes

- Multilocular adipocytes are present in the brown adipose tissue.
- Structure: Multilocular adipocytes are smaller than unilocular adipocytes. They have eccentric round nucleus (not in center). Their cytoplasm contains small pockets of lipid droplets.
- *H&E staining:* Cytoplasm gives a foamy appearance as lipid droplets are washed out and cell shows eccentric round nucleus.^{Identification feature}
- Locations
  - It is mostly found in newborn babies and decreases in adult
  - In adult, it is located in back and neck, scapular region, and posterior abdominal wall
- Functions
  - Brown fat prevents excessive heat loss from body surface. It can generate heat (thermogenesis) by lipid breakdown.^{Viva}
  - Thermoregulation is very essential in newborns for getting adjusted in the new environment outside of the uterus.

Macrophages/Histocytes/Clasmatocytes

Q. Write a short note on macrophages.

- Macrophages/tissue histocytes are derived from circulating monocytes.^{MCQ, Viva}
- The main function of macrophages is phagocytosis of bacteria, damaged tissue, and inorganic particles.
- On *H&E staining*, it is difficult to distinguish macrophages from other cells (Fig. 7.10).
- Macrophages are of two types:
  1. Fixed macrophages: attached to connective tissue fibers
  2. Wandering macrophages: can move
- Fixed macrophage has irregular shape, short branching cytoplasmic processes, and kidney-shaped nucleus.
- Macrophage has numerous lysosomal vesicles that are required for digestion of phagocytosed material.
- *Langhans cell:* Macrophages may fuse to form giant multinucleated cell called Langhans cell (up to 100 nuclei).
- Functions
  1. *Phagocytosis* of unwanted material such as bacteria, damaged tissue, and so on.
  2. Act as an *antigen-presenting* cell and induces immune response.

Mast cells

- Mast cells are also called *histaminocytes* or *mastocytes*.
- They are usually located close to blood vessels in connective tissue.
- Structure
  - These are large, ovoid cells (~20–30 μm in diameter) with small centrally placed nucleus.
  - Cytoplasm has large, *basophilic granules*.

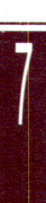

- Granules contain heparin and histamine.*Neet*
- Cell surface shows numerous filopodia (irregular microvilli).
- Staining

 Granules can be stained using: Periodic acid–Schiff stain (magenta-colored), toluidine blue, or alcian blue stain (Fig. 7.10).
- *Metachromasia:* Granules of mast cell look purple to red color when stained with toluidine/alcian blue. Here, dye color is blue, but the structure becomes purple or red. This is called *metachromasia*.*Viva*
- Mast cell identification needs glutaraldehyde fixative.
- Immunoglobulin E is present on the surface of mast cells.
- Functions:*Viva*
  1. Mast cell releases histamine on binding of antigen to immunoglobulin E on its surface.

     Histamine causes contraction of smooth muscles in bronchioles (produces asthma), dilatation of small blood vessels (produces edema), and itching sensation in skin.
  2. Mast cell also releases

     Heparin that acts as an anticoagulant.

     Serine proteases that produce inflammation.

     Leukotriene C that causes bronchospasm due to constrictions of smooth muscles of respiratory tract.

> **Box 7.2:** Mononuclear phagocytic system
>
> - Mononuclear phagocytic system composed of various cells that arise from monocytes.*Viva*
> - All these cells perform antigen presentation.
> - Circulating monocytes enter connective tissue and acquire some specific cells as follows:
>   1. Macrophages: Connective tissue, spleen, lymph node, thymus bone marrow
>   2. Kupffer cells: Liver
>   3. Dust cell: Lungs
>   4. Langerhans cell: Skin
>   5. Monocytes: Blood
>   6. Osteoclast: Bone
>   7. Microglia: Central nervous system
>   8. Dendritic cell: Lymph node, spleen
> - All cells of MPS are capable of phagocytosis, release of lysosomal contents, intracellular digestion in lysosomes.
> - MPS cells have receptor for FC fragments of immunoglobulins.
> - Note: Mast cells are not present in brain and spinal cord.*MCQ*

Lymphocytes

- Lymphocytes are principally involved in immune responses.
- Lymphocyte has deeply staining heterochromatic nucleus and a thin rim of cytoplasm (Fig. 7.10).*Identification feature*
- Lymphocytes are grouped as follows based on the presence of cluster of differentiation (CD) protein/antigen on their plasma membrane:*Viva, MCQ*
  1. *T-lymphocyte:* Play a role in cell-mediated immunity
  2. *B-lymphocyte:* Play a role in antibody-mediated/humoral immunity
  3. *NK (natural killer) cells:* Destroy virus-infected cells and tumor cells.

Plasma Cells/Plasmatocytes

- Plasma cells are derived from B-lymphocytes.*MCQ*

 Structure
  - Plasma cells are ovoid in shape. They have basophilic cytoplasm that contains numerous rough endoplasmic reticulum (required for antibody production) (Fig. 7.10).
  - Nucleus is round and eccentrically placed.
  - Chromatin material gives an analog clock face/*cart-wheel appearance* to the nucleus (Fig. 7.10).*MCQ, Viva*
- *Russell bodies:* Plasma cell may show large homogenous *immunoglobulin-containing* inclusions. These are excessively produced immunoglobulins stored in dilated endoplasmic reticulum. Russel bodies are PAS positive. Plasma cells containing Russell bodies are called *Mott's cells.*ial.*Neet* [William Russell, 1852–1940, Scottish pathologist]
- Function
  - Production of antibodies.

Pigment Cells

- Pigmented cells synthesize melanin pigment. These are called *melanocytes.*
- Locations: Skin, iris, choroid.
- Melanocytes are derived from neural crest cells.
- Melanocytes are star-shaped cells with long branching processes.
- Pigment cells protect deeper cells from exposure to ultraviolet light. (for details, read Chapter 14)

Other Leucocytes

- Leucocytes/white blood cells are derived from bone marrow and some of them migrate to connective tissue.

Table 7.3: White blood cells

White blood cell	Description	Functions
Neutrophil (10–12 μm)	Nucleus: 3–5 lobes Cytoplasm: shows pink or reddish-purple granules	Phagocytosis of microorganism
Basophils (10–12 μm)	Nucleus: segmented Cytoplasm: dark, basophilic granules (contain histamine)	Release histamine, promote inflammation
Eosinophil (10–14 μm)	Nucleus: bilobed Cytoplasm: dark eosinophilic granules	Phagocytose antigen-antibody complexes, induce allergic reactions, and asthma, attack parasites
Lymphocytes (6–14 μm)	Round nucleus, thin rim of cytoplasm	T lymphocytes: cell-mediated immunity B lymphocytes: antibody-mediated immunity NK cells: destroy cancer cells
Monocytes (12–20 μm)	Kidney-shaped nucleus	Phagocytosis Differentiate into mononuclear phagocytic cells (e.g. macrophages)

- Leucocytes are classified as follows (Table 7.3):
  I: Granulocytes
    They have numerous cytoplasmic granules.
    For example, neutrophils, eosinophils, and basophils.
  II: Agranulocytes
    They do not have specific cytoplasmic granules.
    For example, lymphocytes and monocytes.

EMBRYONIC CONNECTIVE TISSUE

- Mesoderm gives rise to embryonic connective tissue.
- There are two subtypes of embryonic connective tissue:
  A. Mesenchyme
  B. Mucous connective tissue

Mesenchyme

- It is found in an embryo.
- It consists of *mesenchymal cells*.
- Mesenchymal cells are small, spindle-shaped cells with fine cytoplasmic processes.*Identification feature*
- Space between mesenchymal cells is occupied by ground substance, reticular fibers, and collagen fibers.
- Processes of adjacent mesenchymal cells are connected with each other by gap junctions.

Mucous Connective Tissue

- Mucous connective tissue is present in umbilical cord.
- It surrounds and supports umbilical vessels (two umbilical arteries and one umbilical vein).
- Mucous connective tissue consists of two components: Cells and Wharton's jelly (Figs 7.11 and 7.12).
- Cells of mucous connective tissue are spindle-shaped with long, thin cytoplasmic processes.*Identification feature*

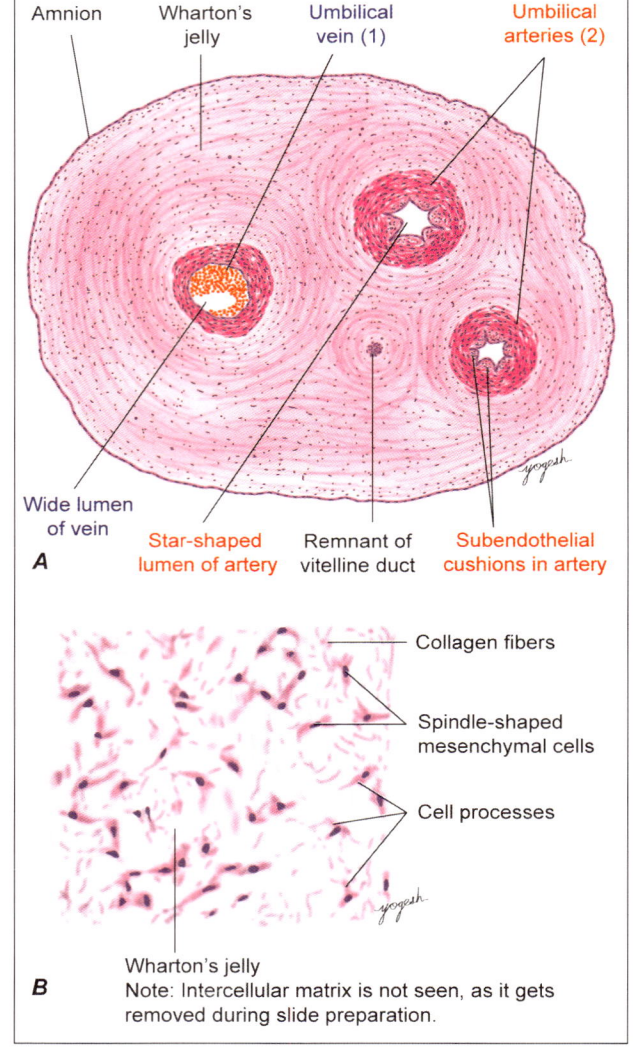

Fig. 7.11: Mucous connective tissue (Wharton's jelly). (A) Transverse section of umbilical cord showing connective tissue, (B) Mucous connective tissue at high magnification (practice figure).

General Connective Tissue

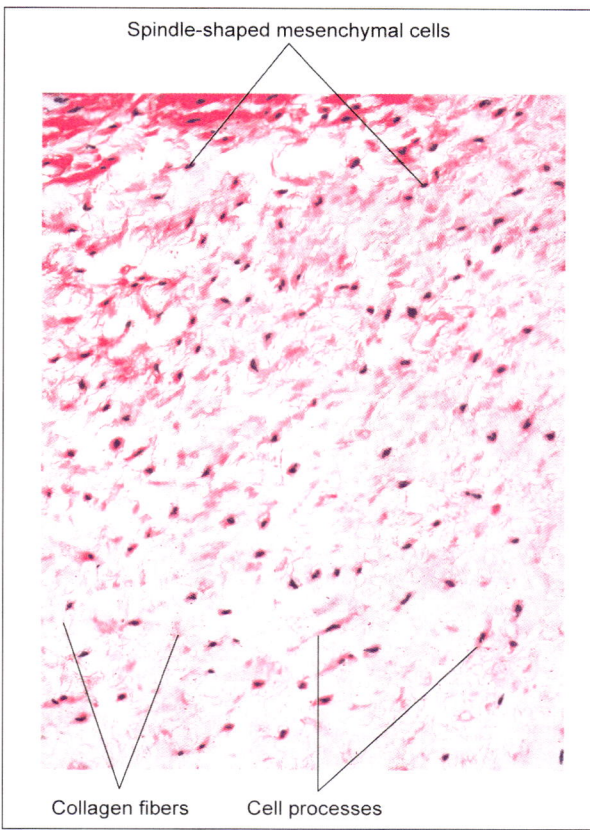

Fig. 7.12: Photomicrograph. Mucous connective tissue (Wharton's jelly). (transverse section of umbilical cord showing mucous connective tissue, *H&E* stain, high magnification).

- *Wharton's jelly*
  - Cells are embedded in gelatin-like ground substance called Wharton's jelly.
  - Wharton's jelly consists of mostly hyaluronic acid.
  - Most of the Wharton's jelly get removed during histological slide preparation. Hence, only spindle-shaped cells with elongated nuclei and fine cytoplasmic processes are seen in mucous connective tissue. *Practical guide*
- Note: Cells isolated from mucous connective tissue (Wharton's jelly of umbilical cord) work as mesenchymal stem cells. Hence, these cells can be used in stem cell therapy. *Clinical fact*

LOOSE CONNECTIVE/AREOLAR TISSUE

- Loose areolar tissue is a widespread connective tissue of body.
- It consists of (Flowchart 7.4, Figs 7.13 and 7.14), the following:
1. Fibers
- It has loosely woven connective tissue fibers.

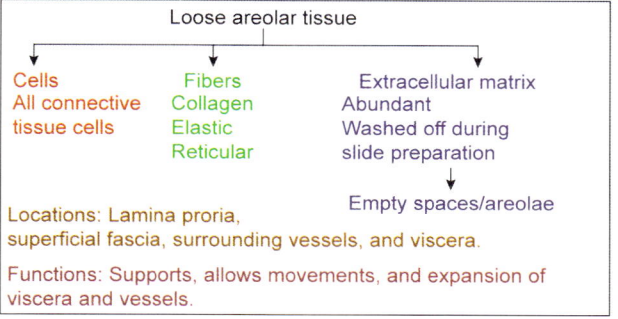

Flowchart 7.4: Loose areolar tissue

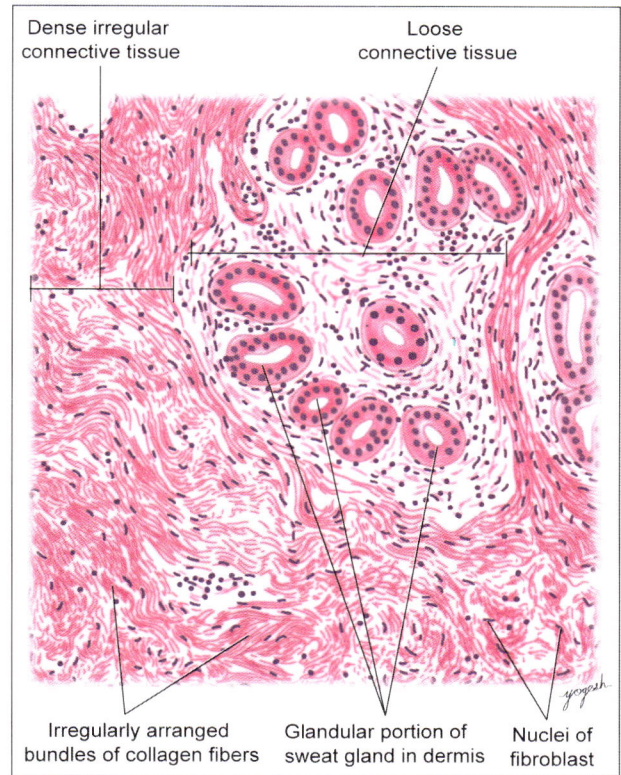

Fig. 7.13: Loose and dense irregular connective tissue (section of dermis at high magnification, practice figure). Note: Reticular and elastic fibers need special stains for visualization (practice figure).

- It has all types of fibers (collagen, elastic, and reticular).
2. Cells:
- It has all types of connective tissue cells such as fibroblasts, macrophages, plasma cells, fat cells, white blood cells, and so on.
3. Ground substance
- Fiber and cells are embedded in abundant viscous, gel-like ground substance. During slide preparation, the ground substance is washed away. In place of

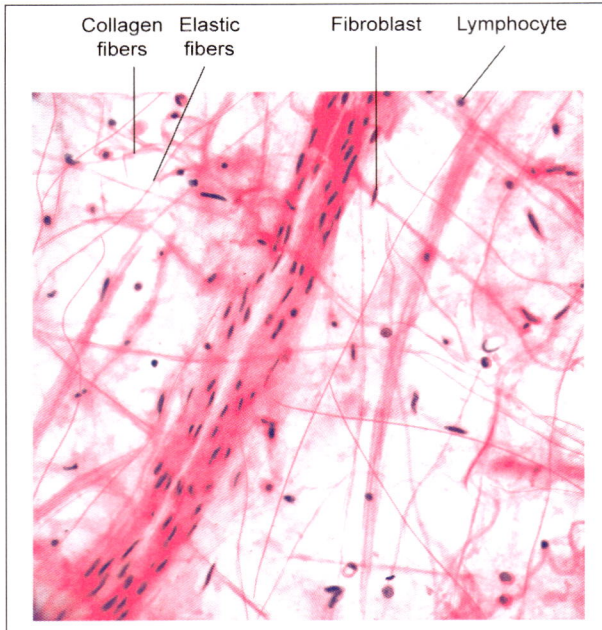

Fig. 7.14: Photomicrograph. Loose connective tissue (mesentery, *H&E* stain, high magnification). Note: Only few types of connective cells can be differentiated on *H&E* staining.

ground substance, empty spaces called *areole* are seen. Hence, it is called loose areolar tissue.*Viva, Practical guide*

Locations
1. Lamina propria: It is present just beneath the epithelium
2. Superficial fascia
3. Surrounding blood vessels, nerves, viscera, muscles, parenchyma of glands
4. In mesentery

Functions
1. It provides support.
2. It provides a plane for movements. For example, superficial facial allows movement of skin over deep fascia.
3. It provides space for expansion of viscera and vessels.

DENSE CONNECTIVE TISSUE

- Dense connective tissue contains large amount of fibers, and less amount of connective tissue cells and ground substance.*Viva*
- Dense connective tissue provides strength tissue and protection to the underlying tissue.
- Dense connective tissue can be grouped into two categories based on orientation of connective tissue fibers as follows:
  1. Dense irregular connective tissue
  2. Dense regular connective tissue

Dense Irregular Connective Tissue

- Dense irregular connective tissue contains mostly collagen fibers and small amount of ground substance (Figs 7.13 and 7.15).
- Cells are mostly fibroblasts.
- Fibers are arranged irregularly or randomly in bundles.
- Locations
  Dermis of skin, dura matter, submucosa of intestinal tract, epineurium, *pericardium*, *periosteum*, tunica albuginea of testis, *sclera*, and *capsules* of various organs.*Neet*
- Functions: Provide strength to the structure and protection to underlying tissue.

Dense Regular Connective Tissue

Q. Write a short note on histology of tendon or ligament.
- Dense regular connective tissue contains predominantly *type I collagen* fibers.
- It contains more collagen fibers and very few cells.
- Fibers are arranged in compact parallel array in thick bundles (regularly).
- Bundles of collagen fibers show wavy appearance.*Identification feature*
- *Regular fibrous tissue* or *white fibrous tissue* is the name given for dense regular connective tissue.
- **Tendon**
  - Tendon is a dense regular connective tissue (Flowchart 7.5, Figs 7.16 and 7.17).

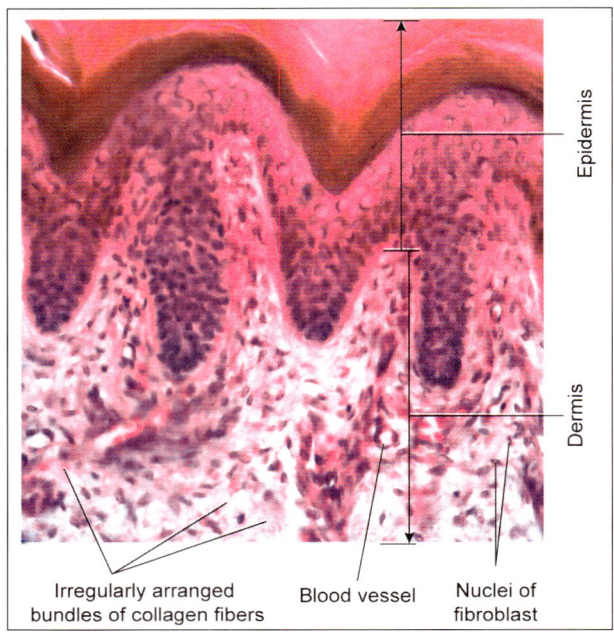

Fig. 7.15: Photomicrograph. Dense irregular connective tissue (section of dermis, *H&E* stain, high magnification).

Flowchart 7.5: Histology of tendon/dense connective tissue

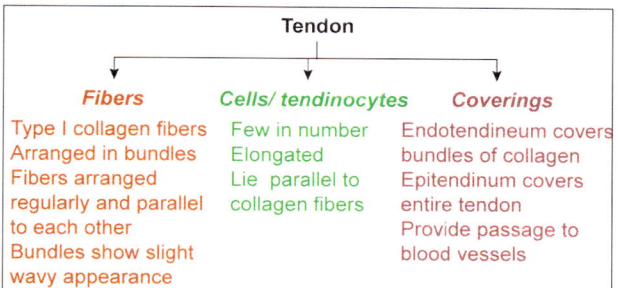

Note: In aponeurosis, bundles of collagen fibers run in layers. Direction of collagen bundle in one layer is arranged at 90° angle to those in adjacent layers (*orthogonal array*).

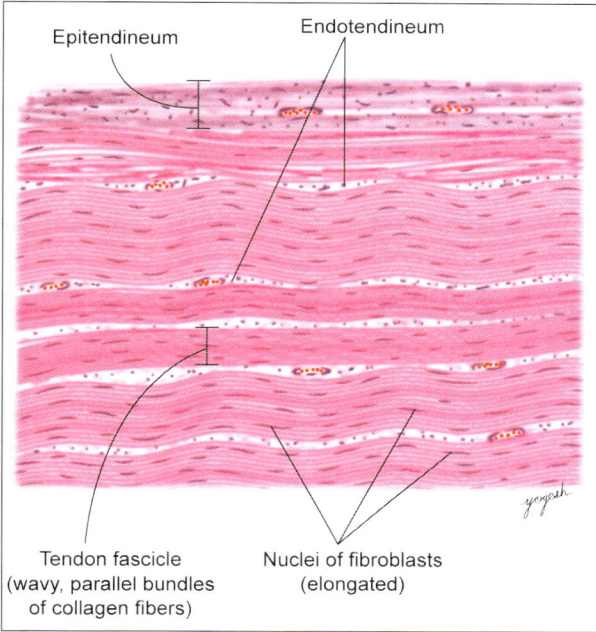

Fig. 7.16: Dense regular connective tissue. Longitudinal section of tendon (practice figure).

- It contains bundles of type I collagen fibers arranged in compact parallel array (*cord pattern*).
- Bundles are separated by vascular connective tissue layer called *endotendineum*. Entire tendon is covered by *epitendineum*.
- In between collagen fibers, *tendinocytes* (cells of tendon) are present. These are elongated cells, oriented along the long axis of collagen bundles.^{Identification feature}

- *Ligament*
  - In ligaments, collagen fibers are arranged in less regular manner than tendon.
  - Ligaments show fibroblasts (similar to tendinocytes) (*sheet pattern* of collagen fibers).

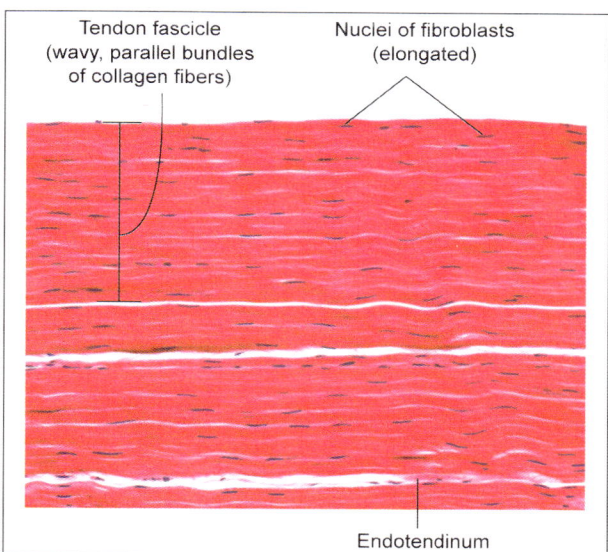

Fig. 7.17: Photomicrograph. Dense regular connective tissue. (longitudinal section of tendon, *H&E* stain).

- Note: Ligamentum nuchae, ligamentum flava contains elastic fibers; hence, they are called as *elastic ligaments*.^{MCQ}

ADIPOSE TISSUE

Q. Write a short note on adipose tissue.
Q. List the differences between yellow and brown adipose tissue.

- Adipose tissue is a specialized connective tissue that play a role in storage of fat.
- Adipose tissue consists of *adipocytes/fat cells*.
- There are two types of adipose tissue (Flowchart 7.6):
  A. White/yellow adipose tissue
  B. Brown adipose tissue

Yellow Adipose Tissue

- It is whitish or yellowish in color.
- Adipose tissue is highly vascular.
- Adipocytes of yellow fat (Figs 7.18 and 7.19):

Flowchart 7.6: Histology of adipose tissue

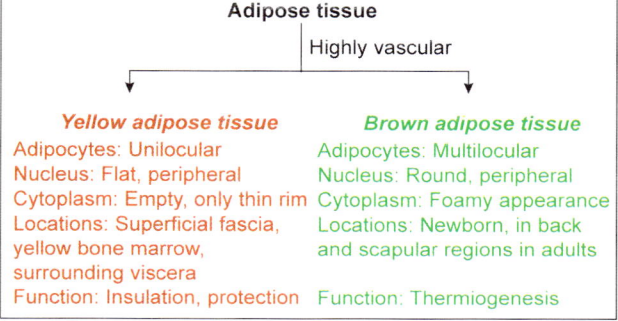

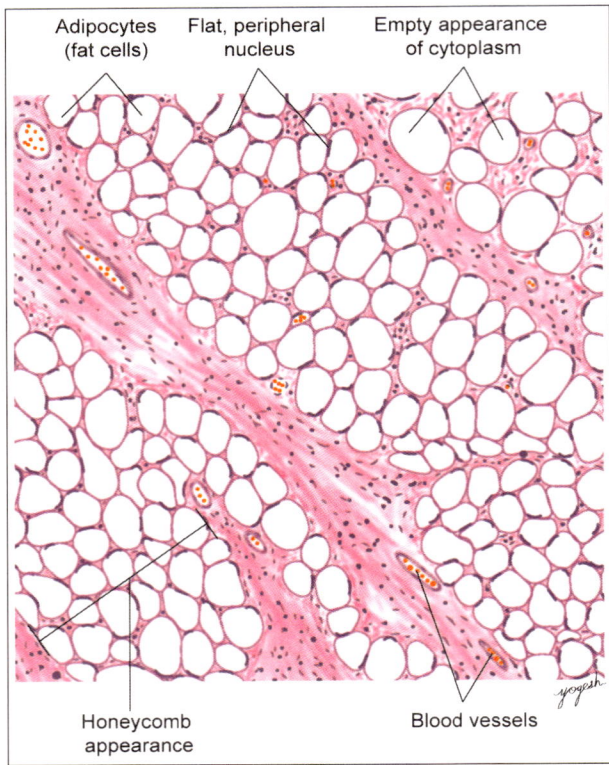

Fig. 7.18: Yellow adipose tissue (high magnification, practice figure).

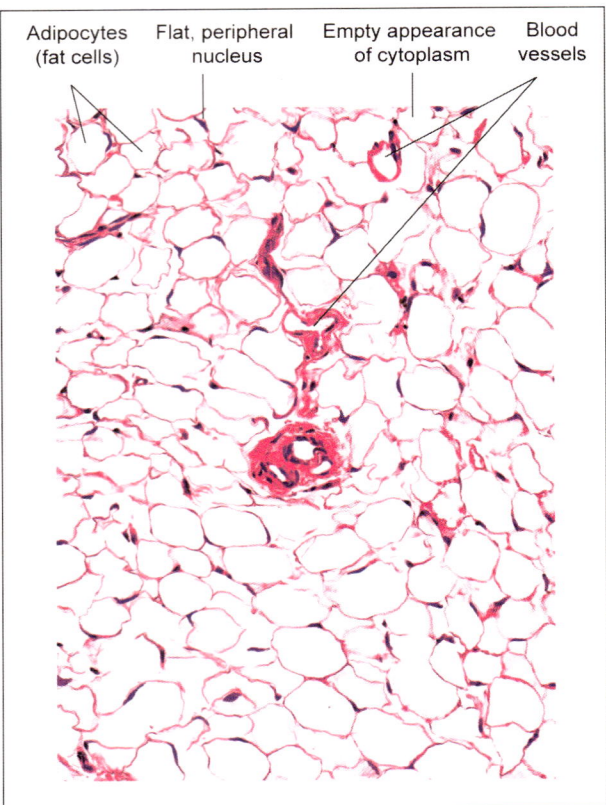

Fig. 7.19: Photomicrograph. Yellow adipose tissue (*H&E* stained, high magnification).

- These are large oval cells.
- Their nuclei are flat and pushed toward one side of the cell.
- They have very thin rim of cytoplasm.
- Cytoplasm contains a single, large lipid droplet; hence, these cells are called unilocular adipocytes. It gives *signet ring appearance* to unilocular adipocytes.*Viva, Identification feature*
- **H&E staining:** As fat gets washed out during tissue processing, cells show empty appearance with thin rim of cytoplasm and peripheral flat nucleus.*Viva, Identification feature*
- **Locations:** Superficial fascia, yellow bone narrow, omentum, mesentery, and around viscera.
- **Functions:** Energy storage, insulation, and protection of viscera.

Brown Adipose Tissue

- It is brownish in color.
- Adipocytes of brown fat:
  - These are smaller than yellow adipocytes.
  - Their nuclei are round and peripherally pushed.
  - Cytoplasm contains multiple small lipid droplets that give foamy appearance to the cell.*Identification feature*
- Locations
  - It is mostly found in newborn babies and its quality decreases in adults.
  - In adults, it is located on back and neck, scapular region, and posterior abdominal wall.
- Functions
  - Brown fat prevents excessive heat loss from body surface. It can generate heat (thermogenesis) by lipid breakdown.*Viva*
  - Thermoregulation is very essential in newborns for getting adjusted in the new environment outside the uterus.

CHAPTER 8

Cartilage

Chapter Outline
- Hyaline cartilage
- Elastic cartilage
- Fibrocartilage

Competency achievement: The student should be able to:

AN71.2 Identify cartilage under the microscope and describe various types and structure-function correlation of the same

INTRODUCTION

- Cartilage is a specialized connective tissue.
- Cartilage consists of two basic components.
  1. Cells (5%)
  2. Extracellular matrix (95%)
- Cells of cartilage are called *chondrocytes*.
- Cartilage is *avascular* tissue that receives its nutrition by diffusion from adjacent tissues.*Viva*
- Glycosaminoglycans (GAGs) and type II collagen fibers of extracellular matrix permit easy diffusion of the nutrients through the cartilage.
- Based on composition and mechanical properties of matrix, cartilages are classified into three types:*Viva*
  1. Hyaline cartilage
  2. Elastic cartilage
  3. Fibrocartilage
- Cartilages are externally supported by a fibrocellular covering called *perichondrium* (except fibrocartilages).

HYALINE CARTILAGE

Q. Write a short note on histology of hyaline cartilage.

- Histologically, hyaline cartilage has glass-like (transparent) matrix. Hence, it is called hyaline cartilage (*hyalos = glass*, in Greek).*Identification feature*
- *Locations*
  - Hyaline cartilage is the most abundant type of cartilage in the human body.
  - It is present at the following locations: Fetal skeleton, articular cartilages, nose cartilage, costal cartilages, laryngeal cartilages (thyroid, cricoid and arytenoids cartilages), trachea and bronchi, and developing bone (epiphyses).

Histology of Hyaline Cartilage

- Histologically, hyaline cartilage consists of cells (chondrocytes), ground substance, and fibers (Figs 8.1, 8.2 and Flowchart 8.1).

Some Interesting Facts

- Avascular cartilage has vascular cartilage canals containing blood vessels that traverse through cartilage substance have been proved by many studies (Wilsman et al., 1972 and many more).
- Chondrocytes receive their nutrition through diffusion.*Viva*
- Mesenchymal tissue differentiates into chondroblast that forms cartilage.
- Hyaline cartilage can undergo ossification (converted into bone) in later age.*Viva*
- Perichondrium has outer fibrous and inner cellular layers.

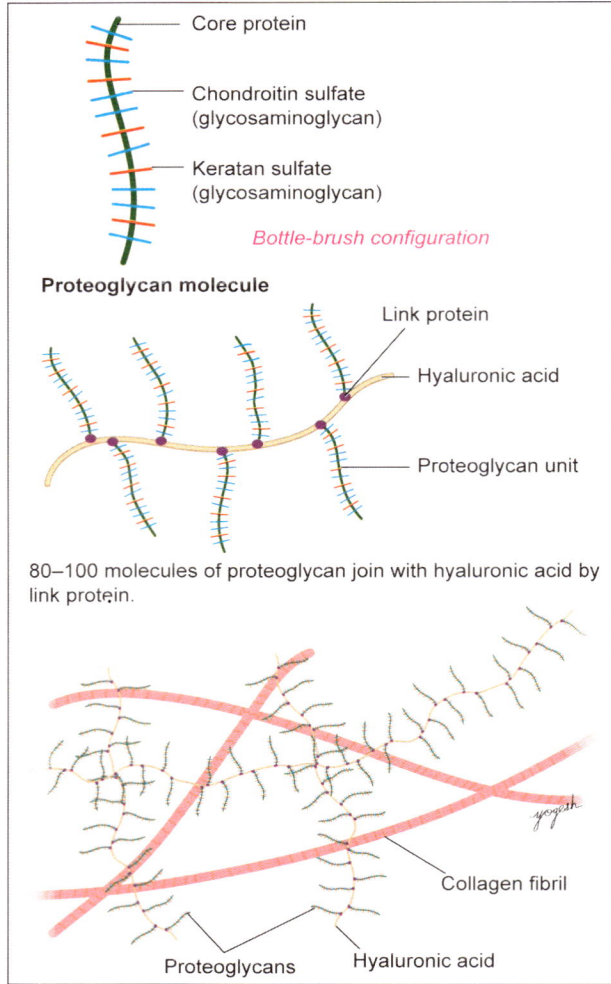

Fig. 8.1: Molecular organization of ground substance of hyaline cartilage.

Matrix
- Matrix of hyaline cartilage has glassy appearance. Hence, the cartilage is called hyaline (*hyalos* = glassy in Greek).
- Matrix shows spaces called *lacunae*. Cells of cartilage (chondrocytes) reside within the lacunae.

Composition
- The hyaline cartilage matrix consists of 60–80% of water, 15% of collagen fibers, approximately 15% proteoglycans and glycoproteins, and 3–5% cells (Fig. 8.1).
- Hyaline cartilage contains mainly *type II collagen fibers* (80%) that form a meshwork in the ground substances. Collagen fibers provide strength and stability to cartilage.^{Neet, Viva}
- Collagen fibers cannot be seen in histological section because refractive indices of the collagen fibers and the ground substance are same. This gives homogenous glassy-appearance to cartilage.^{Viva, Identification feature}
- Ground substance has three types of proteoglycans, namely hyaluronan, chondroitin sulfate, and keratan sulfate.
- These proteoglycans give firmness to cartilage.
- Acidic proteoglycans take hematoxylin (violet) color and hence, matrix of hyaline cartilage looks violet.^{Viva, Identification feature}
- The *aggrecan* is a proteoglycan monomer. It consists of a core protein and peripherally attached chondroitin and *keratan sulfate* molecules in form of *bottle-brush fashion* (Fig. 8.1).

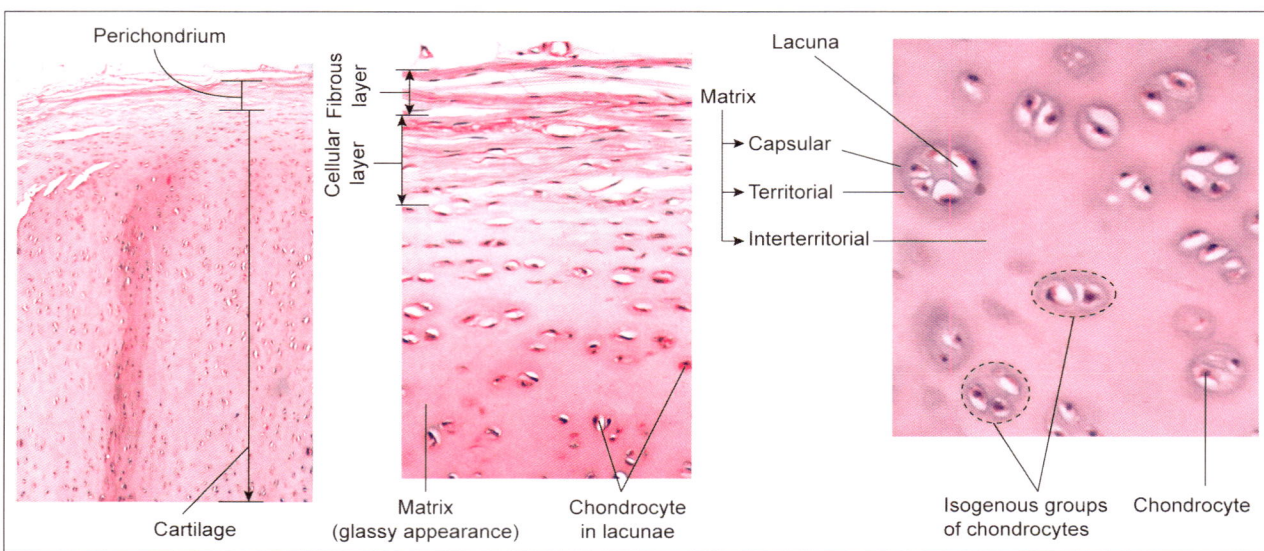

Fig. 8.2: Photomicrograph. Hyaline cartilage.

Cartilage

Flowchart 8.1: Histology of hyaline cartilage

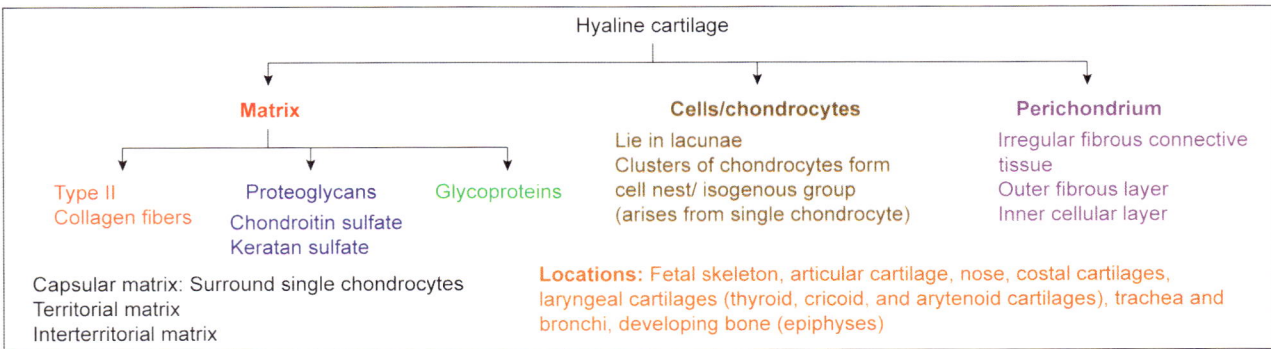

- Aggrecan molecule is negatively charged and hence, it has the capacity to hold water molecules (hydrated matrix).

- Matrix shows multiadhesive glycoproteins that help in the interaction between chondrocytes and matrix.
- Hydrated matrix helps in easy diffusion of metabolites and provide resilience to cartilage.
- Chondrocytes produce sulfated proteoglycans and deposit it in matrix. According to the concentration of sulfated proteoglycans, matrix shows varied property of staining with hematoxylin. Based on this staining, matrix shows *three zones* as follows (Figs 8.3–8.4 and Fig. 8.1): *Viva, Identification feature*

  1. *Capsule/pericellular matrix:* It is a ring of densely staining matrix that surrounds the chondrocytes. It has high content of negatively charged (acidic) sulfated proteoglycans, and type VI collagen fibrils.
  2. *Territorial matrix:* It surrounds capsular matrix. It contains less quantity of sulfated proteoglycans than capsular matrix; hence, stains less intensely than capsular matrix.
  3. *Interterritorial matrix:* It surrounds territorial matrix. It contains less quantity of sulfated proteoglycans; hence stains lighter with

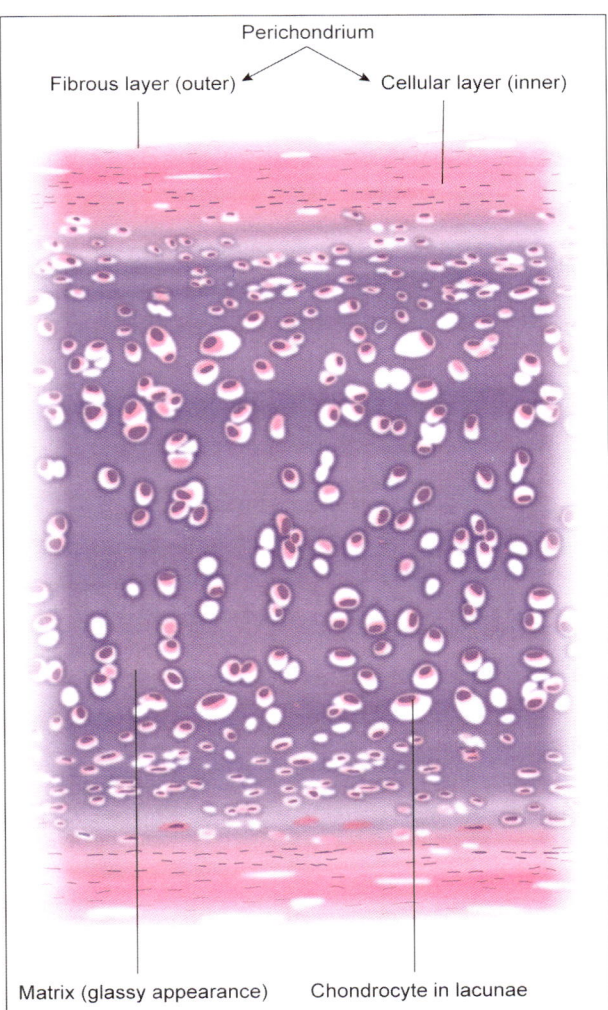

Fig. 8.3: Histology of hyaline cartilage (practice figure).

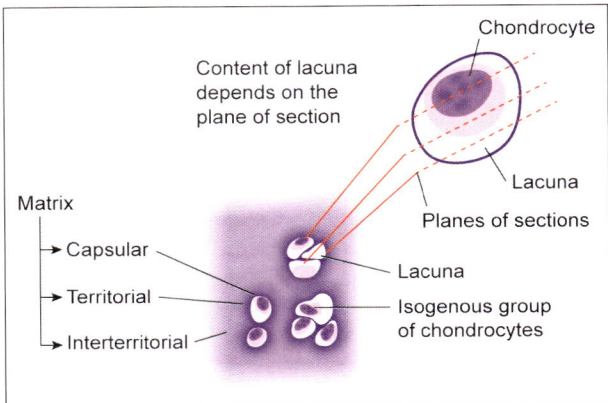

Fig. 8.4: Hyaline cartilage: Matrix and lacunae (practice figure).

hematoxylin (basic dyes) than territorial matrix. *Previous concept:* Capsular and territorial matrices are not separate entities. *New concept:* Territorial matrix surrounds capsular matrix.

Chondrocytes

- Cells of hyaline cartilage are called *chondrocytes.*
- Chondrocytes divide and deposit matrix around them. These chondrocytes occupy lacunae in matrix.
- *H&E staining:* Chondrocytes lie on one side in lacunae and are surrounded by an empty space. This is preparation artifact produced because of shrinkage of chondrocytes. In living state, chondrocyte occupies entire lacunar space. *Viva, Identification feature*
- *Cell nests/ isogenous group:* In developing cartilage, chondrocytes divide to form daughter cells. These newly formed cells lie in a group that is surrounded by territorial matrix. Such a group of daughter chondrocytes raised from a single mother chondrocyte is called *isogenous group*. These isogenous groups form a *cell nest* (group of cells). *Viva, Identification feature*
- Chondrocytes are derived from chondrocytes that divide mitotically. Chondroblasts get trapped in self-produced extracellular matrix, lose their capacity of cell division, and get converted into chondrocytes. *Viva*

Perichondrium

- Free surface of hyaline cartilage is covered by irregular connective tissue (fibrovascular) layer called *perichondrium*. *Viva*
- Perichondrium has two layers: outer fibrous and inner cellular layer.
  1. *Outer fibrous layer* of perichondrium consists of dense irregular fibrous connective tissue.
  2. *Inner cellular layer* has cells that divide and give rise to new chondrocytes.
- *Note:* Fibrous layer of perichondrium has capillaries that provide nutrients to interior of the cartilage through diffusion.
- Perichondrium is absent at the following sites: *Viva, Neet*
  - Articular cartilages.
  - At the site of direct contact of cartilage with bone.

Functions

- Hyaline cartilages maintain patency of trachea and the main bronchi because of the firmness.
- Because of flexibility, costal cartilages provide support and protection to thoracic viscera.
- Articular cartilages provide smooth surface for the movements.

Some Interesting Facts

- Matrix of cartilage is dynamic. Routinely, old matrix is removed, and new matrix is deposited by chondrocytes. This is called *internal remodeling.*
- Internal remodeling depends on stress and strain on the cartilage.
- Cartilage shows limited and slow growth.
- Cartilage shows two types of growth as follows: *Viva*
  - *Interstitial growth:* Its addition of new cartilage on its surface. It takes place before maturation (hardening of matrix) of cartilage. Cartilage cells divide in interstitial growth throughout substance of cartilage.
  - *Appositional growth:* Its formation of new cartilage within the existing cartilage by division of chondrocytes. After maturation, cellular layer of perichondrium deposits new cartilage layers in oppositional growth.
- Cartilage has limited capacity of regeneration.
- Hyaline cartilages may ossify with advancing age, but elastic cartilages do not ossify. *Viva*
- Liver produces *somatomedin C* that stimulates growth of the chondrocytes in epiphyseal cartilage. *Viva*

Clinical Correlation

Osteoarthritis

- Osteoarthritis is one of common joint diseases that occuring due to injury of articular cartilage.
- It mostly occurs by age 65 years.
- Symptoms: Chronic joint pain particularly in weight-bearing joints (hip joint, knee joint).
- Pathology: It occurs due to decrease in proteoglycan content and reduction of water content of the cartilage matrix.
- In osteoarthritis, chondrocytes produce more interleukin 1, and tumor necrotic factor and less type II collagen, and proteoglycans.
- Osteoarthritis has no cure. It usually progresses with age.

Summary (Examination Guide)

- Hyaline cartilage consists of matrix, cells, and covered by perichondrium.
- Matrix is basophilic and shows lacunae for chondrocytes.
- Matrix has intensely stained capsular (around each chondrocyte), less intensely stained territorial (around capsular matrix) and lightly stained interterritorial parts (surround territorial matrix).
- Matrix consists of type II collagen fibers and extracellular

ground substance. Ground substance consists of proteoglycans (chondroitin and keratan sulfates).
- Chondrocytes lie in lacunae. They produce collagen and ground substance.
- Chondrocytes in developing stage divide to form group of cells that lie in form of cell clusters called *isogenous group* or *cell nests*.
- Perichondrium surrounds the cartilage and it has outer fibrous and inner cellular layers.
- Locations: Nasal septum, tracheal rings, articular cartilages, costal cartilages, and fetal skeleton.

ELASTIC CARTILAGE

Q. Write a short note on histology of elastic cartilage.

- Elastic cartilage gives resilience, pliability, and elasticity to the organ.
- Freshly dissected elastic cartilage is yellowish in color; hence, it is also called *yellow elastic cartilage*.
- *Locations:* Elastic cartilage is present in pinna of external ear, walls of external acoustic meatus, auditory tube, *epiglottis*, tips of arytenoids, corniculate, and cuneiform cartilages of larynx.[Neet]

Histology of Elastic Cartilage

- Elastic cartilage contains ground substance, fibers, and cells (chondrocytes). Elastic cartilage is surrounded by perichondrium (Fig. 8.5 and 8.6, Flowchart 8.2).

Fibers

- Elastic cartilage contains a dense meshwork of branching and anastomosing fine elastic fibers. It imparts yellow color to the cartilage.[Viva, Identification feature]

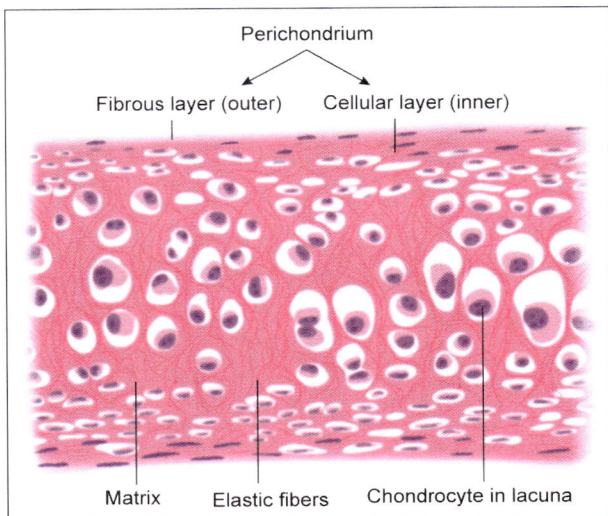

Fig. 8.5: Histology of elastic cartilage (practice figure).

Flowchart 8.2: Histology of elastic cartilage

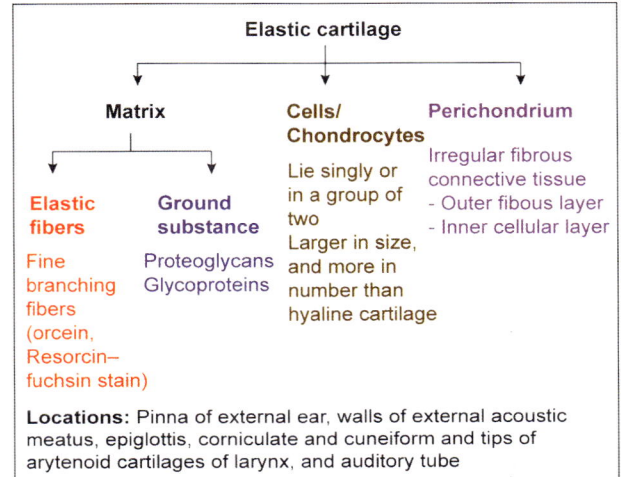

- In addition to elastic fibers, this cartilage also contains few type II collage fibers.
- Elastic fibers cannot be differentiated with H&E staining.[Viva]
- Elastic fibers are well demonstrated with orcein or resorcin-fuchsin staining.[Viva]

Ground Substance

- Similar to hyaline cartilage, elastic cartilage also contains proteoglycans and glycoproteins in matrix.

Chondrocytes

- Chondrocytes (cells of elastic cartilage) occupy lacunae (space within matrix).
- Cells in elastic cartilage are bigger than the cell, in hyaline cartilage.[Viva, Identification feature]
- Cells are surrounded by empty space (lacuna) due to shrinkage of cells during slide preparation (preparation artifacts). In living state, cells occupy complete lacunae.
- Chondrocytes produce elastic fibers, collagen fibers, and ground substance.
- Chondrocytes lie singly or in group of two.[Viva, Identification feature]

Perichondrium

- Free surface of elastic cartilage is covered by irregular connective tissue (fibrovascular) layer called *perichondrium*.
- Perichondrium has two layers: Outer fibrous and inner cellular layer.
  1. *Outer fibrous layer* of perichondrium consists of dense irregular fibrous connective tissue.
  2. *Inner cellular layer* has cells that divide and give rise to new chondrocytes.

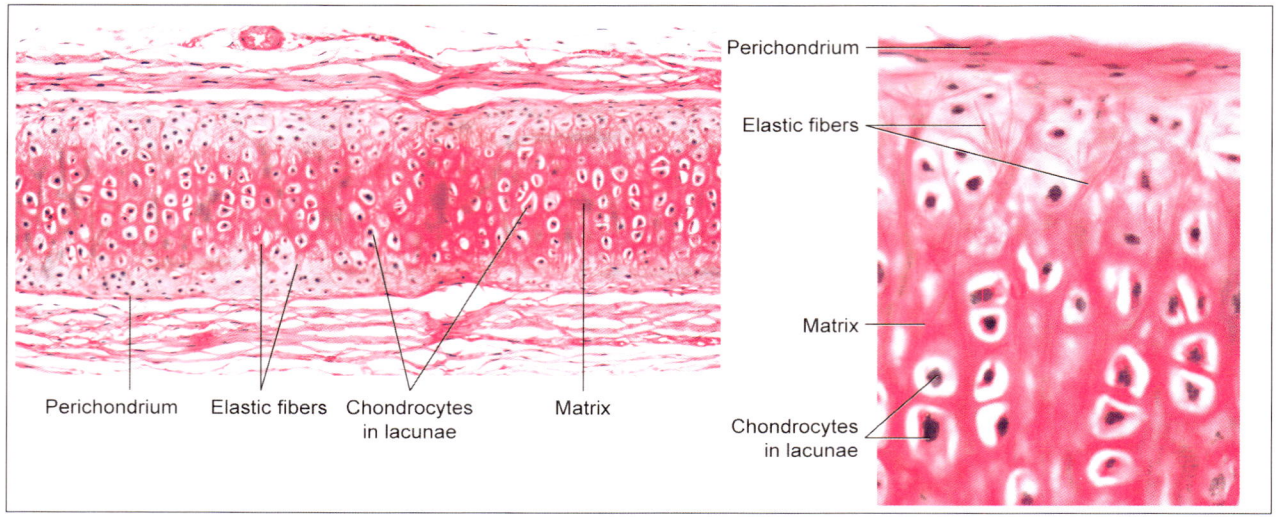

Fig. 8.6: Photomicrograph. Elastic cartilage (low magnification on left and high magnification on right, *H&E* stain).

Functions
- Elastic cartilage provides elasticity, resilience, and firmness to the structure.

> **Summary (Examination Guide)**
> - Elastic cartilage consists of matrix cells and covered by perichondrium.
> - Matrix shows meshwork of branching anastomosing elastic fibers and ground substance that consists of proteoglycans. *Identification feature*
> - Large chondrocytes occupy lacunae in matrix. Chondrocytes lie singly or in group of two. *Identification feature*
> - Perichondrium surrounds cartilage and it has two layers: Outer fibrous and inner cellular.
> - Locations: Pinna of external ear, external acoustic meatus, auditory tube, epiglottis, tips of arytenoids, and corniculate and cuneiform cartilages of larynx.

FIBROCARTILAGE

Q. Write a short note on histology of white fibrocartilage.

- Fibrocartilage contains bundles of thick collagen fibers that give white color to cartilage. Hence, this cartilage is also called **white fibrocartilage**. *Viva*
- Fibrocartilage is combination of dense regular connective tissue and hyaline cartilage. *Viva*
- Locations: *Intervertebral discs,* pubic symphysis, *articular disc* of sternoclavicular and temporomandibular joints, *menisci,* glenoidal labrum, acetabular labrum, articular disc of wrist joint, and at the site of tendon attachment with bones (few places). *Viva, Neet*

Histology of Fibrocartilage
- Histologically, fibrocartilage shows rows of chondrocytes embedded in matrix bundles of thick collagen fibers (Fig. 8.7 and 8.8, Flowchart 8.3).

Fibers
- Fibrocartilage consists of thick collagen fibers that form dense regular connective tissue (similar to tendon). *Identification feature*
- It consists of type I and type II collagen fibers in varying proportions.

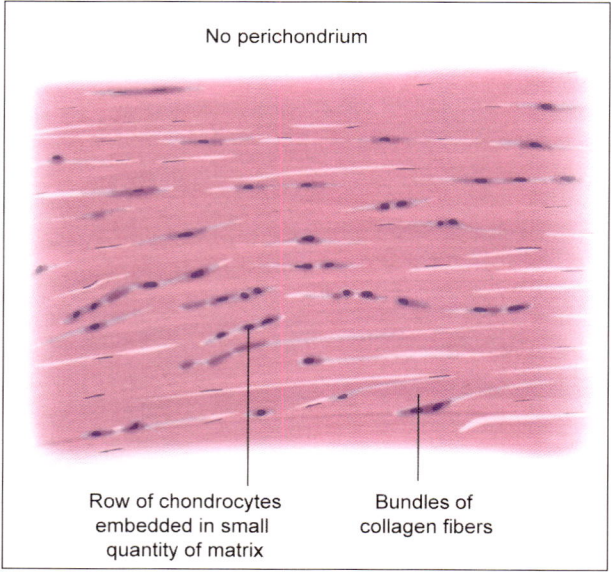

Fig. 8.7: Histology of white fibrocartilage.

Cartilage

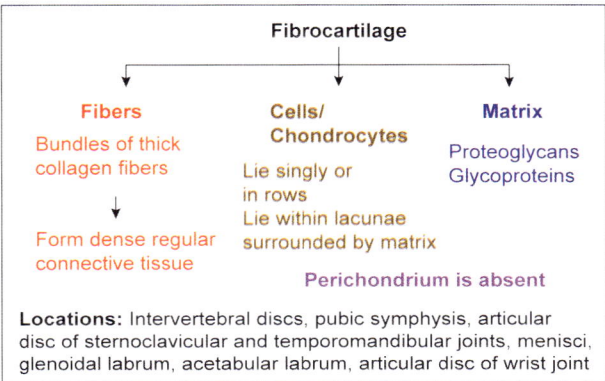

Flowchart 8.3: Histology of fibrocartilage

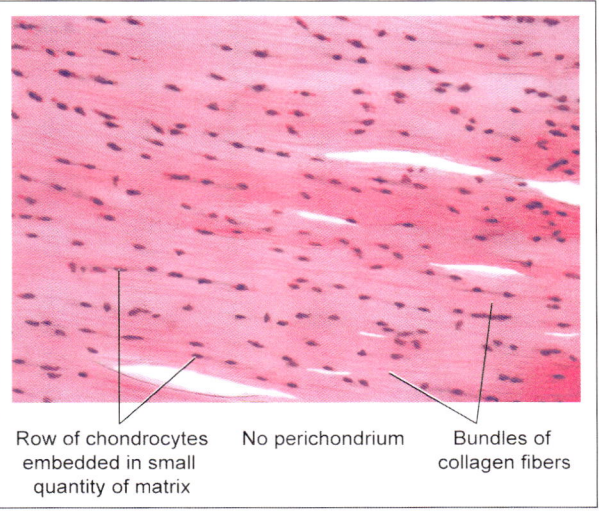

Fig. 8.8: Photomicrograph. White fibrocartilage.

- Some fibroblasts are present among collagen fibers. They have flat elongated nuclei.

Chondrocytes

- Chondrocytes are very few in number in fibrocartilage.
- Chondrocytes lie singly or in isogenous groups in between bundles of collagen fibers.

Matrix

- Chondrocytes lie within the lacunae of the matrix.
- Chondrocytes produce matrix that consists of proteoglycans and glycoproteins.
- Note: Fibrocartilage does not have periosteum.*Viva, Identification feature*
- Note: Histologically, tendon can be differentiated from fibrocartilage on the basis of chondrocytes that are present in fibrocartilage. Fibrocartilage is not covered by perichondrium.*Neet, Identification feature*

Functions

- Fibrocartilage helps in shock absorption.
- Fibrocartilage helps to withstand compression and shearing forces.

Summary (Examination Guide)

- Fibrocartilage consists of dense regular connective tissue with interspaced rows of chondrocytes. It does not have perichondrium.
- It contains type I and II collagen fibrils and few fibroblasts.
- The chondrocytes lie singly or in rows within the lacunae in the matrix.
- Locations: Intervertebral discs, menisci of knee joint, and pubic symphysis.

Some Interesting Facts

- *Note:* Proteoglycans secreted by chondrocytes are aggrecan, whereas proteoglycans secreted by fibroblasts are versican.
- Cartilage has limited capacity of repair because cartilage is an avascular structure. Chondrocytes cannot move to the site of injury because of matrix.
- Perichondral injuries may get repaired easily by formation of scar tissue (dense connective tissue).
- *Calcification of hyaline cartilage:* On aging, calcium salts get deposited in matrix of hyaline cartilage. This calcium reduces diffusion through cartilage and thus, causes death of chondrocytes. Such cartilage segment gets replaced by bone (ossification).
- Chondroclast removes cartilage in many joint diseases such as rheumatoid arthritis.
- *New concept:* Chondroclast (similar to osteoclast) do not remove cartilage during ossification. *Previous concept:* During ossification of hyaline cartilage, chondroclasts remove cartilage.
- *Cellular cartilage:* Cellular cartilage is seen during embryonic life. It consists of numerous cells and minimal matrix.*Viva*
- Differences between hyaline, elastic and fibrocartilages are listed in Table 8.1.

Q. List the differences between hyaline cartilage, elastic cartilage, and fibrocartilage.

Table 8.1: Difference between hyaline, elastic, and fibrocartilages^{Viva}

Features	Hyaline cartilage	Elastic cartilage	Fibrocartilage
Cells	Chondroblasts and chondrocytes	Chondroblasts and chondrocytes	Few fibroblasts, few chondrocytes
Cell occurrence	Lies in groups (cell nests)	Lie single or in a group of two	Lie single or in a row
Fibers	Type II collagen fibers	Elastic fibers and few type II collagen fibers	Type I and type II collagen fibers
Perichondrium	Present	Present	Absent
Production of ground substance	By chondrocytes	By chondrocytes	By chondrocytes and by fibroblasts

Clinical Correlation

- *Achondroplasia/dwarfism*
  - It is an autosomal dominant genetic disorder that is recognized by short legs and arms and normal torso.
  - Cause: Mutation of fibroblast growth factor receptor 3 (FGFR3) gene.
  - Pathogenesis: Defective proteins interfere in the conversion of cartilage in bone.
  - *New concept:* Achondroplasia is transmitted only from father.
- *Chondrosarcoma:* It is a malignant tumor of chondroblasts that develops usually in bones of axial skeleton.

CHAPTER 9

Bone

Chapter Outline

- General features of bone
- Sharpey's fibers
- Composition of bone tissue
  - Cells of bone tissue
  - Bone matrix
- Classification of bones
  - Lamellar bone
  - Woven bone
  - Compact bone
- Interstitial lamellae
- Circumferential lamellae
- Paget's disease
- Formation and growth of bone
  - Formation of bone
  - Intramembranous ossification
  - Endochondral ossification
  - Growth of long bone
- Zones of epiphyseal cartilage

Competency achievement: The student should be able to:

AN71.1 Identify bone under the microscope; classify various types and describe the structure-function correlation of the same

INTRODUCTION

- Bone is the *specialized type of connective tissue* that has extracellular matrix containing calcium salts.
- As bone is a connective tissue, it consists of cells and matrix.
- Mineralized extracellular matrix provides hardness to bones.
- Bone is a *living tissue* that shows dynamic structural changes in response to physical stress and hormonal changes.
- In addition to support and protection of vital organs, bones act as a storehouse for calcium and phosphates.
- Bone also performs hematopoietic function (production of blood cells).

GENERAL FEATURES OF BONE

- Long bone has two ends (*epiphysis*) that are connected by long shaft (*diaphysis*).
- On cross-section, long bone shows diaphysis, epiphyses, and coverings (endosteum and periosteum) (Flowchart 9.1).

Diaphysis/Shaft

- It is a tubular sheath covering a central cavity called *marrow cavity*.
- Tubular sheath does not have visible spaces. This type of bone is called *compact bone*.

Epiphyses

- Ends of long bone show a thin layer of compact bone covering a meshwork of bony plates.

Flowchart 9.1: General features of long bone

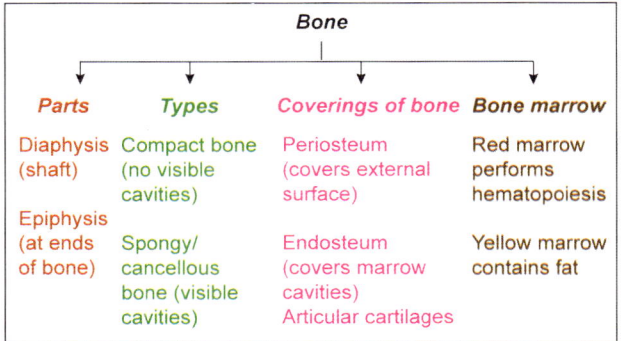

- Meshwork of bony plates shows numerous spaces and looks similar to sponge. Hence, this kind of bone is called *spongy* or *trabecular* or *cancellous bone*.
- Ends of long bone forming articular surfaces are covered by articular (hyaline) cartilage. This cartilage provides smooth, glass-like surface for smooth movements.
- Cavities of the bone are called bone marrow.
- Bone marrows are of the following two types:*Viva*
  - *Red bone marrow:* It is red in color and performs hematopoietic functions.
    Entire bone marrow in fetus and young adult is red bone marrow. In the adults, red bone marrow is present only at ends of long bones, ribs, vertebrae, sternum, and hip bone.*Neet,Viva*
  - *Yellow bone marrow:* With advancing age (in adult), red bone marrow from shafts of long bones get replaced with adipose (fat) tissue (yellow in color). Such a bone marrow is called yellow bone marrow.

Covering of Bone

- Bone has an outer surface and another internal surface that faces marrow cavity. These surfaces have the following coverings:

Periosteum

- Periosteum is a layer of connective tissue that covers external surface of bone except at two places
  1. At muscle attachment
  2. At area covered by articular cartilage *MCQ,Viva*
- Periosteum has two layers: Outer fibrous and inner cellular (osteogenic) layers. Endosteum has only a single layer of osteoprogenitor cells.

Endosteum

- Endosteum is a membranous layer that covers inner surface of bone, facing the marrow cavity, and space of spongy bone.
- Endosteum is thinner than periosteum.
- Endosteum is metabolically the most active layer of bone.*Neet*
- *Note:* Bone is a living, dynamic tissue (organ).
- *Note:* Dried bones are useful for classroom teaching of osteology. These dried bones do not have periosteum, endosteum, articular cartilages, bone marrow, blood vessels, and nerves.*Viva*

> **Box 9.1:** Sharpey's fibers
> - Sharpey's fibers are also called bone fibers or perforating fibers. [William Sharpey, 1802–1880, Scottish anatomist].
> - Usually, collagen fibers in periosteum are arranged parallel to surface of bone.
> - At the site of attachment of ligaments and tendons, collage fibers of periosteum are arranged obliquely or even at right angle to the surface of bone.
> - These fibers are continuous with extracellular matrix of bone. Such perforating fibers in the periosteum are Sharpey's fibers.*Viva*
> - Sharpey's fibers of periodontal ligament help to attach cementum with periosteum of alveolar bone.
> - Sharpey's fibers are part of the outer circumferential lamellae and may extend into the adjacent interstitial lamellae.
> - Sharpey's fibers do not enter osteons.

COMPOSITION OF BONE TISSUE

- Bone is a specialized type of connective tissue. It consists of three basic components as follows (Flowcharts 9.2 and 9.3)

Flowchart 9.2: Cells of bone and their functions

Q. List the cells of bones and their functions.

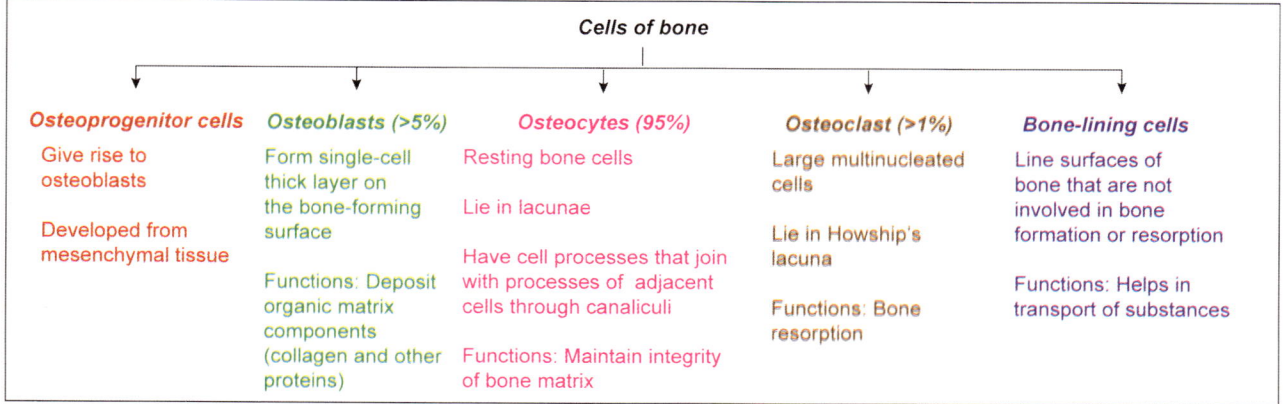

Bone

Flowchart 9.3: Composition of bone tissue

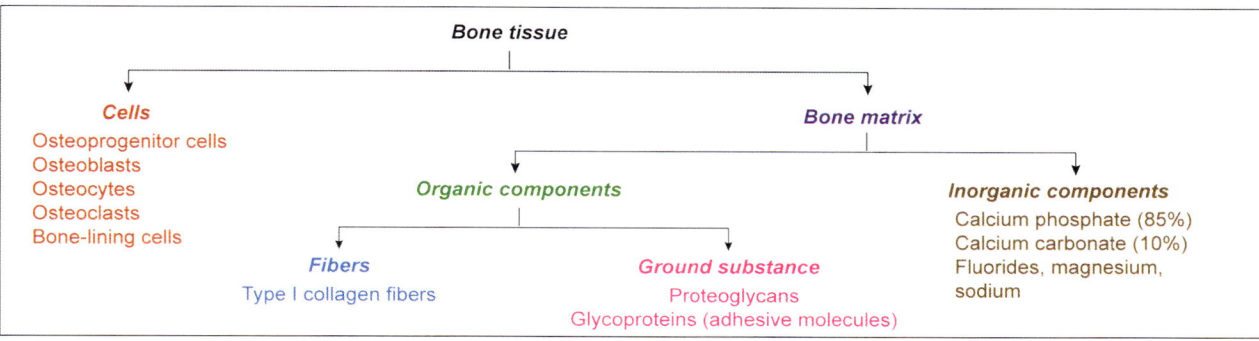

1. Cells
2. Fibers
3. Ground substance

Cells of Bone Tissue

Q. List the cells of bone and their functions.

- Bone tissue consists of five types of cells: Osteoprogenitor cells, osteoblasts, osteocytes, bone lining cells, and osteoclasts (Fig. 9.1 and Flowchart 9.2).

Osteoprogenitor Cells

- These are stem cells arising from mesenchymal tissue.
- They are present in inner cellular layers of periosteum and endosteum, and walls of Haversian and Volkmann's canals.
- Osteoprogenitor cells give rise to osteoblasts that form bone.

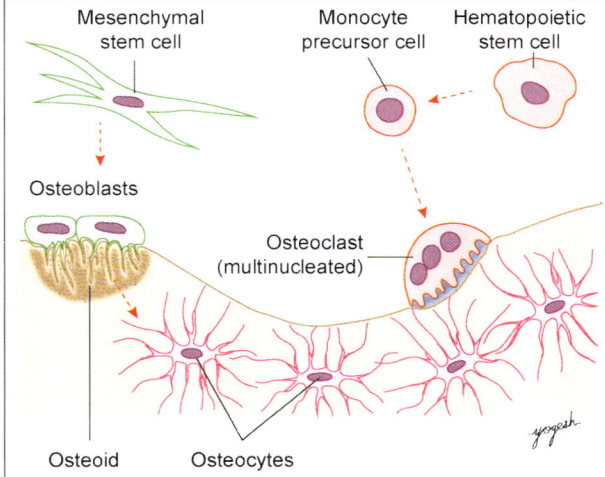

Fig. 9.1: Cells of bone and their origin.

- Osteoprogenitor cells are numerous in fetal life and childhood. Their number decreases with advancing age.
- *Molecular biology:* Insulin-like growth factors and bone morphogenic proteins promote differentiation of osteoprogenitor cells into osteoblasts.
- *New concept:* Electromagnetic field stimulates differentiation of osteoprogenitor cells, and it helps in healing of bone fractures.
- Histology: Osteoprogenitor cells are flattened cells with elongated or ovoal nucleus. These cells resemble fibroblasts.
- Function: To give rise to osteoblasts.

Osteoblasts

- Osteoblasts are bone-forming cells derived from osteoprogenitor cells.
- Histology: Osteoblasts are cuboidal or polygonal cells that lie on the newly formed bone surface. They have oval, euchromatic nucleus, and basophilic cytoplasm.
- Nucleus of osteoblast is placed eccentrically, away from bone-forming surface of these cells.
- Electron microscopy: These cells contain rough endoplasmic reticulum, Golgi apparatus, and secretory vesicles. They have cytoplasmic processes that communicate through gap junctions with similar processes of adjacent osteoblasts.
- Functions
  1. Synthesis of type I collagen fibers.
  2. Synthesis of bone matrix proteins such as calcium-binding proteins (osteocalcin, osteonectin), multiadhesive glycoprotein (bone sialoproteins), and proteoglycans.
  3. These cells secrete alkaline phosphatase.
- Higher serum level of alkaline phosphatase is an indicator of osteoblast and bone-forming activity.[Neet]

- *Note:* Increase alkaline phosphatase is also seen in other conditions; for examples, pregnancy, liver damage, and so on.

Osteocytes

- Osteocytes are the mature bone cells that are trapped in the spaces in the matrix (*lacunae*).
- Osteocytes are derived from osteoblasts.
- Conversion of osteoblasts to osteocytes take three days.
- It involves reduction in cell size and cell organelles.
- On mineralization of the matrix, the cell processes of osteocytes get trapped in the *canaliculi* within the matrix. These cell processes communicate with similar processes of adjacent osteocytes and other bone cells. Such communications help in the transport of nutrients.^Viva
- *H&E staining:* The osteocytes show eosinophilic cytoplasm or lightly stained basophilic cytoplasm due to the presence of small amount of rough endoplasmic reticulum.
- Practical aspects: Because of decalcification processes required prior to slide preparation (before tissue processing), osteocytes are shrunken or even lost.
- *Note:* Canaliculi and cell processes of osteocytes are not seen on *H&E* staining. Canaliculi can be seen on the ground section of dried bone as radiating lines from lacunae.
- Electron microscopy:
  According to needs, mechanical stress, and hormonal changes osteocytes change their form and function. Electron microscopically three forms of osteocytes are seen as follows:
  1. *Quiescent osteocyte* is metabolically less active and has few rough endoplasmic reticula.
  2. *Formative osteocytes* deposit bone matrix and have abundant endoplasmic reticulum and Golgi apparatus.
  3. *Resorptive osteocytes* have conspicuous lysosomes and can cause enzymatic degradation of matrix with the help of matrix metalloproteinases (MMPS). Earlier, this was known as *osteolytic osteolysis*.
- *New concept:* Resorptive osteocytes are responsible for calcium and phosphate homeostasis.
- *Privious concept:* Osteoclast and osteoblast are responsible for calcium and phosphate reabsorption.
- Life span of osteocytes is about 10–20 years.^MCQ
- Functions
  1. Maintenance of integrity of bones
  2. May help in remodeling of bone

Osteoclasts

- Osteoclasts are large, multinucleated cells that remove bone.
- Osteoclasts rest on bone surface where bone resorption takes place.
- *Howship's lacuna* or *resorption bay:* At the site of bone resorption, osteoclast creates a shallow depression called Howship's lacuna.^Viva
- Histology: Osteoclasts are large cells (50–150 μm) having up to 20 or more nuclei and eosinophilic cytoplasm.
- *Clinical fact:* Osteoclast produces acid phosphatase (tartrate-resistant). This is a useful clinical marker for osteoclast activity.^Neet
- Osteoclasts are derived from granulocyte-macrophage progenitor (GMP) cells. GMP cells also give rise to granulocytes and monocytes.
- There are three specialized regions of active osteoclast as follows:
  1. *Ruffled border:* Surface of osteoclast that is in contact with bone shows microvillous-type plasma membrane infoldings. It increases cell surface area for secretion of hydrolytic enzymes.
  2. *Clear zone:* This is the region of osteoclast just adjacent to the ruffled border. It provides attachment to extracellular matrix adhesion proteins and creates a tight-seal compartment for activity of bone resorption.
  3. *Basolateral region:* It lies opposite to the ruffled border. It has nucleus and apparatus for exocytosis of digested endocytosed material. Thus, ruffled border is involved in disintegration (endocytosis), whereas basolateral region is involved in exocytosis of endocytosed matrix material.
- Functions
  1. Bone matrix removal/reabsorption
  2. Synthesis and secretion of hydrolytic lysosomal enzymes (cathepsin K, matrix metalloproteinases)
  3. Creation of acidic environment at the site of bone resorption that initiates degradation of minerals

Some Interesting Facts

- Bisphosphonates and estrogens (drugs) inhibit bone resorption by osteoclast and are useful for osteoporosis treatment.^Clinical fact
- Parathyroid hormone increases osteoclast activity and bone resorption that increases blood calcium level.^Viva
- Calcitonin hormone (secreted by parafollicular cells of thyroid gland) decreases osteoclast activity and decreases blood calcium level.^Viva
- Vitamin D helps in absorption of calcium from intestine.
- Secondary osteons replace primary osteons during remodeling. Haversian canals lie at the center of secondary osteons.^Viva

Bone-lining Cells

- Bone-lining cells cover the surfaces of bone at sites where active bone formation or reabsorption is not taking place.
- These cells form a continuous *epithelium-like layer of flat cells* that lines periosteal surface (called periosteal cells), endosteal surface (called endosteal cells), and canals and canaliculi.
- These cells are derived from osteoblasts.
- These cells regulate movement of calcium, phosphates, and nutrients in and out of the bone.

Bone Matrix

- Bone matrix consists of fibers, ground substance, and minerals.
- Fibers (90%) and ground substance (10%) form organic component of bone matrix, whereas minerals form inorganic components.

Fibers

- Bone matrix contains type I collagen fibers called *osteoid collagen*.^{MCQ}
- These are synthesized by osteoblasts.
- These get embedded into ground substance.
- These fibers are arranged in layers called *lamellae*.
- Fibers in each lamella are parallel to each other but these fibers in adjacent lamellae are perpendicular to each other.
- Functions: Collagen fibers provide tensile *strength/resilience* to bone.^{Viva}

Ground Substance

- Bone has a small quantity of amorphous ground substance.
- Ground substance is made up of proteoglycans-glycosaminoglycans such as hyaluronic acid, keratan sulfate, and chondroitin sulfate.
- Ground substance also contains some adhesive glycoproteins such as osteocalcin, osteonectin, osteopontin, and sialoprotein I and II.
- Osteocalcin captures circulating calcium.

Minerals/Inorganic Ions

- Principal component of bone matrix is crystals of calcium phosphates (85% of total salts in bone).
- It also contains calcium carbonate, calcium fluoride, magnesium, sodium, and so on.
- These minerals form *needle-shaped crystals* called *hydroxyapatite* $(Ca_{10} [PO_4]_6 [OH]_2)$.^{Viva}
- Hydroxyapatite crystals lie parallel to the collagen fibrils in lamellae.

Some Interesting Facts

- Dry bone consists of 65% inorganic salts and 35% of organic components.
- On removal of minerals from a bone (such as fibula) with the help of acids, one can tie a knot of the bone.
- Burning of bone results in destruction of organic components. Such burned bone becomes brittle similar to chalk.
- Elastic cartilage does not ossify.

CLASSIFICATION OF BONES

- Based on various criteria, bones are classified into various groups as follows:

Based on Gross (Naked Eye) Examination of Bone

- Based on naked eye examination, bones are grouped as follows (Fig. 9.2):
  1. Compact bones have no visible cavities
  2. Spongy bones have visible cavities (sponge-like)

Based on Histological Appearance

- Based on histological appearance, bones are grouped as follows (Fig. 9.2):
  1. Woven (immature) bones: These are present in embryonic life and fracture healing.

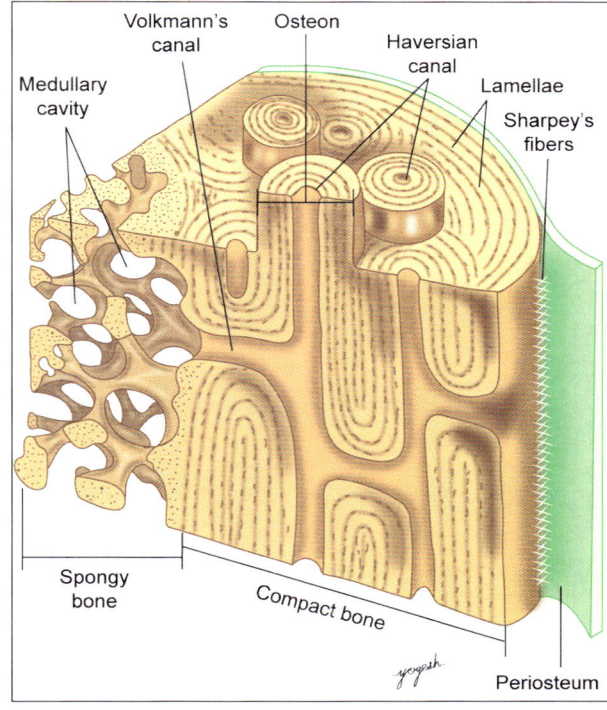

Fig. 9.2: Structure of compact bone.

2. **Lamellar (mature) bones:** These are secondary bones and have lamellar pattern of fiber arrangements.
- For details about the other classifications such as based on shapes (long, short, flat, irregular), read general anatomy book.

LAMELLAR BONE (SECONDARY BONES)

- Bones are made up of thin plates called *lamellae*.
- Lamella consists of parallelly-arranged bundles of type I collagen fibers and mineralized matrix.^{Viva}
- Lamellae are arranged one upon another to form part of the bone.
- Collagen fibers in adjacent lamellae are arranged perpendicular to each other.^{Viva}
- There are small spaces between the adjacent lamellae. These spaces are called *lacunae*.
- Each lacuna contains a single osteocyte.
- Each lacuna is connected with adjacent lacunae by fine *canaliculi*. These canaliculi contain cytoplasmic processes of osteocytes.
- Lamellar bony arrangements are seen in both spongy and compact bones.
- Lamellar bones replace woven (immature/primary) bones; hence, they are called secondary bones.

WOVEN (IMMATURE/PRIMARY) BONES

- These are newly formed bones.
- These are also called as *fibrous bones*.
- Woven bones do not show organized arrangements of collagen fibers as that in lamellar bones.
- In woven bones, fibers run in different directions and form network. Hence, they are called woven bones.

Box 9.2: Paget's disease/osteitis deformans

- Paget's disease involves disorganized bone formation and non-conversion of newly formed woven bones to lamellar bones.
- Cause: Unknown.
- It may affect single or multiple bones, but never the entire skeleton.
- First described by Sir James Paget, British surgeon (1814–1899).
- Other discoveries of Paget
  1. *Paget's disease of nipple:* It is intraductal breast cancer that spreads to skin and nipple.
  2. *Paget-Schroetter disease* is upper limb deep venous thrombosis.
  3. *Paget's abscess* is an abscess that reoccurs at the same site after curing of the abscess.

COMPACT BONES

Q. Write a short note on transverse section of compact bone/ground bone.

Q. Write a short note on longitudinal section of compact bone or ground bone.

- Compact bone does not show visible cavities on gross examination.
- Examples of compact bone are as follows:
  - Diaphysis of long bones
  - Outer thin covering of epiphysis of long bones
  - Outer and inner tables of flat bones (middle spongy bone form diploe)
  - Outer thin layer of all other bones
- In living state, compact bone on its outer surface is covered by *periosteum*, whereas inner surface by endosteum.
- *Note:* In ground section of dry bone, periosteum and endosteum are absent.
- *In compact bone,* lamellae are arranged in three different patterns as follows (Figs 9.3 to 9.9 and Flowchart 9.4):
  - Haversian system of lamellae^{Neet}
  - Interstitial lamellae
  - Circumferential lamellae (outer and inner)

Haversian System of Lamellae (Fig. 9.3)

- *Osteon* is the structural and functional unit of compact bone.
- Each osteon has a central *Haversian canal* and surrounding *concentric lamellae*.^{Idenification feature}
- *Haversian (osteonal) canals* run parallel to the long axis of bone. In living state, each Haversian canal contains loose connective tissue, capillaries, nerves, and lymphatics.
- In ground section (dried bone), Haversian canal may be seen as empty (white) or filled with dirt (black).
- Each Haversian canal is surrounded by 4–15 *concentric lamellae*.
- *Lacunae:* Between adjacent lamellae, small space called lacunae is present. Lacunae contain osteocytes (Fig. 9.5).
- *Canaliculi:* Each lacuna is surrounded by radiating canaliculi that connect adjacent lacunae.^{Viva}
- Canaliculi contain cell processes of osteocytes. With the help of canaliculi nutrients from capillaries of Haversian canal reach to osteocytes that lie away from the canal.
- *Collagen fibers in lamellae:* Collagen fibers in each lamellus are arranged parallel to each other, whereas collagen fibers in the adjacent lamellae are arranged perpendicular to each other.

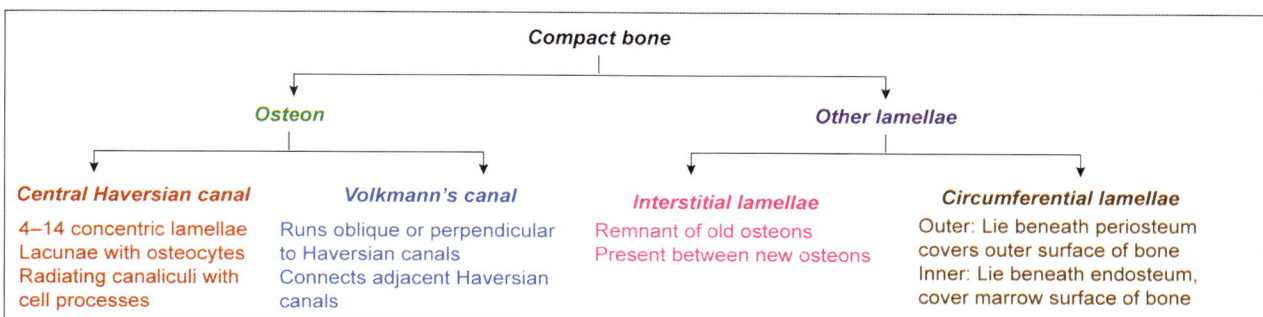

Flowchart 9.4: Histology of compact bone

- There are *two types* of circumferential lamellae
  1. Outer circumferential lamellae: These lie just beneath periosteum on outer surface of bone.
  2. Inner circumferential lamellae: These lie deep to endosteum and encircle marrow cavity.

Periosteum

- Bone is covered externally by a membrane called *periosteum.*
- Periosteum has two layers: Outer fibrous and inner cellular layers.^{Viva}
  - *Outer fibrous layer* is made up of collagen fibers
  - *Inner cellular layer* has osteogenic cells in the young developing bone
- Periosteum is a highly vascular tissue. Vessels and lymphatics from periosteum communicate with the vessels of Haversian canal through Volkmann's canals.

Endosteum

- It is a lining of bone that covers inner surface of bone facing marrow cavities and space of spongy bones.
- Endosteum is lined by a single cell thick layer and consist of osteoblasts, osteoclasts, and resting flat squamous cells.

Summary (Examination Guide)

- Compact bone does not have visible cavities.
- Histologically, T.S. of ground bone shows osteons, interstitial lamellae, and circumferential lamellae.
- Osteon has central Haversian canal surrounded by 4–15 concentric lamellae. Between lamellae, spaces called lacunae (contain osteocyte) are present. Each lacuna is surrounded by radiating canaliculi that contains cell processes of osteocytes.
- Adjacent Haversian canals are connected by Volkmann's canals. Both these canals contain blood vessels, lymphatics, and nerve fibers.

- Interstitial lamellae are present between osteons and they represent remnant of old osteons. Outer and inner bony surfaces are covered by outer and inner circumferential lamellae.
- Cement line covers each osteon. It consists of ground substance (without collagen fibers).

Box 9.3: Preparation of ground section of bone

- For histological section, compact bone (dried) sections cannot be taken with the help of microtome. Using hexa blade (saw), cut the bone into thin slices. This slices further grounded using a grinding stone. Slice takes long time (hours) to become useful for microscopic examination.
- Thin semitransparent slice is then dehydrated using alcohol and treated with xylene to remove alcohol. Then this slice is fixed on the glass slide using DPX mountant and coverslip.
- Ground section of bone does not have the following structures.^{Viva, MCQ}
  - Periosteum, endosteum, cells, blood vessels, and nerves.
  - Cavities of bone include Haversian canals, Volkmann's canals, bone marrow, and canals for nutrient vessels.

SPONGY BONE

Q. Write a short note on histology of spongy bone.

- It is also called *cancellous bone* or *trabecular bone.*
- Examples: Inner core of epiphysis of long bones, short bones, flat, and irregular bones.
- All spongy bones have a thin covering of compact bone.

- On gross examination, spongy bone shows sponge-like appearance having numerous cavities between irregular plates of bones. These bony spicules, plates, or rods are called trabeculae.*Identification feature*
- Trabeculae do not have Haversian system.*MCQ*
- In trabeculae, osteocytes lie in cavities called lacunae.*Identification feature* Fine radiating canaliculi connects adjacent lacunae. Canaliculi contain cell processes of osteocytes (Figs 9.10, 9.11 and Flowchart 9.5).
- As trabeculae are thinner (<0.4 mm in thickness), there is no need of Haversian system. Osteocytes in trabeculae can receive blood supply from marrow cavity.
- Trabeculae are covered by endosteum, osteoblasts, osteoclasts, and osteoprogenitor cells.

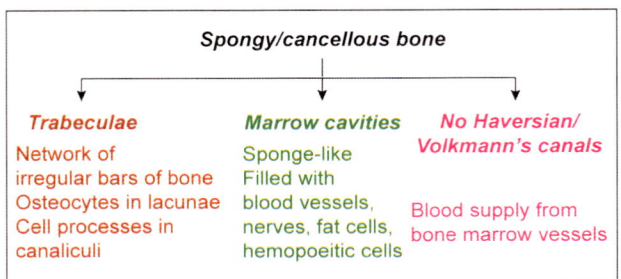

Flowchart 9.5: Histology of spongy bone

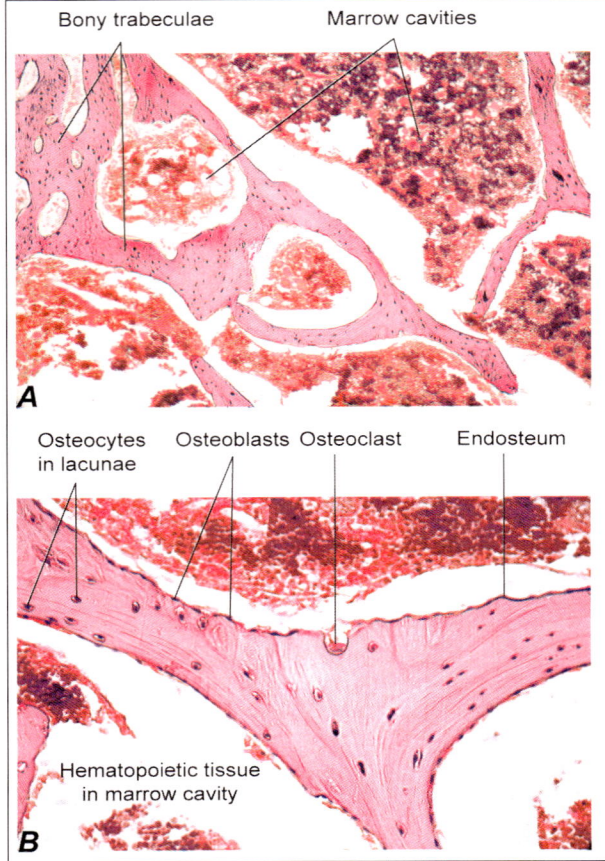

Fig. 9.11: Photomicrograph. Cancellous bone with trabeculae and bone marrow cavities. (A) Low magnification, (B) High magnification.

FORMATION AND GROWTH OF BONE (For further reading)

Formation of Bone

- Bones are mesodermal derivative (except facial skeleton–formed by neural crest contribution).
- Process of formation of bone is called *ossification.*
- Ossification may be
  1. *Intramembranous ossification* that involves direct conversion of mesenchymal tissue to bone.
  2. *Endochondral (cartilaginous) ossification* that involves conversion of mesenchyme to cartilage that later gets replaced by bone.

Intramembranous Ossification

- In intramembranous ossification, mesenchymal tissue forms bone.
- Bones formed by membranous ossification are called *membranous bones.*

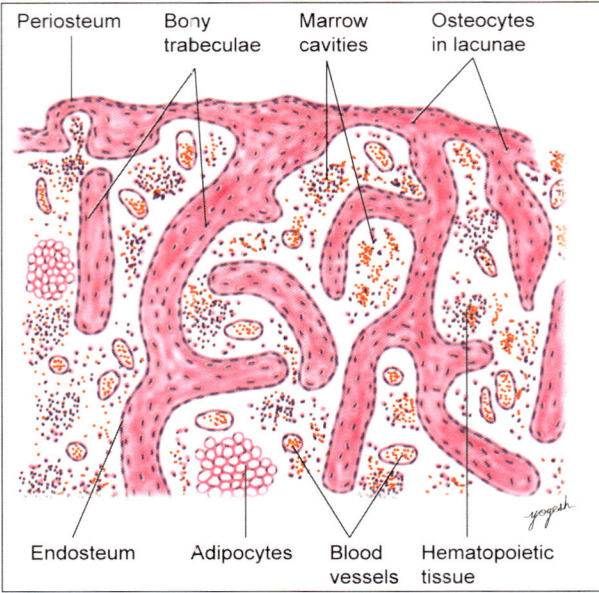

Fig. 9.10: Cancellous bone with trabeculae and bone marrow cavities (low magnification, practice figure).

- Examples: Bones of skull vault, mandible, clavicle (partly).

Steps of Formation (Fig. 9.12 and Flowchart 9.6)

- Mesenchymal condensation: Star-shaped mesenchymal cells condense and differentiate to spindle-shaped fibroblasts that form a fibrous membrane.
- Osteoid formation: Fibroblasts differentiate to osteoblasts that laydown collagenous early bone matrix and form *uncalcified bone (osteoid).*^{Viva}
- Calcification of osteoid: Osteoblasts deposit calcium salts in intercellular matrix, and thus convert osteoid into calcified bony spicules.
- Formation of woven bone: Trapped osteoblasts in the matrix get differentiated into osteocytes. Bony spicules fuse with each other to form plates of compact bone. Arrangement of collagen bundles running in different directions produces woven bone appearance.
- Formation of Haversian system: Waves of calcification and trapping of osteocyte processes in bony canaliculi forms Haversian system.
- Stage of bone modeling and remodeling: Fusion of progressively growing bone gives a primitive

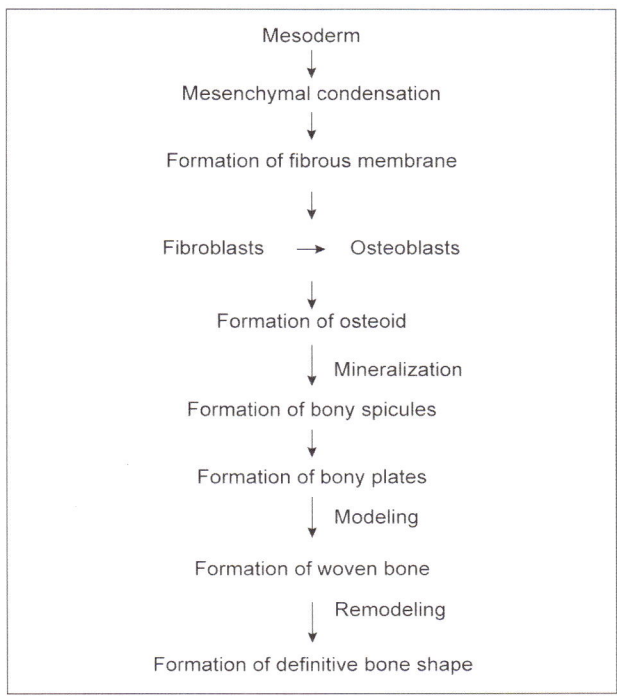

Flowchart 9.6: Intramembranous ossification (Source: Textbook of Human Embryology, Yogesh Sontakke, 1st edn., CBS Publishers)

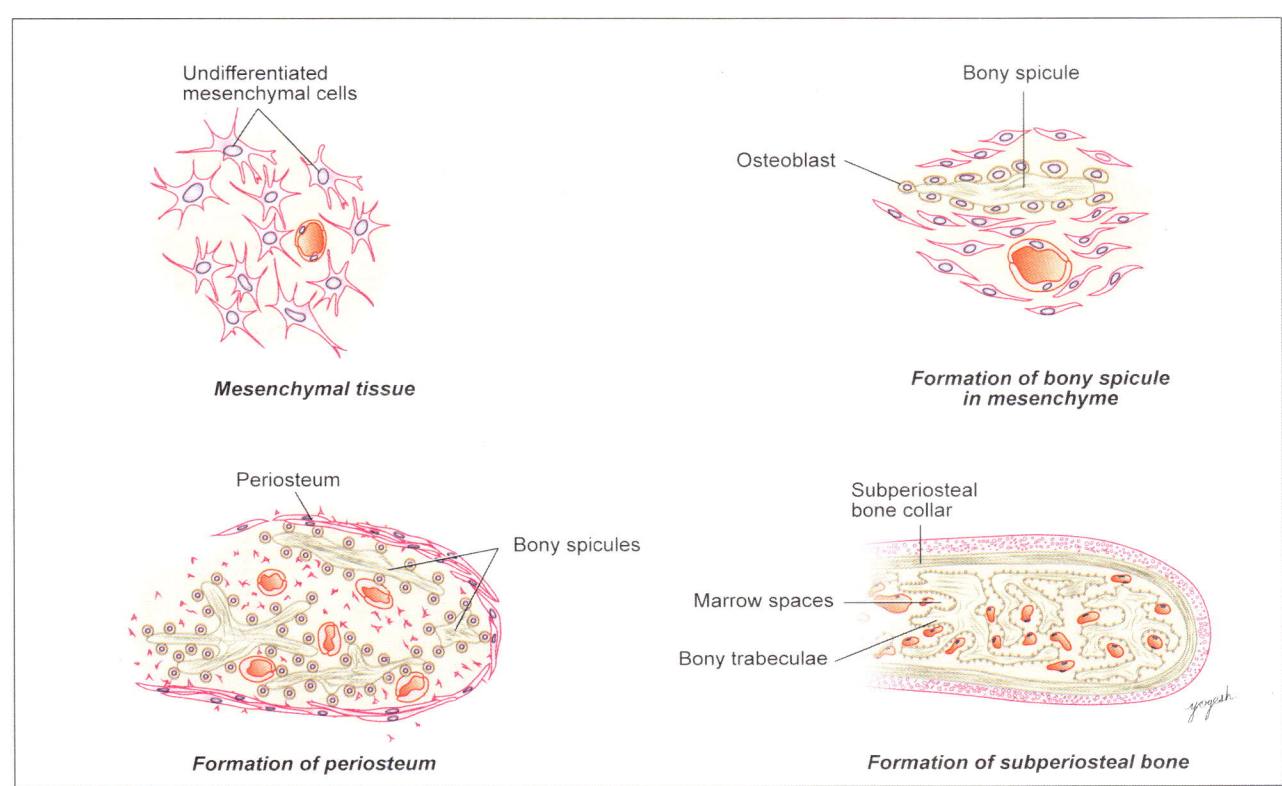

Fig. 9.12: Intramembranous ossification (Source: Textbook of Human Embryology, Yogesh Sontakke, 1st edn., CBS Publishers).

shape to the bone model. Continuous deposition and resorption of bone give definitive shape to the bone.

Endochondral Ossification (Fig. 9.13 and Flowchart 9.7)

- Endochondral/cartilaginous ossification involves conversion of mesenchymal tissue into cartilage that later gets replaced by bone.
- Bones developed by cartilaginous ossification are called *cartilaginous bones.*
- *Examples:* All long bones (except clavicle), base of skull, vertebrae, ribs.

Stages of Endochondral Ossification[Neet]

- Mesenchymal condensation: Mesenchymal cells form condensed mesenchymal tissue at the site of bone formation.
- Formation of cartilaginous model: At the site of mesenchymal condensation, chondroblasts appear and deposit hyaline cartilage. This cartilage is surrounded by vascular mesenchyme that forms perichondrium.
- Stage of cartilage hypertrophy: At the site of bone formation, cells of cartilage increase in size (hypertrophy).
- Stage of calcification: Hypertrophied cartilaginous cells start secretion of *alkaline phosphatase* and deposit calcium in intercellular matrix. Soon, chondrocytes lose nutritional source and die because of calcified matrix to leave behind *primary areole.*
- Formation of periosteal bud: Perichondral vessels and osteogenic cells invade calcified matrix to form periosteal bud.
- Formation of secondary areolae: Periosteal bud removes calcified matrix from the wall of primary areola and forms large cavities called *secondary areolae.*
- Formation of osteoid: Osteogenic cells (osteoblasts) form a gelatinous matrix along wall of secondary areolae. This newly formed mass is called ***osteoid.***

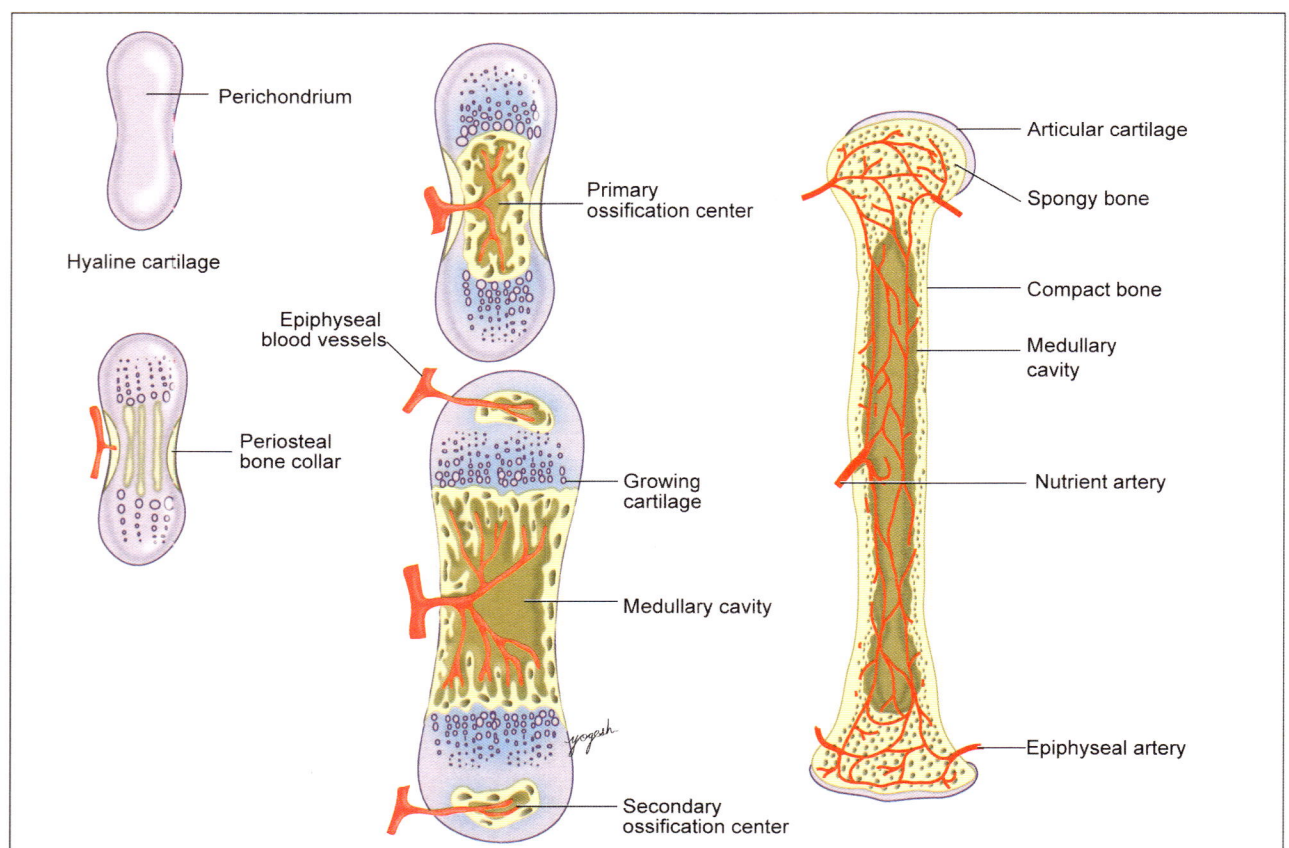

Fig. 9.13: Endochondral ossification (Development of long bone) (Source: Textbook of Human Embryology, Yogesh Sontakke, 1st edn., CBS Publishers)

Flowchart 9.7: Endochondral ossification (Source: Textbook of Human Embryology, Yogesh Sontakke, 1st edn., CBS Publishers)

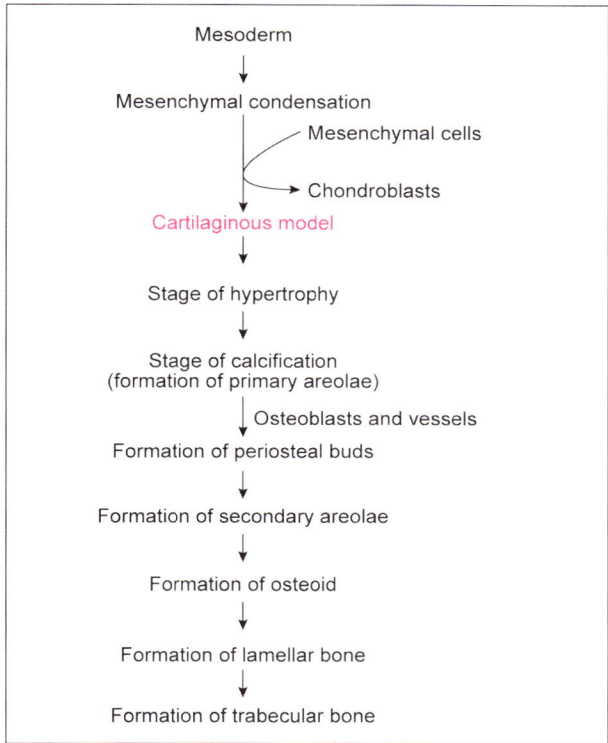

- Formation of bone lamella: Intercellular gelatinous matrix of osteoid gets calcified to develop a lamella of bone.
- Formation of trabecular bone: Osteoblasts lay another lamella over the first one and so on. Osteoblasts trapped in lamellae form osteocytes. The multilamellar portion is called *trabecular bone*.

Growth of Long Bone

- Calcification in cartilaginous model of long bones starts in shaft at *primary center of ossification* (diaphysis).
- On appearance of the primary center of ossification, periosteum produces a calcified bone on surface of cartilage by intramembranous ossification. This periosteal bone is called *periosteal collar*.^Viva
- After birth, cartilages at end of long bones start ossification (*secondary centers*) to form epiphyses.
- Diaphysis and epiphyses are separated by a plate of *epiphyseal cartilage*.
- Increase in thickness and formation of bone marrow: Periosteal collar increases in thickness by deposition of more layers on outer surface of bone. Simultaneously, osteoblasts remove lamellae from inner surface of bone leaving behind a marrow cavity.
- Increase in length: Length of bone increases by lengthening of epiphyseal cartilage and its simultaneous conversion into new bone
- In developing bone, epiphyseal cartilage shows zone of resting cartilage, zone of proliferation, zone of calcification and zone of ossification
- Terminal portion of diaphysis (active site of bone formation) is called *metaphysis*.
- When bone growth gets completed, epiphyseal cartilage stops proliferation and epiphysis fuses with diaphysis.

Box 9.4: Zones of epiphyseal cartilage

Q. Write a short note on zones of epiphyseal cartilage
Q. List the zones of epiphyseal cartilage.

- Epiphyseal cartilage is site of long bone growth (lengthening). It begins at about 12th week of gestation and continues till early adulthood.
- During bone growth, vascular endothelial growth factor (VEGF) stimulates replacement of vascular epiphyseal cartilage with vascular bony tissue.
- At the site of bone formation, epiphyseal cartilage shows the following zones (Figs 9.14, 9.15 and Flowchart 9.8):
1. *Zone of reserve cartilage:* This is resting cartilage portion. It shows small chondrocytes that lie singly in the lacunae.
2. *Zone of proliferation:* Cells of this zone undergo cell division. Chondrocytes of this zone are larger and more in number than that of zone of reserve cartilage.
3. *Zone of hypertrophy:* Cells of this zone are bigger in size (hypertrophic). They have clear cytoplasm. These cells get arranged in columns.
4. *Zone of calcified cartilage:* In this zone, calcium gets deposited in cartilage matrix. It results in apoptosis and loss of cartilage cells. Calcified cartilage zone forms temporary supporting framework for deposition of a new bone.
5. *Zone of resorption:* In this zone, small blood vessels and osteoprogenitor cells from marrow cavity invade zone of calcified cartilage. In the zone of resorption, portion of calcified cartilage is present in the form of longitudinal spicules. On surface of longitudinal spicules, osteoblasts start depositing bone, and thus form mixed spicules later, mixed spicules get anastomosed with each other to form bony trabeculae.

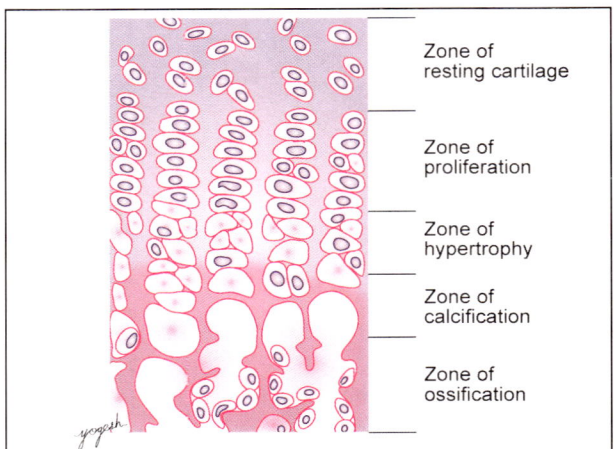

Fig. 9.14: Epiphyseal cartilage of a developing bone (Source: Textbook of Human Embryology, Yogesh Sontakke, 1st edn., CBS Publishers)

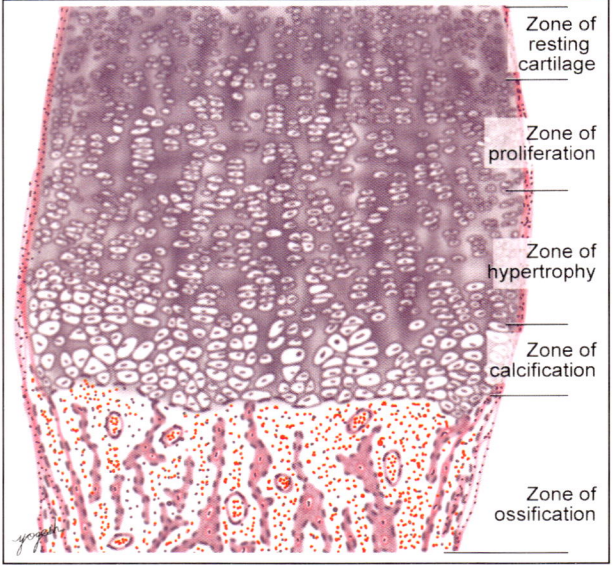

Fig. 9.15: Histology of developing bone (practice figure).

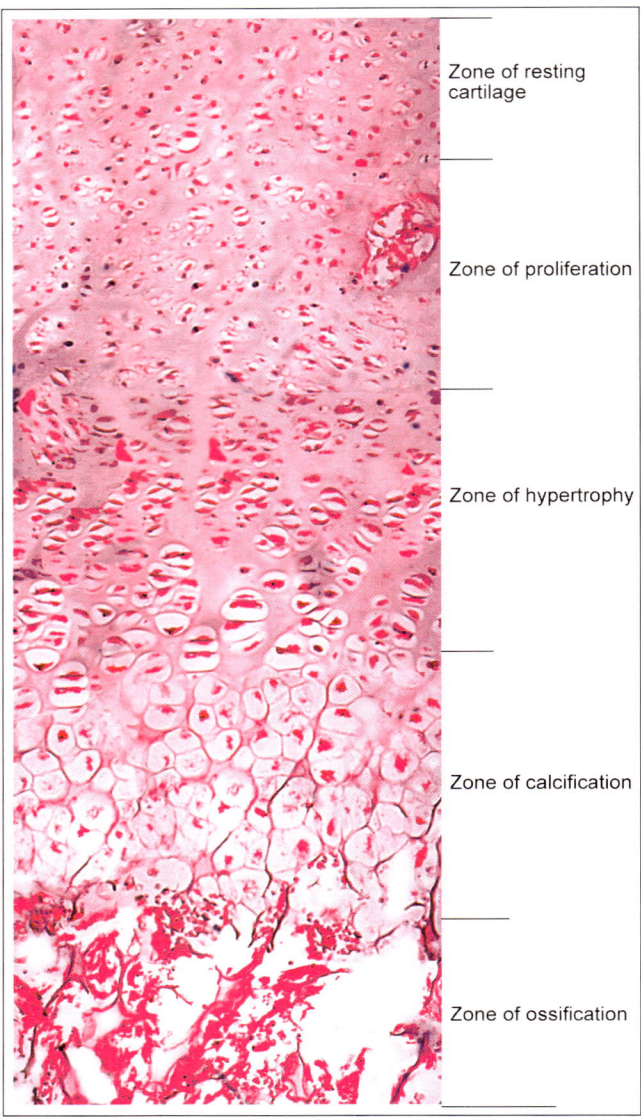

Fig. 9.16: Photomicrograph. Developing bone (low magnification, combined image).

Flowchart 9.8: Zones of epiphyseal plate and their characteristic features

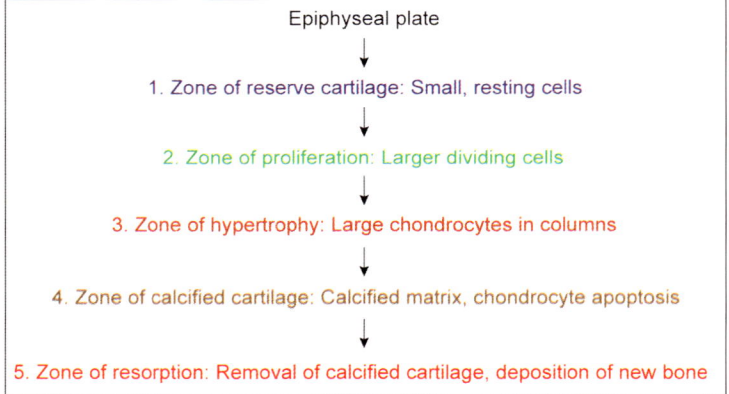

Clinical Correlation

- *Osteogenesis imperfecta/brittle-bone disease:* It involves lack of collagen type I fibers and defective calcification. Hence, bones break easily. Other symptoms include short height, hearing loss, blue sclera, and loose joints.[Neet]
- *Scurvy:* Deficiency of vitamin C results in inadequate synthesis of collagen fibers and organic matrix. In scurvy, spongy bones show reduced number of trabeculae, whereas compact bone show thinner cortex.
- *Rickets:* Vitamin D deficiency in rickets causes reduced mineralization of bone matrix in young individuals. It causes bowing of long bones.[Viva]
- *Osteoporosis:* It mostly occurs in old age, especially in postmenopausal women because of reduced estrogen level. There is increased bone resorption in osteoporosis.
- *Osteoma* is a benign tumor of osteoblasts, whereas osteosarcoma is a malignant tumor arising from osteoblasts. Note: Benign tumor does not spread; malignant tumor can spread to distinct sites.

CHAPTER 10

Muscle Tissue

Chapter Outline

- Skeletal muscle
  - Histology of skeletal muscle
  - Ultrastructure of skeletal muscle
- Details of skeletal muscle
  - Muscle contraction
  - Relaxation of muscle fiber
  - Types of skeletal muscle fibers
  - Nerve supply of skeletal muscle
  - Sarcoplasmic reticulum and T-tubules
  - Muscle spindle
- Cardiac muscle
- Intercalated disc
- Smooth muscle

Competency achievement: The student should be able to:

AN67.1 Describe and identify various types of muscle under the microscope
AN67.2 Classify muscle and describe the structure-function correlation of the same
AN67.3 Describe the ultrastructure of muscular tissue

INTRODUCTION

- In human, all the body cells have a property of the contractility to some extent. The property of contractility is well developed in muscular tissue.
- *Myocytes* (muscle fibers): The cells of muscular tissue are called *myocytes*. As the myocytes are elongated or spindle shaped, they are also called *muscle fibers*.
- Muscles are derived from mesoderm.
- In muscle,
  - Sarcolemma is plasma membrane.
  - Sarcoplasm is cytoplasm.
  - Sarcoplasmic reticulum is endoplasmic reticulum.
  - Sarcosome is mitochondria [*sarcos* = flesh, *plasma* = thing in Greek].
- Histologically, the muscles are classified into three groups: *Viva*
  1. Skeletal muscle
  2. Cardiac muscle
  3. Smooth muscle
- Some authors classify the muscles as *striated muscles* (skeletal and cardiac muscles) and *non-striated muscles* (smooth muscles).
- Striated muscles show transverse striations in their cytoplasm because of specific arrangement of contractile proteins in their sarcoplasm (cytoplasm). *Viva*

- Physiologically, muscles are classified as *voluntary* (skeletal muscles) and *involuntary* (cardiac and smooth muscles). Voluntary muscles are under control of our will, whereas involuntary muscles are not under our control.

SKELETAL MUSCLE

- Skeletal muscles are also called *striated muscles* (because of striations) as well as *voluntary muscles* (under our will).
- Because of skeletal attachment, these muscles are responsible for the locomotion.
- *Visceral striated muscles*: These are microscopically identical to the skeletal muscles, but they are confined to the viscera such as tongue, pharynx, peripheral part of diaphragm, and upper two-third of esophagus. *Viva* Visceral striated muscles are involved in speech, breathing, swallowing, and coughing.

Histology of Skeletal Muscle

- Microscopically, skeletal muscle consists of muscle cells called *myocyte* or *muscle fiber* (Flowchart 10.1, Figs 10.1 and 10.2).
- Muscle fiber is a **multinucleated syncytium** of varied length (few millimeters to meter) (Figs 10.1 and 10.2). *Identification feature*

Muscle Tissue

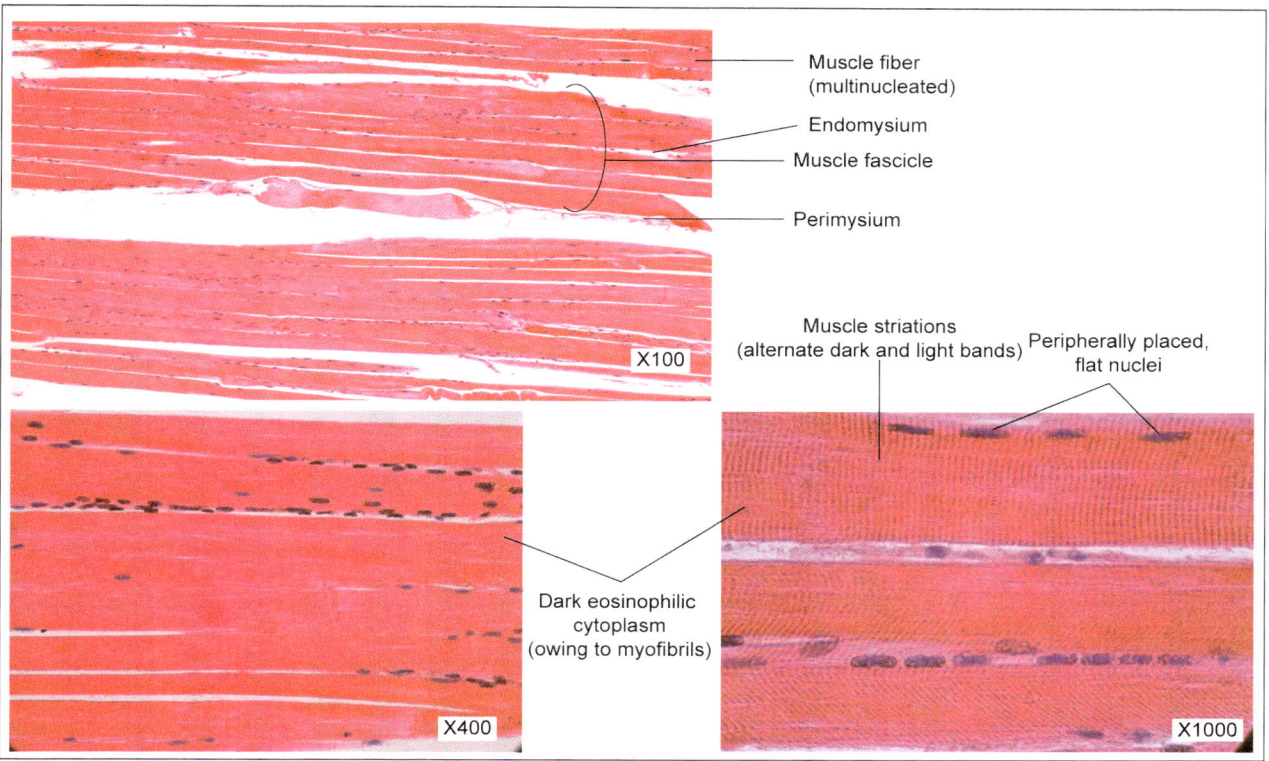

Fig. 10.1: Photomicrograph of skeletal muscle (longitudinal section).

Flowchart 10.1: Histology of skeletal muscle

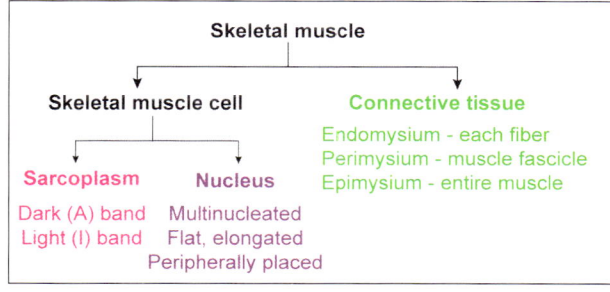

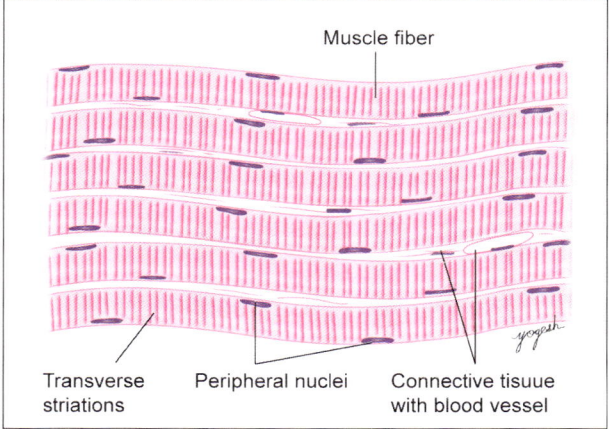

Fig. 10.2: Histology of skeletal muscle.

- *Note*: Muscle fiber is a cell, whereas connective tissue fibers are extracellular, nonliving material
- Each muscle fiber is elongated, unbranched cell.
- Nuclei are flat and located in the periphery of the cell just beneath the sarcolemma (plasma membrane). *Identification feature*
- On *H&E staining*, the skeletal muscle fiber shows transverse (cross) striations of alternate dark and light bands. *Identification feature*
- Connective tissue of skeletal muscle consists of endomysium, perimysium and epimysium.
- *Endomysium* is a layer of reticular fibers that cover an individual muscle fiber.
- *Perimysium* covers a bundle of muscle fibers (fascicle).
- *Epimysium* covers the entire skeletal muscle.
- Blood vessels and nerve fibers are present in all these layers of connective tissue.
- Motor end plate is the point of contact between the terminal end of axons of motor neurons and muscle fibers.
- Dark band is called A (anisotropic) band and light band is I (isotropic) band because of their power to refract the light in polarized light microscopy. *Viva*

Summary (Examination Guide)

- Skeletal muscle consists of multinucleated, long, non-branching muscle fibers.
- The muscle fiber shows many flat nuclei that are placed at the periphery.
- The muscle fiber shows alternate dark and light bands (striations); hence, called striated muscle.
- Each muscle fiber is surrounded by connective tissue, endomysium.
- Group of fibers form bundle or fascicle. Each fascicle is surrounded by perimysium; whereas entire muscle is surrounded by epimysium.

Ultrastructure of Skeletal Muscle

Myofibril

- Myofibrils are the structural and functional subunits of muscle fiber (Fig. 10.3).
- Myofibrils are arranged longitudinally in the muscle fiber and runs in the entire length of muscle fiber.
- Myofibrils consists of bundles of *myofilaments*.
- Each myofilament consists of *thick* (myosin II protein) filaments and *thin* (actin and its associated proteins).
- Arrangements of thick and thin filament give striated appearance to muscle fiber when observed unstained under phase contract or polarizing microscope and on H&E staining under light microscope.^{Viva}
- In polarized microscopy, the polarized light passing through dark band gets diffracted and does not reach the observer. Hence, this part of muscle fiber looks dark (no light) and called *anisotropic* or **A-band** (Flowchart 10.2, Fig. 10.3).
- In polarized microscopy, light band do not diffract the light. Hence light band is called *isotropic* or **I-band** (Flowchart 10.2).
- In the center of light (I) band, a dark line is present called **Z-line**, Z-disc or Zwischenscheibe line [Zwischenscheibe = between discs in German].
- In the center of dark (A) band, a narrow lighter zone is present call **H-band** (*hell* = light, in German).
- In the center of H-band, a central dense line is present called **M-line** (*mittle* = middle in German).
- **Sarcomere**
  – It is the structural and functional unit of myofibrils.^{Viva}
  – Length: 2–3 μm.
  – Sarcomere lies between two adjacent Z-lines.^{Viva}

Flowchart 10.2: Polarized microscopy of skeletal muscle fiber.

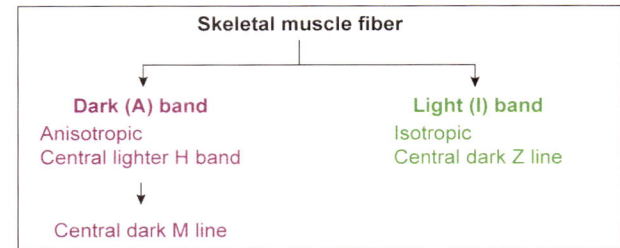

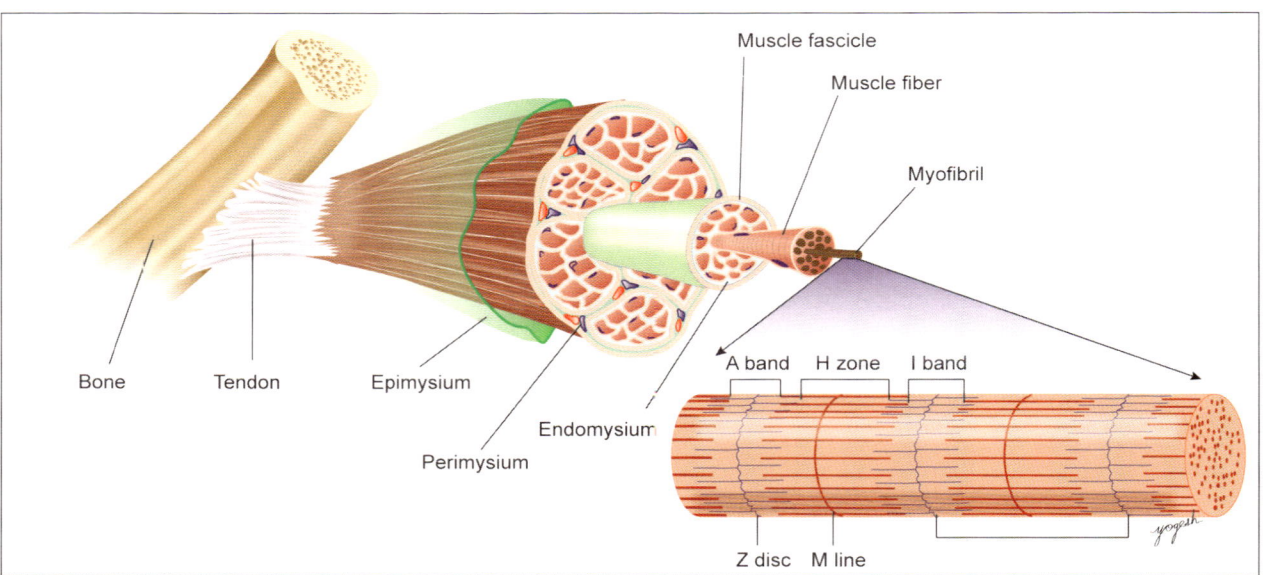

Fig. 10.3: Structure of skeletal muscle. Entire skeletal muscle is covered by epimysium. Perimysium covers a bundle of muscle fibers called fascicle, whereas endomysium is a layer of reticular fibers that cover an individual muscle fiber.

DETAILS OF SKELETAL MUSCLE (FOR FURTHER READING)

Molecular Details of Myofibrils (Figs 10.4 and 10.5)

- In sarcomere, there are two types of myofibrils:
  1. Thick myosin filaments and
  2. Thin actin filaments.

Thin Filament

- Its diameter is 5–6 nm.
- Each thin filament consists of a double-stranded helix of F-actin and actin associated proteins such as tropomyosin, troponin, pomodulin and nebulin.
- *F-actin chain*: It consists of two chains of *G-actin* protein. Each G-actin protein has an active binding site for myosin. This active myosin binding site remains covered (masked) tropomyosin protein chain during relaxation of muscle.
- *Tropomyosin* is a polypeptide chain that runs parallel to F-actin chain and masks the myosin binding sites of G-actins.
- *Troponin* is a key protein molecule for muscle contraction. It consists of three subunits:
  1. Troponin C (TnC) binds with Ca^{++}.
  2. Troponin T (TnT) binds with tropomyosin.
  3. Troponin I (TnI) binds with F-actin.
- *Tropomodulin* – It is attached to the free end of thin filament. Tropomodulin regulates the length of the actin filament.
- *Nebulin* – It anchors thin filament to Z-lines.
- *Dystrophin* – It links external lamina of skeletal muscle to actin filaments. Absence of dystrophin result in Duchenne's muscular dystrophy.

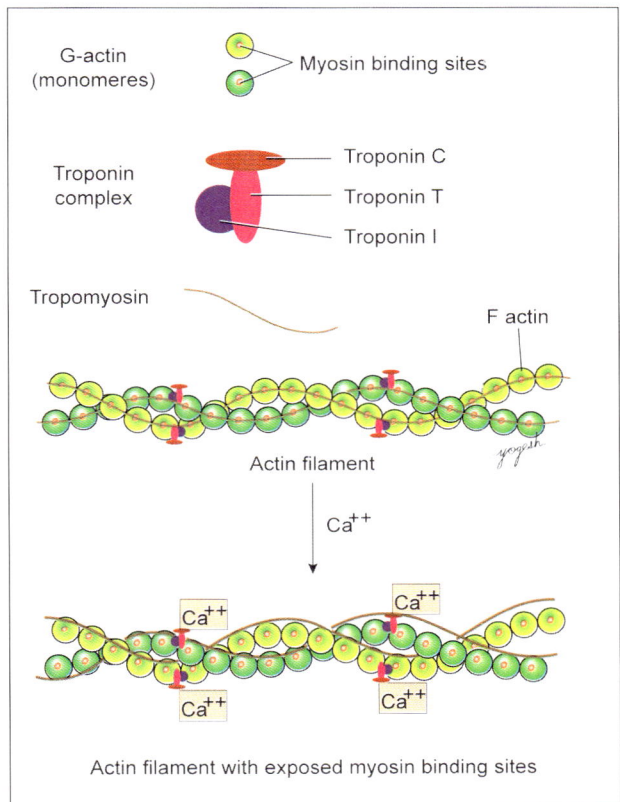

Fig. 10.5: Structure of thin filament. Actin consists of polypeptide chain of G-actin monomers. In relaxed stage, tropomyosin covers the active binding sites of F-actin for myosin. Ca^{++} ions bind with troponin C and it result in release of tropomyosin from F-actin. Thus, Ca^{++} exposes myosin-binding sites of actin.

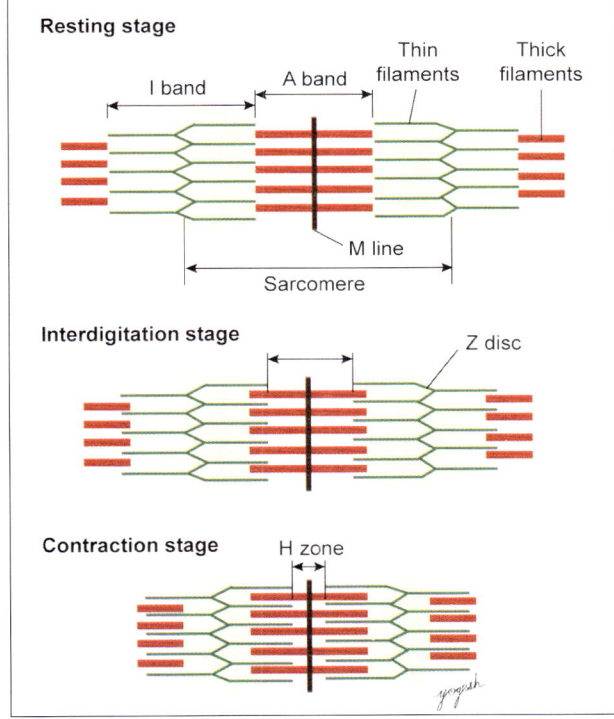

Fig.10.4: Sarcomere length in different stages of muscle contraction.

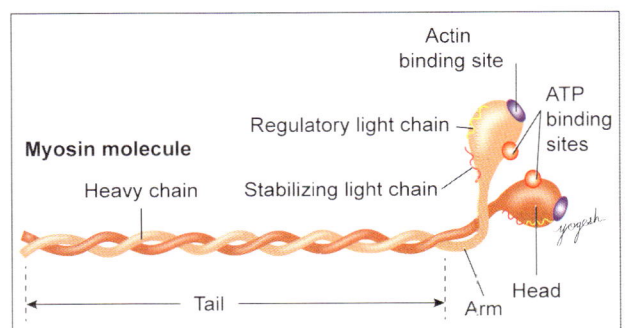

Fig. 10.6: Structure of myosin II molecule.

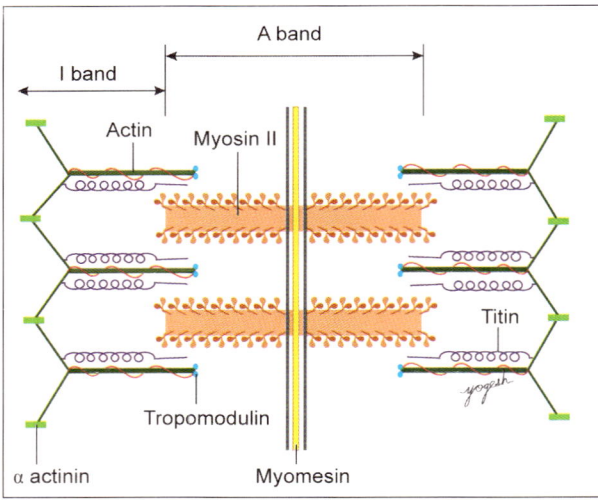

Fig. 10.7: Actin and myosin associated proteins.

Thick Filament

- Thick filament mainly consists of myosin II protein, chains (Figs 10.4 and 10.6).
- Each myosin II molecule consists of two heavy polypeptide chain and four light chains.
- Heavy chains spiral around each other.
- Each heavy chain shows (Fig. 10.6):
  1. Main part
  2. Peripheral globular heads (S1 region) – motor domain
  3. Arms (S2 region) that connects heads with main part.
- Each heavy chain in the arm is surrounded by two light chains:
  1. Essential light chain (ELC)
  2. Regulatory light chain (RLC) – stabilizes the arm.
- Head of heavy chain has two binding sites: one for ATP and another for actin.
- Myosin molecules forms assembly that shows projecting myosin heads and central core of myosin filaments. The assembly has middle bare zone (devoid of projecting myosin heads).
- Myosin assembly binds with adjacent assemblies at M line with the help of M line proteins.

Accessory Proteins

- In addition to the above-mentioned proteins, accessory proteins are present that help in structural formation and functions of thick and thin filaments.
- These proteins include (Fig. 10.7):
  1. Titin (spring-like filament that prevent excessive stretching of sarcomere).
  2. α-actinin: It anchors thin filaments to Z-line.
- *Desmin* anchors Z-line with plasma membrane.

Muscle Contraction

- During contraction of a muscle fiber (Fig. 10.4)
  1. Overlapping of thick and thin filament increases.
  2. Length of sarcomere shortens
  3. Length of I (light) band shortens
  4. A (dark) band do not change
  5. H band narrows because of encroaching thin filaments.

Sliding Filament Theory (Flowchart 10.3)

- This theory can be explained by actomyosin cross-bridge cycle.
- *Relaxed state* – Tropomyosin covers the active myosin binding sites of F-actin.
- Nerve stimulation induces Ca^{++} ion release in the sarcoplasm.
- This Ca^{++} ion binds with troponin C and it result in release of tropomyosin from F-actin. Thus, Ca^{++} exposes myosin-binding sites of actin.

Flowchart 10.3: Mechanism of muscle contraction (actomyosin cross-bridging cycle)

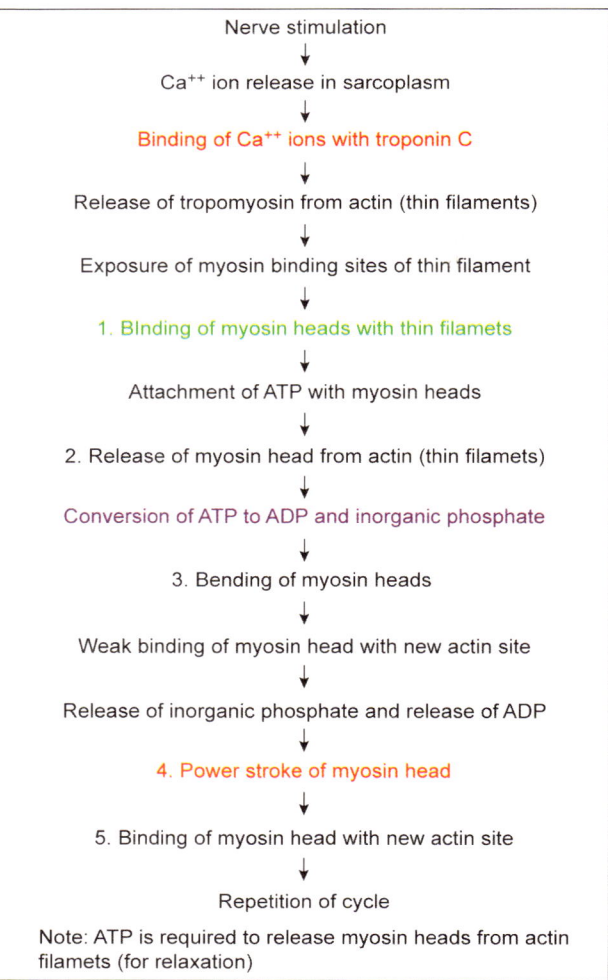

- The cross-bridge cycle helps in movement of myosin heads and sliding of actin over myosin.
- Actomyosin cross-bridge cycle takes place in five steps as follows:
  1. *Attachment*: Myosin heads attach to exposed sites of actin filament.
  2. *Release of myosin heads*: ATP binds with myosin heads and it results in release of myosin heads from actin/thin filament.
  3. *Bending of myosin head (recovery stroke)*: Conversion ATP into ADP and inorganic phosphate causes rotation of myosin heads by about 5 nm. Thus, rotated myosin head assumes pre-power stroke position.
  4. *Stage of power stroke of myosin head*: On rotation, the myosin head reaches near the newer binding site of actin (thin) filament. Meanwhile, myosin heads bind weakly with thin filament at new binding site. Release of inorganic phosphate form myosin head causes straightening of myosin head and movement of thin filament (sliding). It is called ***power stroke***. ADP gets detached from myosin during power stoke.
  5. *Stage of reattachment*: Myosin heads form tight bond with actin till the attachment of ATP.
- All these 5 steps together produce movement of the thin filament over thick filament.

> **Box 10.1: Sarcoplasmic Reticulum and T-tubules**
>
> - Sarcoplasmic reticulum of the muscle fiber consists of longitudinally oriented multiple tubules (Fig. 10.8).
> - Sarcoplasmic reticulum serves as the reservoir of calcium (Ca^{++}) ions. *MCQ*
> - Tubules of sarcoplasmic reticulum forms network of anastomosing tubules.
> - ***Terminal cistern:*** In the skeletal muscle, at the junction of dark (A) and light (I) band, tubules of sarcoplasmic reticulum form dilated part called terminal cistern. *Viva, MCQ*
> - ***T-tubules*** (transverse/tubules): T-tubule is the invagination of the plasma membrane (sarcolemma). *Viva*
> - T-tubules are oriented transverse to the long axis of the muscle fibers.
> - T-tubules communicates with extracellular fluid.
> - In the skeletal muscle, at the junction of dark (A) and light (I) band, T-tubules are present.
> - ***Triad:*** Each T-tubule on either side is related to one terminal cistern of sarcoplasmic reticulum. These two terminal cisterns with central T-tubule form triad that lies at the junction of dark band with light band.

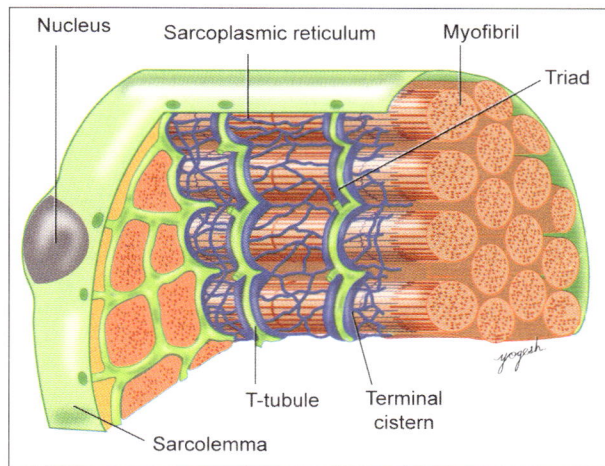

Fig. 10.8: Skeletal muscle: Organization of sarcoplasmic reticulum, T tubules and terminal cisterns. Two terminal cisterns and T tubule form a triad at the junction of A and I bands.

> **Function**
> - The depolarization wave is carried deep inside the sarcoplasm. It stimulates adjacent terminal cisterns for release of Ca^{++} ions and thus, initiate rapid muscle contraction through Ca^{++} ions.

Relaxation of Muscle Fiber
- During muscle contraction, calcium ions bind with troponin C and induce muscle contraction.
- Calcium-activated ATPase pump transport Ca^{++} ions from sarcoplasm to sarcoplasmic reticulum in 30 milliseconds.
- Decreased Ca^{++} ion concentration, deactivates troponin C and it results in binding of tropomyosin with myosin-binding site of actin filament.
- Finally, myosin cannot bind with actin and muscle fiber undergo relaxation.

Types of Skeletal Muscle Fibers
- Based on the diameter and color of the muscle fiber, the skeletal muscle fibers are grouped into three types: red, white and intermediate.
- *Note*: These types are based on the appearance of fibers in the body (*in vivo*) and not on histological basis by *H&E* staining.
- *Newer nomenclature*
  1. Red fibers are also called type I fibers or slow oxidative fibers.
  2. Intermediate fibers are called type IIa fibers or fast oxidative fibers.

3. White fibers are also called type IIb fibers or fast glycolytic fibers.
- Rate and speed of contraction of muscle fiber depend of the following factors:
  - Velocity of myosin ATPase to break down ATP molecules during contraction.
  - Rate of regeneration of ATP molecule in muscle by oxidative phosphorylation or glycolysis.
- Muscle contain myoglobin. It is oxygen binding protein (resembles hemoglobin). It has ferrous ions (Fe^{++}) that help in storage of required oxygen for oxidative phosphorylation.

Type I Fibers
- These are red fibers.
- They contain large amounts of myoglobin (red colored) and mitochondria.
- These fibers show strong positive immunohistochemical reaction for succinic dehydrogenase and nicotinamide adenine dinucleotide-tetrazolium (NADH-TR).
- These are slow-twitch fibers because they contract slowly.
- These are resistant to fatigue.
- They generate less force of contraction but produce prolonged contractions.
- Examples: postural muscles, muscles of limbs and back.

Type IIa Fibers
- These are intermediate fibers.
- These are medium sized fibers having large amount of glycogen. These fibers can undergo anaerobic glycolysis.

Type IIb Fibers
- These are white fibers.
- These are thick fibers.
- They contain less amount of myoglobin, and mitochondria and high amount of glycogen.
- These fibers are high-twitch fibers that can generate strong force of contraction.
- They mostly generate energy from anaerobic glycolysis, hence, fatigue rapidly.
- Examples: Type IIa fibers (white) fibers are present in the muscle that requires more precision and fast actions. For example, muscle of eyeball and fingers.[Neet]
- The differences between red fibers and white fibers are listed in Table 10.1.

Nerve Supply of Skeletal Muscle
- The muscle fibers are supplied by alpha-efferent fibers arising from multipolar anterior horn neurons of spinal cord.
- These are myelinated, large diameter fibers.
- *Motor unit*: It is consisting of one anterior horn neuron and all the muscle fibers supplied by it. Small motor unit are present in precision acting muscles (muscles of eyeball), whereas large motor units are present in postural muscles.
- *Motor end plate:* It is the junction between muscle fiber and nerve terminal.
- Muscle spindles are the sensory organs located in the muscle. Muscle spindles are supplied by myelinated gamma efferent fibers that arise from gamma motor neurons of anterior horn of spinal cord.

Q. List the differences between red fibers and white fibres.

Table 10.1: Differences between red fibers and white fibers

Characteristic	Red Fibers	White fibers
Another name	Type I or slow oxidative fibers	Type IIb or fast glycolytic fibers
Fiber diameter	Small	Large
Colour in living	Red	Light pink
Myoglobin quantity	More	Less
Mitochondria	More	Less
Force of contraction	Weak	Strong
Mode of contraction	Slow-twitch	Fast-twitch
Fatigability	Resistant to fatigue	Easily fatigued
Mode of energy generation	Oxidative phosphorylation	Anaerobic glycolysis
Glycogen content	Less	More
Examples	Postural and limb muscles	Precise, rapid muscles: muscles of eyeball, fingers
Blood supply	Rich	Poor
Nerve supply	Small nerve fibers	Large nerve fibers

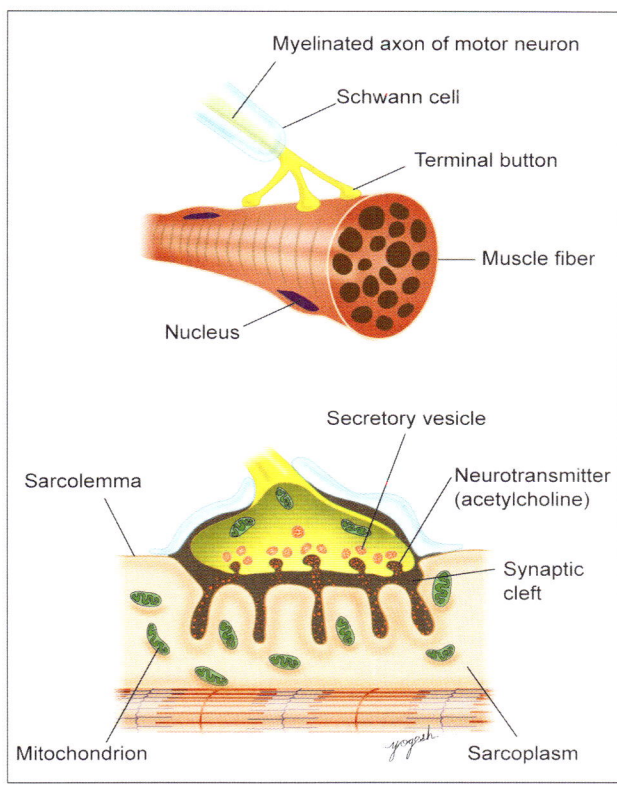

Fig. 10.9: Neuromuscular junction.

Neuromuscular Junction/Motor End Plate

- It is the junctional complex of the axon terminal and muscle fiber (Fig. 10.9).
- At the terminal end, axon lose its myelination and divide into many terminal branches. Each terminal branch expands at its end (terminal button) and form junctional zone of muscle fiber at soloplate (part of sarcolema).
- *Terminal button* of axon contain secretory vesicles containing acetylcholine and number of mitochondria.
- *Soloplate* or *motor end plate* forms number of folding that contains many receptors for acetyl choline.
- *Synaptic cleft* is the narrow gap (40–100 nm) between axonal terminal button and motor end plate. Neurotransmitter needs to cross synaptic cleft.
- Acetyl cholinesterase (AChE) is the enzyme that destroys acetylcholine quickly.

Clinical Correlation

- **Myasthenia gravis**
  It is autoimmune diseases in that antibodies are found against acetyl choline receptors (AChR).
  These antibodies damage progressively acetyl choline receptors and muscle slowly becomes weak (nonresponsive to acetyl choline).
  Note: *myasthenia* = weakness of muscle, *gravis* = serious.

- **Neurotoxins**
  Many snake venoms contain neurotoxins that bind with acetylcholine receptors.
  It may cause paralysis of respiratory muscle and death of the individual.
- **Stretch reflex**
  It is a myotatic reflex. It can be elicited by a blow upon a muscle tendon that in reflex induces muscle contraction. Blow using hammer on a tendon of muscle causes stretching of muscle spindles that through sensory inputs stimulate alpha motor neurons and finally produce muscle contraction. Example, biceps reflex.

Box 10.2: Muscle spindle

- Muscle (neuromuscular) spindle is a spindle-shaped sensory end organ of skeletal muscles (Fig. 10.10).
- Length: 5–10 mm
- Diameter: 100 μm.

Structure (Fig. 10.10)
- It consists of capsules, sensory neuron, gamma motor neurons, and intrafusal muscle fibers.
- Capsule: Muscle spindle is enclosed within fusiform connective tissue fibers.
- Intrafusal muscle fibers: Muscle spindle has intrafusal muscle fibers that are enclosed within the capsule.
  Note: Extrafusal fibers from main bulk of the muscle.

There are two types of intrafusal fibers
1. *Nuclear bag fibers*: Many nuclei are located in the middle of the fiber.
2. *Nuclear chain fibers*: Nuclei are arranged in a single row.
   Nuclear bag fibers are long and extend outside the capsule up to the endomysium of adjacent extrafusal fibers.
- Nerve supply of muscle spindle:
  – Muscle spindle is supplied by gamma motor neurons and sensation is carried by sensory afferent nerve fibers (type Ia and II).
    Note: Extrafusal (main muscle) fibers are supplied by alpha motor neurons.
  – Type Ia fibers have annulospiral nerve endings that surrounds central area of nuclear chain and bag fibers.
  – Type II fibers have floral spray endings that are present in peripheral part of bag fibers.
  – The sensory neurons get stimulated on stretching of muscle fibers.

Functions
- During muscle contract on stretching of muscle spindle stimulates sensory nerve fibers (type Ia and type II).
- These sensory fibers provide inputs to the CNS about muscle stretch and help modulate the activity of motor neurons supplying same muscle.

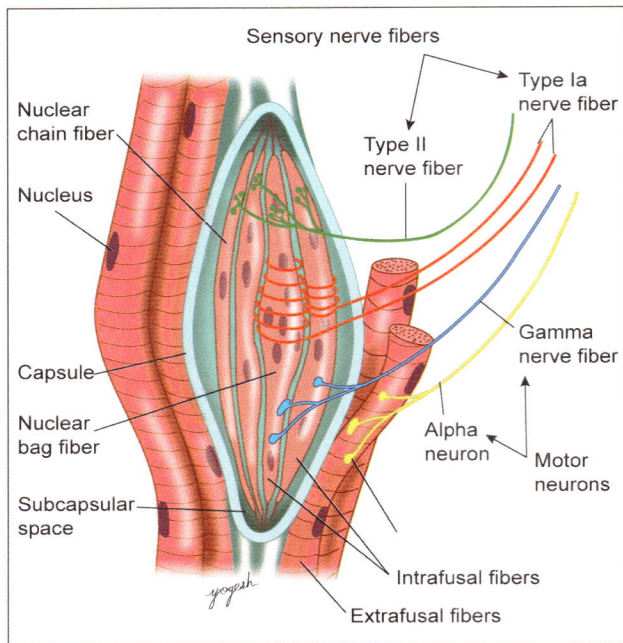

Fig. 10.10: Muscle spindle. Extrafusal (main muscle) fibers are supplied by alpha motor neurons. Muscle spindle is supplied by gamma motor neurons. Sensation is carried by type Ia fibers (annulospiral nerve endings) from central area of nuclear chain and bag fibers, whereas by type II fibers (floral spray endings) from peripheral part of bag fibers. The sensory neurons get stimulated on stretching of muscle fibers.

CARDIAC MUSCLE

- Cardiac muscle also shows striations, but it is involuntary in action (***striated involuntary muscle***).
- Cardiac muscle fibers are located in the heart.
- They show following peculiarities:
  1. Cardiac muscle fibers have *autorhythmicity* (contract on their own without any stimulation): Hence, it can work as *pace maker*.
  2. Cardiac muscle fibers show cytoplasmic striations.
  3. Cardiac muscle fibers are supplied by autonomic nervous system (sympathetic stimulates and parasympathetic inhibits its activity).
  4. Cardiac myocytes are connected with each other by densely staining cross bands called ***intercalated discs***.

Histology of Cardiac Muscle

Cardiac Myocytes and Muscle Fibers

- Cardiac muscle consists of long, thick, branching muscle fibers (Fig. 10.11).*Identification feature*
- Each muscle fiber shows various number of cardiac myocytes that are joined with other by intercalated discs.
- Each *cardiac myocyte* measure about 50–100 µm in length and about 15 µm in thickness.
- Each cardiac myocyte has a *single, centrally placed, large, oval nucleus.*^{Identification feature} (*Note*: Skeletal muscle has long, multinucleated muscle fiber with peripherally placed, flat nuclei).

Cell Organelles

- Cardiac myocyte shows a biconical juxtanuclear region (perinuclear halo on *H&E staining*).
- Most of the cell organelles are arranged in this region. It is devoid of myofibrils.
- This region contains numerous mitochondria that supply required energy to cardiac myocytes.
- It also shows Golgi apparatus, glycogen (stored form of glucose), lipofuscin pigments.
- Atrial cardiac myocytes show *atrial granules* containing two polypeptide hormones: atrial natriuretic factor and brain natriuretic factor.*MCQ*

Some Interesting Facts

Atrial natriuretic factor and brain natriuretic factor
- These are polypeptide hormones secreted by cardiac myocytes of atrium.
- These act on kidney and inhibit reabsorption of sodium and inhibit secretion of renin.
- These act on adrenal gland and inhibit secretion of aldosterone.
- Thus, finally, they reduce blood pressure by causing vasodilation.

Intercalated Disc

- The adjacent cardiac myocytes are connected with each other by a specialized zone called ***intercalated disc***.
- Light microscopy (*H&E staining*): Intercalated discs are dark staining transverse line running across the muscle fibers.*Viva, Identification feature*
- It consists of short segments that are arranged in a 'steps'.*Viva*
- For details, read Box 10.3.

Muscle Tissue

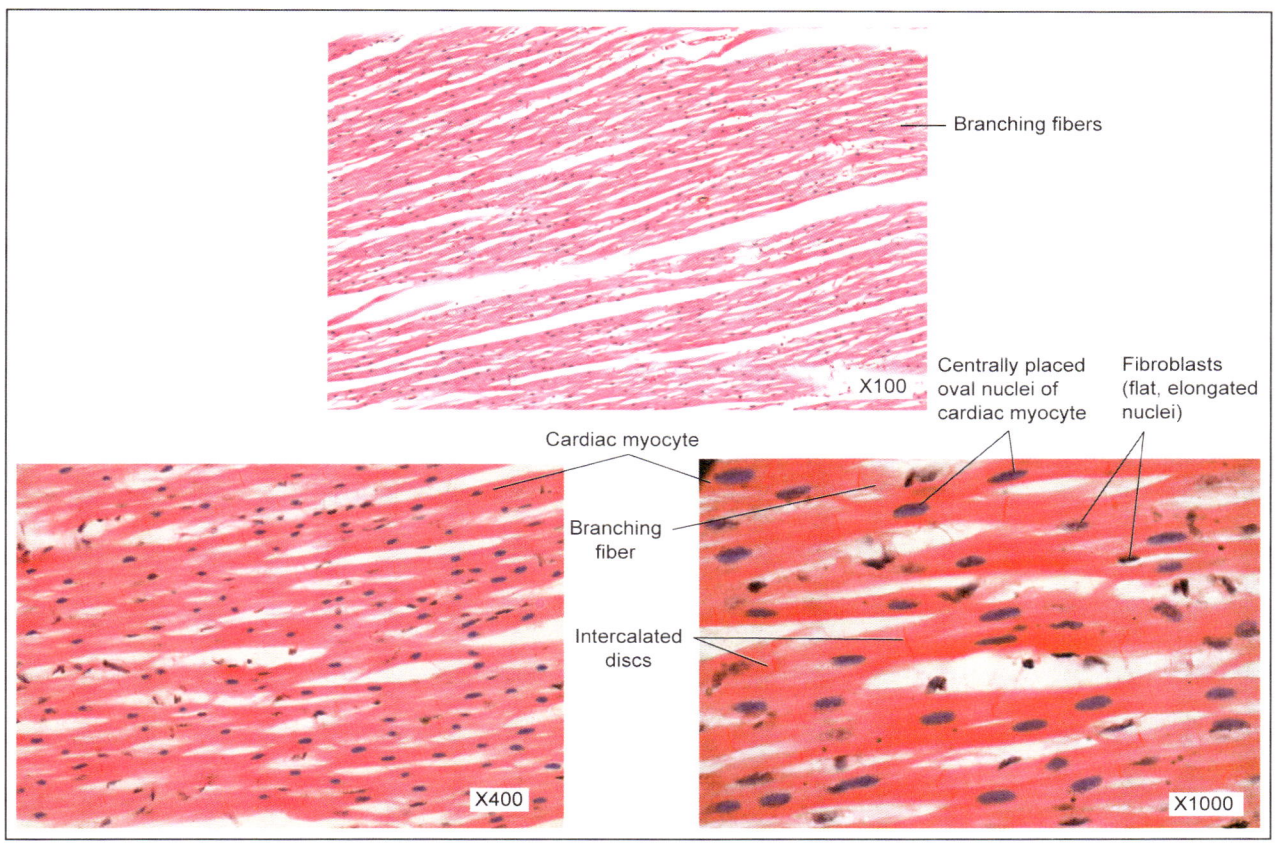

Fig. 10.11: Photomicrograph of cardiac muscle (longitudinal section).

Myofibrils and Striations

- Cardiac muscle shows *less number of myofibrils* (thick and thin filaments) than that of skeletal muscle. Hence, *striations are less prominent* in cardiac muscle fibers.
- Cardiac muscle fiber accommodates more amount of sarcoplasm and mitochondria.
- Myofibrils are arranged similar to skeletal muscle fibers. It also shows dark (A) and light (I) bands, Z lines, and H hands.

T-tubules and Sarcoplasmic Reticulum

- Smooth endoplasmic (sarcoplasmic) reticulum of the cardiac muscle is not well organized. It is well organized in skeletal muscle).
- T-tubules (extension of sarcolemma) penetrate the cardiac muscle at the level of Z-lines thus cardiac muscle has only one T-tubule per sarcomere (Fig. 10.12).
- *Diad*: Each T-tubule in cardiac myocyte is surrounded by a small cistern (dilatations of sarcoplasmic reticulum. Thus, a small cistern and T-tubule form diad at the level of Z-line (*Note*: triad in skeletal muscle).^Neet

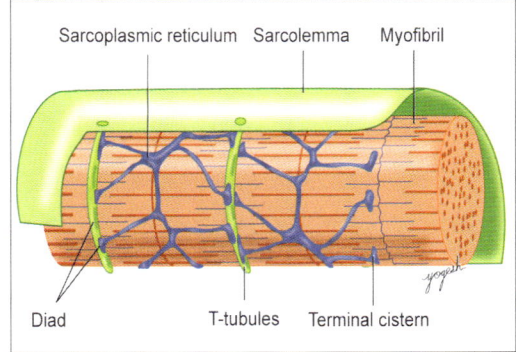

Fig. 10.12: Cardiac muscle: Organization of sarcoplasmic reticulum, T tubules and terminal cisterns. A small terminal cistern and a T tubule form a diad at Z lines.

Box 10.3: Intercalated disc

Q. Write a short not on intercalated disc.

- Intercalated discs are specialized cell junctions between adjacent cardiac myocytes (Fig. 10.13).
- It consists of fascia adherence, macula adherents, and gap junctions.
- Light microscopy (*H&E staining*): Intercalated discs are dark staining transverse line running across the muscle fibers.^Viva, Identification feature

- Intercalated disc shows two components:
  1. *Transverse component* that lies perpendicular to myofibrils, in stairway manner.
  2. *Lateral (longitudinal) component* that lies parallel to the myofibrils. It is not visualized in light microscopy.
- Transverse component consists of fascia adherens and desmosomes, whereas lateral component shows gap junctions.

1. *Facia adherens*
   - It is present in transverse component of intercalated disc and forms its major portion.
   - It takes dark-staining.
   - It is similar to zonula adherens of epithelium.
   - It binds adjacent myocytes with each other to form a cardiac muscle fiber.
   - It consists of electron-dense material that fills intercellular space.
   - It gives attachment to thin filaments of terminal sarcomere.

2. *Desmosomes (maculae adherents)*
   - They are also present in both transverse and lateral components of the intercalated disc.
   - They bind adjacent myocytes with each other.

3. *Gap junctions*
   - These are present in the lateral component of the intercalated discs.
   - They provide *'ionic-continuity'* in cardiac myocytes and help in the rapid spread of action potential from one cell to another.
   - They make the cardiac muscle as *physiological syncytium*.

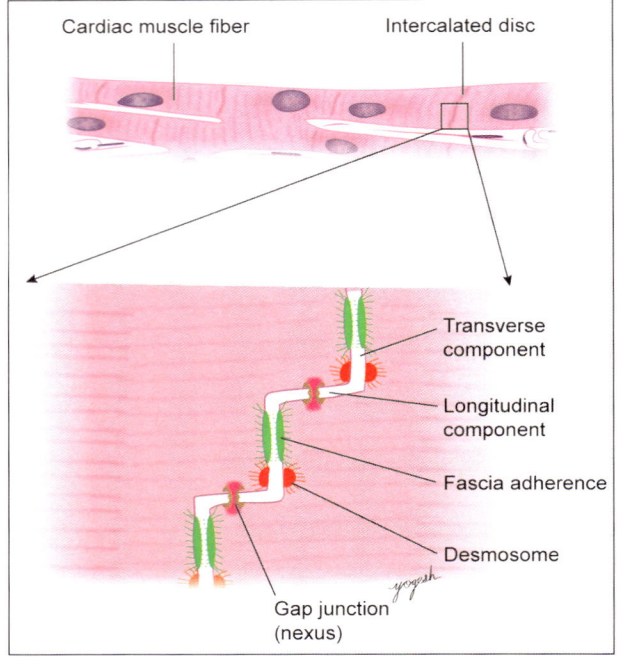

Fig. 10.13: Intercalated discs are specialized junctions between adjacent cardiac myocytes. Intercalated disc shows transverse and longitudinal components. Transverse component consists of fascia adherences and desmosomes, whereas lateral component shows gap junctions.

Summary (Examination Guide)
Q. Write a short note on histology of cardiac muscle.
- Cardiac muscle consists of single nucleated, short, branching muscle fibers (Flowchart 10.4 and Fig. 10.14).
- Each muscle cell shows a single, oval nucleus that is place centrally.
- Muscle fiber shows alternate dark and light bands (striations); however, less prominent than skeletal muscle.
- The muscle fibers are connected with each other by dark stained intercalated discs.

Some Interesting Facts
- Nodal cells (SA node, AV node) and conducting fibers of heart are called **Purkinje fibers**. These fibers are *larger* than other cardiac muscle cells. These fibers show perinuclear glycogen and peripherally placed myofibrils. *Purkinje fibers do not have T-tubules.*
- *Myocardial infarction* is the damage to the cardiac muscle cells due to lack of blood supply.
- On healing, damaged cardiac muscle cells get replaced by fibrous tissue.
- *Previous concept*: Cardiac myocyte cannot divide. *New concept*: Cardiac myocyte can undergo mitosis.
- *Hypertrophy*: Due to increased workload (high blood pressure or regurgitation of blood or stenosis of values), the cardiac muscle undergo hypertrophy (only increased size of muscle fibers). *Viva*

Flowchart 10.4: Histology of cardiac muscle

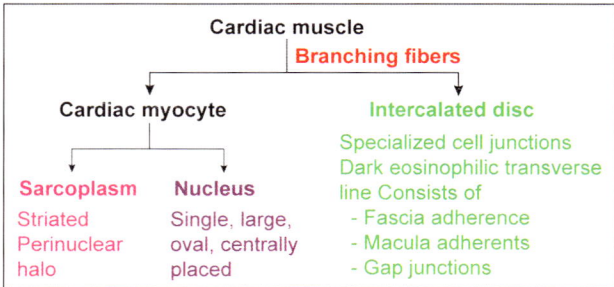

Muscle Tissue

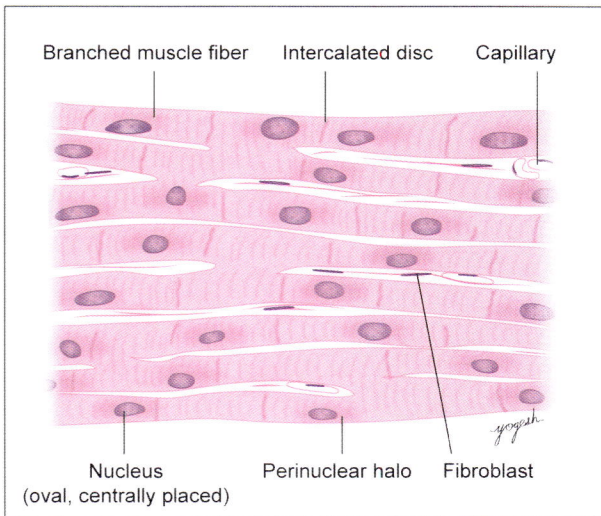

Fig. 10.14: Histology of cardiac muscle (practice figure).

SMOOTH MUSCLE

- Smooth muscles are non-striated, involuntary muscle.
- These are supplied by autonomic nerves (sympathetic and parasympathetic).
- *Locations*: Wall of gastrointestinal tract, blood vessels, respiratory tract, urinary tract, arrector pili muscle.

Structure of Smooth Muscle

- Smooth muscle consists of elongated, spindle shaped muscle cells.
- *Size*: It varies according to location.
  Smooth muscle cells in the wall of blood vessel: 15 µm long.
  Uterine smooth muscle cells during pregnancy: 500 µm.

H&E Staining

- *Longitudinal section*: The cells are elongated *spindle shaped*. The *cytoplasm stains dark eosinophilic (pink)* because of myofilaments. Nucleus is elongated, lightly stained with hematoxylin (violet). *Identification feature* The cells are arranged parallel to each other and placed so closely that it is difficult to differentiate between adjacent cells (Fig. 10.15, 10.17).

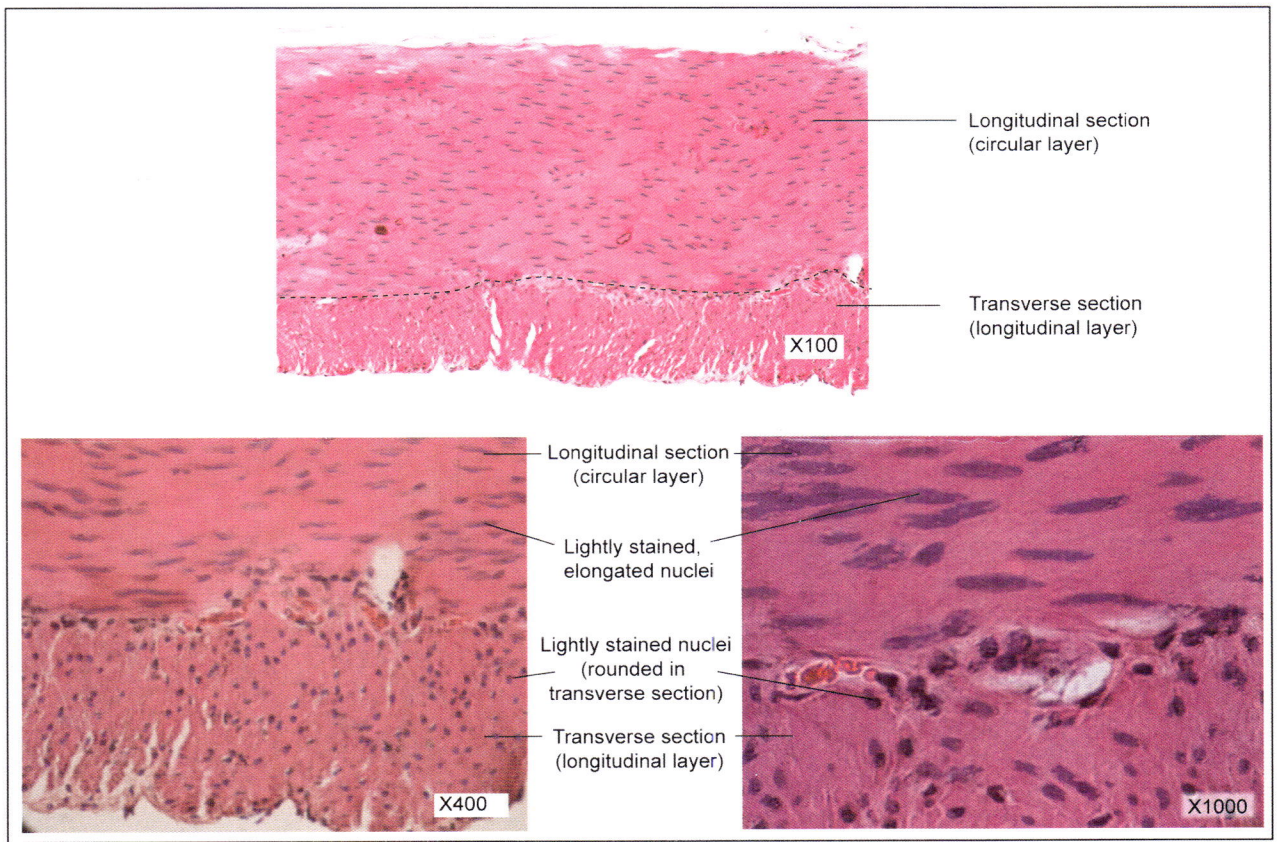

Fig. 10.15: Photomicrograph of smooth muscle.

- *Transverse section*: The smooth muscle cells stains dark eosinophilic and show centrally placed nuclei.
- In most of the organ the smooth muscle cells are arranged in bundles these bundles may be longitudinally or concentrically oriented to the long axis of the organ.
- In bundles the cells are arranged tightly so that the central thick part of one cells lies adjacent to the tapering part of other cells.

Electron Microscopy

- Each smooth muscle cell is bounded by a plasma membrane.
- This plasma membrane is externally surrounded by basal lamina and delicate layer of reticular fibers.
- Adjacent smooth muscle cells are connected with each other through *gap junctions*. It helps in simultaneous contraction of adjacent cells.^{Viva}
- Smooth muscle cells do not have T-tubules.^{MCQ}
- Smooth muscle cell contains actin (thin) and myosin (thick) filaments (1:15).
- These filaments are not arranged in orderly manner (unlike skeletal muscle). Hence, smooth muscles do not show cross-striations.^{Viva}
- Smooth muscle cell contains *dense bodies* in the cytoplasm. The dense bodies are attached to sarcolemma through intermediate filaments (Fig. 10.16).
- Dense bodies give attachment to actin (thin) filaments.
- During contraction, actin filament slides over myosin filament and pull the adjacent dense bodies with sarcolemma closer to each other. Thus, it results in shortening of muscle cell.

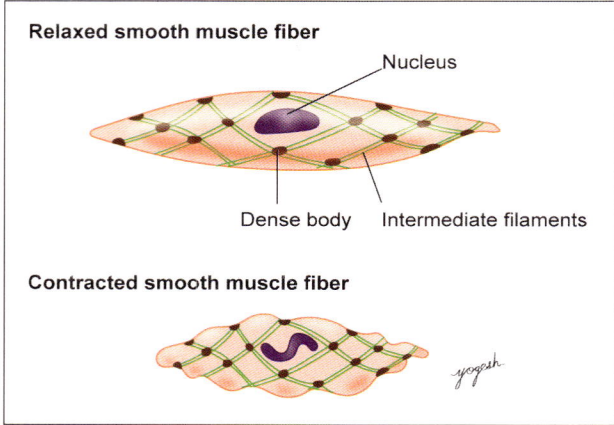

Fig. 10.16: Internal structure of smooth muscle cell. Dense bodies give attachment to actin filaments and dense bodies are attached with each other and with sarcolemma by intermediate filaments.

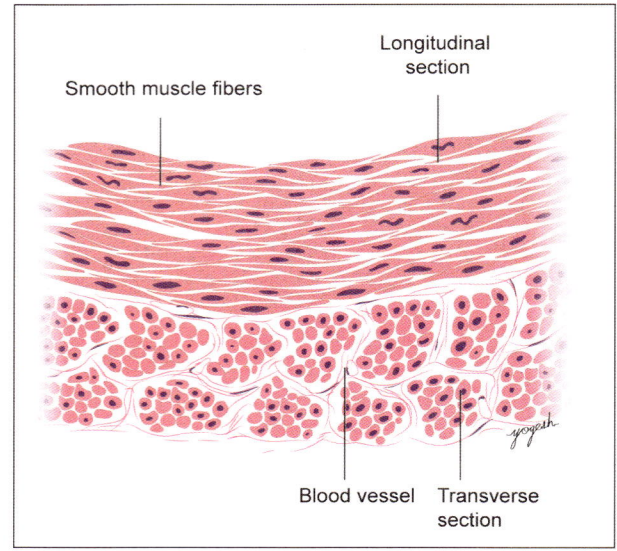

Fig. 10.17: Smooth muscle. In longitudinal muscle cells are elongated spindle shaped. The cytoplasm stains dark eosinophilic (pink) because of myofilaments. Nucleus is elongated, lightly stained with hematoxylin (violet). In transverse section, cells show centrally placed nuclei (practice figure).

Some Interesting Facts

- Smooth muscle produces slow and prolonged contraction.
- Smooth muscle cells produce extracellular matrix, type IV and type III collagen fibers. In blood vessels, smooth muscle cells produce elastic laminae.^{MCQ}
- Smooth muscle cells can divide and undergo hyperplasia (increased cell number). It can undergo hypertrophy (increased cell size).^{Viva}
- Special example of muscle cells:
  1. Vascular pericytes located within basal lamina of capillaries and post-capillary venules.
  2. Myofibroblast appears in healing wound.
  3. Myoepithelial cells in sweat gland, salivary glands, and mammary glands.
  4. Myoid cells in testis.
- Smooth muscle cells respond to hormones of adrenal medulla (adrenalin and noradrenalin) and posterior pituitary hormone (oxytocin).
- The differences between skeletal, cardiac and smooth muscles are listed in Table 10.2.

Q. List the differences between skeletal, cardiac and smooth muscles.

Table 10.2: Differences between skeletal, cardiac and smooth muscles

Characteristic feature	Skeletal muscle	Cardiac muscle	Smooth muscle
Muscle fiber	Very long, unbranched cylindrical	Small, branched cylindrical	Small, unbranched spindle shaped
Nuclei	Multinucleated, peripherally placed, flat	Single, centrally placed, oval	Single, centrally placed, elongated
Striations	Well defined cross-striations	Poorly defined cross-striations	Absent
Sarcoplasmic reticulum	Form triads	Form diads	Not well organized
T-tubules	Present at A-I junction	Present at Z lines	Absent
Cell junction	Absent	Intercalated discs	Gap junctions
Function	Voluntary	Involuntary	Involuntary
Innervations	Motor nerves	Autonomic nerves	Autonomic nerves
Mitosis	None	None (new concept: limited)	Present
Regeneration after injury	Limited	None	Present
Locations	Skeletal muscles, tongue, esophagus, diaphragm	Heart, superior and inferior vena cava, pulmonary veins	Vessels, tubular viscera, and organs

CHAPTER 11

Lymphoid Tissue

Chapter Outline
- Lymphatic tissue
- Cells of lymphoid system
  - Lymphocytes
  - Antigen-presenting cells
  - Reticular cells
- Lymph
- Lymphatic vessels
- Lymphatic nodule
- Lymph node
- Thymus
- Epithelioreticular cells
- Blood-thymic barrier
- Spleen
- Palatine tonsil

Competency achievement: The student should be able to:

AN43.2 Identify, describe and draw the microanatomy of tonsil.
AN70.2 Identify the lymphoid tissue under the microscope and describe microanatomy of lymph node, spleen, thymus, tonsil and correlate the structure with function

INTRODUCTION

- Lymphatic system provides protection to individuals by imparting immunity.
- *Immunity* is ability of organism to resist a particular infection or toxic substance with the help of antibodies or activated white blood cells.
- There are two types of immunity: Innate and acquired immunity (Flowchart 11.1).
  1. *Innate/native immunity* is present at birth. Innate immunity provides nonspecific protection against all type of infections.

Flowchart 11.1: Immunity

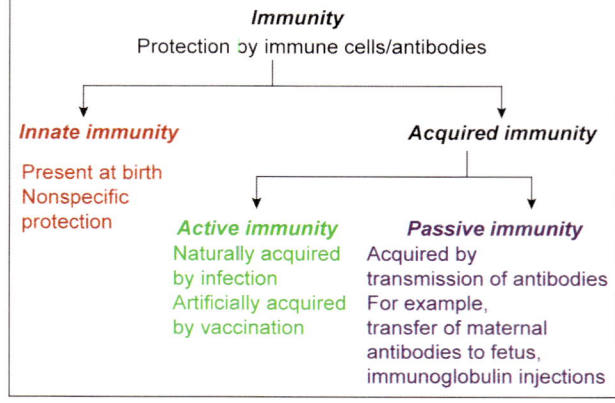

  2. *Acquired or adaptive immunity* is acquired by an individual throughout the life.
- Acquired immunity is of two types:^{Viva}
  A. *Active immunity:* It is acquired by an individual on exposure of antigenic agents, toxins or microorganisms. During exposure, immune cells get activated and impart acquired immunity.
  B. *Passive immunity:* It is acquired by an individual by the transfer of readymade antibodies (immunoglobulin injections).

LYMPHATIC TISSUE

Q. List the primary and secondary lymphoid organs.

- Lymphatic tissue is a specialized form of connective tissue that consists of immune cells (lymphocytes and plasma cells), meshwork of reticular fibers and cells.
- Lymphoid tissue identifies foreign antigens and dead/old cells of body and removes them by phagocytosis or by producing antibodies.
- Lymphoid organs are classified as primary and secondary lymphoid organs (Flowchart 11.2).

Primary Lymphoid Organs

- These are also called *central lymphoid organs.*
- These organs produce immature lymphocytes from stem cells or immature cells.
- For example, thymus, and bone marrow^{Neet}

Flowchart 11.2: Lymphoid organs[Neet]

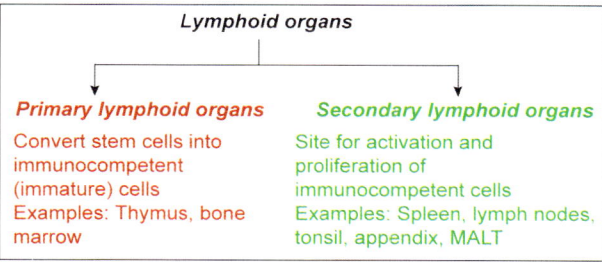

Secondary Lymphoid Organs

- These organs provide exposure to foreign antigen and convert immature lymphocytes into active lymphocytes.
- For example, spleen, lymph nodes, tonsils, appendix, and payer's patches
- Histologically lymphoid tissues are grouped as follows (Flowchart 11.3).
  A. Diffuse lymphoid tissue
  B. Dense lymphoid tissue

Diffuse Lymphoid Tissue

- Lymphocytes are distributed throughout mucosa of gastrointestinal tract, respiratory, urinary, and reproductive tracts. This type of lymphoid tissue is called *diffuse lymphoid tissue.*
- As this lymphoid tissue is associated with mucosa, it is also called *mucosa-associated lymphoid tissue* (MALT). Ileum is the most common site of MALT.[Neet]
- It protects and provides immunity against microorganisms coming in contact with mucosa.
- Diffuse lymphoid tissue is not enclosed within capsule.[Identification feature]
- Some authors consider MALT as a dense lymphoid tissue.

Dense Lymphoid Tissue

- Dense lymphoid tissue is enclosed by a well-defined capsule.[Identification feature]
- It includes discrete lymphoid organs such as lymph nodes, spleen, thymus, and tonsils.

CELLS OF LYMPHOID SYSTEM

Q. List the cells of lymphoid tissue.

- Lymphoid tissue consists of lymphocytes and other supporting cells such as reticular cells, epithelio-reticular cells.
- Some cells of immune system also form part of lymphoid system. They include monocytes, macrophages, neutrophils, basophils, dendritic cells, and so on (Flowchart 11.4).
- Differentiation of cells of lymphoid tissue depends on presence of specific molecules on their surface. These molecules are called *cluster of differentiation (CD)* molecules or markers.

Lymphocytes

- Lymphocyte is a subtype of white blood cells that forms a major component of lymphoid tissue.

Flowchart 11.3: Lymphoid tissue

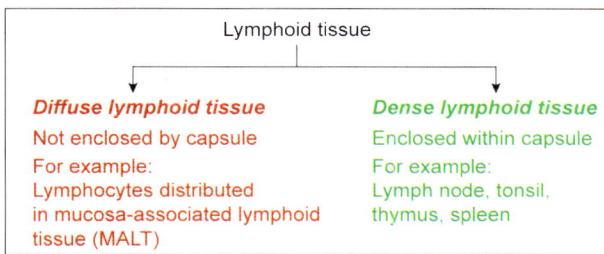

Flowchart 11.4: Cells of lymphoid system

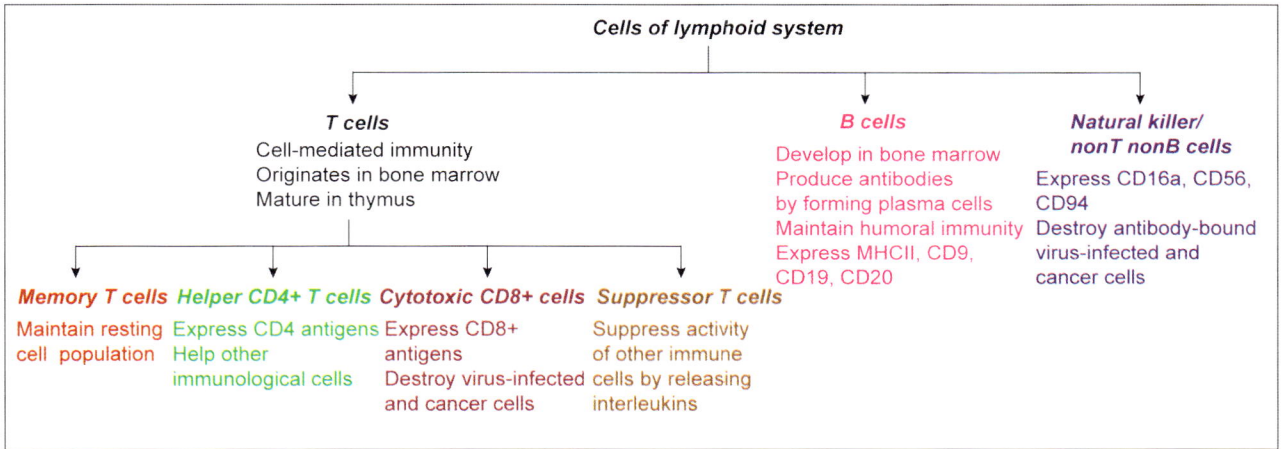

- They have a central round nucleus and thin rim of cytoplasm. Nucleus is densely stained (heterochromatic).*Identification feature*
- Size: Small lymphocytes: 7–10 μm and large lymphocytes: 14–20 μm. Histologically, lymphocytes cannot be differentiated into subtypes.
- Based on the presence of specific CD molecules, lymphocytes are grouped into three types: T lymphocytes, B lymphocytes, and natural killer (NK) cells.*MCQ*
- All lymphocytes originate from bone marrow. T lymphocytes also originate from bone marrow (Fig. 11.1).

T Lymphocytes (T Cells)

- Undifferentiated lymphocytes originate from bone marrow and enter thymus. In thymus, they get differentiated into mature T lymphocytes (Fig. 11.1).
- They maintain *cell-mediated immunity*.*Viva*
- T cells have a specific *T cell receptor* (TCR).
- TCR recognizes antigens bound to cell membrane proteins called *major histocompatibility complex* (MHC) molecules.
- Exposure of T cells to specific MHC molecules converts T cells into effector or memory T cells.
- *Memory T cell* maintains population of T cells that get easily activated on reinfection by the same microorganism. These cells persist for a long time.

- Effector T cells are grouped into three subtypes as follows (based on presence of specific CD antigen):
  1. *Helper T cell (T4 cells)/CD4+ T lymphocytes*
     - These cells have CD4 glycoprotein molecules on their surface.
     - These cells help other immunological cells, such as B cells, plasma cells, cytotoxic T cells for their activation and functions.
     - Helper T cells secrete interleukins for activation of other cells.
  2. *Cytotoxic T cells/CD8+ lymphocytes*
     - These cells have CD8 glycoprotein molecules on their surface.
     - CD8+ lymphocytes kill virus-infected cells, cancer cells, other cells infected with parasite, and transplanted cells.*Viva*
  3. *Suppressor/regulatory T cells*
     - These cells suppress immune response against foreign and self-antigens.

B Lymphocytes (B Cells)/Plasma Cells

- B lymphocytes were first recognized in the bursa of Fabricius in birds; hence, called B cells.
- In human, B cells originate from bone marrow (Fig. 11.1).
- They maintain *humoral immunity,* that is, immunity by antibodies.*Viva*
- *Antibodies* are immunoglobulins.
- B cells have membrane-bound *B cell receptors* on their surface.
- On activation, B cell differentiates into *plasma cells* or memory B cell. Plasma cell continues secretion of antibodies against specific antigens.*Viva*
- B cell marker includes CD9, CD19, and CD20.*MCQ*
- B cell expresses major histocompatibility complex II (MHCII) molecules on their surface.

Natural Killer Cells

- Natural killer cells (NK cells) are the variety of lymphocytes that are neither T nor B cells.
- NK cells originate from bone marrow.
- They constitute 5–10% of circulating lymphocytes.
- NK cells kill cancer cells and virus-infected cells similar to cytotoxic CD8+ T cells.
- Specific markers for NK cells are CD16a, CD56, and CD94.
- NK cells destroy antibody-bound cells. This is called *antibody-dependent cellular cytotoxicity* (ADCC).

Antigen-Presenting Cells

- Antigen-presenting cells (APC) present antigens with the help of MHCII molecules to helper CD4+ T cells.

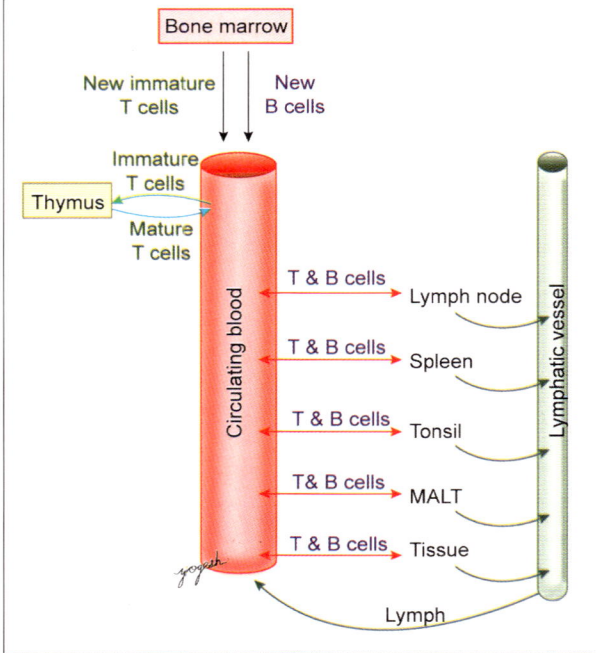

Fig. 11.1: Development and circulation of T and B cells (MALT, mucosa-associated lymphoid tissue).

- APC include macrophages, perisinusoidal Kupffer cells in liver, Langerhans's cells in epidermis, dendritic cells in spleen and lymph nodes, epithelio-reticular cells (type II or III) in thymus, and B lymphocytes.^MCQ
- APC process the antigen (digest the bacteria or foreign material in lysosomes) and display small peptides of digested antigen on the cell surface using MHC-II molecules.

Note: Mononuclear phagocytic system (MPS) and macrophages are described in Chapter 7.

Reticular Cells

- Reticular cells form the structural framework of reticular fibers in spleen, lymph node, and tonsil.
- These reticular cells secrete type III collagen/reticular fibers and ground substance.
- Reticular cells are elongated cells with long fine cell processes.

LYMPH

- Lymph is a fluid that flows through lymphatic vessels and lymph nodes.
- It is a pale fluid that is generated from transudate (extravascular fluid) and contains plasma proteins.
- Lymph also contains white blood cells, predominantly lymphocytes.
- Lymph also contains large fat molecules called *chylomicrons* that are absorbed from intestine. Such lymph containing large amount of fat molecules looks similar to milk; hence, it is also called *chyle*.
- Lymph may also contains cancerous cells, viruses, bacteria, and foreign material (dyes).

LYMPHATIC VESSELS

- Lymphatic vessels carry large molecules and excess extracellular fluid to main bloodstream. Lymphatic vessels include lymph capillaries, large lymphatic vessels, and thoracic duct.

Lymph Capillaries

- Lymph capillaries begin in tissue as blind-ended sacs.
- Similar to the endothelium of blood capillaries, lymphatic capillaries are lined by *lymphatic endothelium*.
- Lymphatic capillaries are more permeable than blood capillaries, thus they permit entry to absorbed larger lipid molecules in intestine.
- Most of the tissues have lymph capillaries.
- Lymph capillaries are **absent in** the following structures: Epidermis, cornea, cartilage, hair, nails, splenic pulp, bone narrow, choroid, internal ear, meninges, and nervous tissue.^Neet
- Most of the lymph capillaries carry lymph toward lymph nodes through *afferent lymph vessels*. Lymph leave the lymph nodes through *efferent lymph vessels*.

Larger Lymph Vessels

- Lymph capillaries join to form lymph vessels.
- Larger lymph vessels include thoracic duct, right lymphatic duct, jugular lymph trunk, subclavian trunk, broncho-mediastinal trunk, intestinal lymph trunks, and lumbar lymph trunks.
- Larger lymph vessels show tunica intima, media, and adventitia (similar to veins).
- Differences of lymphatic vessels from veins are as follows:
  – Elastic fibers are present in all layers of lymphatic vessel.
  – Circular smooth muscles are present in both tunica media and adventitia of lymphatic vessels.
  – In thoracic duct, smooth muscles are arranged longitudinally.^Viva

LYMPHATIC NODULE/FOLLICLE

- Lymphatic nodule/follicle is a well-circumscribed concentration of lymphatic cells.^Viva
- Lymphatic nodule is **not surrounded by capsule.**
- Lymphatic nodule is a spherical or ovoid mass.
- Lymphatic nodules are present in all dense lymphoid tissues **except thymus.**^Viva
- There are two types of lymphatic nodules: primary and secondary.^Viva.

Primary Nodules

- It shows uniform type of cells.
- Primary nodules are present before birth and get converted into secondary nodules on antigen exposure.

Secondary Nodules

- Secondary nodules do not show uniform type of cells.
- Secondary nodules show germinal center.^Viva
- *Germinal center* lies at center of lymphatic nodule. It contains large immature lymphocytes called *lymphoblasts* and *plasmoblasts*. Cells of germinal center are **lightly stained** and have larger nuclei.^Viva, Identification feature
- Germinal center is surrounded by small cells with dense nucleus (mature lymphocytes); this zone is called *corona* or mature zone.
- Germinal center also possesses *follicular dendritic cells* (FDCs) that help in proliferation of lymphocytes.

LYMPH NODE

- Lymph node is a small kidney-shaped structure that filters the lymph.
- Lymph node has convex surface and concave area (hilum) (Fig. 11.2).
- Each lymph node receives lymph through many *afferent lymphatic vessels*.
- Each lymph node has *efferent lymphatic vessels* through which filtered lymph leave through hilum.
- Lymph node receives blood vessels through hilum.

Histology of Lymph Node

- Section of a lymph node shows capsule, subcapsular sinus, outer cortex, paracortex, and medulla (Flowchart 11.5, Figs 11.3 and 11.4). *Viva*

Capsule

- Lymph node is covered by connective tissue capsule. It is made up of dense connective tissue.
- Trabeculae extend from capsule in the substance of lymph node.

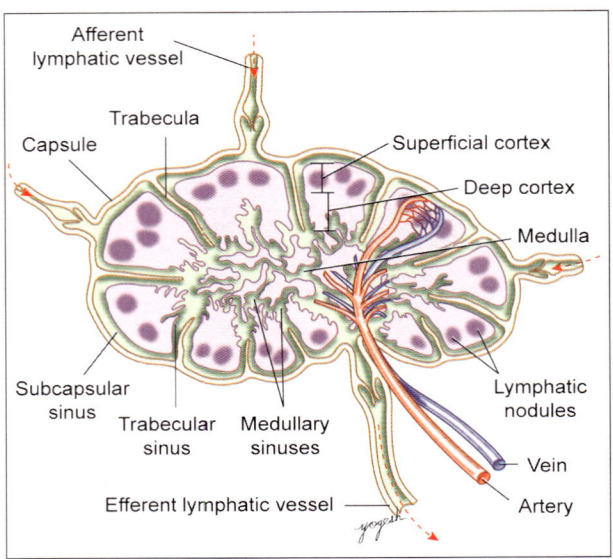

Fig. 11.2: Structure of the lymph node (sectional view).

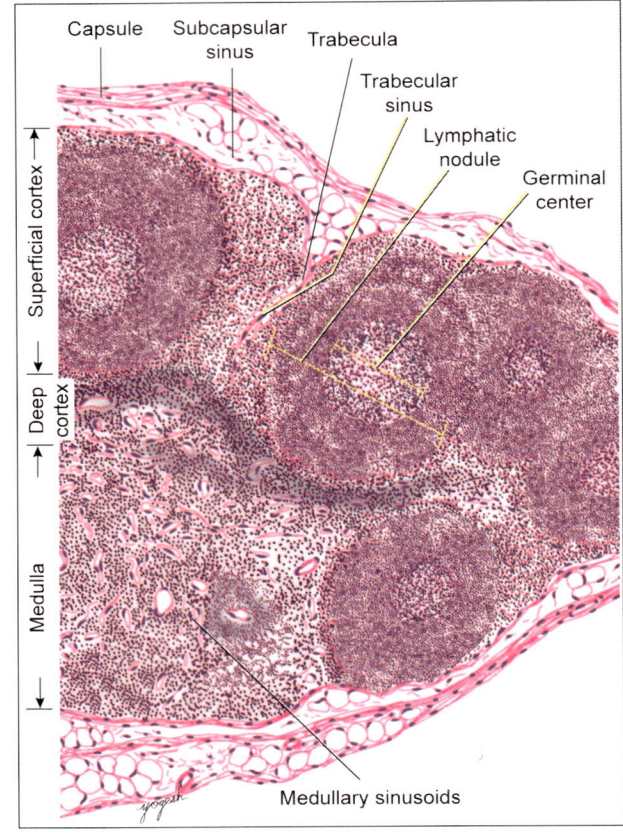

Fig. 11.3: Histology of lymph node (low magnification, practice figure).

Flowchart 11.5: Histology of lymph node

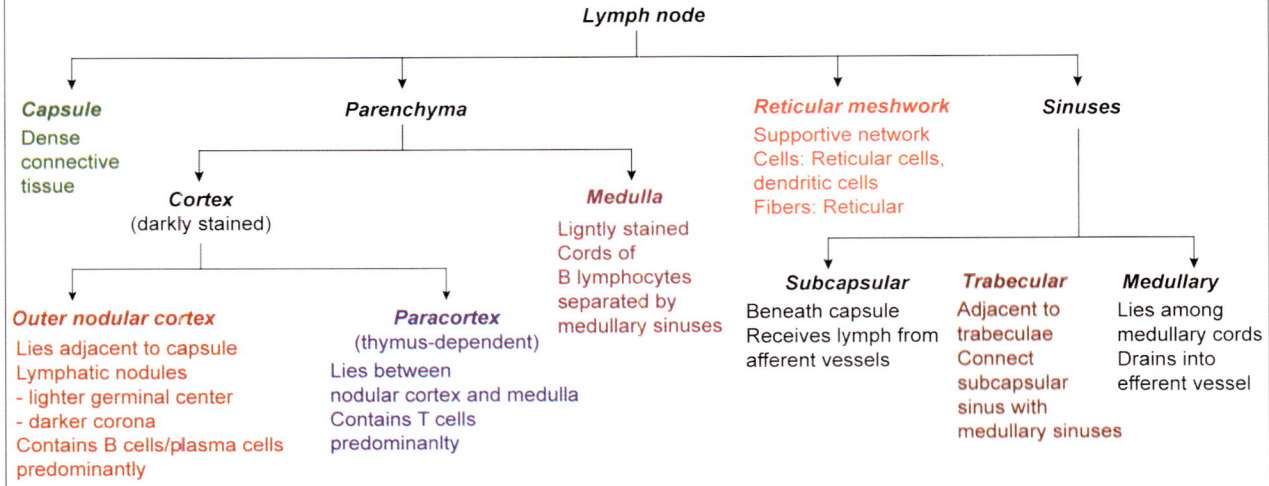

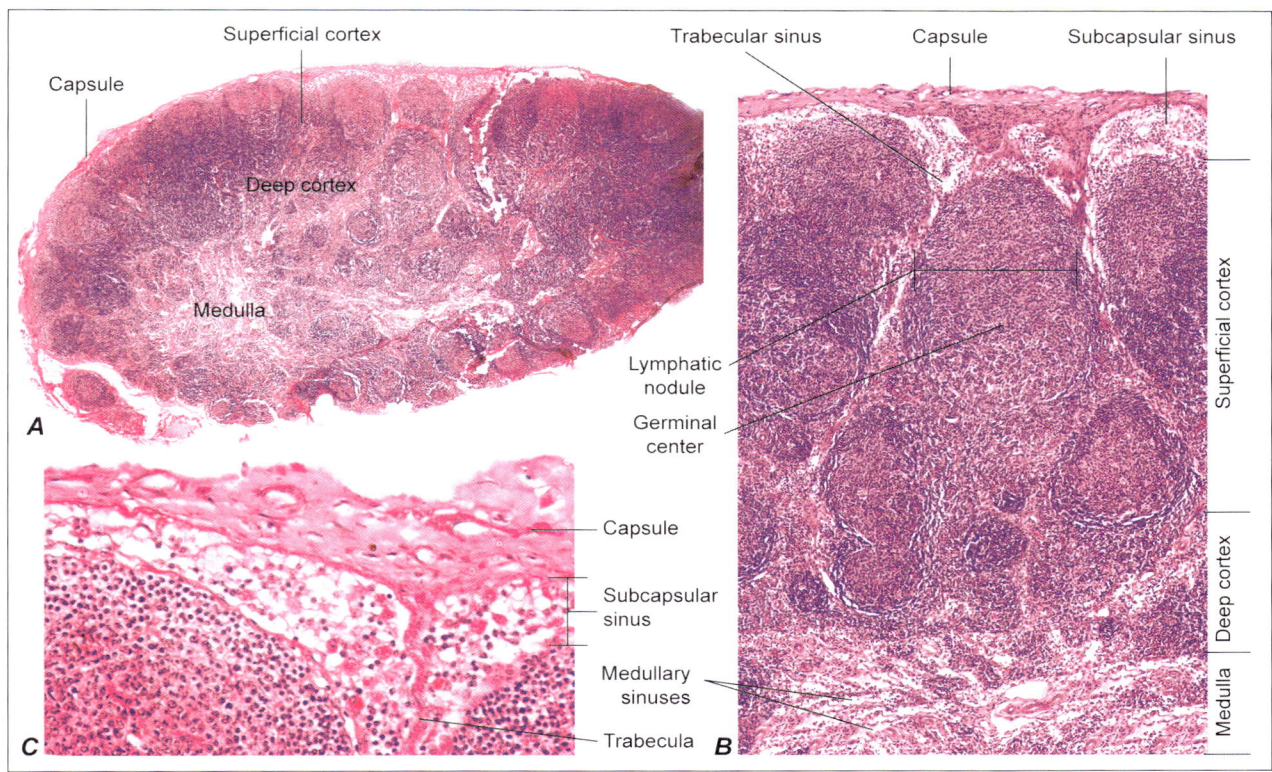

Fig. 11.4: Photomicrograph. Structure of the lymph node. (A) Panoramic view; (B) Low magnification; (C) High magnification showing subcapsular sinus (*H&E* stain).

- Reticular meshwork
  - Reticular tissue forms supporting meshwork.
  - Reticular tissue consists of reticular cells, *follicular dendritic cells*, macrophages, and reticular fibers.[Neet]
  - Reticular cells synthesize type III collagen/reticular fibers.
  - Reticular cells are elongated cells with fine cytoplasmic processes.
  - Dendritic cells are antigen-presenting cells that present antigens to T-cells.

Parenchyma of Lymph Node

- Parenchyma of lymph node shows:
  A. Outer darkly stained cortex
  B. Inner lightly stained medulla
- *Cortex*
  - It is darkly stained outer part of parenchyma.
  - It consists of
    1. *Superficial nodular cortex:* It shows presence of numerous lymphatic follicles.[Neet]
    2. *Deep cortex or paracortex:* It lies between nodular cortex and medulla.
  - Nodular cortex contains mainly B lymphocytes.[Neet]
  - Lymphatic nodules have central lightly stained germinal center and outer darkly stained corona or mantle zone. Germinal center is the zone of B cell proliferation.
  - Paracortex mainly consists of T cells; hence, it is also called *thymus-dependent cortex*.[Neet]

Sinuses of Lymph Node[Viva]

- There are the following three types of sinuses in lymph node:
  1. Subcapsular sinus/cortical sinus
     - Just beneath the capsule, a zone called subcapsular sinus is present.[Neet, Identification feature]
     - It receives lymph from afferent lymphatic vessels.
  2. Intermediate/trabecular sinuses
     - Trabecular sinuses are present adjacent to trabeculae.
     - Trabecular sinuses connect subcapsular sinus with medullary sinuses.
  3. Medullary sinuses
     - Medullary sinuses lie among the anastomosing medullary cords. They receive lymph from trabecular sinus and drain it into efferent lymph vessels.
- Sinuses are filled with reticular meshwork that helps in filtration of lymph, trapping of cellular debris and microorganisms, and antigen presentation to immune cells.

Medulla

- Medulla is an inner part of the lymph node. It consists of
  - Medullary cords: These are anastomosing cords of lymphocytes, macrophages, and plasma cells.
  - Medullary sinuses: These are spaces that separate adjacent medullary cords. They converge at hilum and form efferent lymphatic vessels.
  - Medullary cords mainly consist of *B cells*, in addition to plasma cells and macrophages.*Viva*

Circulation through Lymph Node*Viva*

- Lymph node receives lymph through afferent vessels (Fig. 11.5).
- Afferent vessels pour lymph into subcapsular sinus.
- This lymph enters trabecular sinus and finally medullary sinus.
- All medullary sinuses converge towards hilum and drain into efferent vessel that exits the lymph node through hilum.
- These sinuses are lined by endothelium and reticular cells.
- Arteries enter lymph node through hilum and form a capillary network in cortex and medulla. Veins leave lymph node through hilum.

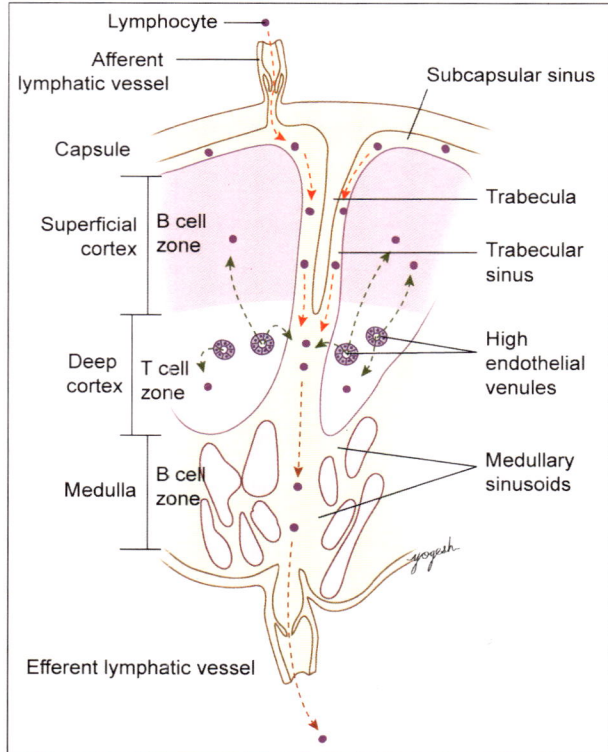

Fig. 11.5: Circulation of lymphocytes through lymph node and specific lymphocytes-dependent zones of lymph node.

Some Interesting Facts

- Lymphocytes enter lymph node from two sources:
  1. Through afferent lymphatic vessels
  2. High endothelial venules
- *High endothelial venules* are present in deep cortex (paracortex) of lymph node. These are postcapillary venules that are lined by cuboidal or columnar epithelium.
- Function of high endothelial venules:
  1. Provide channel for entry of T and B lymphocyte into lymph node
  2. Reabsorption of water from lymph
- Lymph nodes become palpable only after they get enlarged in infection or cancerous conditions.*Viva*

Functions of Lymph Node

1. Filtration of lymph
2. Presentation of antigens to T cells
3. Activation and proliferation of B cells
4. Conversion of B cells into plasma cells and production of antibodies

Thus, removal of bacteria, support of humoral and cell-mediated immunity are the major functions of lymph nodes.

Clinical Correlation

Lymphadenitis
- Inflammation of lymph node is called lymphadenitis.
- In lymphadenitis, lymph node becomes enlarged due to proliferation of lymphocytes.
- Causes: Infection, spread of cancer cells to lymph nodes (metastasis)
- Symptoms: Swollen, painful lymph nodes, and fever

Metastasis to lymph nodes
- Loose cancer cells from primary cancer lesion get trapped in lymph nodes. These cancer cells multiply in lymph node and form secondary cancer lesion.

Summary (Examination Guide) (Flowchart 11.5)

- Lymph node is covered by connective tissue capsule.
- Lymph node has darkly stained cortex and lightly stained medulla.
- Cortex is divided into
  I. Outer nodular cortex showing lymphatic nodules with B cells
  II. Thymus-dependent paracortex with T cells.
- Medulla consists of cords of B lymphocytes separated by anastomosing medullary sinuses.

Lymphoid Tissue

- Lymph node shows three sinuses:
  i. Subcapsular sinus lies beneath the capsule
  ii. Trabecular sinuses connect subcapsular sinus with medullary sinuses
  iii. Medullary sinuses drain into efferent vessels

THYMUS

- Thymus and bone marrow are primary lymphoid organs.
- Thymus or thymic gland is a bilobed structure located in the anterior part of superior mediastinum.
- Embryologically, thymus develops from *third pharyngeal pouch* and mesoderm contributes thymocytes and connective tissue.
- Thymus continues to grow from birth till puberty and then undergo gradual *atrophy* called *thymic involution*.*Viva*

Histology of Thymus

- Thymus has capsule, cortex, and medulla (Flowchart 11.6, Figs 11.6 to 11.8).

Capsule and Septa

- Thymus is covered by thin connective tissue capsule.
- Trabeculae/septa extend into parenchyma of thymus and divide it into incomplete thymic lobules. Each lobule consists of outer darker cortex and inner lighter medulla.*Identification feature*
- As septa are shorter (do not traverse through entire parenchyma), medulla of adjacent thymic lobules is continuous with each other.*Identification feature*
- Note: Do not get confused with lymphatic nodule (outer darker corona and inner lighter germinal center). Thymus do not have lymphatic nodules *Viva, Practical guide*

Cortex

- Cortex is a peripheral darker/basophilic zone of thymus.
- It contains closely packed T lymphocytes (thymocytes).
- Thymocytes are supported by meshwork of epithelioreticular cells.

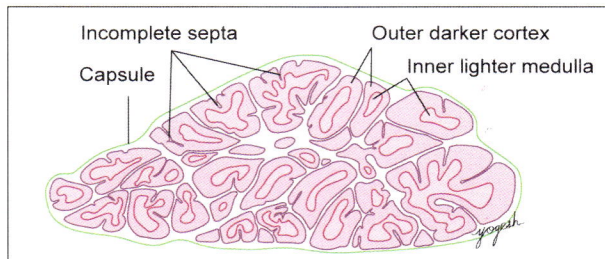

Fig. 11.6: Architecture of thymus.

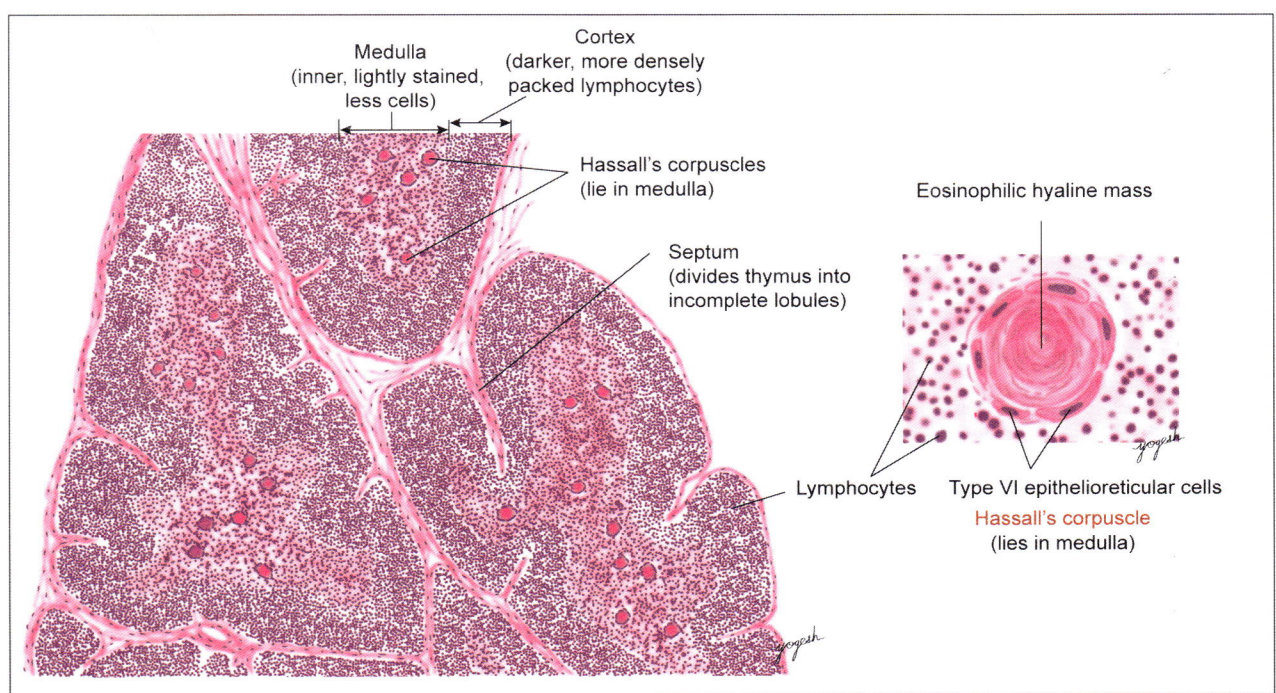

Fig. 11.7: Histology of thymus (low magnification on left, Hassall's corpuscle at high magnification on right, practice figure).

Flowchart 11.6: Histology of thymus

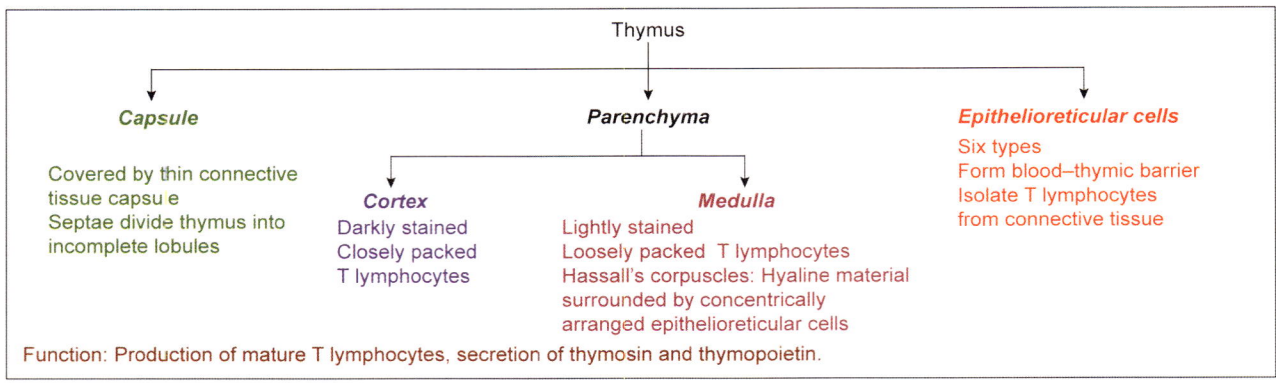

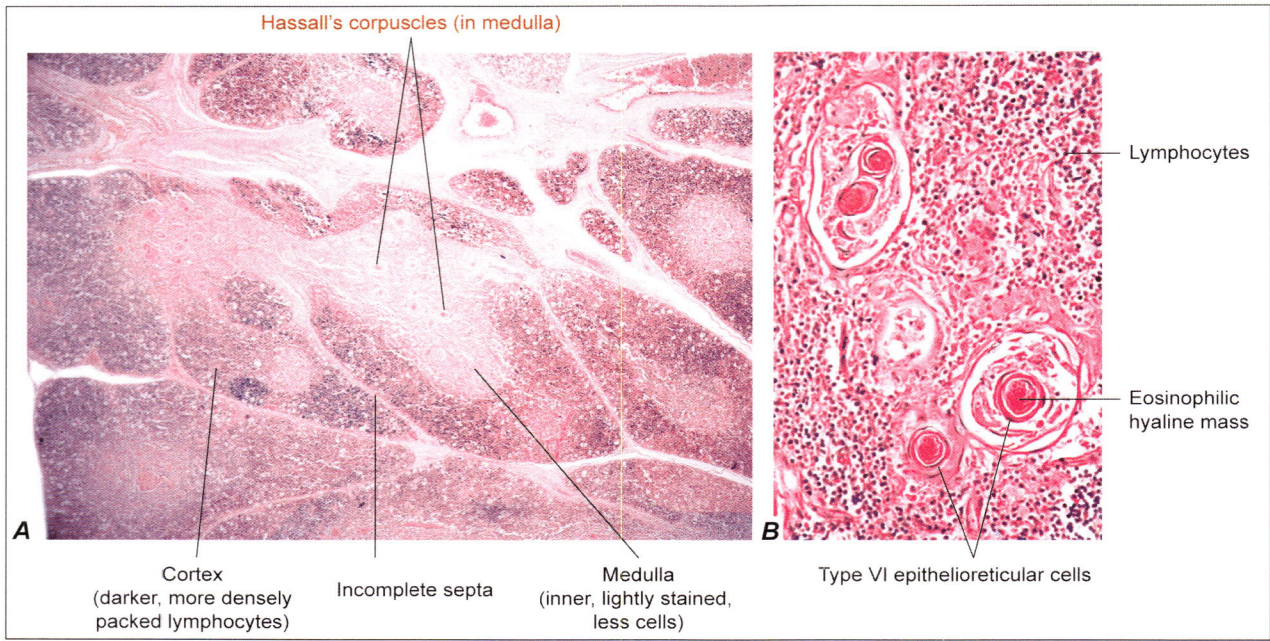

Fig. 11.8: Photomicrograph. Histology of thymus. (A) Low magnification. (B) Hassall's corpuscles at high magnification (*H&E* staining).

- These *epithelicreticular cells/epitheliocytes* are derived from third *pharyngeal pouch*.^{Neet}
- Cortex also contains few macrophages that phagocytose degenerating lymphocytes.

Medulla

- Medulla is an inner lighter zone of thymus.
- Medulla of each thymic lobule is continuous with medulla of adjacent lobules.
- Medulla has less density of thymocytes; hence it is lightly stained.^{Identification feature, Viva}
- Medulla also contains epithelioreticulocytes in addition to thymocytes.
- Unique feature of thymic medulla is *Hassall's corpuscles*.^{Identification feature, Viva}

Hassall's/Thymic Corpuscles^{Viva, Neet}

- These are small rounded or ovoid structures present in medulla.
- It consists of eosinophilic hyaline mass at the center that is surrounded by concentrically arranged type VI epithelioreticular cells.^{Neet}
- Hassall's corpuscle represents degenerating thymocytes and their number increases with age.^{Neet}
- Type VI epithelioreticular cells secrete IL-4 and IL-6 that help in thymocyte maturation.
- Thymic corpuscles produce thymosin and thymopoietin hormones.
- Immature thymocytes mature in cortex and migrate to medulla; finally mature thymocytes leave thymic medulla and enter systemic circulation.

> **Box 11.1: Epithelioreticular cells**
>
> - Epithelioreticular cells/*epitheliocytes* form supporting meshwork in thymus.^{Viva}
> - These cells are derived from third pharyngeal pouch.
> - These cells are also called *nurse cells* as they provide required microenvironment for the differentiation and maturation of T cells.^{Viva}
> - There are six types of epithelioreticular cells in thymus.^{Viva}
> - They are numbered as type I, type II, ..., type VI
> - First three types are present in thymic cortex, whereas last three types are found in thymic medulla.
>
> Type I: They isolate lymphocytes from connective tissue capsule, trabeculae, and blood vessels. These cells are connected with each other by occluding junctions.
>
> Type II: These cells create an isolated compartment for developing T cells and educate T cells.
>
> Type III: These cells create a functional barrier between cortex and medulla.
>
> Type IV: These cells are located adjacent to type III cells. Along with type III cells, they form corticomedullary junction.
>
> Type V: These cells form a cellular framework in medulla.
>
> Type VI: These cells form concentric layers in Hassall's corpuscles. These cells secrete IL-4 and IL-6 that help in thymocyte maturation. Thymic corpuscles produce thymosin and thymopoietin hormones.

Functions of Thymus

1. Education and maturation of T lymphocytes.
2. To provide isolated environment for T lymphocyte maturation.
3. Secretion of thymopoietin by epithelioreticular cells.
4. Thymopoietin stimulates T cell production.
5. Thymus is essential for development of immunity in early life. After puberty, thymus gets atrophied.

Blood–Thymic Barrier^{Viva}

- Immature T lymphocytes mature in thymus in an isolated environment (Fig. 11.9).
- They are prevented from exposure to antigens by blood–thymic barrier.
- Components: Blood–thymic barrier has the following components:^{Viva}
  1. Capillary endothelium with basal lamina and few pericytes
  2. Perivascular connective tissue with few macrophages
  3. Type I epithelioreticular cells^{Neet}

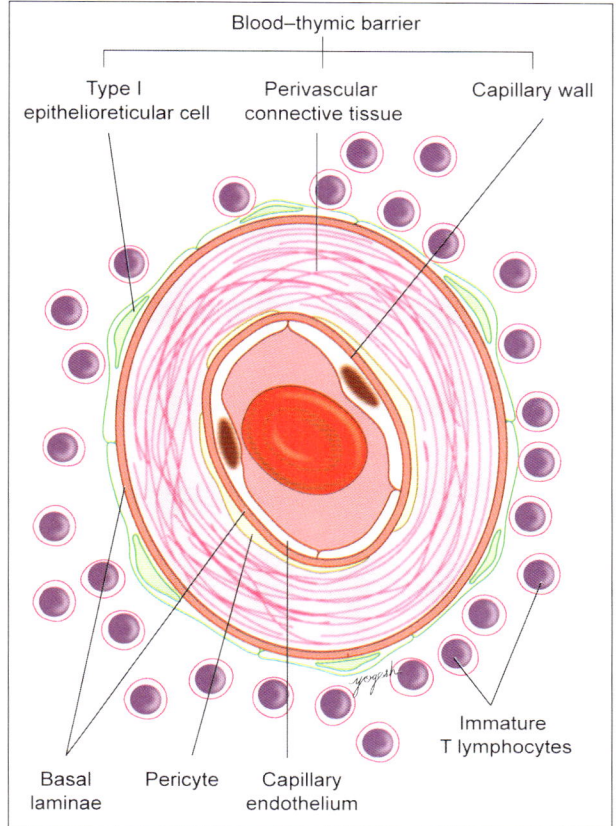

Fig. 11.9: Blood–thymic barrier.

- Cells of capillary endothelium and type I epithelioreticular cells show occluding junctions.
- Blood–thymic barrier isolates T cells from circulating blood and antigens in it.

> **Clinical Correlation**
>
> *Myasthenia gravis*^{Viva}
> - It is a rare autoimmune disease.
> - It is associated in 70% cases of *thymoma* (tumor of epithelioreticular cells).
> - In myasthenia gravis, antibodies slowly destroy cholinergic receptors from skeletal muscle and cause weakness of muscles. It results in double vision (eye muscles), dropping of eyelid, dysarthria (muscles of throat), and so on.
>
> *DiGeorge syndrome*
> - It is *22q11.2 deletion syndrome* caused by deletion of segment of chromosome 22.^{MCQ}
> - It is characterized by *absence of thymus* and parathyroid glands.
> - Patient does not have T lymphocytes; hence, there is no cell-mediated immunity.^{Viva, Neet}

- Patient usually dies at an early age because of infections.
- Absence of parathyroid gland may produce tetany.
- These patients may also have congenital heart defects, cleft palate, and developmental delay.

Summary (Examination Guide) (Flowchart 11.6)

Q. Write a short note on histology of thymus.
- Thymus is surrounded by a thin connective tissue capsule.
- Thymus is divided into number of incomplete lobules by septa arising from capsule.
- Thymus has outer darkly stained cortex and inner lightly stained medulla.
- Medulla of adjacent lobules is continuous with each other.
- Medulla shows Hassall's corpuscles: A central pink hyalinized material surrounded by type VI epithelioreticular cells.
- Epithelioreticular cells (type I-VI): Form meshwork, form blood–thymic barrier, and secrete thymosin and thymopoietin.

SPLEEN

Q. Write a short note on histology of spleen.
- Spleen is the largest lymphoid organ.
- Spleen filters blood and helps to remove old RBCs and maintain immunity.
- Spleen is located in upper part of abdomen.
- It has lateral diaphragmatic surface and medial visceral surface.
- Visceral surface has hilum. Through hilum, splenic vessels enter spleen.

Gross Section of Spleen
- A slice of fresh spleen specimen shows while pulp and red pulp.
- *White pulp* is grayish white areas that are scattered throughout substance of the spleen.
- *Red pulp* surrounds the white pulp.
- Microscopically, it is observed that white pulp shows aggregation of lymphocytes and looks basophilic (blue) on *H&E* staining. Red pulp shows presence of many blood-filled (RBCs) sinusoids.

Histology of Spleen
- Histologically, spleen shows capsule, white pulp and red pulp (Flowchart 11.7, Figs 11.10 and 11.11).^(Viva, Identification feature)
- Spleen does not have afferent lymphatics.^(Viva, MCQ)

Capsule and Trabeculae
- Spleen is covered by a dense connective tissue *capsule*.
- *Trabeculae* arise from capsule and enter into the parenchyma of spleen.
- Trabeculae divide repeatedly.
- *Reticular cells* and reticular fibers form a meshwork in spleen.
- Connective tissue of spleen also contains *myofibroblasts* that contract the capsule and trabeculae and helps to discharge stored blood from the spleen.^(Viva)

White Pulp
- Based on the color of fresh section, parenchyma of spleen has two regions–white pulp and red pulp.
- White pulp consists of lymphoid tissue.^(Viva)

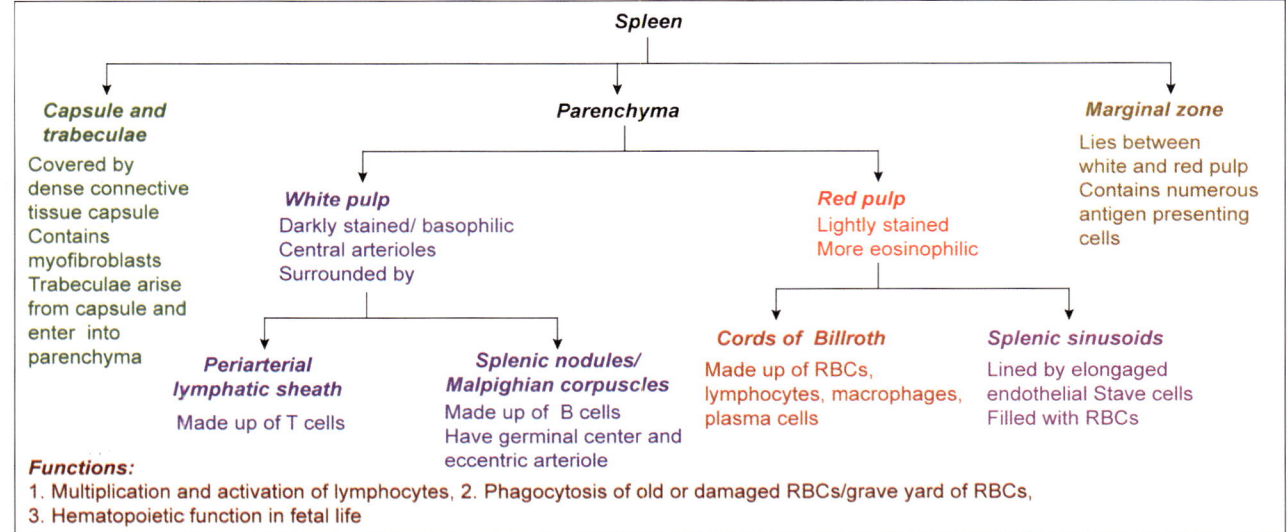

Flowchart 11.7: Histology of spleen

Lymphoid Tissue

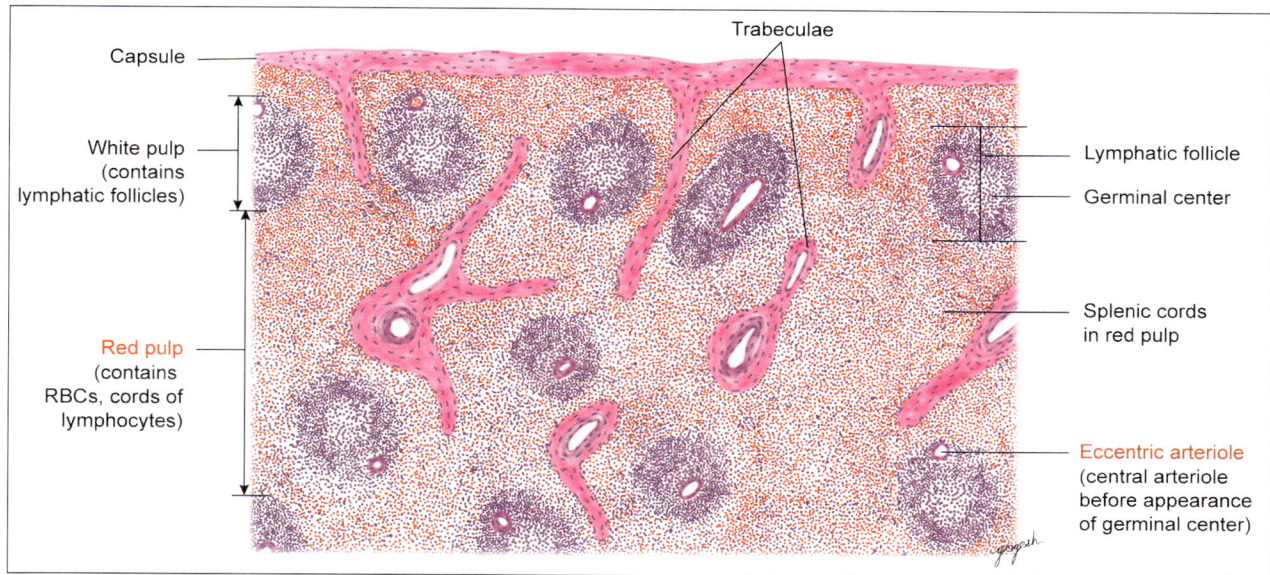

Fig. 11.10: Histology of spleen (low magnification, practice figure).

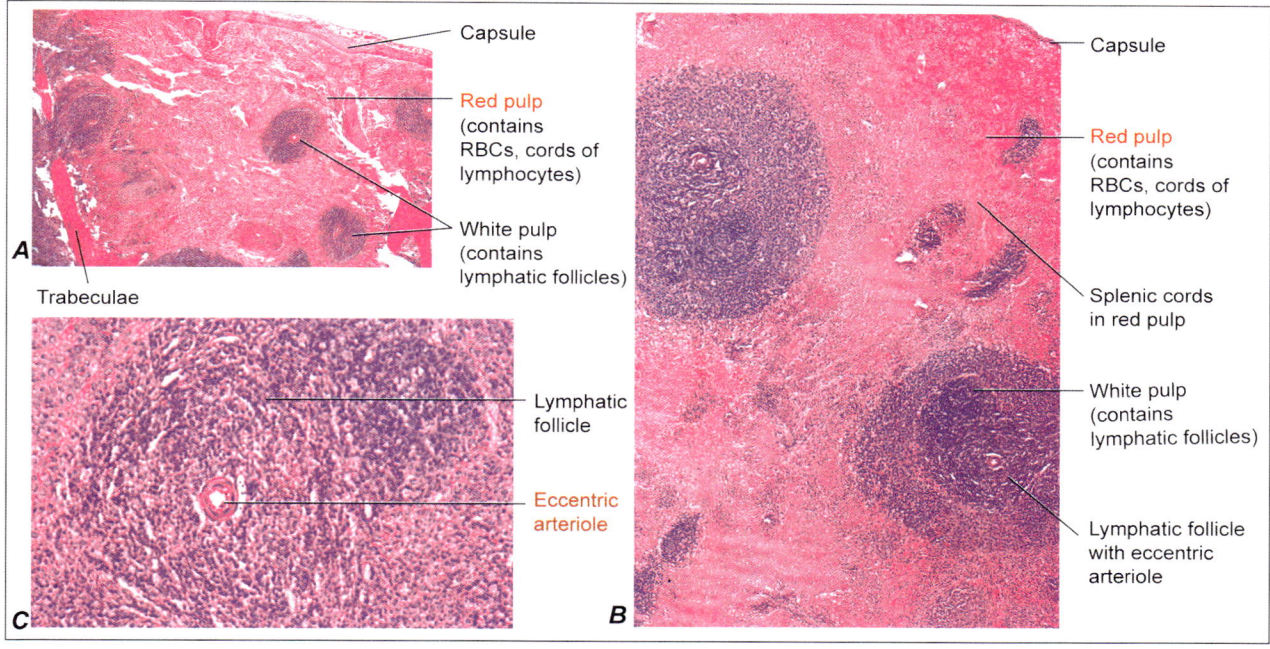

Fig. 11.11: Photomicrograph. Histology of spleen. (A) Low magnification, (B) High magnification, (C) Eccentric arteriole at X1000 magnification (H&E stain).

- Trabecular branches of splenic artery give rise to *central arterioles* that enter into parenchyma of spleen. *Viva*
- White pulp forms sheaths of lymphoid tissue surrounding central arterioles. These are called *periarterial lymphatic sheaths* (PALS).
- PALS are cylindrical masses that runs along the long axis of central artery.
- In cross section, PALS looks like a mass of lymphoid tissue surrounding central artery. *Identification feature*
- PALS contains T cells; hence, form thymus-dependent zone of spleen.
- *Splenic nodule/Malpighian corpuscles:* At some places, B cells proliferate in PALS on exposure of antigen and develops germinal center. Such nodules are called splenic nodules or Malpighian corpuscles. They have *eccentric arteriole* (central arteriole pushed to one side) because of formation of germinal centers.

Red Pulp

- White pulp is surrounded by red pulp.
- Red pulp forms a major part of the splenic parenchyma.
- Red pulp consists of two components
  1. Cords of Billroth
  2. Sinusoids[Viva]
- *Cords of Billroth:* (Christian Billroth, 1829–94, Austrian surgeon)
  - Cords of Billroth or splenic cords are irregular anastomosing cords.[Neet]
  - Splenic cords are made up of reticular cells, reticular fibers, lymphocytes, macrophages, plasma cells, and large number of RBCs.
- *Splenic sinusoids*[Neet]
  - Cords of Billroth are separated by splenic sinusoids.
  - Splenic sinusoids have wide lumen.
  - Splenic sinusoids are lined by elongated endothelial cells that lie parallel to the longitudinal axis of sinusoids. Basal laminae of sinusoids are discontinuous.
- Adjacent endothelial cells are separated by larger intercellular space that allows blood cells to pass through.
- Wall of splenic sinusoids does not have pericytes or smooth muscle cells.
- As red blood cells are present within sinusoids as well as in splenic cords, it is difficult to distinguish splenic sinusoids.

Marginal Zone

- The zone of red pulp that lies immediately surrounding the white pulp is called marginal zone.
- It consists of reticular or network of blood sinusoids, lymphocytes, numerous *antigen presenting cells, and macrophages.*[MCQ]
- Function of marginal zone: Antigen presenting cells bring circulating antigens in contact with lymphocytes in spleen and induce required immune response.

Splenic Circulation

- *Splenic artery* enters spleen through hilum.
- Splenic artery divides to form *trabecular arteries* that run in splenic trabeculae.
- Trabecular arteries give rise to numerous *central arterioles* (Fig. 11.12).
- Central arterioles run through sleeves of while pulp (PALS).[MCQ]
- Central arteriole finally enters the red pulp and divide into numerous *penicillar arterioles* that follows straight course.

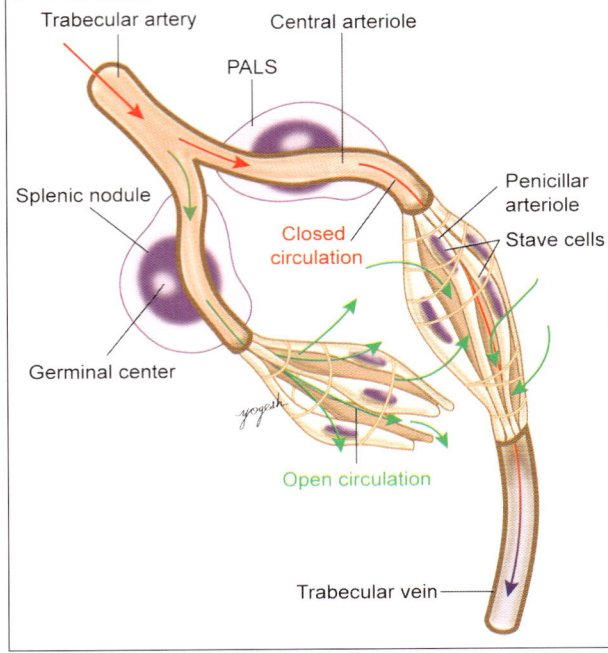

Fig. 11.12: Splenic circulation.

- Penicillar arterioles continue as *sheathed capillaries/ellipsoids.*[Neet] These sheathed capillaries are surrounded by macrophages.
- There are two concepts of splenic circulation:[Viva]
  1. *Open circulation:* Sheathed capillaries open into red pulp and blood passes through cords of red pulp and finally enter into splenic sinusoids.
  2. *Closed circulation:* Capillaries open directly into splenic sinusoids.
- Note: In humans, only open circulation is present in spleen; whereas, in dogs and rats, closed circulation is present.[Viva]
- *Splenic sinusoid* drains the blood into *trabecular veins.*
- Trabecular veins join to form *splenic vein*.
- Splenic sinusoids are lined by elongated (banana-shaped) endothelial cells called *stave cells*.[Neet,Viva] Cytoplasmic fibrils of stave cells help in opening and closeing intercellular gaps, and thus plays a major role in trapping of aged/damaged RBCs.[Neet]

Functions of Spleen[Viva]

Spleen performs immune system functions as well as hematopoietic functions as follows:
1. Spleen activates lymphocytes by using antigen presenting cells and induces immune response.
2. Spleen is the site for proliferation of T and B lymphocytes.
3. Spleen helps in the destruction of old and damaged RBCs and platelets.[MCQ]

4. In embryonic life, spleen acts as the hematopoietic organ.^MCQ
5. Spleen stores small quantity of blood.

Clinical Correlation
Splenomegaly
- Splenomegaly is the enlargement of spleen.
- Causes: It occurs because of immunological or hematological causes such as:
  - Abnormal RBCs (thalassemia, sickle cell anemia)
  - Immune disorders and infections (malarial infection, splenic abscess, typhoid fever, rheumatoid arthritis)
  - Cancerous conditions (leukemia)
  - Obstruction to venous blood (cirrhosis of liver, obstruction of portal vein)

Splenectomy
- It is surgical removal of spleen.
- Indications: Injury to spleen, cancerous conditions (leukemia), severe hemolytic anemias, and so on.
- Patients after splenectomy do not respond properly to the infections.^Viva

Summary (Examination Guide)
- Spleen is covered by dense connective tissue capsule that sends trabeculae into the parenchyma of spleen (Flowchart 11.7).

Spleen shows:
- *White pulp:* It consists of central arterioles surrounded by periarterial lymphatic sheaths of T lymphocytes
- *Splenic nodules/Malpighian corpuscles* consist of B cells aggregates with germinal center around eccentric arterioles.
- *Red pulp:* It consists of cords of Billroth (made up of RBCs, lymphocytes, macrophages, and plasma cells).
- Red pulp has sinusoids that are lined by elongated Stave cells (endothelial cells).
- *Marginal zone* lies between red and white pulp and contains numerous antigen presenting cells.

PALATINE TONSIL

Q. Write a short note on histology of tonsil.
- Tonsils are collection of lymphoid tissue near the junction of oral and nasal cavity with pharynx.
- Aggregation of tonsils forms Waldeyer tonsillar ring [Heinrich von Waldeyer, 1836–1921, German anatomists].
- Waldeyer ring includes pharyngeal tonsil, tubal tonsil, palatine tonsil, and lingual tonsil (Fig. 11.13).
- Palatine tonsil is the largest tonsil in the group of tonsils.

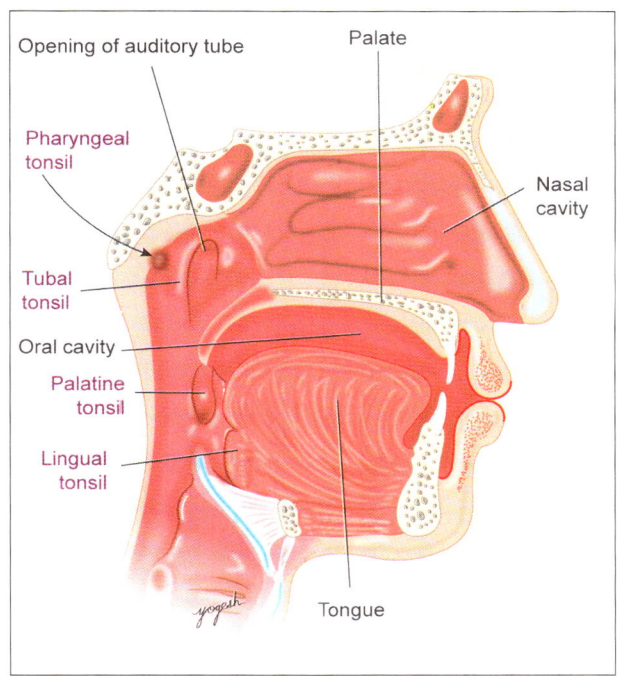

Fig. 11.13: Tonsils forming Waldeyer ring.

- Palatine tonsil (commonly called tonsils) are located on either side of oropharyngeal isthmus between palatoglossal arch and palatophargyngeal arches of soft palate.
- Tonsils form a part of *mucosa-associated lymphoid tissue* (MALT).

Histology of Palatine Tonsil
- A section of palatine tonsil shows (Flowchart 11.8, Figs 11.14 to 11.16):
  1. Lining epithelium

Flowchart 11.8: Histology of palatine tonsil

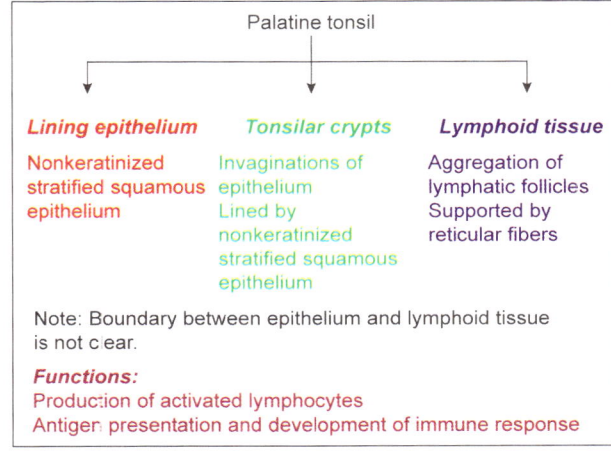

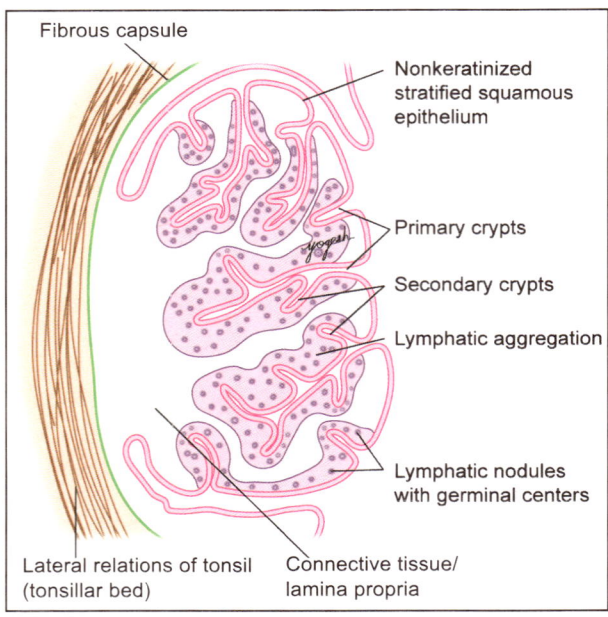

Fig. 11.14: Cross section of palatine tonsil.

2. Tonsillar crypts
3. Lymphatic follicles

- *Lining epithelium:* Oral surface of the palatine tonsil is covered by *nonkeratinized stratified squamous epithelium.* *Neet, Identification feature*
- *Tonsillar crypts:* The epithelium invaginates internal surface of tonsil and forms tonsillar crypts. *Identification feature,Viva*
- Tonsillar crypts are lined by nonkeratinized stratified squamous epithelium. Epithelium and even lumen of crypts may show invaginated lymphocytes.
- Note: It is difficult to find boundary between epithelium and lymphoid tissue.
- Laterally, tonsil is bounded by connective tissue *capsule* and has some efferent lymphatic vessels.
- *Lymphoid tissue:* Just beneath epithelium, palatine tonsil shows dense aggregation of lymphatic follicles. Lymphatic follicles are supported by meshwork of reticular fibers.

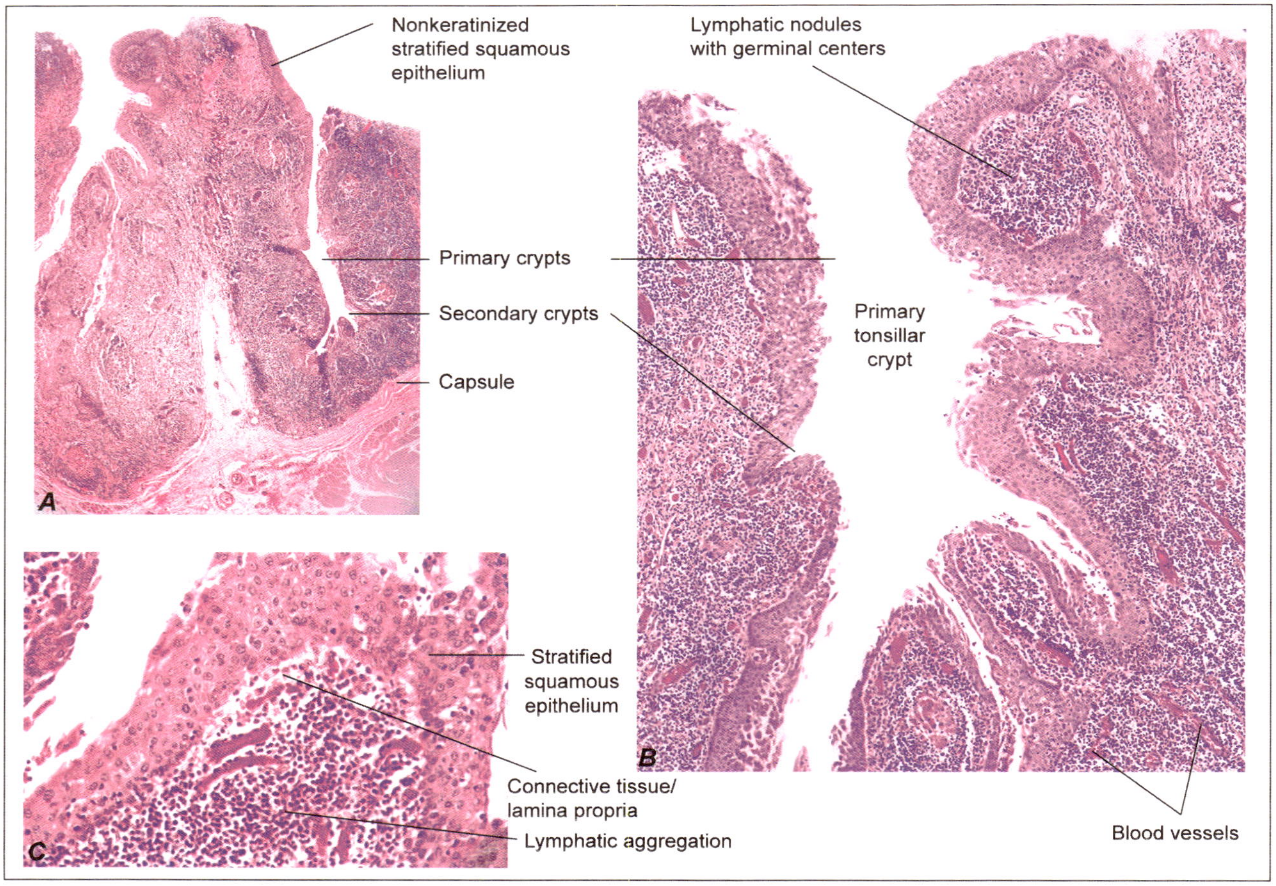

Fig. 11.15: Photomicrograph. Histology of palatine tonsil. (A) Low magnification, (B) High magnification, (C) Tonsillar crypt lined by stratified squamous epithelium.

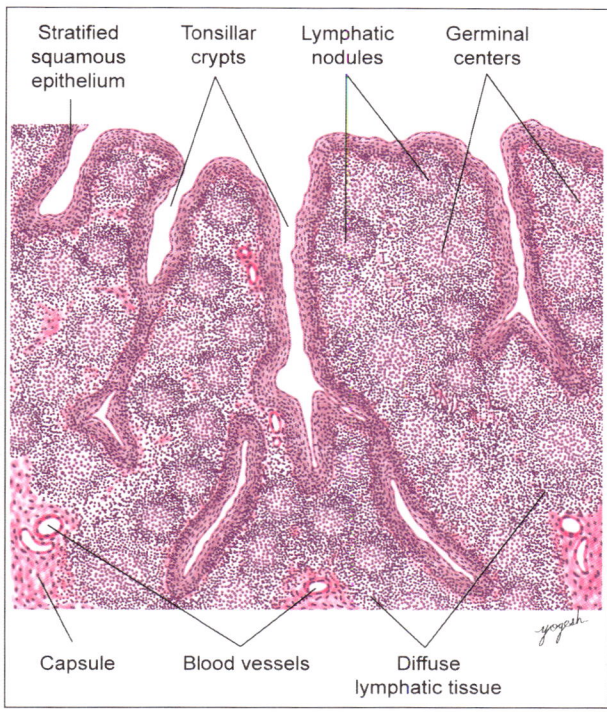

Fig. 11.16: Histology of palatine tonsil (practice figure).

Functions of Tonsil

1. Production of lymphocytes.
2. Antigen presentation and development of immune response.

Clinical Correlation

Tonsillitis
- It is an inflammation of tonsil.
- It is caused by viral or bacterial infections.

Tonsillectomy
- Surgical removal of tonsil is tonsillectomy.
- It is usually required in children who have recurrent tonsillitis (repeated infections).

Salivary corpuscles
- In palatine tonsil, few lymphocytes and desquamated epithelial cells mix with the saliva to form salivary corpuscles. *Viva*

CHAPTER 12

Nervous Tissue

Chapter Outline
- Neuron
- Classification of neurons
- Neuroglia
- Myelin sheath
- Synapse
- Peripheral nerve
- Ganglion

Competency achievement: The student should be able to:
- **AN68.1** Describe and identify multipolar and unipolar neuron, ganglia, peripheral nerve
- **AN68.2** Describe the structure-function correlation of neuron
- **AN68.3** Describe the ultrastructure of nervous tissue

INTRODUCTION

- Nervous tissue is a specialized tissue that shows property of irritability and conductivity. Because of these properties, nervous tissue can receive information about external and internal environment and transmit it to another tissue.
- Anatomically, nervous system is divided into central nervous system and peripheral nervous system (Flowchart 12.1).
- *Central nervous system* (CNS) includes brain and spinal cord (Chapter 6).
- *Peripheral nervous system* (PNS) includes cranial, spinal, and peripheral nerves and ganglia.
- A collection of nerve cell bodies outside the central nervous system is called *ganglia*.
- Functionally, nervous system is divided into somatic and autonomic nervous system.
- Somatic nervous system is under conscious control, whereas *autonomic nervous system* works involuntarily.
- Autonomic nervous system is divided into two components: Sympathetic and parasympathetic nervous system.
- Autonomic nervous system controls smooth muscles, cardiac muscles, and glandular epithelium (for secretions).

Constituents of Nervous Tissue

- Nervous tissue consists of two components: Neurons and neuroglia.

- *Neuron* (nerve cell) is the structural and functional unit of the nervous system. It has body and processes (axon and dendrites).*Viva*
- Supporting cells (neuroglial cells) are not involved in impulse transfer (nerve conduction). These are only supportive cells. They are ependymal cells, astrocytes, oligodendrocytes and microglia in CNS and Schwann cells, and satellite cells in PNS.*Neet*
- Neuroglial cells also maintain blood–brain barriers.

Flowchart 12.1: Classification of nervous system

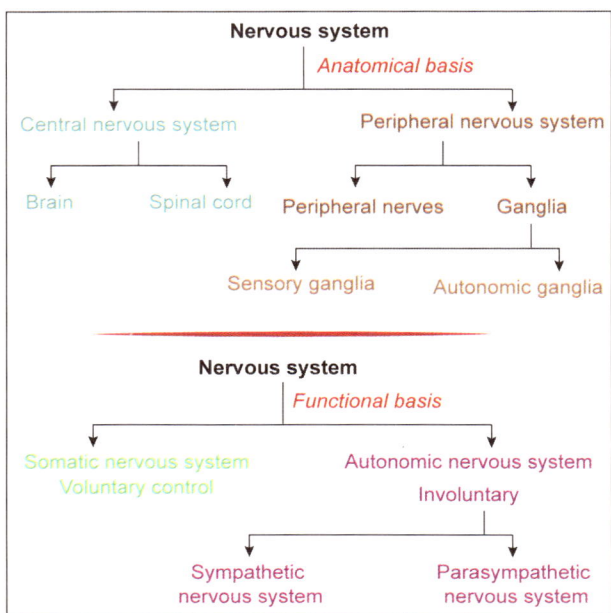

NEURON

- Neuron is the structural and functional unit of nervous system.
- Human nervous system has more than 10 billion neurons.
- Neurons are grouped as sensory neurons (carries information toward nervous system), motor neurons (carries information away from nervous system), and interneurons (communicates information from sensory to motor neurons).
- More than 99% neurons are interneurons (intercalated neurons).

Structure of Neuron

- Neuron has body, axon, dendrites, and synaptic junctions (Fig. 12.1).

Body/Perikaryon

- Cell body of neuron is also called perikaryon or soma.
- It consists of nucleus, perinuclear cytoplasm, and cell membrane.

Cytoplasm

- Cytoplasm contains a large central vesicular nucleus, numerous mitochondria, rough endoplasmic reticulum, and Golgi complex.
- Nucleus is euchromatic (lightly stained) with 1–2 nucleoli.
- **New concept:** Neurons have centrioles, but they cannot divide.^Viva (Previous concept: Neurons do not have centrioles).
- Cytoplasm shows presence of *Nissl bodies*.

Nissl bodies/substance/granules:^Viva

- Cytoplasm of neurons shows presence of granular *basophilic* cytoplasmic material (blue colored on *H&E staining*) called Nissl bodies.^Neet,Viva
- On electron microscopy, Nissl bodies are stacks of rough endoplasmic reticulum.^Viva, MCQ
- Neuron contains many *neurofibrils* (microtubules and microfilaments). Centrioles may help in the production of neurofibrils.^Viva
- Some of the neurons also contain melanin pigment (substantia nigra) and lipofuscin pigments.^MCQ

Neurites

- Processes arising from cell body of a neuron are called *neurites*. They are axons and dendrites.

Dendrites

- Dendrites are multiple, short, thick, tapering processes.

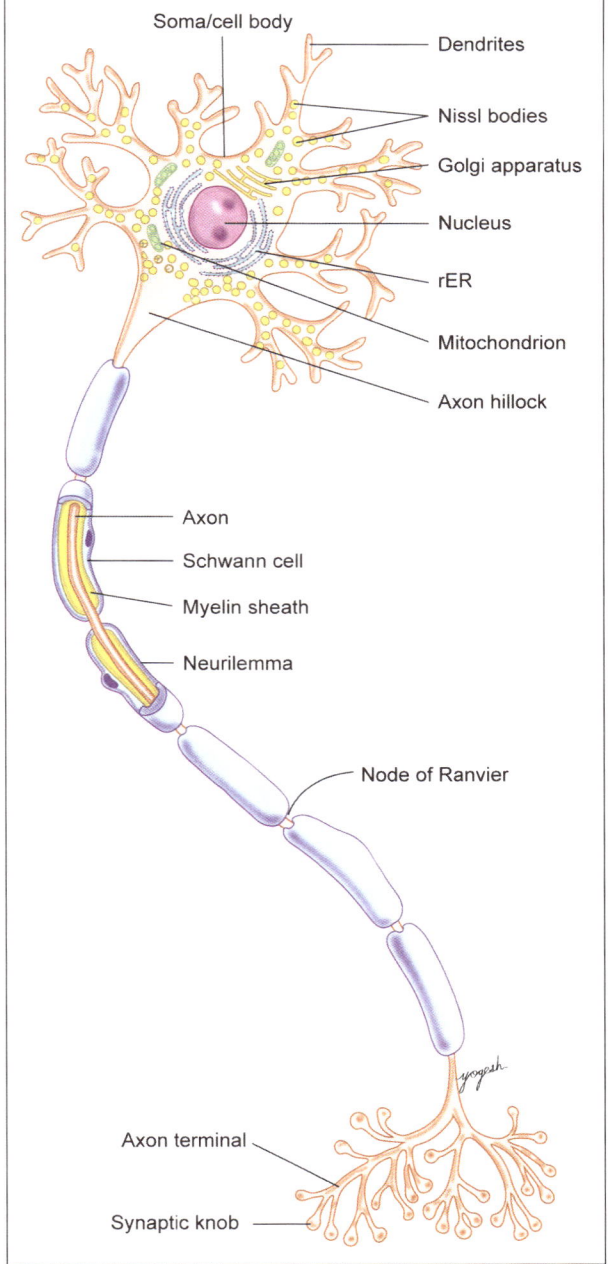

Fig. 12.1: Parts of neuron. (Note: Axon collateral and microtubules are not shown in the figure to maintain clarity of image.)

- Nissl granules extend into the dendrites.
- Branching pattern of dendrites (*arborization*) is called *dendritic trees*. Dendrites receive information and carry it toward the body of cell.

Axons

- Axon is a single, long, and thin process of neuron.
- Axons carry information away from the neuron body and have a uniform diameter.

- Axon is devoid of Nissl granules.^MCQ
- *Axoplasm* is cytoplasm in axon and *axolemma* is its cells membrane.
- *Axoplasmic transport* (Axonal transport system): As axons do not contain rough endoplasmic reticulum, protein synthesized in the cell body needs to be transported across axon.
- New concept: Peri-axoplasmic plaques: These are axon terminals that have protein synthesis machinery (rER). These are involved in the process of neuronal cell memory.^Neet
- *Axon hillock:* It is a part of cell body that is devoid of Nissl granules and gives rise to axon.
- New concept: Some cells of olfactory bulb and dentate gyrus of hippocampus are neural stem cells and they can generate new neurons. [Paulina, Histology, 7th edition].
- *Initial segment:* It is the initial *unmyelinated* part of axon between axon hillock and myelinated part of axon. An action potential is generated at initial segment.
- The differences between axons and dendrites are listed in Table 12.1.

Classification of Neurons (Flowchart 12.2)

Q. Classify the neurons.

A. Based on Number of Processes

- Neurons are classified as unipolar, pseudounipolar, bipolar, and multipolar depending on number of processes (Fig. 12.2).
  1. *Unipolar neurons:* Unipolar neurons have only one cell process, mostly dendrite. Example: Neurons of mesencephalic nucleus of trigeminal nucleus and some neurons during embryonic life.^MCQ
  2. *Pseudounipolar neurons:* These neurons have only one process (axon) that divide into two branches, peripheral and central. Examples, Dorsal root ganglia, sensory nerve ganglia.^Neet
     New concept: Unipolar and pseudounipolar neurons are under same category [Pawlina, Histology, 7th edition].
  3. *Bipolar neurons:* They have two processes: One axon and another dendrite. Examples: Retina,

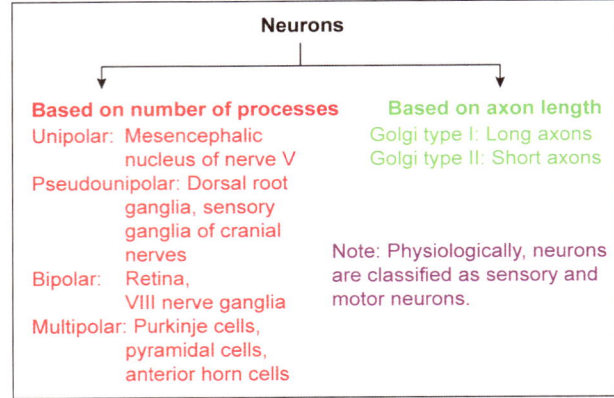

Flowchart 12.2: Classification of neurons^Viva, Neet

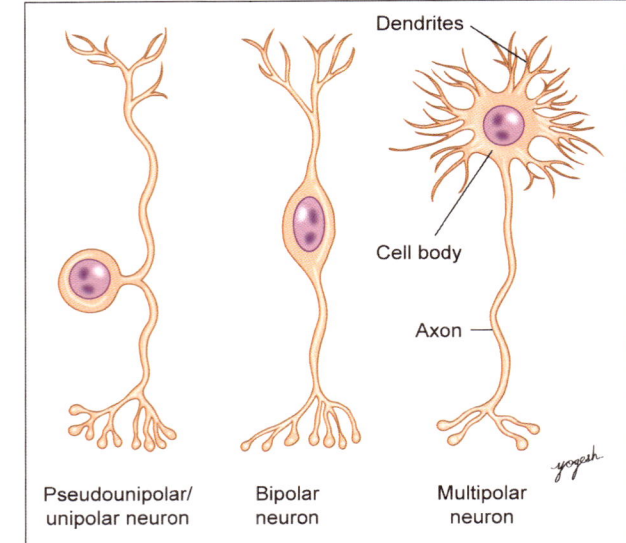

Fig. 12.2: Types of neurons.

ganglionic cells of vestibular and spiral ganglia (VIII cranial nerve).
  4. *Multipolar neurons:* They have multiple processes: One axon and many dendrites. Examples: Stellate (star-like) cells, Purkinje (flask-shaped) cells, pyramidal (triangular) cells. These are present in spinal cord, cerebellum, and cerebrum as *motor neurons* and *interneurons*.^Neet

Q. List the difference between axon and dendrites.

Table 12.1: Differences between axon and dendrites

Axon	Dendrites
It is a single, long, thin process of neuron	These are multiple, short, thick processes of neuron
It carries signal away from nerve cell body	It carries signal toward nerve cell body
Axon rarely branches. Branches of axon form axon terminals	Branches of dendrite form dendritic tree
Diameter: uniform	Diameter: tapper toward distal end (away from neuron)
Does not contain Nissl granules	Contain Nissl granules

B. Based on Length of Axon

- Based on length of axon, neurons are grouped as Golgi type I and Golgi type II neurons.
  1. *Golgi type I neurons* have long axons. Example: Pyramidal cells of motor cortex in cerebrum.
  2. *Golgi type II neuron* has short axons. Example: Neurons of cerebral and cerebellar cortex.

C. Physiological Classification

- Based on function, neurons are classified as sensory and motor neurons.
  1. *Sensory neurons:* They receive impulses and carry signals to the nervous system.
  2. *Motor neurons:* They carry impulses from nervous system to muscles and glands.

NEUROGLIA

Q. List the types of neuroglia.

- Supporting cells of nervous system are called *neuroglia or glia*.
- Neuroglia are grouped as follows (Flowchart 12.3 and Fig. 12.3):

1. Central neuroglia (neuroglia of central nervous system)
2. Peripheral neuroglia (neuroglia of peripheral nervous system)

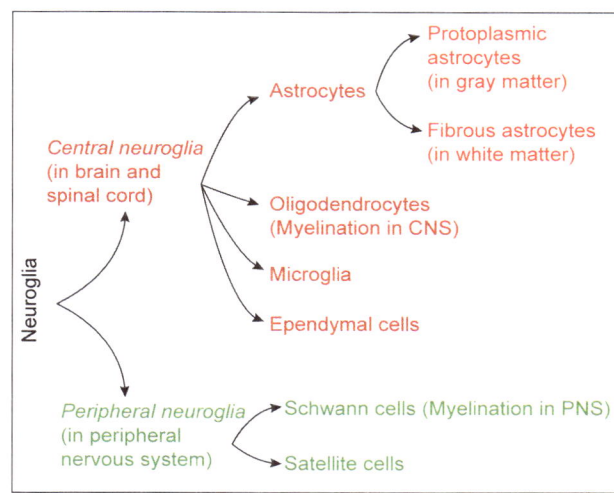

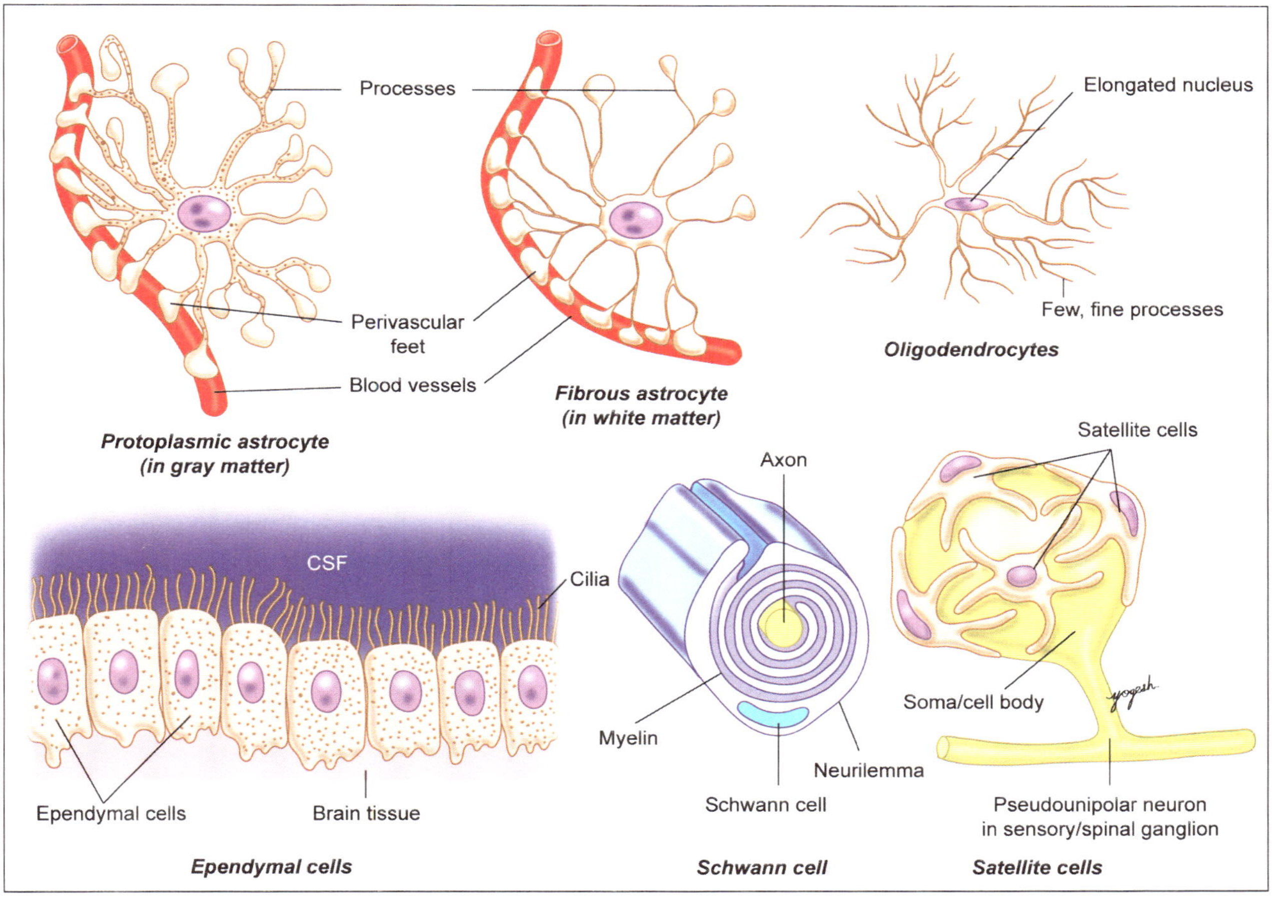

Flowchart 12.3: Types of neuroglia

Fig. 12.3: Varoious neuroglial cells.

Central Neuroglia

- These are supporting cells of central nervous system.
- There are four types of central neuroglia: Astrocytes, oligodendrocytes, microglia, and ependymal cells.
- On routine *H&E staining*, only nuclei of neuroglial cells can be identified. Their cell processes can be demonstrated using immunohistochemistry or heavy metal staining.
- Neuroglial cells support embryonic (developing) neurons as well as provide physical support after development.
- Radial glial cells direct migration of neurons during development.*Neet*

Astrocytes

- These are star-shaped cells (largest neuroglia) and they have numerous processes.
- There are two types of astrocytes: Fibrous and protoplasmic.
- *Fibrous astrocytes:* They have fewer and thin processes and mostly found in white matter of CNS.
- *Protoplasmic astrocytes:* They have numerous, short, thick, branching cytoplasmic processes. They are mostly found in gray matter.
- Both the astrocytes have glial fibrillary acidic protein (GFAP). Antibodies to GFAP are specific for astrocytes.*Neet*
- **Functions of astrocytes**
  - They provide physical support to neurons.
  - They maintain a favorable metabolic environment for neurons by removing neurotransmitters from synapses. They store glycogen.
  - They help in maintenance of blood–brain barrier.
  - *Glial limitans* is the membrane-like barrier on external surfaces of brain and spinal cord. It is produced by protoplasmic astrocytes.
  - Astrocytes maintain K^+ ion concentration in extracellular spaces of brain and spinal cord by potassium spatial buffering.
  - *Gliosis* is proliferation of astrocytes to heal the damaged zones of nervous tissue.*Neet*
  - *Fibrous astrocytoma* (tumor) account for about 80% of brain tumors in adults.

Oligodendrocytes

- Oligodendrocytes are small rounded cells and have few cytoplasmic processes (*oligo* = scanty, in Greek).
- Oligodendrocytes produce myelin in CNS.*Neet*
- One oligodendrocyte myelinate many adjacent axons or sometimes same axons at different places.
- Gap between adjacent processes of oligodendrocytes that myelinate an axon is called node of Ranvier [Louis-Antoine Ranvier, 1835–1922, French physician-anatomist].
- Myelin sheath in CNS differs from that of PNS in protein expression.
- In CNS, proteolipid protein (PLP), myelin oligodendrocyte glycoprotein (MOG), and oligodendrocyte myelin glycoprotein (OMgp) are specific to myelination. Myelin in CNS has fewer *Schmidt-Lanterman clefts* because astrocytes provide favorable metabolic environment to neurons.*Neet*
- Oligodendrocytes do not have external lamina (as it is present in Schwann cells).
- *Note:* Unmyelinated neurons are not enclosed by processes of oligodendrocytes in CNS.
- *Function:* Oligodendrocyte produces myelin sheaths in CNS.*Viva, MCQ*

Microglia

- These are smallest neuroglial cells.
- These are involved in phagocytosis when they become active (reactive microglial cells).*Viva, MCQ*
- Microglia are derived from mesoderm (bone marrow).*Neet*
- They are small cells with few cytoplasmic processes and elongated nuclei.
- *Function:* Microglia are phagocytic cells. They proliferate specifically in nervous tissue injuries and diseases. Microglia form a part of mononuclear phagocytic system in CNS.*Viva*
- *Current update:* Microglia removes bacteria, cancer (neoplastic) cells, and dead nerve cells.
- *Gitter or Hortega cell* is a lipid-laden microglial cell observed at the edge of healing brain infarcts. It is also called compound granule cell, gitterzelle, mesoglea or perivascular glial cell.*Neet*

Ependymal Cells

- The cavities of the nervous system are lined by epithelium-like *ependymal cells.*
- Ependymal cells are cuboidal to columnar in shape and arranged in single layer.
- Ependymal cells are derived from neural tube.*MCQ*
- There are three types of ependymal cells: ependymocytes, choroid epithelial cells, and tanycytes.
- Most of the cavities are lined by ependymocytes except at:
  1. Choroid plexuses are lined by *choroid epithelial cells* that secrete cerebrospinal fluid.
  2. Floor of third (not fourth)*Neet* ventricle is lined by *tanycytes* (specialized ependymal cells). These cells are *sensitive to changes in glucose concentration* and monitor levels of metabolites.*Neet*

- *Functions*
  1. Exchange of substances between brain and cerebrospinal fluid at brain–CSF barrier.
  2. Choroid plexus secretes CSF.
  3. Tanycytes: Responds to glucose concentration changes.

Peripheral Neuroglia

Schwann Cells (Theodor Schwann, 1810–1882, German physiologist):

- Schwann cells are also called *neurolemmocytes*.
- These are present only in peripheral nervous system.
- Schwann cells are flattened cells with flattened nucleus that is surrounded by abundant cytoplasm.
- Schwann cells are derived from neural crest cells.[Neet]
- *Functions*
  Schwann cells produce myelin in peripheral nervous system.[Neet]

Satellite Cells

- In ganglia (collection of neuronal cells bodies outside the CNS), neuronal bodies are surrounded by a layer of flat cuboidal cells called satellite cells.
- These cells work similar to Schwann cells but do not produce myelin.
- *Satellite cell capsule* gives passage to nerve cell processes.
- In sensory ganglia, satellite cell capsule is nearly complete as sensory neurons do not synapse in ganglia.
- In autonomic ganglia, satellite cell capsule is not complete as autonomic neurons have synapse in the ganglia.
- *Function:* Protection and support ganglionic neurons.

MYELIN SHEATH

Q. Write a short note on myelin sheath.

- Myelin is an insulating sheath surrounding the axons of myelinated nerve cells.[Viva]
- Myelin is produced by oligodendrocytes in CNS and Schwann cells in PNS.[Neet, Viva]

Formation of Myelin Sheath (Fig. 12.4)

- In process of myelination, axon initially lies in a groove of Schwann cell.
- Cell membrane of Schwann cell is converted into three zones:
  - *Abaxonal plasma membrane* – that is exposed to external environment

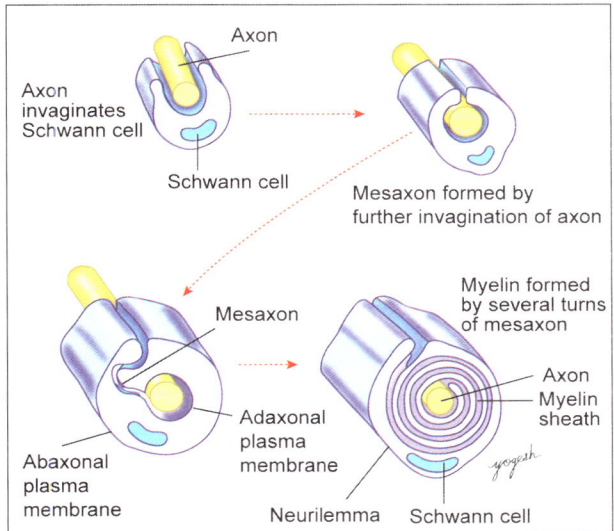

Fig. 12.4: Process of myelination.

  - *Adaxonal/periaxonal plasma membrane* – that lies in contact with axon
  - *Mesaxon* is a double membrane fold that connects abaxonal and adaxonal membranes
- Sheet-like extension of mesaxon surrounds axon spirally and cytoplasm of mesaxon gets squeezed. Thus, it results in the formation of myelin sheath (lipid-layer) around axon.
- Outside the myelin sheath, thin layer of cytoplasm of Schwann cell is present along with surrounding cell membrane of Schwann cells, now called *neurilemma* or *neurilemmal sheath*.

Composition of Myelin

- Myelin consists of lipids (80%), proteins, and water.
- *Schmidt-Lanterman clefts:* These are the small pockets of cytoplasm in inner layers of myelin sheath. Usually, cytoplasm gets squeezed out of myelin sheath during wrapping of mesaxon around the axon.[Neet]
- Unmyelinated axons are covered by Schwann cells in PNS. Single Schwann cell is invaginated by multiple unmyelinated axons.

Functions of Myelin Sheath

1. Protection and physical support to axons
2. Insulation of axons
3. Increases nerve conduction by saltatory conduction
4. Neurilemmal sheath plays a major role in nerve regeneration

Some Interesting Facts

- In myelin sheath, myelin-specific proteins are present. These include protein O (PO), peripheral myelin protein 22 (PMP22), and myelin basic protein. These proteins can be used in immunohistochemistry for staining of myelin.
- Protein O is adhesion molecule in mesoaxonal folding of myelin sheath. Mutation of PO gene produces demyelinating diseases such as *Guillain-Barré syndrome* and *multiple sclerosis*.^{MCQ}
- One Schwann cell can produce a myelin sheath around a small segment of one axon. One Oligodendrocyte can produce a myelin sheath around many axons.^{Neet} Hence, *neurilemmal sheath* is present only in peripheral nervous system (cell membrane of Schwann cell) and not in CNS as a single oligodendrocyte does not cover one axon. Because of absence of neurilemmal sheath in CNS, regeneration of neuron is not possible in CNS.^{Viva}
- Around a single axon, many Schwann cells form myelin sheath. The gap between the segment of myelin and between adjacent Schwann cells is called *nodes of Ranvier* or *incisura myelini* (Louis Antoine Ranvier, 1835–1922).
- Nodes of Ranvier increases rate of nerve conduction by saltatory conduction.
- *Internode* is segment of myelin sheath between adjacent nodes of Ranvier.
- Thickness of myelin sheath depends on axon diameter and not on Schwann cell.^{MCQ} Myelin sheath thickness is regulated by neuregulin (NRG1) growth factor that is expressed on axolemma of axon.
- A single Schwann cell protects many unmyelinated axons (Fig. 12.5).

SYNAPSE

- Neuron conveys messages to another cell (neuron/effector cell) through a synapse.
- Synapse is junction between neurons.

Morphological Classification (Flowchart 12.4)

Depending on components of synapse, they are classified as follows (Fig. 12.6):

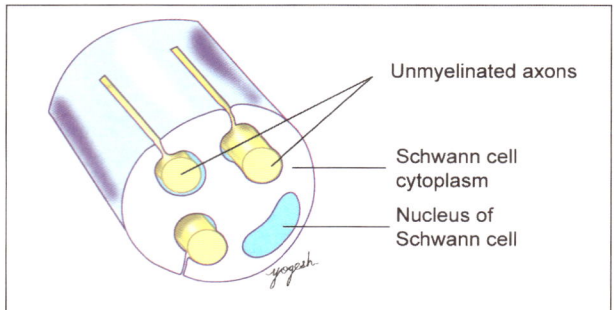

Fig. 12.5: Role of Schwann cell in protection of unmyelinated axon. Note: One Schwann cell surrounds multiple unmyelinated nerve fibers.

1. *Axodendritic synapse:* It is the most common type of synapse. In axodendritic synapse, axon of one neuron synapse with dendrite of another neuron.
2. *Axosomatic synapse:* Axon covey impulse to soma (body) of another neuron.
3. *Axoaxontic synapse:* It is synapse between two axons.
4. *Dendroaxonic synapse:* It is synapse between dendrite of presynaptic neuron and axon of postsynaptic neuron. It is seen in some part of thalamus.

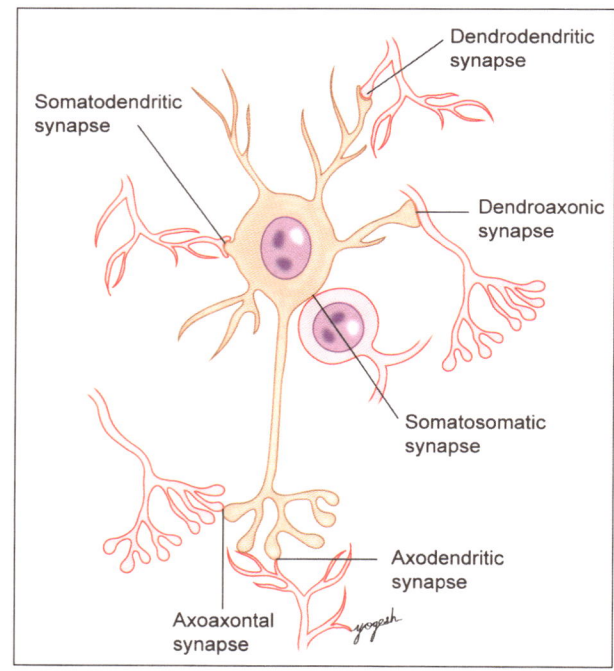

Fig. 12.6: Types of synapse.

Flowchart 12.4: Morphological classification of synapse

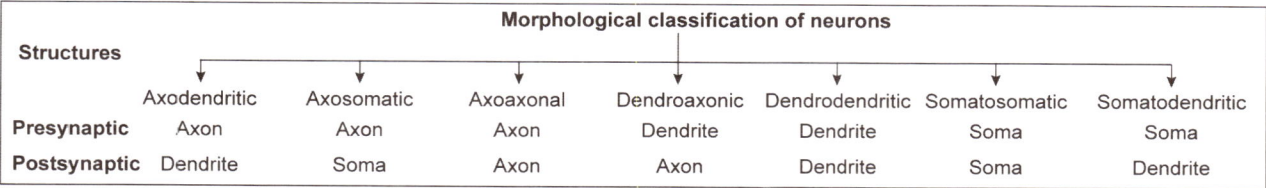

Structures	Morphological classification of neurons						
	Axodendritic	Axosomatic	Axoaxonal	Dendroaxonic	Dendrodendritic	Somatosomatic	Somatodendritic
Presynaptic	Axon	Axon	Axon	Dendrite	Dendrite	Soma	Soma
Postsynaptic	Dendrite	Soma	Axon	Axon	Dendrite	Soma	Dendrite

5. *Dendrodendritic synapse:* It is synapse between two dendrites.
6. *Somatosomatic synapse:* It is synapse between bodies of neurons.
7. *Somatodendritic synapse:* It is synapse between soma and dendrite of postsynaptic neurons.
   - Synapse is not distinguishable on *H&E staining*.
   - *Boutons en passant:* Presynaptic neuron makes several contacts with postsynaptic neuron. These contacts are called boutons en passant (means *buttons in passing* in French).
   - Silver staining (Golgi method): Synapse is visible as oval bodies.
   - *Bouton terminal:* Enlarged terminal end of axon is called bouton terminal (means *terminal button* in French).

Chemical and Electric Synapses (Flowchart 12.5)

Based on mechanism of conduction of nerve impulses, synapses are classified as chemical or electrical.

Chemical Synapses
- Chemical synapse involves release of chemical (neurotransmitter) from preganglionic neurons for conduction of impulse.

Flowchart 12.5: Classification of synapse based on mode of transmission

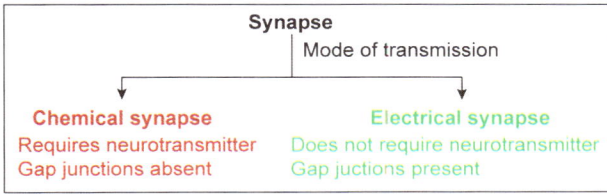

Structure of chemical synapse (Fig. 12.7)
- Components of chemical synapse are as follows:
  1. *Presynaptic element (presynaptic knob):* It is the part of presynaptic neuron that releases neurotransmitter. Presynaptic element stores neurotransmitter in synaptic vesicles.
  2. *Synaptic cleft:* It is narrow gap (20–30 nm) between presynaptic and postsynaptic neurons. Neurotransmitter needs to cross synaptic cleft.
  3. *Postsynaptic membrane/process:* It is a membrane of postsynaptic neuron that has receptors for neurotransmitters.
- New concept: *Porocytosis* is a process of secretion of neurotransmitter through pores created by calcium ions between secretory vesicles and presynaptic membrane. (Privous concept: Secretory vesicle fuses with presynaptic membrane for the release of neurotransmitter).

Electrical Synapses
- Electric synapse involves passage of electric signal from one cell to another cell by gap junctions.
- Electrical synapses do not involve neurotransmitter release.
- Examples: Gap junctions of cardiac and smooth muscles.

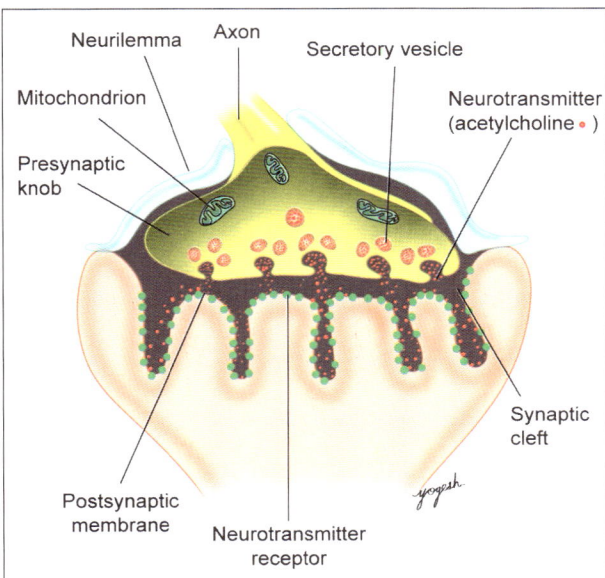

Fig. 12.7: Structure of synapse.

Some Interesting Facts
- Merkel epidermal cells, auditory receptors, and taste buds are epithelial receptors, whereas olfactory epithelium is a neuroepithelial receptor.*Neet*
- Neurotransmitter once released in synaptic cleft may be degraded by enzymes or may be taken back (uptake) by presynaptic neurons.

For example:
- Catecholamine action is terminated by their uptake. *Clinical fact:* Amphetamine and cocaine inhibit catecholamine uptake and prolong their actions.
- Acetylcholine is degraded by acetylcholine esterase. *Clinical fact:* Many poisons (pesticides) and other drugs inhibit action of acetylcholine esterase and cause prolonged muscle contraction.

PERIPHERAL NERVE

Q. Write a short note on histology of peripheral nerve (TS).
Q. Draw a well-labeled diagram for section of nerve stained by osmium tetroxide.

- Peripheral nerve is collection of many nerve fibers held together by connective tissue.
- Concept of nerve fiber is confusing as it does not mean a connective tissue fiber.

- Nerve fiber indicates:
  1. *Motor or efferent nerve* fibers are axons that carry impulses from CNS to muscle or glands. Cells bodies of motor neurons lie in CNS, especially in gray matter of spinal cord and brain stem.
  2. *Afferent or sensory nerve* fiber are nerve processes that carry impulses or information toward CNS. Nerve cell bodies of afferent fibers lie in sensory ganglia.
- *Ganglion* is a collection of nerve cell bodies outside the CNS. Examples: Dorsal root ganglion, autonomic ganglion.

Basic Structure of Peripheral Nerve
(Flowchart 12.6 and Figs 12.8 to 12.11)

- *Nerve fiber* with Schwann cells and basal lamina is the basic structural unit of peripheral nerve.
- Each single *nerve fiber* is surrounded by a thin connective tissue called *endoneurium*.
- *Endoneurium* consists of the loose connective tissue with collagen fibril, few fibroblasts, occasional mast cells and macrophages.
- Note: In peripheral nerve section, 90% of nuclei are of Schwann cells and only 10% belongs to connective tissue cells.

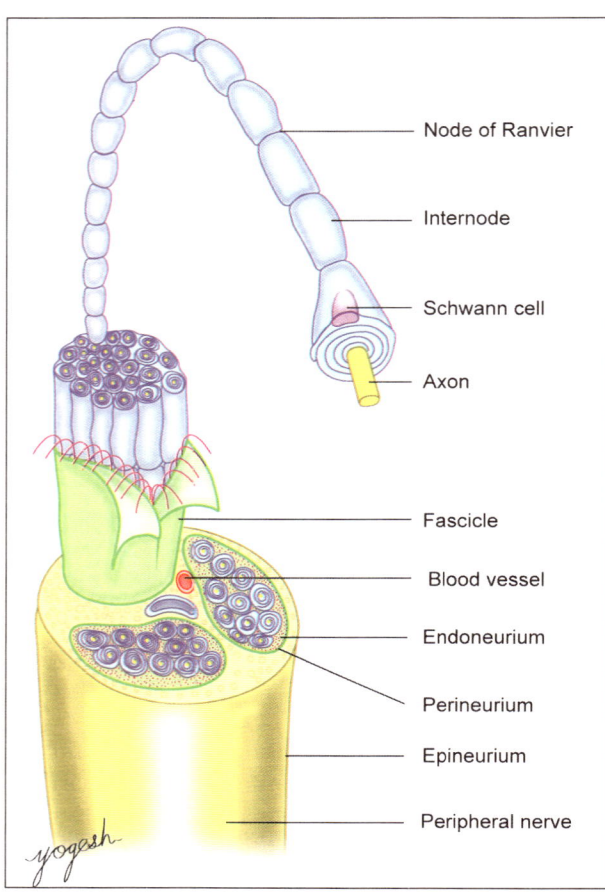

Fig. 12.8: Structure of peripheral nerve.

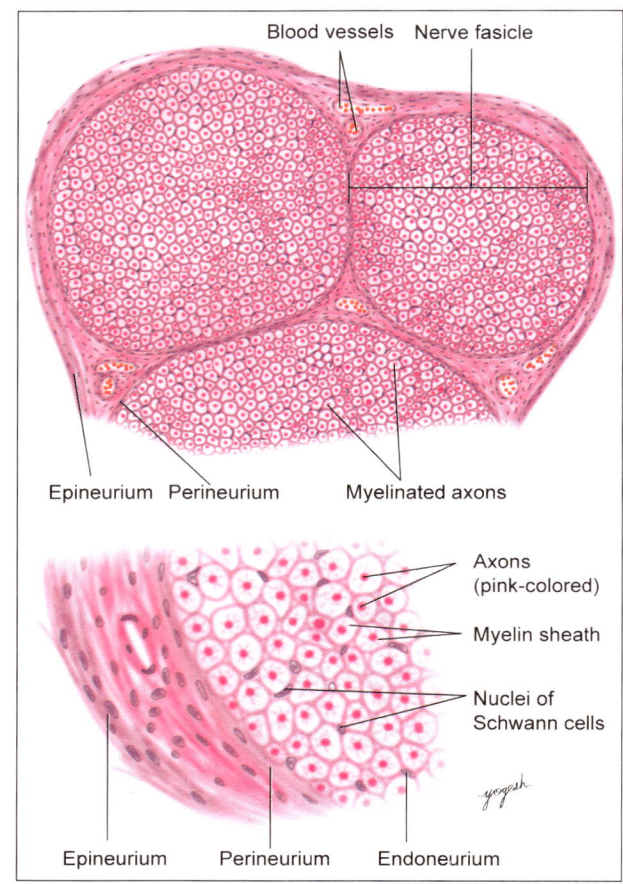

Fig.12.9: histology of peripheral nerve (transverse section, *H&E* stained, low magnification above, high magnification below, practice figure).

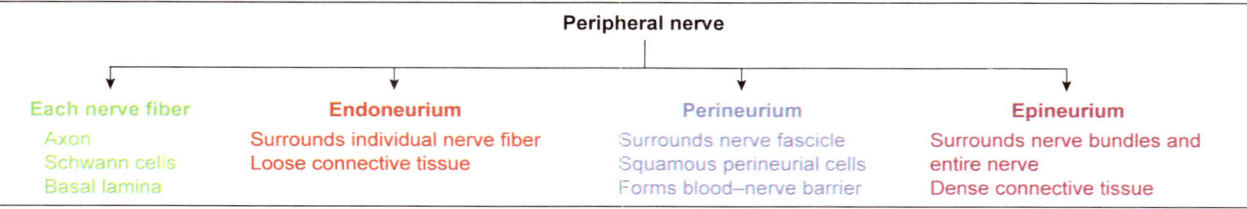

Flowchart 12.6: Peripheral nerve

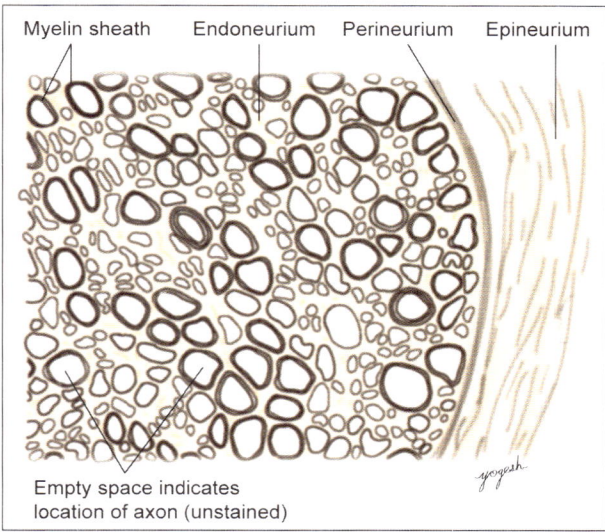

Fig. 12.10: Transverse section of peripheral nerve (fixed in osmium tetroxide that stains lipid/myelin black, practice figure).

- A group of nerve fibers form a nerve fascicle or bundles.
- Each *nerve fascicle* is surrounded by layer of specialized connective tissue called perineurium.
- *Perineurium* is made up of flattened (squamous) perineurial cells. They may be arranged in two or more perineurial cell layers and externally covered by a *basal lamina*.
- Perineurial cells are connected with each other by tight junctions and hence, form a *blood-nerve barrier*.
- Many fasciculi are held together by dense irregular connective tissue called epineurium.
- *Epineurium* surrounds entire peripheral nerve. It contains blood vessels that supply the nerve.
- Note: Blood vessels (*vasa nervorum*) are present only in epineurium and perineurium. Endoneurium does not have blood vessels. Nerve fibers receive nutrition by diffusion through endoneurium.*Neet, Viva*

Osmium Staining for Myelin (Figs 12.10, and 12.12)

- Osmium tetroxide is a special stain used for myelin.*Viva*
- Myelin is washed away during preparation for *H&E stain*. Hence, osmium tetroxide staining method is used.
- In this method, myelin sheath stains black.*Viva*
- Note: *H&E staining:* Axons, endoneurium, perineurium, and epineurium is stained. Myelin gives empty appearance.*Viva*

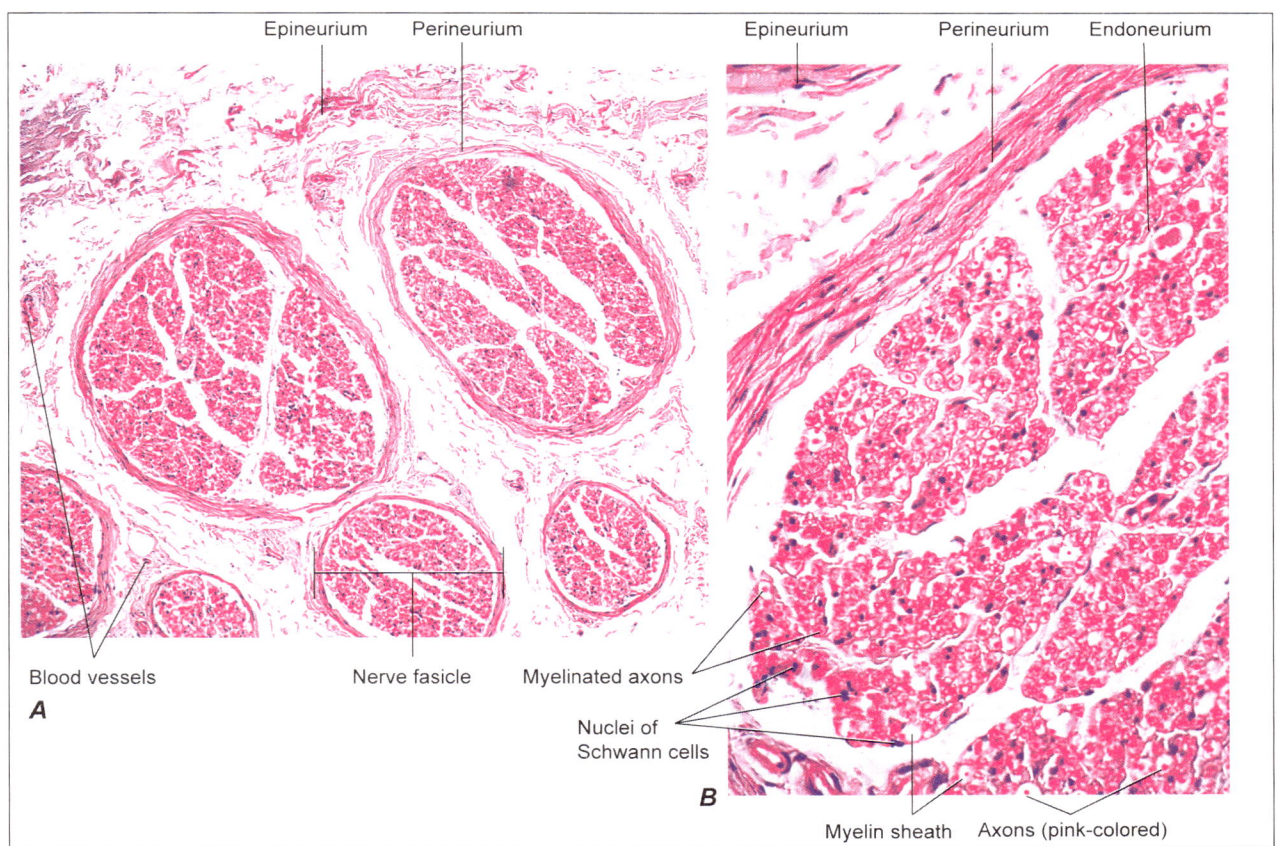

Fig. 12.11: Photomicrograph. Histology of peripheral nerve (transverse section, *H&E* stain, (A) Low magnification, (B) High magnification).

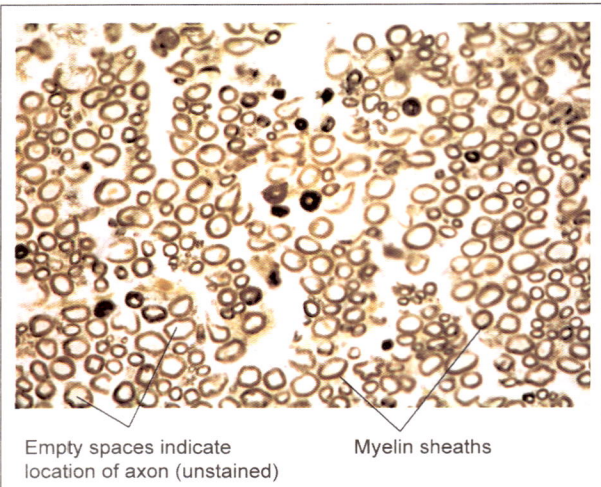

Fig. 12.12: Photomicrograph. Transverse section of peripheral nerve (fixed in osmium tetroxide that stains lipid/myelin black).

> **Summary (Examination Guide)**
> - Each peripheral nerve consists of nerve fibers and connective tissue coats.
> - Each nerve fiber consists of axon, Schwann cells, and basal lamina. On *H&E staining,* myelin gives empty appearance. *Identification feature*
> - Connective tissue coats: *Identification feature*
>   1. *Endoneurium* is loose connective tissue that surrounds a single nerve fiber.
>   2. *Perineurium* is the layer of perineurial cells that surrounds nerve fascicles and form blood–nerve barrier.
>   3. *Epineurium* is the layer of dense connective tissue that surrounds bundles of nerve fascicles and entire nerve.
> - Note: Blood vessels are present only in perineurium and epineurium.
> - Osmium tetroxide stains myelin black. *Identification feature*

Flowchart 12.7: Histology of sensory/dorsal root ganglion Dorsal root ganglion

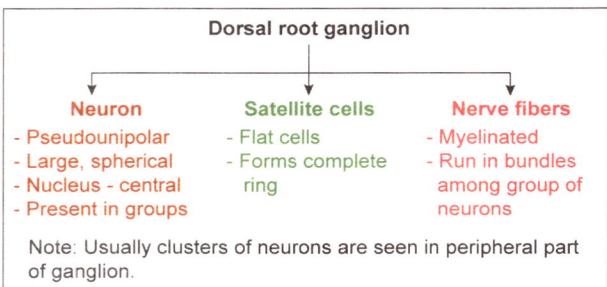

GANGLION

- Ganglion is the aggregation of cell bodies of neurons outside central nervous system.
- Ganglia are of two types: Sensory and autonomic.

Sensory Ganglia

Q. Write a short note on histology of sensory ganglia.

- Sensory ganglia are present just outside the CNS.
- Neurons of sensory ganglia carry impulses toward CNS.
- Examples:
  1. Dorsal root ganglia of spinal nerves
  2. Sensory ganglia of cranial nerves: Trigeminal, facial, vestibulocochlear, glossopharyngeal, and vagus nerve

Structure of Sensory Ganglia (Flowchart 12.7, Figs 12.13 and 12.14)

- Sensory ganglia have *pseudounipolar neurons* (except vestibulocochlear ganglia that has bipolar neurons). *Next*

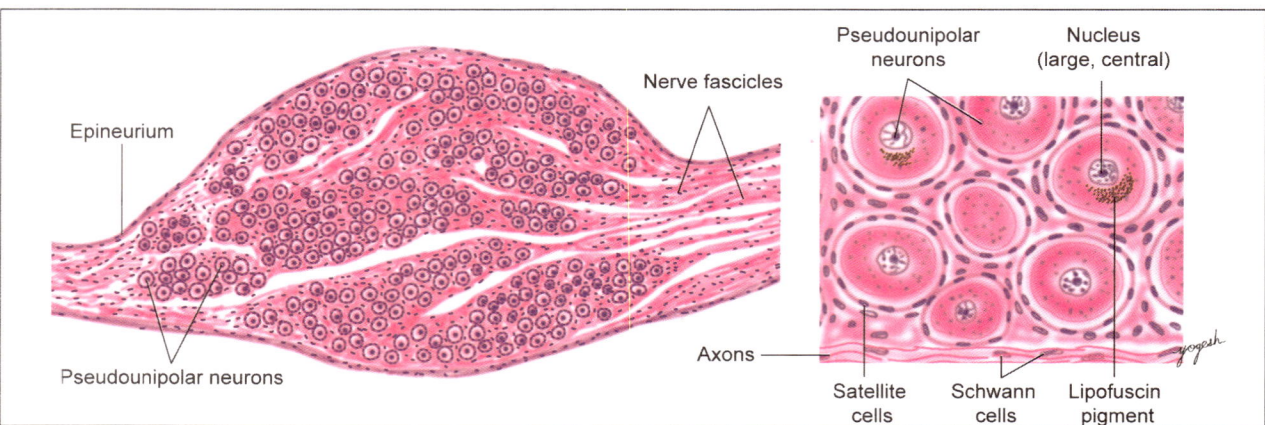

Fig. 12.13: Histology of dorsal root/sensory ganglion (low magnification on left, high magnification on right, practice figure).

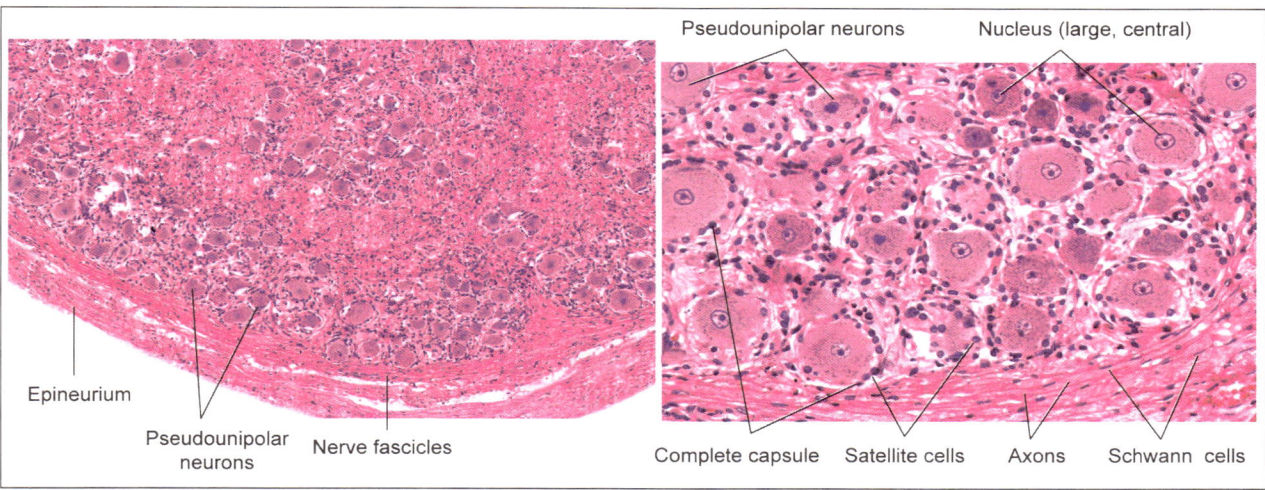

Fig. 12.14: Photomicrograph. Histology of dorsal root/sensory ganglion (low magnification on left, high magnification on right, H&E stain).

- Pseudounipolar neurons have a peripheral process that carries information from sensory receptor and a central process that pass received information to CNS.
- A section of sensory ganglia shows *large neurons that are present in groups,* mostly at the periphery of ganglia. *Identification feature*
- *Nuclei* of neurons are large, vesicular, and *centrally placed.*
- Group neurons are separated by bundles of myelinated nerve fibers.
- *Satellite cell/capsular cells:* Each neuronal body is surrounded by a *complete capsule* of satellite or capsular cells. *Identification feature*
- Satellite cells are flattened cells (low cuboidal)
- The ganglion is covered by fine connective tissue capsule.

Autonomic Ganglia

Q. Write a short note on histology of autonomic or sympathetic ganglion.

- Autonomic ganglia supply smooth muscles and glands.
- Autonomic nervous system shows two neurons:
  1. *Preganglionic neuron:* It lies in CNS and their axons extend from CNS up to autonomic ganglia.
  2. *Postganglionic neuron:* It lies in autonomic ganglia and its axon supplies smooth muscle cells and glands.
- Examples:
  1. *Sympathetic ganglia:* Sympathetic trunk, paravertebral ganglia (celiac, superior mesenteric, inferior mesenteric, and aorticorenal ganglia), and adrenal medulla.
  2. *Parasympathetic ganglia:* Ciliary ganglion, submandibular ganglion, otic ganglion, pterygopalatine ganglion, and terminal ganglia that lies near the organs.

Structure of Autonomic Ganglia (Flowchart 12.8, Figs 12.15 and 12.16)

- Usually, sympathetic ganglion is easy to obtain and sufficiently large for teaching purpose; hence, its slide (section) is given for practical demonstration as a prototype of autonomic ganglia.
- Autonomic ganglia are smaller than the sensory ganglia.
- On *H&E staining:* Multipolar postganglionic neurons of autonomic ganglia are scattered throughout ganglion. *Identification feature*
- These neurons are separated from each other by discrete bundles of nerve fibers (unmyelinated and thin).
- *Nuclei* of neurons are large, pale-staining with prominent nucleolus, and *eccentrically placed* in the cytoplasm. *Identification feature*

Flowchart 12.8: Histology of autonomic/sympathetic ganglion

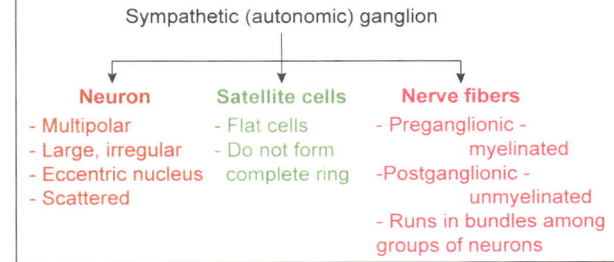

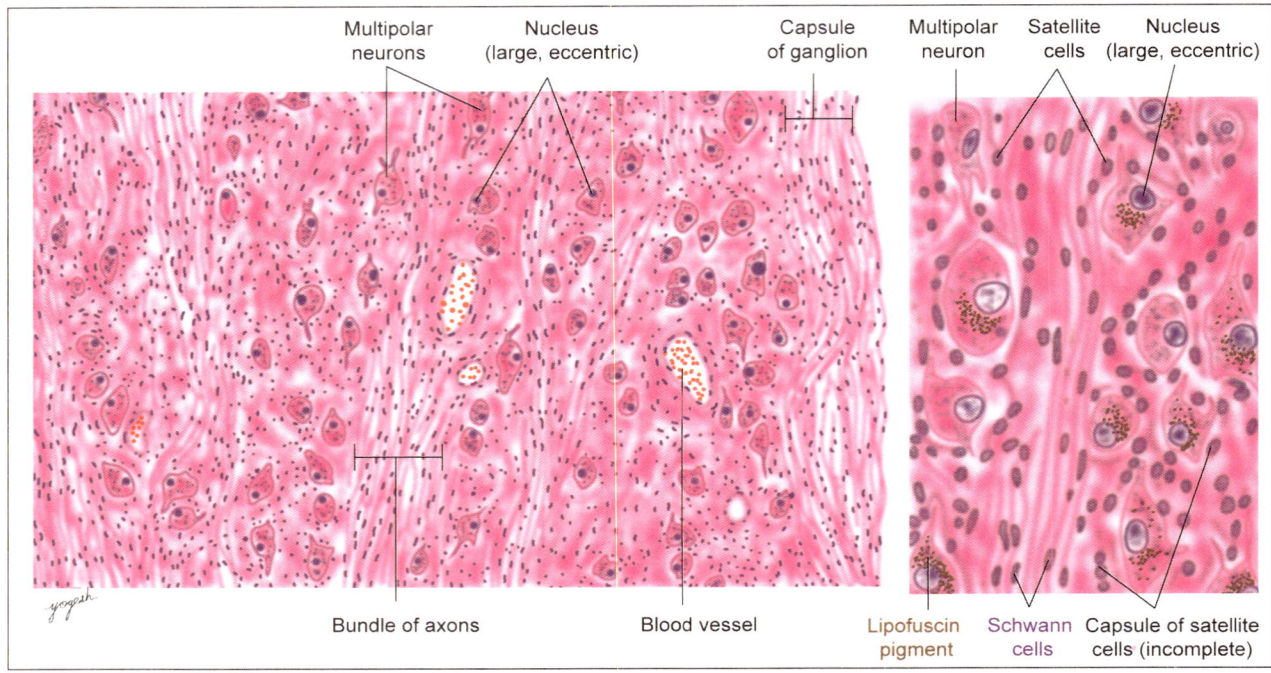

Fig.12.15: Histology of autonomic/sympathetic ganglion (low magnification on left, high magnification on right, practice figure)

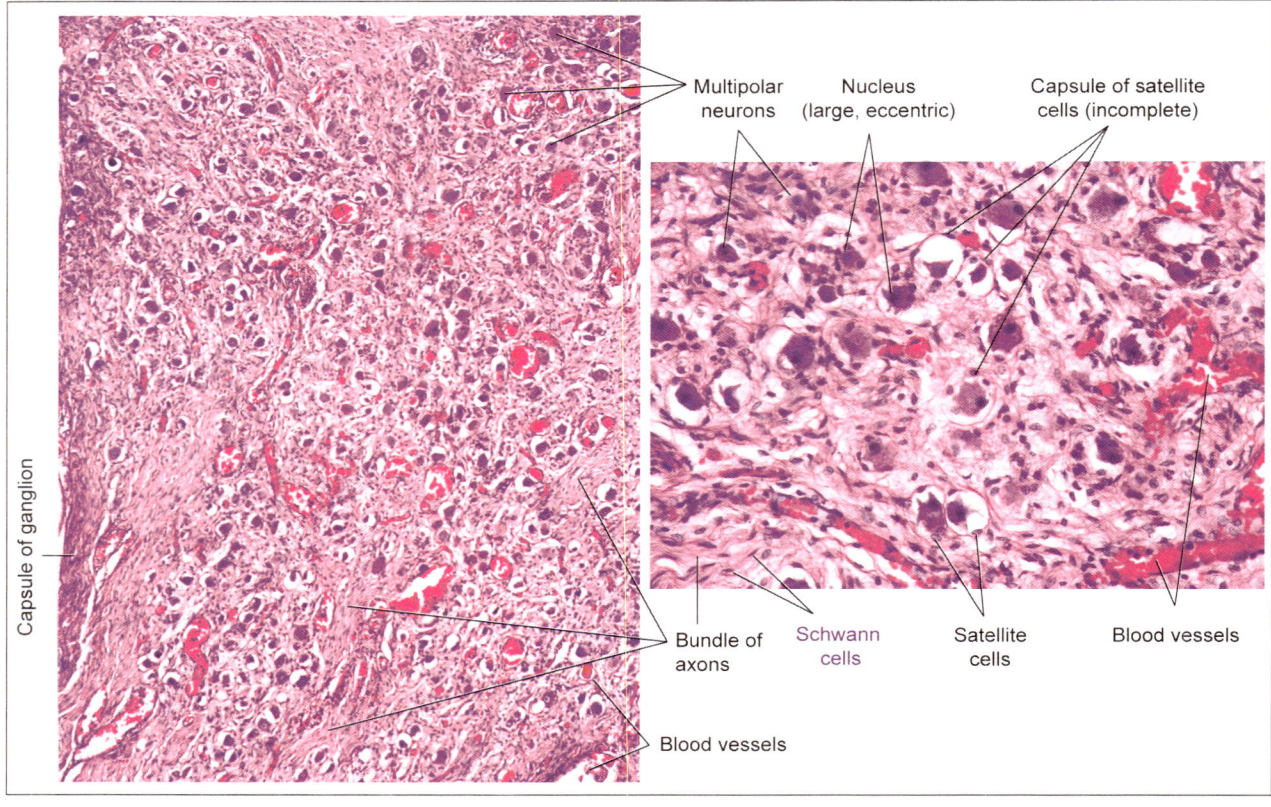

Fig. 12.16: Photomicrograph. Histology of autonomic/sympathetic ganglion (low magnification on left, high magnification on right, *H&E* stain).

Q. List the differences between dorsal root ganglion and sympathetic ganglion.

Table 12.2: Differences between sensory and autonomic ganglia

	Sensory (Dorsal root) ganglion	Autonomic (sympathetic) ganglion
Neuron	Pseudounipolar *Neet*	Multipolar *Neet*
Neuron–body shape	Large spherical	Small irregular
Types of neuron	Sensory	Postganglionic autonomic/sympathetic neuron
Nucleus	Large, vesicular, centrally placed *Neet*	Large, vesicular, eccentrically placed *Neet*
Satellite cells	Complete ring around neuronal body	Few satellite cells, do not form complete ring around neuronal body
Neuronal groups	Neurons present in groups (clusters) *Neet*	Neurons are scattered *Neet*
Nerve fibers	Nerve fibers are present in bundles that separate clusters of neurons	Nerve fibers are present between scattered neurons

- *Satellite/capsular cells:* Few satellite cells are seen to surround each nerve cell body, but these cells *do not form a complete capsule*. Reason: Automimic neurons are multipolar, their numerous processes break the continuity of capsule, and autonomic neurons have synapse in the ganglia. In sensory ganglia, satellite cell capsule is nearly complete as sensory neurons do not synapse in ganglia. *Identification feature*
- The ganglion is surrounded by connective tissue capsule.
- As postganglionic autonomic neurons synthesize catecholamines, Nissl granules are prominently seen in their cytoplasm.
- Silver staining is useful for better visualization of processes of neurons.

The difference between sensory and autonomic ganglia are listed in Table 12.2.

Note: For histology of cerebrum, cerebellum, spinal cord and brain stem, refer Chapter 26.

Summary (Examination Guide) of Ganglion

- Ganglion is surrounded by connective tissue capsule.
- **Dorsal root ganglion**
  - Pseudounipolar neuronal bodies: They are arranged in clusters (groups). They are large, spherical in shape with large, vesicular, and centrally placed nuclei. Neurons are present on one side of ganglion. *Identification feature*
  - Nerve fibers (myelinated) are arranged in bundles that separate groups of neurons.
  - Satellite cells: Flattened satellite cells form a *complete* ring around body of each neuron. *Identification feature*

- *Autonomic/sympathetic ganglion*
  - Multipolar neuronal bodies: They are scattered among nerve fibers. They are large, irregular shaped. Nuclei of neurons are large, vesicular, and eccentrically placed. *Identification feature*
  - Nerve fibers are arranged in bundles that run between scattered neurons.
  - Satellite cells: Few flat satellite cells surround each nerve cell body but do not form a complete ring. *Identification feature*
  - Nerve fibers are both myelinated (preganglionic) and unmyelinated (postganglionic).

CHAPTER 13

Cardiovascular Tissue

Chapter Outline

- Endothelium
- Basic structure of blood vessels
- Classification of blood vessels
- Elastic arteries
- Muscular arteries
- Arterioles
- Capillaries
  - Continuous capillaries
  - Fenestrated capillaries
  - Sinusoids
- Arteriovenous anastomosis
- Veins
  - Venules and small veins
  - Medium veins
  - Large veins
- Difference between artery and vein

Competency achievement: The student should be able to:
AN69.1 Identify elastic and muscular blood vessels, capillaries under the microscope
AN69.2 Describe the various types and structure-function correlation of blood vessel
AN69.3 Describe the ultrastructure of blood vessels

INTRODUCTION

- Cardiovascular system transports blood to and from various tissues of the body.
- Cardiovascular system consists of heart and blood vessels. Blood vessels include arteries, capillaries, and veins. Some authors consider lymphatic vessels as part of cardiovascular system.
- Heart is a muscular organ that pumps the blood into the arterial system. Heart receives blood from veins.
- Blood vessels form a network of pipe system that transport blood from heart to tissues and back to heart.
- Blood vessels can be grouped as follows (Flowchart 13.1):
  - *Arteries* carry blood away from the heart.
  - *Arterioles* are the smallest arteries that deliver blood to capillaries.
  - *Capillaries* are the smallest vessels that exchange nutrients between blood and tissue.
  - *Venules* are the smallest veins that receive blood from capillaries.
  - *Veins* carry blood toward heart.
- There are several types of circuits in body that distributes blood. For example, systemic circulation, pulmonary circulation, portal circulation, and so on.
- Pulmonary and systemic circulation has only single plexus of capillaries.
- In portal circulation, portal vein forms another (second) set of capillary plexus. Examples of portal circulations: Hepatic portal system, hypothalamo-hypophyseal portal system.
- All blood vessels, irrespective of their size and type, are lined by endothelium.

ENDOTHELIUM

- Vascular endothelium is a lining epithelium of internal surface of cardiovascular system (Fig. 13.1).
- Vascular endothelium is a *simple squamous epithelium.*
- Endothelium consists of *endothelial cells.*
- Endothelial cells are flattened, elongated and polygonal cells.
- The long axis of endothelial cell is parallel to the axis of blood flow.
- *H&E staining:* In transverse section, endothelial cell shows small quantity of cytoplasm and elongated, flat, densely stained nucleus.
- *Electron microscopy:* Cytoplasm contains endoplasmic reticulum, mitochondria, and microfilaments. Adjacent endothelial cells are connected with each other by *tight junctions.* Endothelial cells rest on basal lamina that can be visualized by periodic acid-Schiff staining method.

Cardiovascular Tissue

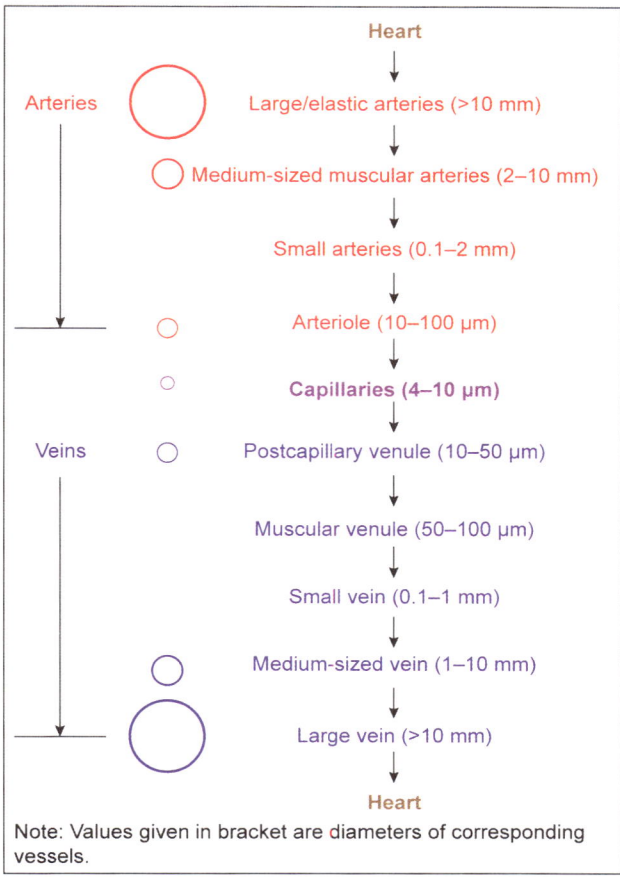

Flowchart 13.1: Blood circulation through vessels

Note: Values given in bracket are diameters of corresponding vessels.

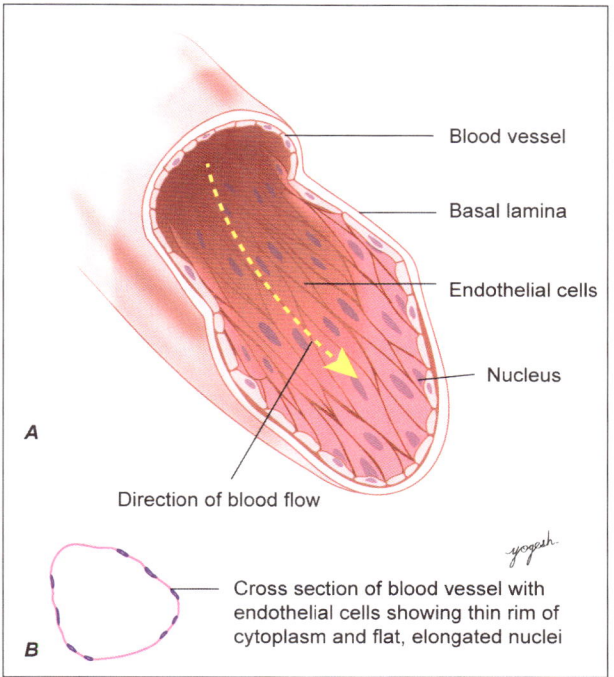

Fig. 13.1: (A) Endothelial cells. Note: Long axis of endothelial cells lies parallel to the direction of blood flow. (B) Practice figure for endothelial cells.

Functions of Endothelium (Table 13.1)

Q. List the functions of endothelium.

- *Smooth surface:* Endothelium provides a smooth nonadherent surface for flowing blood columns.
- *Selective permeability barrier:* Endothelium allows movement of selected substances across it through simple diffusion, pinocytosis, and receptor-mediated endocytosis. Transport of substance mainly depends on its size and charge.
- *Release of von Willebrand Factor* (plasminogen-activator inhibitor): Damaged endothelium release von Willebrand factor that induces platelet aggregation and clot formation [Erik Adolf von Willebrand, 1870–1949, Finnish physician].
- *Release of nitric oxide* (NO) and prostacyclin: These are vasodilator agents.
- *Release of endothelin, angiotensin-converting enzyme* (ACE): These are vasoconstrictor agents. With the help of vasodilator and vasoconstrictor agents, endothelium controls blood flow through the vessels.
- *Hormone synthesis:* Endothelium synthesizes and secretes many growth factors such as colony-stimulating factors, fibroblast growth factors, platelet-derived growth factors.
- *Release of endothelial-derived relaxing factor* (EDRF): EDRF produces vasodilatation with the help of nitric oxide (NO).
- *Synthesis of type IV collagen fibers* that are responsible for the formation of basal lamina.

Table 13.1: Function of endothelium[Viva]

1. Prevention of clotting
2. Selective permeability barrier
3. Release of von Willebrand Factor
4. Release of nitric oxide (NO) and prostacyclin
5. Release of endothelin, angiotensin-converting enzyme (ACE)
6. Hormone synthesis: colony-stimulating factors, fibroblast growth factors, platelet derived growth factors
7. Release of endothelial-derived relaxing factor (EDRF)
8. Synthesis of type IV collagen fibers

Some Interesting Facts

1. In atherosclerosis, macrophages endocytose low-density lipoproteins and form foam cells in the wall of blood vessels.
2. *Histamine* increases permeability of vascular endothelium. Thus, during an allergic reaction, histamine increases vascular permeability and causes extravasation of the fluid into extracellular spaces. Accumulation of excess tissue fluid in extracellular spaces is called *edema.*
3. Endothelial nitric oxide synthase is essential for production of *nitric oxide.*
4. Functions of nitric oxide:
   - Acts as a vasodilator
   - Enhances synthesis of vascular endothelial growth factors
   - Acts as an anti-inflammatory agent
   - Acts as a potent neurotransmitter in many parts of brain
   - Regulates apoptosis
   - Activates macrophages and induce immune response
5. *Endothelin* produced by vascular endothelial cells produces vasoconstrictions. Snake venom of *Israeli burrowing asp* binds with endothelium receptors and causes death due to intense coronary vasoconstriction.

BASIC STRUCTURE OF BLOOD VESSELS

- Histologically, blood vessels show three basic layers in their transverse section: Tunica intima, tunica media and tunica adventitia (*tunica* = coat) (Fig. 13.2 and Flowchart 13.2). *Viva*
- Presence and thickness of these layers depend on size and type of the blood vessel.

Tunica Intima

- *Tunica* intima is the innermost layer of blood vessel.
- Tunica intima consists of endothelium, subendothelial connective tissue, and internal elastic lamina (inside outwards).

Flowchart 13.2: Structure of blood vessel

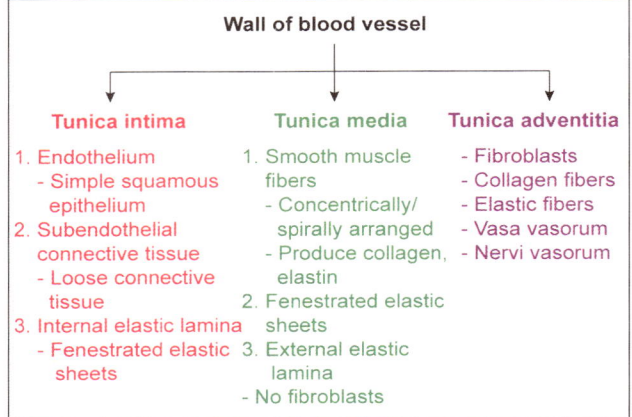

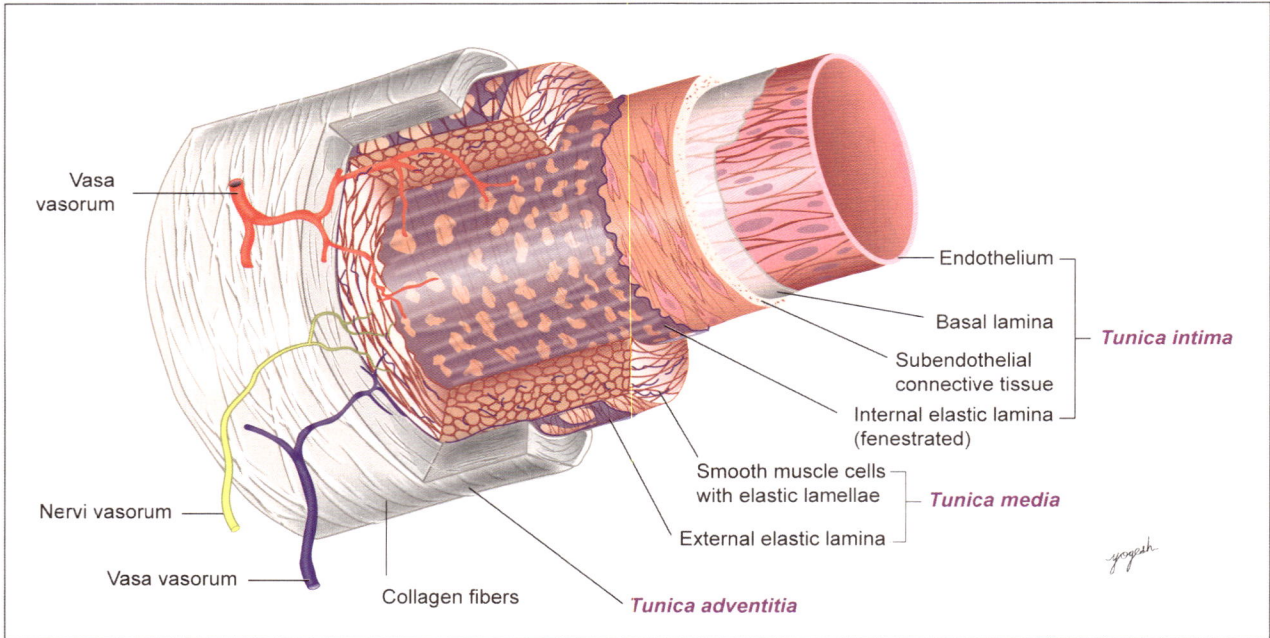

Fig. 13.2: General structure of blood vessel.

- *Endothelium* consists of *simple squamous epithelium* (endothelial cells/endotheliocytes) resting on *basal lamina*.
- Endotheliocytes are flat, elongated polygonal cells that are oriented parallel to the direction of blood flow.
- *Subendothelial connective tissue* consists of loose connective tissue containing collagen and elastic fibers.
- *Internal elastic membrane* consists of many fenestrated elastic sheets.
- Presence of fenestrations of elastic sheets permits transmission of nutrients to the outer wall of blood vessels from its lumen.

Tunica Media

- It is *middle* layer of blood vessels.
- It consists of concentric layers of spirally oriented *smooth muscles.*
- Smooth muscles show elongated nucleus.
- Apart from vasoconstriction, these smooth muscles produce elastic fibers, collagen fibers, and ground substance (proteoglycans).*Neet*
- Elastic fibers are present in the form of fenestrated sheets.
- Tunica media of arteries are thicker and contains more smooth muscles than that of veins.
- External elastic lamina separates tunica media from tunica adventitia. External elastic lamina is thinner than internal elastic lamina.
- Tunica media do not contain fibroblasts.*Neet*
- Smooth muscle cells of tunica media can
  - produce contraction or relaxation under autonomic neuronal control.
  - grow under the control of endothelium-derived growth factors.

Tunica Adventitia

- Tunica adventitia is the *outermost* layer of blood vessels.
- Tunica adventitia is a connective tissue layer that consists of collagen fibers, few fine elastic fibers, fibroblasts, and occasional macrophages.
- *Vasa vasorum* consist of fine network of small blood vessels that supply wall of blood vessel.*Neet*
- *Nervi vasorum* consist of unmyelinated postganglionic sympathetic nerve fibers that release norepinephrine and produce vasoconstriction.*Neet*

Some Interesting Facts

- Inner part (one-third) of blood vessel is supplied by diffusion from luminal blood. In thicker vessels (>0.5 mm), outer portion (two-thirds) of vessel wall is supplied by vasa vasorum.
- Coronary arteries are analogous to vasa vasorum for myocardium of heart.*Viva*

CLASSIFICATION OF BLOOD VESSELS

- Blood vessels are grouped into three groups: Arteries, capillaries, and veins (Flowchart 13.3).
- Arteries carry blood away from heart, capillaries nourish the tissue, whereas veins carry blood toward heart.

Arteries

- Arteries are classified into groups based on characteristics of tunica media as follows:
  1. *Elastic or large arteries* (conducting arteries) have multiple layers of vascular smooth muscles and elastic lamellae in tunica media
  2. *Muscular arteries* (medium-sized arteries) have more smooth muscles and less elastic lamellae
  3. *Small arteries* have up to 8 smooth muscle layers in tunica media
  4. *Arterioles* have only a single layer of smooth muscles

Capillaries

- Capillaries form a network of vessels in tissue and are sites for exchange of nutrients.
- Capillaries are classified into three groups based on continuity of wall and basal lamina as follows:
  1. *Continuous capillaries* have continuous endothelial cells and basal lamina.
  2. *Fenestrated capillaries* have fenestrated endothelial cells but continuous basal lamina.
  3. *Sinusoid* or *sinusoidal capillaries* have fenestrated endothelial cells and discontinuous basal lamina.
- Note: Some authors consider sinusoid as a separate group of vessels.

Veins

- Veins are grouped into four groups based on their size as follows:
  1. Venules (diameter 10–100 µm): They receive blood from capillaries

Flowchart 13.3: Classification of blood vessels*Viva*

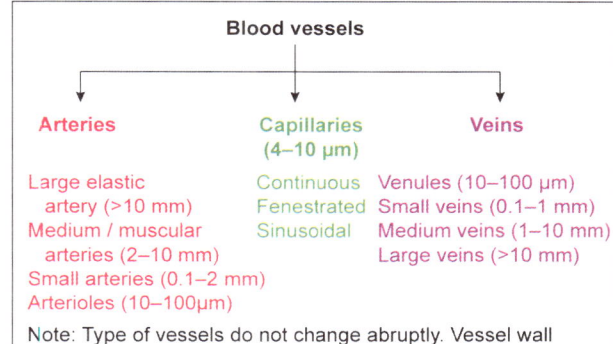

2. Small veins (diameter 0.1–1 mm)
3. Medium-sized veins (diameter 1–10 mm): They accompany arteries
4. Large veins (diameter >10 mm)

ELASTIC ARTERIES

- Elastic artery is also called *large arteries* or *conducting arteries*.
- Examples: Aorta, pulmonary trunk, brachiocephalic artery, common carotid artery, subclavian artery, common iliac artery, pulmonary artery.^{MCQ, Viva}
- Diameter is more than 10 mm.
- These arteries convey blood from heart to muscular arteries; hence, also called *conducting arteries*.
- Function as a *diastolic pump*: During ventricular systole, elastic arteries dilate to acquire a sudden rush of blood from ventricles (accommodate blood). During ventricular diastole (relaxation), because of *elastic recoil*, these arteries push the blood into medium-sized arteries and maintain continuous blood flow. Thus, elastic arteries pump blood during diastole of ventricles.^{Viva}

Flowchart 13.4: Histology of elastic/large artery

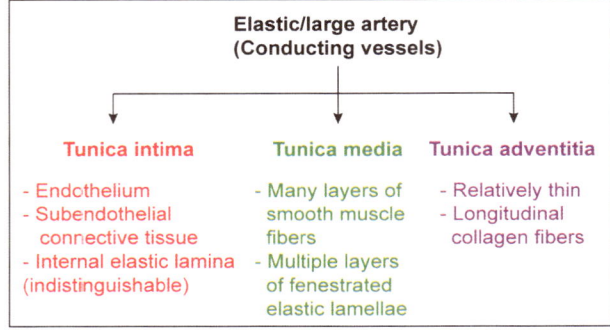

Structure of Elastic Artery

- Histologically, wall of elastic artery shows three layers: Tunica intima, tunica media, and tunica adventitia (Flowchart 13.4, Figs 13.3 to 13.5).

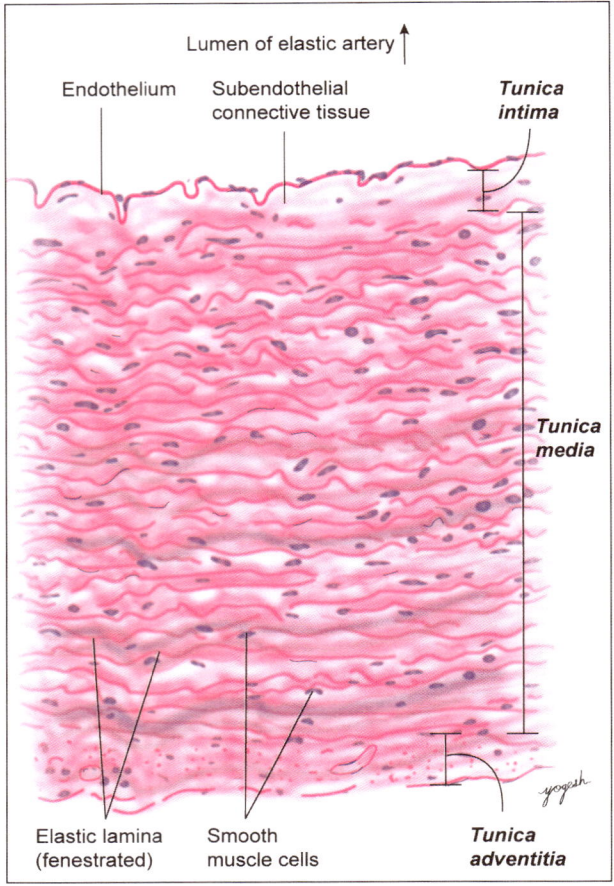

Fig. 13.3: Elastic artery (practice figure).

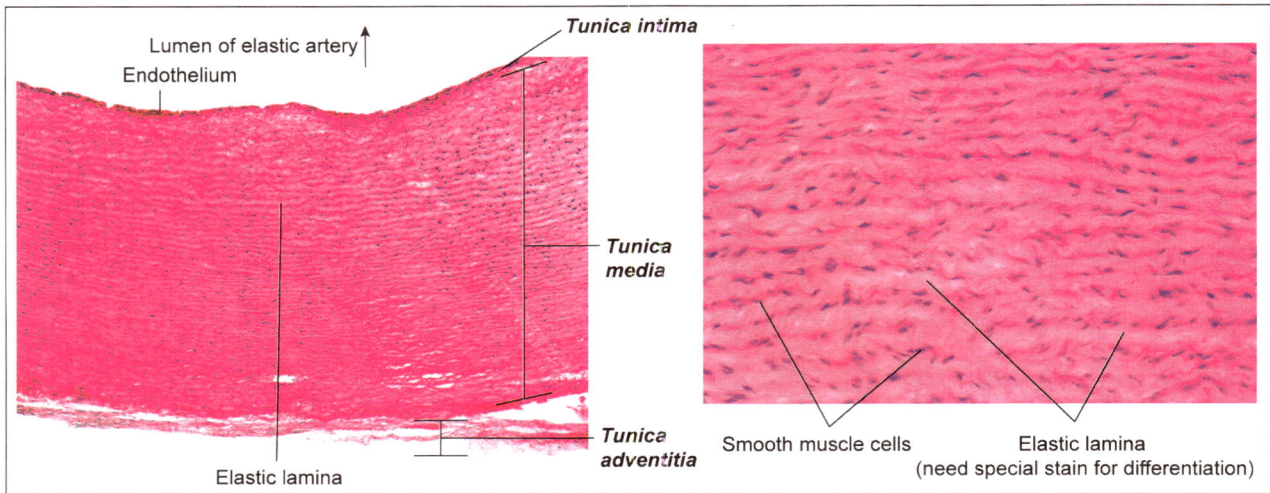

Fig. 13.4: Photomicrograph. Elastic artery (low magnification on left, high magnification of tunica media on right, *H&E* stain).

Cardiovascular Tissue

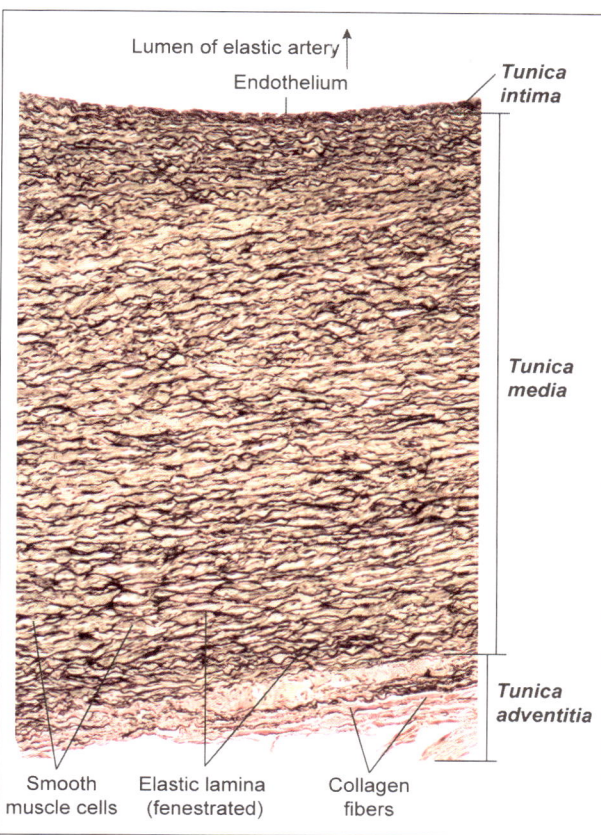

Fig. 13.5: Photomicrograph. Elastic artery (Verhoeff-van Gieson stain, low magnification).

Tunica Intima

- Tunica intima consists of endothelium, subendothelial connective tissue, and internal elastic lamina.
- *Endothelium* is a simple squamous epithelium that rests on basal lamina. Endothelial cells are flat and elongated and lie parallel to the direction of blood flow.
- *Subendothelial connective tissue* consists of few smooth muscle fibers, collagen, and elastic fibers. *Identification feature*
- *Internal elastic lamina* consists of fenestrated sheets of elastin. In large arteries, it is not easily differentiable because of presence of multiple elastic sheets in tunica media. *Identification feature*

Tunica Media

- It is the *thickest layer* in wall of arteries. *Identification feature*
- It consists of many layers of vascular *smooth muscles* and *fenestrated elastic lamellae* (sheets).
- Vascular smooth muscles form many concentric layers. These are spindle-shaped cells with an elongated nucleus and are oriented spirally.
- Vascular smooth muscles produce elastin and collagen.
- Layers of smooth muscle fibers are separated from each other by concentric fenestrated sheets of elastin. *Identification feature*
- In adult human aorta, about 40–70 elastic lamellae are present.
- Both internal and external elastic lamellae are not clearly differentiated from other elastic lamellae of tunica media.

Tunica Adventitia

- Tunica adventitia of elastic artery is relatively thin.
- It consists of *longitudinally running collagen fibers.*
- It also shows fibroblasts, macrophages, and fine elastic fibers.
- It also consists of the following:
  - Vasa vasorum: Small vessels that supply the outer part of wall of the blood vessel.
  - Nervi vasorum: Autonomic nerves that supply vascular smooth muscles.

Summary (Examination Guide)

Q. Write a short note on histology of elastic/large artery.

- Elastic (large/conducting) artery consists of tunica intima, tunica media, and tunica adventitia.
- *Tunica intima* shows vascular endothelium (simple squamous epithelium), subendothelial connective tissue and indistinguishable internal elastic lamella.
- *Tunica media* shows many layers of spindle-shaped vascular smooth muscle fibers. These fibers are separated from each other by many thick sheets of fenestrated elastic lamellae.
- *Tunica adventitia* is relatively thin.
- Examples: Aorta, brachiocephalic, common carotid and subclavian arteries, pulmonary trunk, pulmonary arteries.

MUSCULAR ARTERIES

- These are also called *medium-sized arteries* and have a diameter of 2–10 mm.
- These arteries distribute blood to tissues; hence, also called *distributing arteries.*
- The prominent feature of muscular arteries is presence of more number of *smooth muscles* and less amount of elastic material in tunica media. *Identification feature*
- Because of less amount of elastic material in tunica media, internal elastic lamina (part of tunica intima) can be easily identified. *Identification feature*
- Smooth muscles regulate amount of blood flow through these arteries by contraction (vasoconstriction) and relaxation (vasodilatation).

Structure of Muscular Arteries

- Elastic arteries gradually change into muscular arteries; this change mainly includes
  1. Decrease in diameter
  2. Decrease in number of elastic fibers
  3. Increase in amount of smooth muscle in tunica media
- Structurally, muscular artery consists of tunica intima, tunica media, and tunica adventitia (Figs 13.6 to 13.8 and Flowchart 13.5).

Tunica Intima

- It consists of endothelium, subendothelial connective tissue, and internal elastic lamina.
- *Endothelium* is a simple squamous epithelium that rests on basal lamina.
- *Subendothelial connective tissue* is sparse (very less).
- *Internal elastic lamina* is prominent (clearly visible as a wavy structure) just adjacent to endothelium because of scanty subendothelial connective tissue. *Identification feature*

Tunica Media

- Tunica media (predominantly) consists of concentric smooth muscle fibers. *Identification feature*

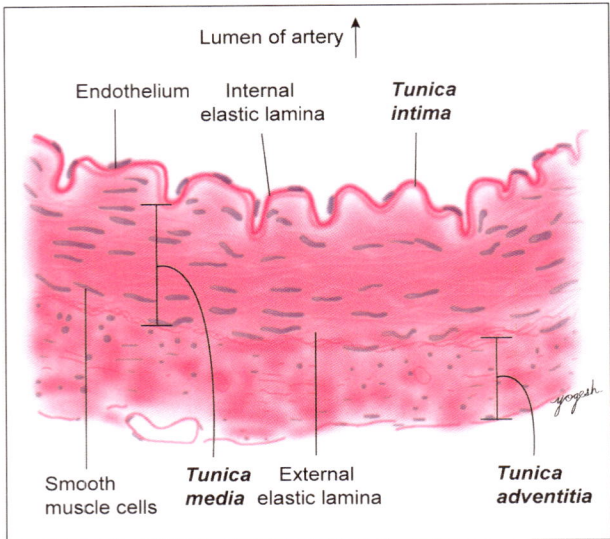

Fig. 13.6: Medium-sized/muscular artery (practice figure).

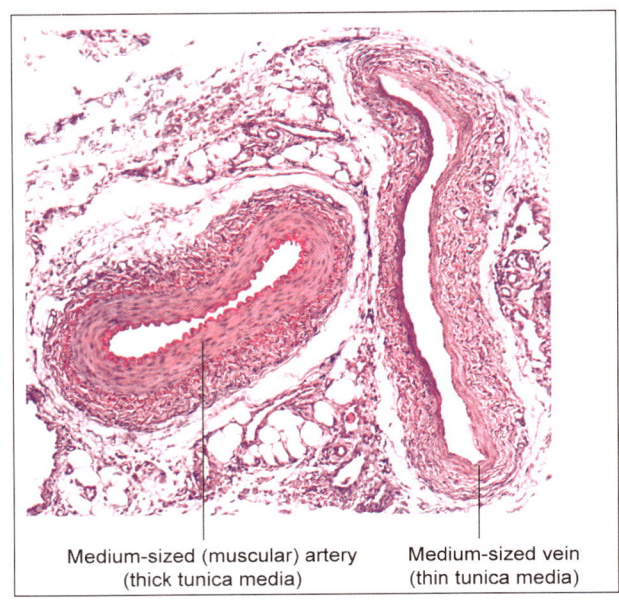

Fig. 13.7: Photomicrograph. Medium-sized artery (muscular artery) and medium-sized vein (H&E stain, low magnification).

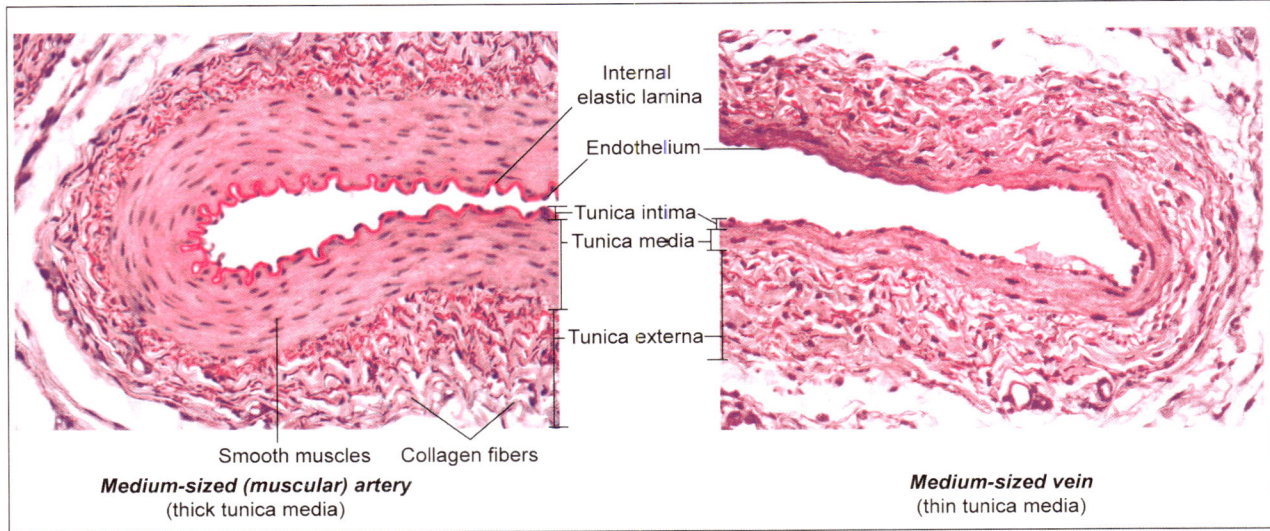

Fig. 13.8: Photomicrograph. Layers of medium-sized artery (muscular artery) and medium-sized vein (H&E stain, high magnification).

- Smooth muscle fibers are spindle-shaped cells that are arranged spirally and are responsible for maintenance of blood pressure.
- Tunica media contains a small number of elastic fibers and collagen fibers.
- Tunica media does not contain fibroblasts.^MCQ
- Smooth muscle cells are connected to each other by gap junctions for rapid and coordinated contraction.
- At junction of tunica media with adventitia, elastic fibers may form external elastic lamina.

Tunica Adventitia

- It consists of connective tissue.
- Tunica adventitia of muscular artery is relatively thicker than elastic arteries.
- Tunica adventitia also shows vasa vasorum and nervi vasorum.

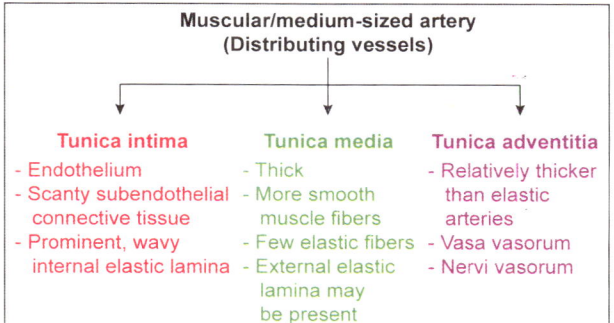

Flowchart 13.5: Structure of medium-sized/muscular artery

> **Summary (Examination Guide)**
>
> **Q. Write a short note on histology of muscular arteries.**
>
> - Muscular (medium-sized/distributing) artery consists of tunica intima, tunica media, and tunica adventitia.
> - Tunica intima has endothelium (simple squamous epithelium), scanty subendothelial connective tissue, and *prominent internal elastic lamina*.
> - Tunica media shows more layers of smooth muscle cells and a few elastic fibers.
> - Tunica adventitia is relatively thick.
> - Examples: Brachial artery, femoral artery, and other arteries of limbs.

> **Some Interesting Facts**
>
> - *Weibel-Palade bodies:* These are rod-like cytoplasmic inclusions in endothelial cells. Weibel-Palade bodies contain von-Willebrand factor (involved in platelet aggregation) and p-selection (involved in neutrophil migration) [Ewals Weibel, Swiss biologist; George Palade, 1912–2008, Romanian American cell biologist: Weibel ER, Palade GE. New cytoplasmic components in arterial endothelia. *J Cell Biol* 1964;23(1):101–12.]
> - Tunica media does not contain fibroblasts.
> - Vascular smooth muscles produce elastin, collagen fibers, and ground substances.
> - In hypertension, number and thickness of elastic lamellae increase significantly.
> - Differences between elastic artery and muscular artery are listed in Table 13.2.

ARTERIOLES

- Muscular arteries divide and redivide to give rise to a vessel called *arterioles* (diameter 10–100 μm).
- Distally, arterioles form capillary plexuses.
- Arterioles are grouped as
  - *Muscular or large arterioles:* Diameter 50–100 mm.
  - *Terminal arterioles:* Diameter less than 50 μm.
- Arterioles regulate flow of blood through capillary plexus and maintain blood pressure.

Q. List the differences between elastic artery and muscular artery.

Table 13.2: Differences between elastic artery and muscular artery^Viva

Layer	Elastic artery	Muscular artery
Tunica intima	Significant amount of subendothelial connective tissue is present. Internal elastic lamina is not clearly identifiable	Subendothelial connective tissue is scanty. Internal elastic lamina is clearly visible
Tunica media	Many thick fenestrated elastic laminae are present. Smooth muscles are present intermittently between elastic laminae	Very less amount of elastic fibers present. Many layers of smooth muscles are present
Tunica adventitia	It is relatively thin layer of connective tissue	It is relatively thick layer of fibroelastic connective tissue
Examples	Aorta, carotids, and subclavian arteries	Brachial artery, femoral artery

Structure of Arteriole

- Arteriole consists of tunica intima, tunica media, and tunica adventitia (Figs 13.9 and 13.10).

Tunica intima
- It consists of vascular endothelium (simple squamous epithelium) that rests on small amount of subendothelial connective tissue.
- Internal elastic lamina is mostly absent in arterioles.

Tunica media
- It consists of 1–3 cell layer thick, circularly arranged smooth muscle cells.
- Muscular arterioles may have 2–3 layers of smooth muscle layers, whereas in terminal arteriole there is only one layer of smooth muscle layer.
- *Precapillary sphincter:* It consists of vascular smooth muscle cells that surround terminal arterioles at their junction with capillaries. Pre-capillary sphincter regulates entry of blood into capillary plexus.^{Viva}
- *Vascular resistance:* Smooth muscles of arterioles generate resistance to blood flow and regulates the blood pressure.

Tunica adventitia
- It is a thin connective tissue layer that separates arteriole from adjacent structure. It may not be clearly distinguishable.

Functions
- Arterioles regulate blood flow through capillary plexus with the help of precapillary sphincters.
- Arteriole increases vascular resistance to blood flow and enhances blood pressure.

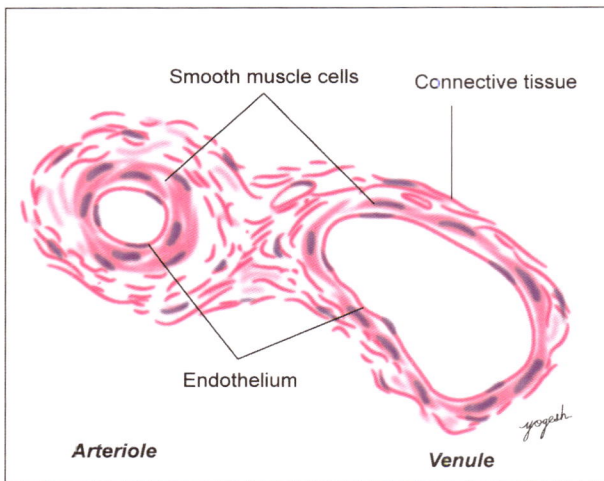

Fig. 13.9: Arteriole and venule (practice figure).

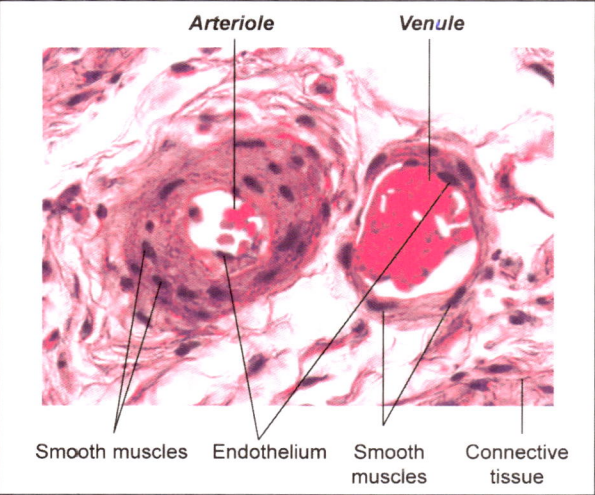

Fig. 13.10: Photomicrograph. Arteriole and venule (H&E stain, high magnification).

Clinical Correlation
- *Atherosclerosis:* Atherosclerosis is disease of artery that narrows lumen because of *plaque* (*sclerosis* means hardening, in Greek). In atherosclerosis, a thick layer of fibrous connective tissue/atheromatous plaque gets accumulated in tunica intima.^{MCQ} Plaque consists of smooth muscle cells, macrophages, foam cells, collagen fibers, and cholesterol crystals. Atherosclerosis causes narrowing of blood vessel lumen, and reduced blood supply to viscera. It may even lead to heart attack (myocardial infarction) or paralysis (stroke).
- *Hypertension:* Hypertension is the sustained diastolic pressure above 90 mm Hg or sustained systolic blood pressure above 140 mm Hg. It affects most of the elderly people because of increased vascular resistance, atherosclerotic changes, increased vascular smooth muscle cells, decreased amount of elastic fibers, and increased amount of collagen fibers in vessel walls.
- *Aneurysm:* It is a sac-like dilatation of arterial wall because of its weakness (*aneurysm* means *dilatation*, in Greek). Aneurysm is associated with replacement of elastic fibers with collagen fibers. Aneurysm is usually seen in old age because of atherosclerosis, syphilis, Marfan syndrome and Ehlers-Danlos syndrome.
- **Syphilis** is sexually transmitted disease caused by *Treponema pallidum* bacteria. Marfan syndrome is an autosomal dominant disorder. Ehlers-Danlos syndrome is a genetic connective tissue disorder [Edvard Ehlers, Danish dermatologist, 1863–1937; Henri-Alexandre Danlos, French dermatologist, 1844–1912].

Cardiovascular Tissue

Some Interesting Facts
- *Metarterioles* are arterioles that supply blood capillaries (Fig. 13.11).
- In meta-arterioles, vascular smooth muscle layer is not continuous (muscle cells are present at intervals).
- Metarterioles can increase or decrease blood supply as per need. For example, during physical exercise, arterioles in skeletal muscle dilate to enhance blood supply.

CAPILLARIES

Q. Write a short note on capillaries.
- Capillaries are the smallest blood vessels.
- Capillaries form a network that connects arteriole with venule and nourishes tissue.
- Capillary has an average diameter of 8 μm (4–10 μm).
- Human body has ~50,000 miles of capillaries.
- Capillary lumen at some place is narrower than the diameter of RBCs (7.2 μm). RBCs need to get folded on themselves for passage through such capillaries.
- Capillaries consist of endothelium and its basal lamina.*MCQ*
- Note: There is *no tunica media and tunica adventitia* in capillaries.*MCQ*
- In some capillaries, *pericytes* are present.
- Pericytes lie embedded in basal lamina of endothelium.*Viva*
- Pericyte has long oval euchromatic nuclei and several cytoplasmic processes that clasp capillary.
- Pericyte can get differentiated into smooth muscle cell or fibroblast.*MCQ*

Classification of Capillaries

- On the basis of morphology, capillaries are classified into three types: continuous capillaries, fenestrated capillaries, and sinusoids or discontinuous capillaries (Flowchart 13.6 and Fig. 13.12).*Viva*
- Some authors consider sinusoids as a separate type of vessel.

Continuous Capillaries (Somatic)

- In continuous capillaries, edges of endothelial cells fuse completely with adjoining cells by *tight junctions* (uninterrupted vascular endothelium) (Figs 13.12 and 13.13).
- Basement membrane completely surrounds the endothelium (*continuous basal lamina*).
- In continuous capillaries, exchange of nutrients takes place through cytoplasm of endothelial cells.

Flowchart 13.6: Classification of capillaries

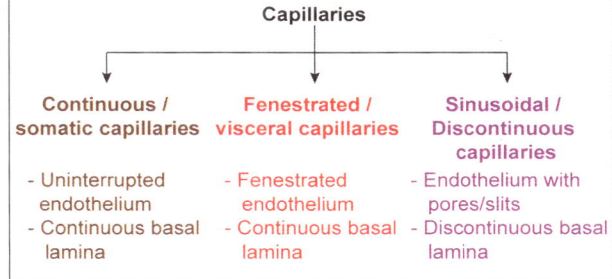

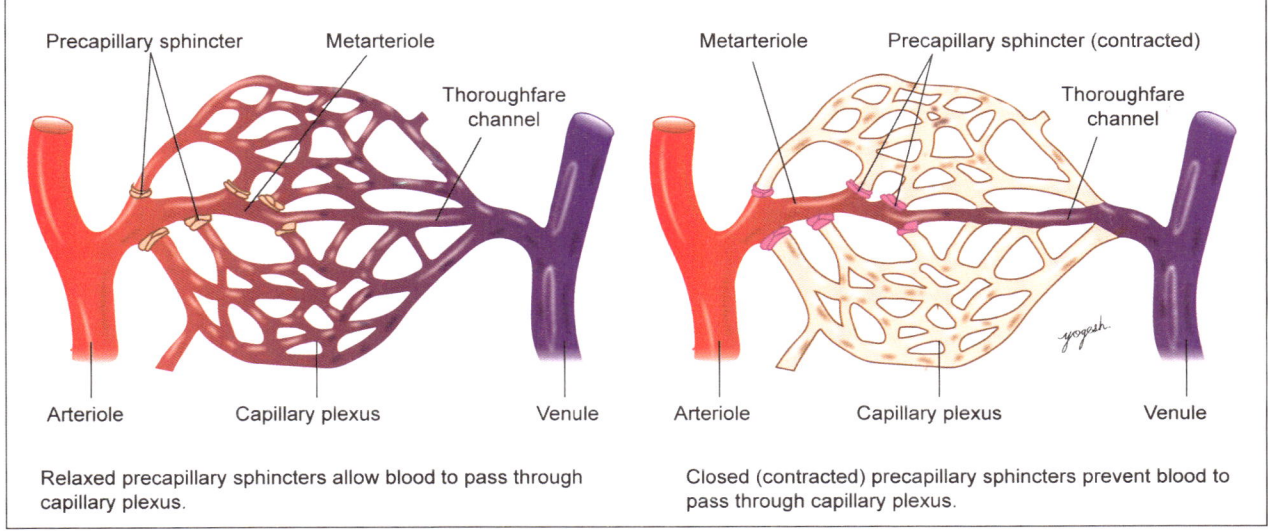

Fig. 13.11: Microcirculation and role of precapillary sphincter and metarteriole.

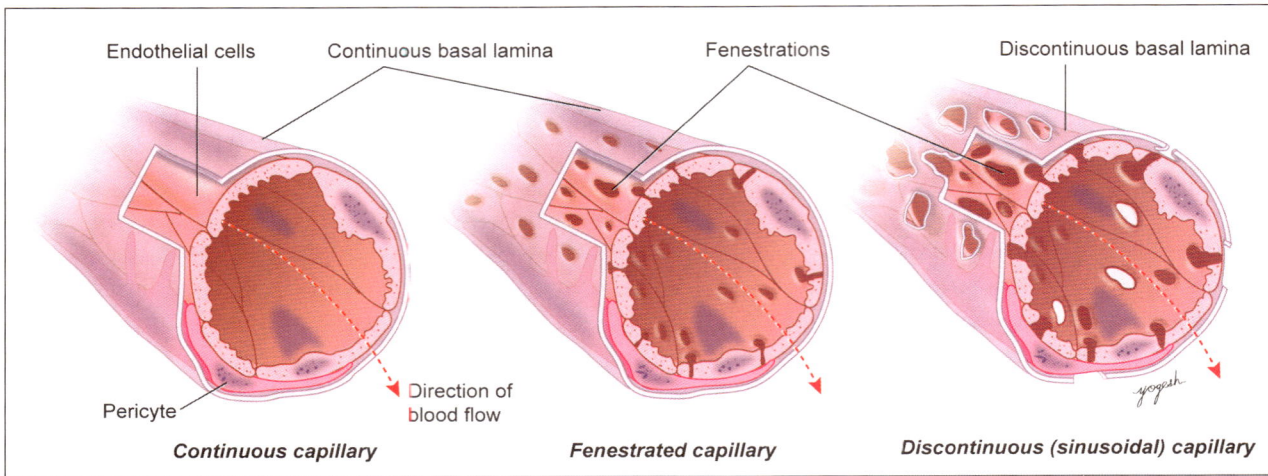

Fig. 13.12: Classification of capillaries.

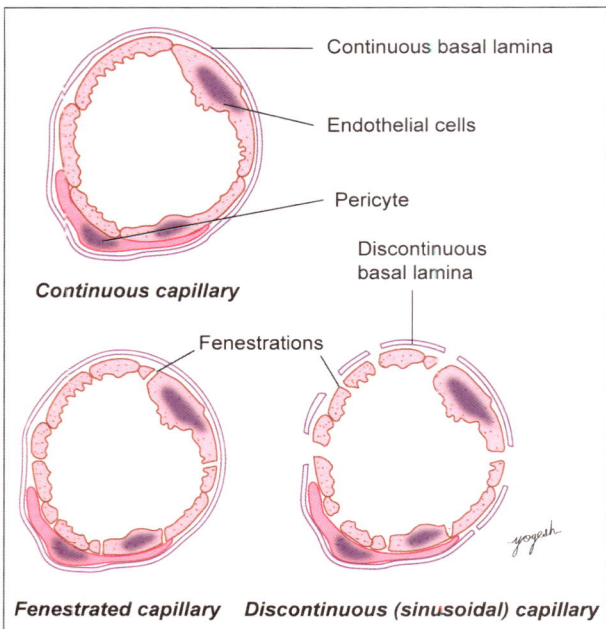

Fig. 13.13: Classification of capillaries (practice figure).

- *Transcytosis:* Endothelial cells of continuous capillaries show pinocytic vesicles in the cytoplasm (*mode of transepithelial transport*).
- Tight junction restricts passage of large molecules (>10 kDa).
- *Locations:* Continuous capillaries are found in connective tissue, muscles, skin, lungs, and central nervous system.^{MCQ, Viva}

Fenestrated Capillaries (Visceral)

- In fenestrated capillaries, endothelial cells have numerous circular openings called fenestrations (*fenestrations* = aperture or pores) (Figs 13.12 and 13.13).
- Size of fenestrations: 50–80 nm.
- Basal lamina is continuous and covers entire capillary.
- *New concept:* Fenestrations are developed because of pinched off process of pinocytosis. Thin endothelium loses its portion on pinocytosis leaving behind a fenestration (gap).
- *New concept:* Fenestrations are closed by a nonmembranous diaphragm that consists of thin layer of cytoplasm and basal lamina. Diaphragm closes filtration pores or fenestrations.
- *Locations:* Fenestrated capillaries are present in renal glomeruli, pancreas, endocrine glands, intestinal villi, choroid plexus, ciliary process of eye, and gallbladder.^{MCQ, Viva}

Sinusoids (Discontinuous Capillaries)

Q. Write a short note on sinusoids.

- In discontinuous or sinusoidal capillaries, large, irregular gaps are present in the wall (Figs 13.12 and 13.13).
- Endothelial cells have large pores or slits. Most of these pores are not closed by basal lamina (*discontinuous basal lamina*).
- Because of sluggish blood flow, sinusoids provide a chance of exchanging of bigger molecules easily.
- *Locations:* Liver, spleen, lymph nodes, bone marrow, endocrine glands (adrenal cortex, hypophysis cerebri, parathyroid gland), and carotid bodies.^{Neet, Viva}
- In liver, sinusoidal wall shows two special cells
  1. Kupffer cells – Phagocytic (macrophages) cells
  2. Ito cells – Vitamin A storing cells^{Neet}
- In spleen, endothelial cells have unique elongated shape and have gaps between adjacent cells.

Some Interesting Facts

- Pericytes are also called Rouget cells or mural cells. Pericytes are contractile cells that respond to nitric oxide released from endothelial cells.
- Pericytes are undifferentiated mesenchymal cells that can get differentiated into adipocytes, fibroblasts, chondrocytes, osteocytes, and skeletal muscle cells.
- During angiogenesis in embryo, in wound healing, and in pathological neovascularization (diabetic retinopathy), pericytes give rise to new endothelial cells and smooth muscle cells.
- Vascular endothelium in capillaries can produce endothelin I (produce vasoconstriction) and prostacyclin (produces vasodilatation).

Box 13.1: Arteriovenous (AV) shunts/anastomosis

Q. Write a short note on AV shunts

- Arteriovenous shunt connects arteriole to venule and *bypasses capillary network.*
- It helps to divert blood from capillaries (short-circuit).
- **Locations:** Skin of fingertips, nose, lips, erectile tissue of penis and clitoris.

Structure

- AV shunts may be straight or coiled.
- Wall of AV shunt is lined by endothelium and several layers of smooth muscle cells. Contraction of these smooth muscle cells closes AV shunt and enhances blood supply to capillary plexus.

Function

- *Thermoregulation:* In skin, opening of AV shunts helps to bypass capillary plexus and help to conserve heat.
- *Erectile function:* In erectile tissue, AV shunts divert blood to cavernous spaces and initiate erection.
- AV shunts of newborn are not well formed and in old age, number of AV shunt decreases. Hence, thermoregulation is not good in newborns and old.*Clinical fact*
- *Glomus* is a specialized form of AV shunt that is formed by rounded bunch of vessels. It is found in skin, at the tip of finger and toes, lips, and tip of the tongue and nose. Smooth muscle cells lining connecting vessels in glomus are epithelioid cells because they appear as epithelial cells.

VEINS

- Veins carry blood toward the heart.
- Based on diameter, veins are classified as: Venules, small veins, medium-sized veins, and large veins.

Venules and Small Veins

- The smallest veins are called venules. They collect blood from capillaries (Fig. 13.9).
- Diameter of venule is 0.1 mm or less.
- Venules are of two types:
  1. *Post-capillary venules* (10–50 μm diameter): They receive blood from capillaries. They are lined by endothelium and pericytes.
  2. *Muscular venules* (50–100 μm diameter): They are lined by endothelium, 1–2 layers of smooth muscles and surrounded by thick layer of connective tissue.

Some Interesting Facts

- Histamine and serotonin act mainly on postcapillary venules and cause extravasation of white blood cells during inflammation and allergic reactions.
- *High endothelial venules* are specialized postcapillary venules in lymphoid tissue.*MCQ* High endothelial venules are lined by *cuboidal endothelial cells.* Locations: Lymph nodes, tonsils, lymph nodules. High endothelial venules are not present in spleen.*MCQ*
- Small veins (0.1–1 mm diameter) drain blood from muscular venules. They are lined by endothelium, 2–3 layers of smooth muscle cells, and connective tissue adventitia.
- The differences between artery and vein are listed in Table 13.3.

Medium-Sized Veins

Q. Draw well-labeled diagram of histology of medium-sized vein.

- Medium-sized veins (1–10 mm diameter) show poorly identifiable three layers of vessels: Tunica intima, tunica media, and tunica adventitia (Figs 13.14, 13.7 and 13.8).
- *Tunica intima* consists of endothelium, basal lamina, thin subendothelial connective tissue, and discontinuous internal elastic lamina.
- *Tunica media* is thin and consists of few layers of smooth muscle cells.
- *Tunica adventitia* is a thick layer of connective tissue containing collagen and elastic fibers.
- Medium-sized veins accompany medium-sized arteries. For example, radial vein, tibial vein, popliteal vein, and so on.
- Medium-sized veins show presence of valves in their lumen to prevent retrograde (backward) flow of blood. Venous valves are more in veins of lower limb to counteract effect of gravity.

Q. List the differences between artery and vein

Table 13.3: Differences between artery and vein^Viva

Feature	Artery	Vein
Wall	Thicker than vein	Thinner than artery
Lumen	Oval, circular, patent (open)	Collapsed, irregular
Internal elastic lamina	Well defined in medium and small arteries	Absent or not well defined
Tunica media	Thicker than veins.	Thinner than arteries.
	Thicker than adventitia of arteries	Thinner than adventitia of veins
	Consists of many layers of smooth muscle cells and elastic fibers	Consists of a few layers of smooth muscle cells, collagen fibers, and fibroblasts
Tunica adventitia	Consists of connective tissue	Consists of longitudinal smooth muscle cells and elastic fibers (especially in large veins)
Layers	All three layers of vessel are well defined	In small and medium-sized veins, all three layers of vessel are not clearly identified

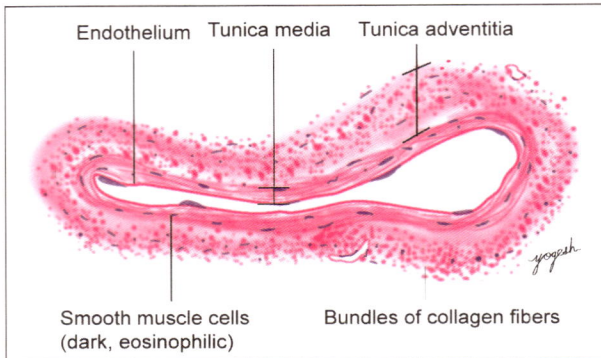

Fig. 13.14: Medium-sized vein.

Large Veins

Q. Write a short note on histology of large vein.

- Large vein (>10 mm diameter) shows presence of three layers of vessels: Tunica intima, tunica media, and tunica adventitia (Flowchart 13.7, Figs 13.15 and 13.16).

Tunica intima

- Tunica intima consists of vascular endothelium, basal lamina, and thin subendothelial connective tissue.

Flowchart 13.7: Histology of large vein

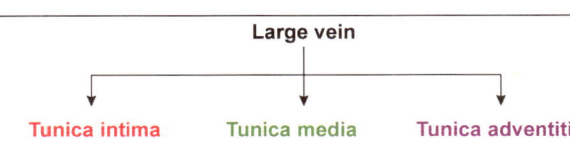

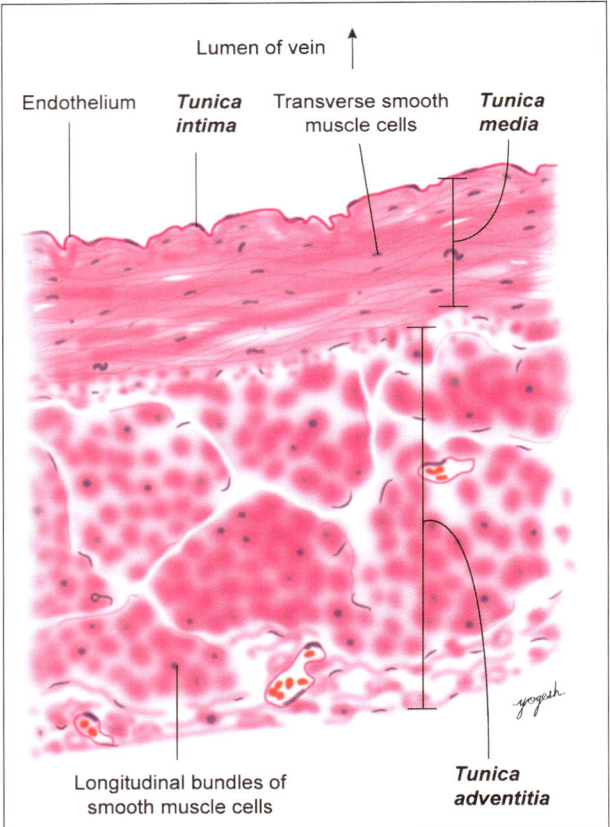

Fig. 13.15: Large vein (practice figure).

- Subendothelial connective tissue contains few smooth muscle cells.

Tunica media

- It consists of concentrically arranged smooth muscle cells, collagen fibers, and fibroblasts.
- Boundary between tunica media and tunica intima is difficult to decide.

Cardiovascular Tissue

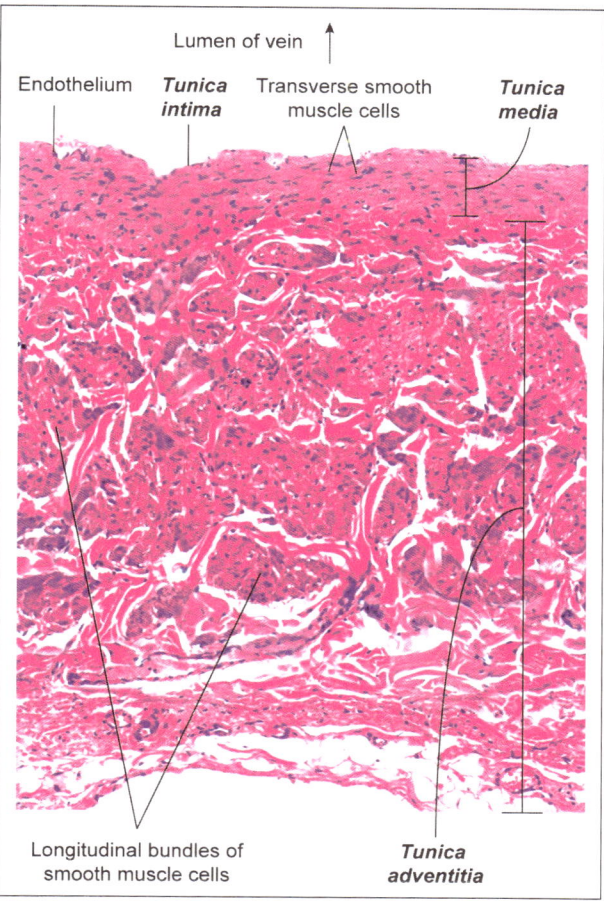

Fig. 13.16: Photomicrograph. Large vein (low magnification, H&E stain).

Tunica adventitia
- It is the thickest layer of large vein.*Identification feature*
- It consists of *longitudinally* arranged smooth muscle cells.*Identification feature*
- It also contains collagen fibers, elastic fibers, and fibroblasts. Examples: Superior vena cava, interior vena cava.

Clinical Correlation
- Deep venous thrombosis (DVT): In medium-sized veins, especially of lower limb, thrombus may form. This condition is called deep venous thrombosis. It is especially seen in patients with prolonged bed rest and in orthopedic cases with casts for treatment of fractures. Part of such clots may get separated, enter pulmonary circulation and forms blockage (pulmonary embolism).
- Varicose veins: These are abnormally dilated veins. It is especially seen in the veins of lower limbs in older people because of
  - Failure of valves
  - Decreased vascular smooth muscle tone
  - Prolonged standing
- Varicose veins are also present in the form of piles (hemorrhoids) in together esophagus and anal canal.

Some Interesting Facts
- Myocardial sleeves: These are atrial myocardial extensions in tunica adventitia of superior and inferior vena cava and pulmonary trunk. Myocardial sleeves may cause atrial fibrillation.
- Coronary arteries are medium-sized arteries.*Neet*
- Atherosclerotic changes in coronary artery cause reduced blood supply to heart (ischemic heart disease)
- Dural venous sinuses are lined by endothelium. They are devoid of vascular smooth muscles.*MCQ*
- Great saphenous vein is called muscular vein because of presence of numerous smooth muscles in its all tunics.
- Central adrenomedullary vein contains several longitudinally oriented smooth muscle cushions in tunica media.*Neet*

CHAPTER 14

Skin and its Appendages

Chapter Outline

- Introduction
- Structure of skin
  - Epidermis
  - Dermis
- Cells of epidermis
- Blood supply and nerve supply of skin
- Panniculus carnosus
- Sensory receptors of skin
- Appendage of skin
  - Hairs
  - Sebaceous glands
  - Sweat glands
  - Nails
- Arrector pili muscle
- Nail clubbing

Competency achievement: The student should be able to:

AN72.1 Identify the skin and its appendages under the microscope and correlate the structure with function

INTRODUCTION

- Integumentary system consists of skin and its appendages as follows:
  - Skin consists of two layers epidermis and dermis
  - Hair follicles and hairs
  - Sweat glands
  - Sebaceous glands
  - Nails
  - Mammary glands
- Hypodermis consists of adipose tissue that lies deep in to the dermis (*hypodermis* = subcutaneous fascia).
- Skin forms the outer covering of body.
- Skin-covering is supported by appendages or derivatives of skin such as hairs, nails, sebaceous glands, and sweat glands.
- Skin is the largest organ of body constituting about 16% (15–20%) of total body weight.*Viva*
- Skin has two layers: Superficial epidermis and deep dermis.

Types of Skin

- There are two types of skin depending on thickness of epidermis:
  1. *Thick skin:* Thick skin has very thick layer of epidermis. Its epidermis shows thick stratum corneum. Thick skin is also called *glabrous skin*. Thick skin does not have hairs. Locations: Skin of palm of hand and sole of feet.*Viva*
  2. *Thin (hairy) skin:* In thin skin, epidermis is thin. Thin skin shows hairs. Locations: Skin covering all parts of body except palm and soles.*Viva*
- For detailed differences between thick and thin skin, refer Table 14.1.

Structure of Skin

- Histologically, skin consists of two layers:
  1. *Epidermis:* It is a superficial layer that consists of keratinized stratified squamous epithelium.
  2. *Dermis:* It is deep layer that is made up of connective tissue.

Epidermis

- Epidermis consists of keratinized stratified squamous epithelium.*MCQ, Viva*
- Epidermis shows five layers of cells as follows (Figs 14.1 to 14.5):*Neet, Viva*
  1. Stratum basale
  2. Stratum spinosum
  3. Stratum granulosum
  4. Stratum lucidum (only in thick skin)
  5. Stratum corneum

Skin and its Appendages

Q. List the differences between thick and thin skin.

Table 14.1: Differences between thin and thick skin[Viva]

	Thick skin	Thin skin
Stratum lucidum	Present	Absent
Thickness of epidermis	0.6–4.5 mm	0.01–0.15 mm
Epidermal ridges	Present	Absent
Hair follicles	Absent	Present
Arrector pili muscle	Absent	Present
Sebaceous glands	Absent	Present
Sweat glands	Many	Few
Sensory receptors/Merkel's cells	More	Less
Location	Skin of palm and sole	Skin except of palm and sole

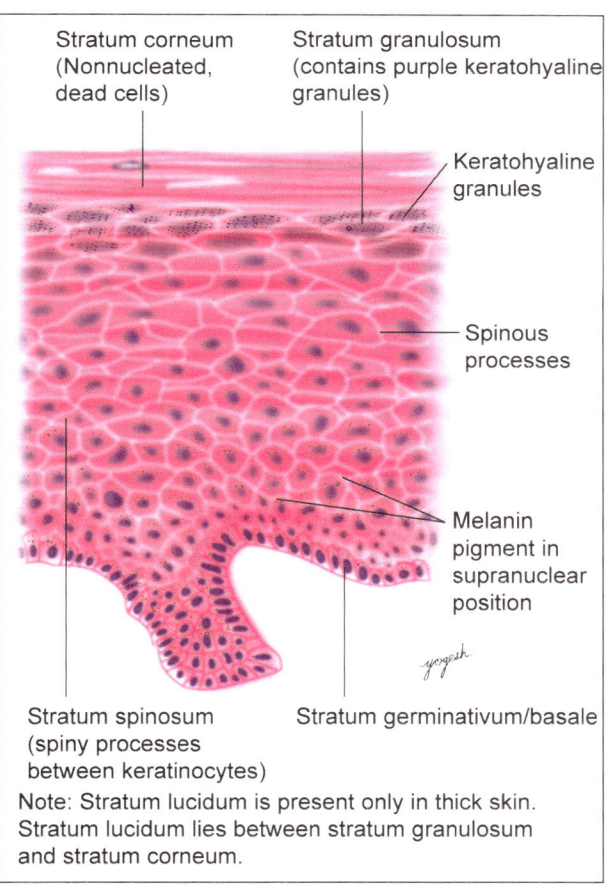

Fig. 14.1: Layers of epidermis.

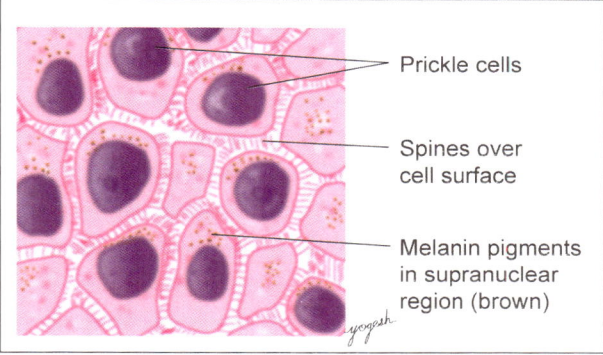

Fig. 14.2: Stratum spinosum of epidermis.

Some Interesting Facts
- *Thickest skin of body* is present in upper part of the back. Here, thin skin covers extremely thick dermis.
- Skin of eyelid is the *thinnest skin of body*. It is devoid of fat.
- *Cutaneous root for drug delivery:* Lipid-soluble drugs can be absorbed by skin when applied as ointment, spray, or patches.
- Cells of skin undergo specialized form of apoptosis. Stratum basale cells divide and migrate toward superficial layers. During migration, these cells show nuclear apoptotic changes and accumulation of intracellular keratin protein.

1. Stratum Basale (Stratum Germinativum)
- Stratum basale is the deepest layer of epidermis.
- Cells: It consists of a *single layer of cuboidal (low columnar) cells* that rest on basal lamina.
- H&E staining: Cells show basophilic cytoplasm and *melanin pigments.*
- Functions: These cells divide mitotically to give rise to keratinocytes (cells of skin) that form superficial layers of skin. Hence, stratum basale is also called stratum germinativum.[Viva]

2. Stratum Spinosum (Malpighian Layer, Prickle Cell Layer) (Figs 14.2, 14.5 and 14.6)
- Above the stratum basale, several layers of thick *stratum spinosum* are present.

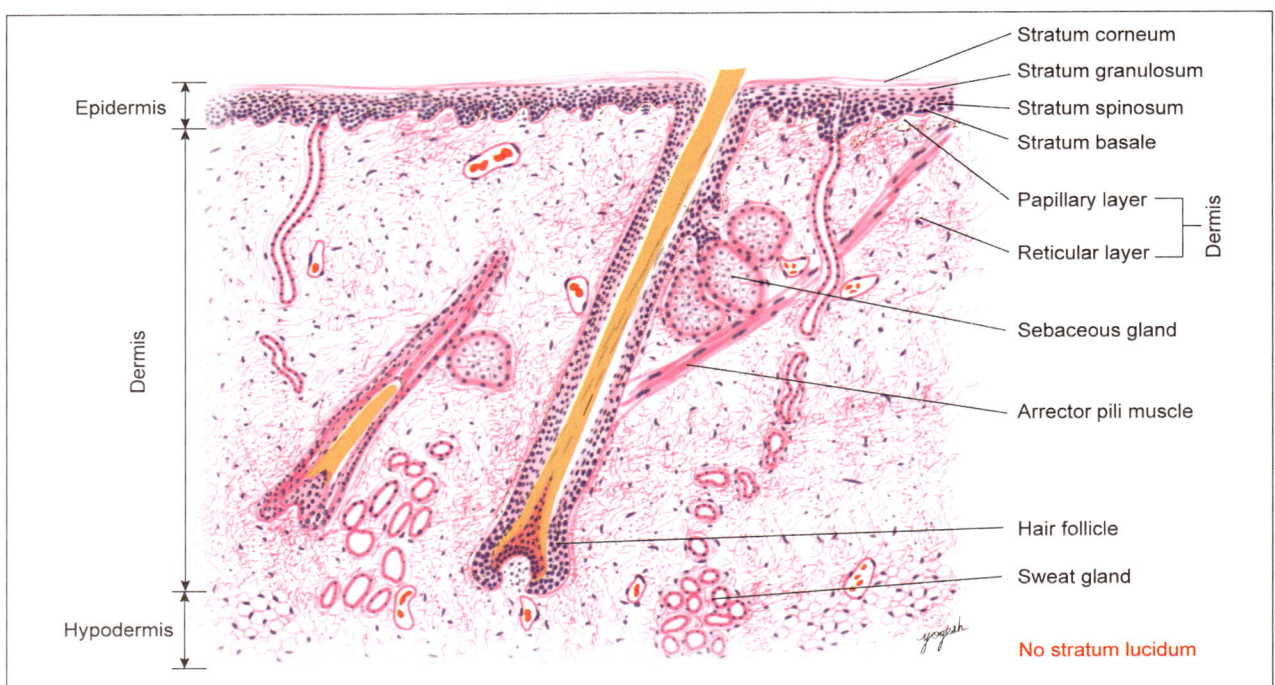

Fig. 14.3: Histology of thin skin (practice figure).

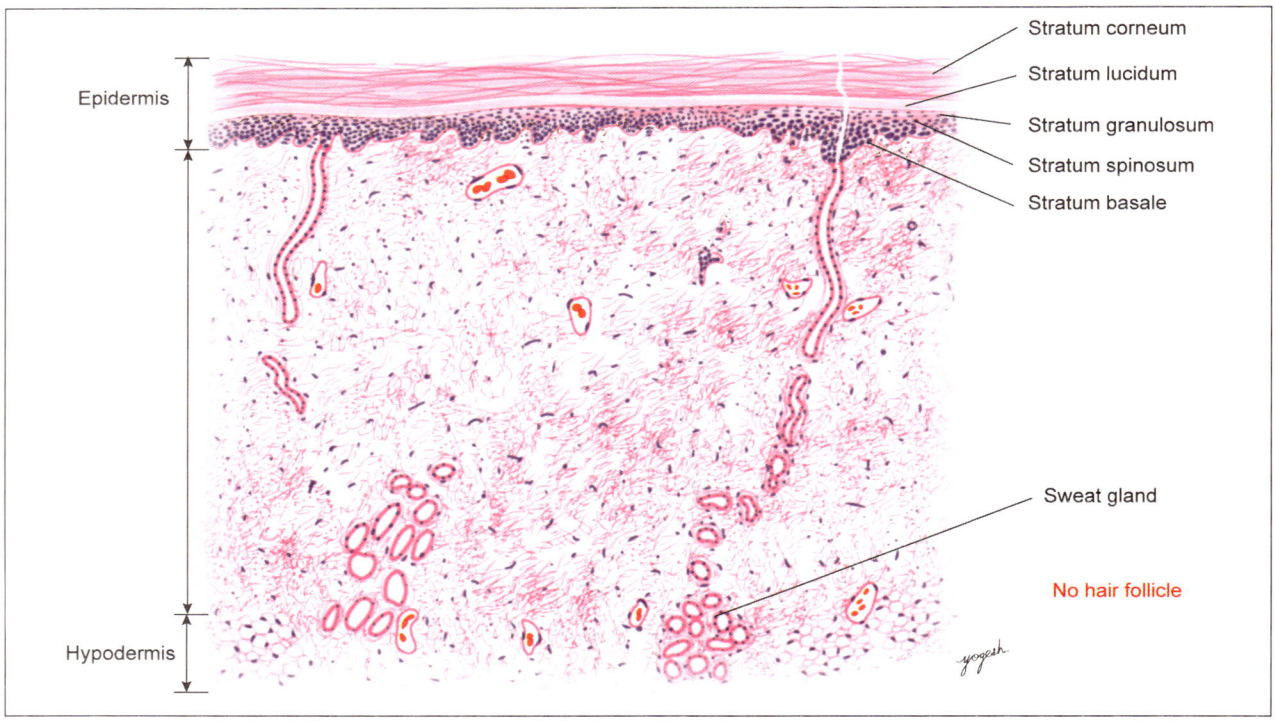

Fig. 14.4: Histology of thick skin (practice figure).

- Keratinocytes of stratum spinosum are *polygonal cells* that are connected with adjacent cells by *desmosomes*.
- *Spines are artifact:* During preparation of tissue for sectioning, cells often shrink. But these keratinocytes

Skin and its Appendages

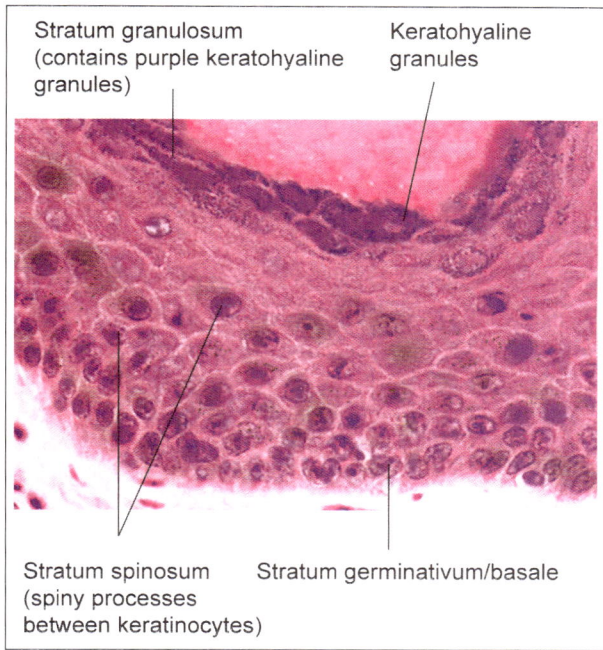

Fig. 14.5: Photomicrograph. Layers of epidermis.

(*prickle cells*) remain adherent with each other at the site of desmosomes. It creates spines over the surface of these cells at the site of desmosomes.^{Viva}
- Some cells of stratum spinosum may undergo mitosis; hence, stratum spinosum and stratum basale together can be considered as germinative zone.
- *Node of Bizzozero:* It is a site of thickened zone of desmosomes on light microscopy. [Giulio Bizzozero, Italian physician, 1846–1901].

3. Stratum Granulosum
- Stratum granulosum consists of 1–3 cells thick layer of keratinocytes.
- Cells of stratum granulosum contain granules of keratohyalin protein; hence, the name stratum granulosum.
- Keratohyalin is a precursor of filaggrin protein that on aggregation forms keratin filaments.
- *H&E stationing:* Cells of stratum granulosum are *intensely basophilic* because of keratohyalin granules.

4. Stratum Lucidum (Lucid = Clear)
(Figs 14.4 and 14.7)
- Stratum lucidum is present only in thick skin.^{MCQ}
- *H&E staining:* The cells of stratum lucidum are stained lightly with eosin and appears homogenous. Their cell boundaries are indistinct. The nuclei and cell organelles become disrupted and disappear toward superficial layer.
- *Cells of stratum lucidum contain eleidin.* It is a clear intracellular protein derived from keratohyalin and gets stained with hematoxylin. Later, eleidin gets converted to keratin in stratum corneum.^{Viva}
- *Note:* Some authors consider stratum lucidum as a part of stratum corneum.

5. Stratum Corneum
- This is the most superficial layer of epidermis.
- Cells of stratum corneum are *nonnucleated*, flat, scale-like (squamous) *cells* (dead cells) and they do not have cells organelles.

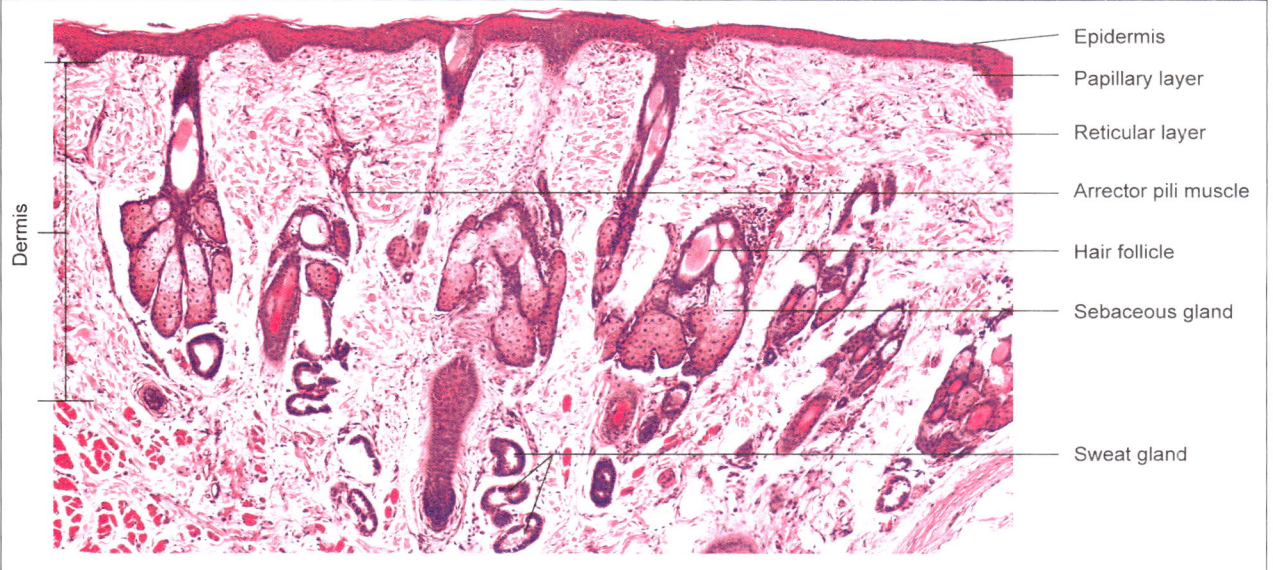

Fig. 14.6: Photomicrograph. Thin skin (low magnification, *H&E* stain).

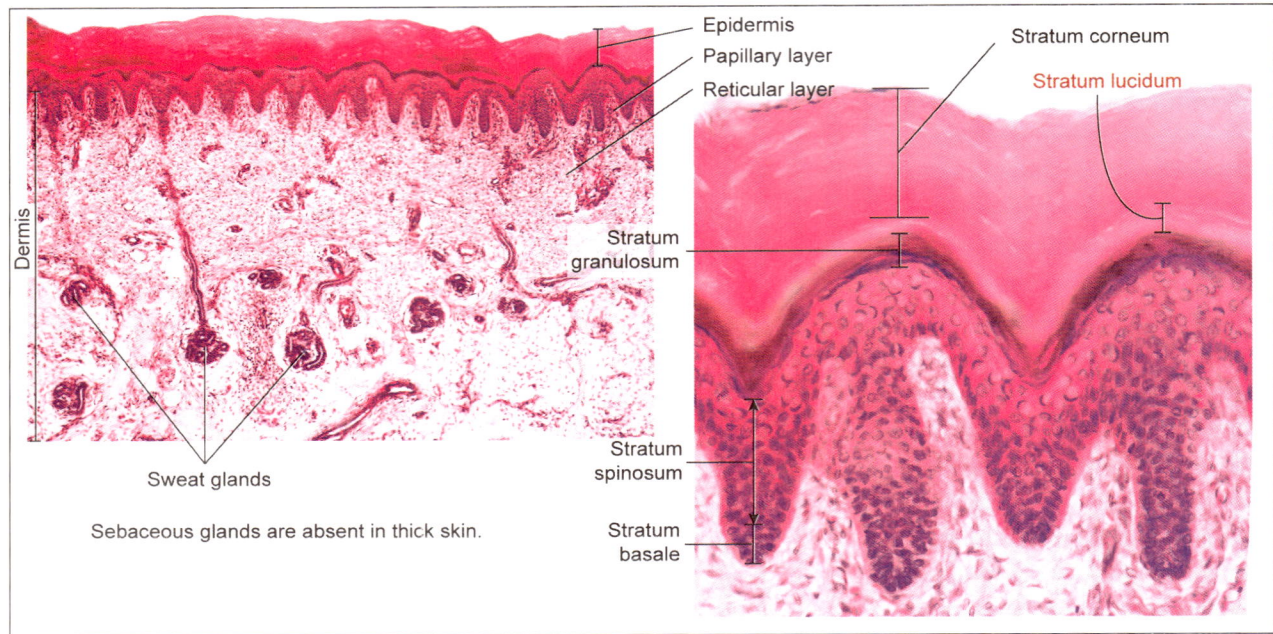

Fig. 14.7: Photomicrograph. Thick skin (low magnification on left, high magnification on right, *H&E* stain).

- Cells of stratum corneum are filled with keratin filaments.
- These cells are held together by extracellular lipid and carbohydrates that form a glue-like substance.
- Extracellular lipids make skin water impermeable.
- Thickness of stratum corneum depends on the amount of friction to which skin is exposed. Stratum corneum is very thick in palms and soles.
- Superficial cells of stratum corneum are being constantly shed off and are replaced by proliferation of stratum germinativum.

Clinical Correlation

- *Basal cell carcinoma:* It is the most common skin cancer. It arises from trichoblast or folliculosebaceous-apocrine germ.^{Neet} It begins as painless skin elevations. It rarely metastasizes (spreads to distinct locations). Basal cell carcinoma occurs in hairy skin (mostly on face).
- *Squamous cell carcinoma* (epidermoid carcinoma): It arises from squamous cells of skin, part of respiratory tract, and gut. Squamous cell carcinoma of skin usually arises in sun-exposed parts (UV light exposed) in older people and mostly on face, ears, back of hands, scalp, and lips.

Dermis

- Dermis is made up of connective tissue containing collagen bundles, blood vessels, lymphatics, and nerve fibers.
- Dermis has two layers:^{Viva}
  1. Papillary layer
  2. Reticular layer

1. Papillary Layer of Dermis

- It lies just deep to basal lamina of epidermis.
- It consists of loose connective tissue.^{Viva}
- It shows finger-like projections into the under surface of epidermis. These projections are called *dermal papillae*.^{Viva}
- Epidermis also protrude into dermis in the form of *epidermal ridges, rete ridges,* or *rete pegs*.^{Viva}
- Dermal papillae and epidermal ridges are longer in skin where mechanical stress is more. For example, skin of palm and dorsum of hand.
- Dermal papillae create superficial elevations on the surface of epidermis called *dermal ridges*. Pattern of dermal ridges is unique to each individual and genetically determined. *Dermatoglyphics* or finger-print patterns form the basis for study of many genetic disorders.
- *Transmission electron microscopy:* Hemidesmosomes attach basal cells of epidermis with basal lamina.
- *Immunohistochemistry:* Papillary layer contains type I and type III collagen fibers.
- Blood vessels of papillary layer do not penetrate epidermis. *Note:* Epidermis is avascular and receives nutrition by diffusion.^{Viva}
- Nerves from papillary layer may terminate in the basal layer of epidermis.

2. Reticular Layer

- Reticular layer of dermis lies deep to papillary layer and it is a dense irregular connective tissue.*Viva*
- Reticular layer is thicker and less cellular than papillary layer.
- It consists of thick, irregular bundles of type I collagen fibers and elastic fibers.

Some Interesting Facts

- *Langer's lines:* These are tension lines of skin. These lines correspond to natural orientation of collagen and elastic fibers in reticular layer of skin.
- Skin incisions made parallel to these lines heals with least scarring. [Karl Langer, Austrian anatomist, 1819–1887].

Box 14.1: Panniculus carnosus

- It is a part of subcutaneous connective tissue.
- It consists of a layer of striated muscles just deep to subcutaneous facia or hypodermis.
- It is well developed in lower animals.
- In human, examples of panniculus carnosus include:
  1. Muscles of facial expression including platysma
  2. Palmaris brevis in hand
  3. Dartos muscle in scrotum.

CELLS OF EPIDERMIS

- Skin has four types of cells: keratinocytes, melanocytes, Langerhans cells, and Merkel's cells.*Viva*

Keratinocytes (85%)

- Keratinocytes constitute approximately 85% of cells of skin (predominant cell type).*Viva*
- Germinal cells of stratum basale divide mitotically and give rise to keratinocytes.
- The major functions of these cells include production of keratin and formation of epidermal water barrier.
- Deeper layers of keratinocytes are basophilic because of presence of rough endoplasmic reticulum. It is required for synthesis of keratins (proteins).
- Keratin assemble to form keratin filaments or tonofilaments (intermediate filaments).
- Keratin filaments form bundles of tonofibrils in the superficial layers of keratinocytes. These superficial cells do not have nuclei and cell organelles. These cells give acidophilic or eosinophilic appearance.
- Appearance of keratohyalin granules and its associated proteins (filaggrin) is a clinical marker for initiation of apoptosis.*Neet*

- *Keratinization:* Keratinocyte synthesizes keratohyalin granules. Later, keratohyalin granules release keratin filaments into the cytoplasm. These filaments get aggregated with the help of filaggrin and trichohyalin proteins. This process is called keratinization.
- Lamellae of stratum spinosum produces ovoid, membrane-bound organelles called *lamellar bodies.* These bodies contain lipids that get released in to the extracellular spaces. This lipid is involved in formation of epidermal water barrier and also act as glue to hold keratinocytes.

Some Interesting Facts

- *Desquamation of surface keratinocytes:* Surface keratinocytes are held together by desmosomes. Released proteolytic enzymes (Kallikrein-related serine peptidases) break desmosomes in superficial layers of epidermis and produces desquamation.
- There is an equilibrium in the production of keratinocytes and desquamation of keratinocytes.
- Total time required for formation of keratinocyte till its desquamation is approximately 47 days.*MCQ*
- *Psoriasis:* It is a skin disorder showing a patch of skin covered by silvery white scales. It occurs because of rapid turnover of keratinocytes (~8–10 days).

Melanocytes (Fig. 14.8)

- Melanocytes are the derivatives of neural crest cells.*MCQ*
- Melanocytes are present in stratum germinativum/basale.
- Melanocytes show dendrite-like processes arising from a rounded cell. Processes of melanocytes lie between the keratinocytes.
- *Premelanosomes* are tyrosine filled vesicles that are site of melanin synthesis.*Viva*
- Melanocyte synthesizes melanin and transfers it to melanin nonproducing cells through cell processes. This melanin transfer is an example of *cytocrine secretion.*
- *Melanophores* are cells that receive melanin from melanocytes.*Viva*

Box 14.2: Melanin

- Melanin is a brown pigment.
- Melanin is present in melanocytes, keratinocytes of skin, pigmented epithelium of retina, pigmented cells of vascular zone of eyeball (choroid, ciliary body, and iris), and in some neurons of brain.

Synthesis

- Tyrosine amino acid is converted into dihydroxyphenylamine (DOPA) by tyrosinase. This DOPA is converted into melanin by tyrosinase.
- Synthesis of melanin is under control of melanocyte stimulating hormone (MSH) of intermediate lobe of pituitary gland.
- On synthesis of melanin, it forms membrane-bound granules called **melanosomes**.
- *Color of skin:* It depends on three factors
  1. Amount of melanin in epidermal cells
  2. Carotene pigment (yellow color) of skin
  3. Vascularity of skin
- Role of melanin: *Melanosomes* acquire supranuclear position in keratinocytes and protect nuclei from ultraviolet ray induced damage.
- *Albinism:* It is inborn error of metabolism that makes melanocytes incapable of melanin synthesis. It occurs because of *absence of tyrosinase enzyme.*[MCQ]
- *Vitiligo:* It occurs on destruction of melanocytes, mostly because of autoimmune reactions. It produces patchy depigmentation of skin.
- *Moles/naevocellular naevi:* These are dark, slightly elevated or flat lesions of skin. These are present almost in all individuals either at birth or appears in later life because of hormonal influence.
- *Malignant melanoma:* It is an invasive tumor arising from melanocytes. It may spread locally or throughout the body through blood or lymphatics. It may occur because of excessive exposure to sunlight.

Dendritic Cells of Langerhans (Fig. 14.8)[Neet]

- These are *antigen presenting cells of epidermis.*[Neet, Viva]
- They arise from lymphoid precursor cells of bone marrow.
- These cells lie in stratum spinosum of skin, oral mucosa, vagina, and thymus.
- *Langerhans bodies* or *Birbeck bodies:* These are elongated vacuoles seen under electron microscope in Langerhans cells. Langerhans bodies are *tennis-racket-shaped bodies.*[Neet, Viva]
- Langerhans cells phagocytose bacteria and present bacterial antigens to T-lymphocytes. Thus, Langerhans cells constitute a part of mononuclear phagocytic system.
- Langerhans cells undergo malignant transformation to form *histiocytosis X*. It is a group of immune disorders.
- Langerhans cells are responsible for delayed type of hypersensitivity reaction.
- In AIDS patients, Langerhans cells may show presence of HIV virus. And may act as reservoir of HIV virus.

Cells of Merkel (Fig. 14.8)

- These are sensory cells responsible for cutaneous sensation.
- These are located in stratum basale.
- Merkel cells are *mechanoreceptor (faithfully represents the Braille text/characters – useful for blind people).*[Neet]
- Sensory nerve endings are present in relation to Merkle cells.
- These cells are more abundant in fingertips, oral mucosa, and hair follicles.
- Merkel cell carcinoma is a rare condition. It is highly aggressive skin cancer.

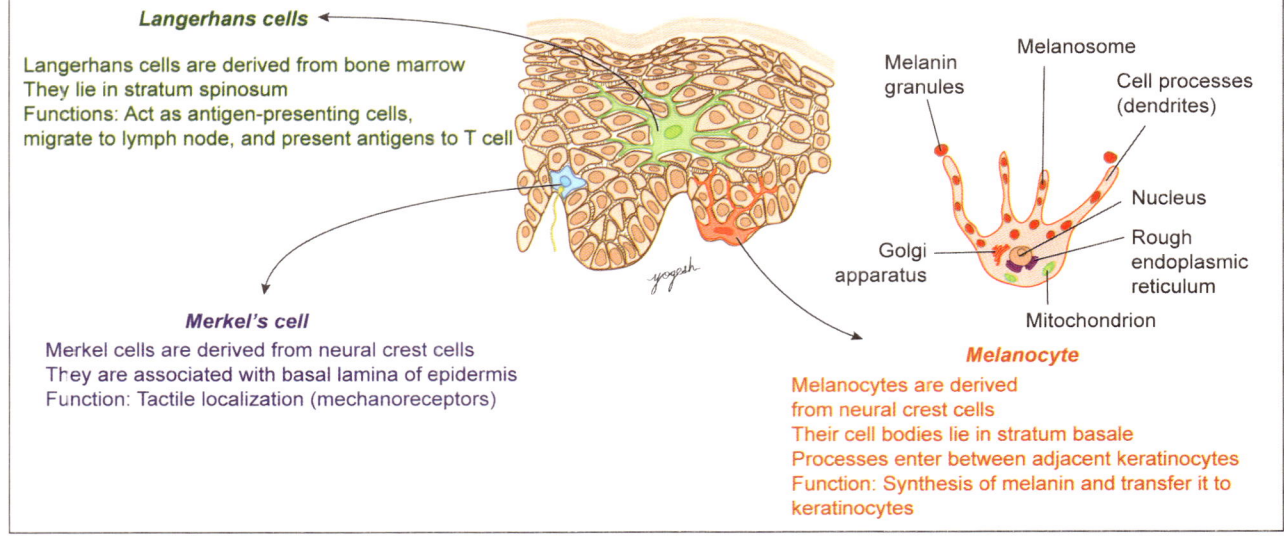

Fig. 14.8: Migrated cells in epidermis and their functions.

BLOOD SUPPLY AND NERVE SUPPLY OF SKIN

Blood Supply

- Epidermis is *avascular*. It derives its nutrition by diffusion.^{Viva}
- Skin receives its blood supply by the following arterial plexuses:
  1. *Rete subapapillare or papillary plexus:* It is located just below dermal papillae.^{Viva}
  2. *Rete cutaneum or reticular plexus:* It lies just below dermis.
  3. *Deepest plexus:* It lies over deep fascia.
- There are numerous *arteriovenous anastomoses* in skin that regulate blood flow through capillary plexuses of skin. Decreased blood flow to these capillaries conserve body temperature, whereas increased blood flow decreases body temperature.^{Clinical fact}

Nerve Supply

- Skin is supplied by cutaneous nerves that carry sensation from free nerve endings, Meissner's corpuscles, Pacinian corpuscles, and Ruffini end organs.
- Blood vessels of skin receive autonomic supply. Sympathetic stimulation produces vasoconstriction and divert the blood away from skin.
- Autonomic nerves in skin increse secretions of sweat gland (contraction of myoepithelial cells) and produce contractions of arrectors pilorum muscles.

Summary (Examination Guide) (Flowchart 14.1)

- Skin has two layers: Superficial epidermis and deep dermis.

Epidermis: It consists of the following layers:

- *Stratum basale:* It is a single layer of low columnar cells that divide mitotically to form keratinocytes.
- *Stratum spinosum:* It is several layers thick. Deeper layer cells are polygonal with spherical nucleus. Upper layer cells are flat. These cells are connected with each other by spinous processes (desmosomes). These cells synthesize keratin granules.
- *Stratum granulosum:* It is 4–5 layers thick, flattened cells. These cells contain keratin filaments.
- *Stratum lucidum (only in thick skin):* It is translucent, narrow layer. The cells do not show nuclei and cytoplasmic organelles.
- *Stratum corneum:* It is 15–20 cells thick. Cells are flat and dead.

Dermis: It consists of

- Superficial *papillary layer* of loose connective tissue. It shows dermal papillae that invaginate epidermis.
- Deep *reticular layer* of dense irregular connective tissue.

Box 14.3: Sensory receptors of skin

- Skin is enriched by free nerve endings, Pacinian corpuscles, Meissner's corpuscles, and Ruffini corpuscles (Fig. 14.9).
- *Free nerve endings:* Free nerve endings terminate in stratum granulosum of epidermis and surround most of the hair follicles. These carry fine touch, heat, cold, pain sensation, and hair-movement senses. Free nerve endings are not covered by Schwann cells.
- *Pacinian corpuscles:* These are large, oval structures present in deeper part of dermis and in hypodermis. Pacinian corpuscles in transverse section looks-like hemisection of onion. Nerve ending in Pacinian corpuscle is surrounded by concentric lamellae of flat, fibroblast-like supportive cells. Pacinian corpuscles carry deep pressure and vibration sense.
- *Meissner's corpuscles:* These are located within dermal papillae of hairless skin. In Meissner's corpuscle, nerve ending is surrounded by perpendicularly arranged supporting cells. *H&E staining:* Meissner's corpuscle resembles a loose, twisted skein of wool because of orientation of Schwann cells. Meissner's corpuscles are responsible for light touch sensation.
- *Ruffini corpuscles:* These are elongated fusiform corpuscles. It consists of a single myelinated nerve fiber that is surrounded by fluid-filled space enclosed in a capsule. The nerve fiber arborizes into fine axonal

---

Flowchart 14.1: Histology of skin

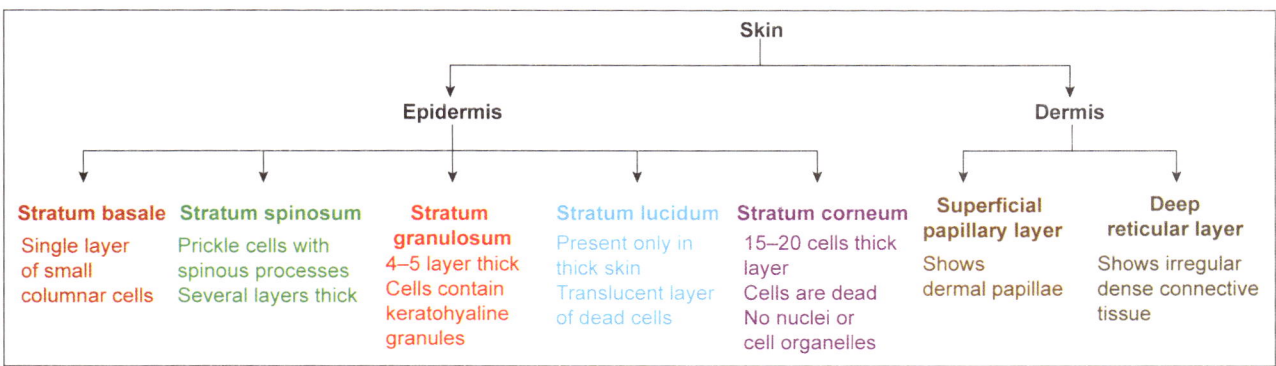

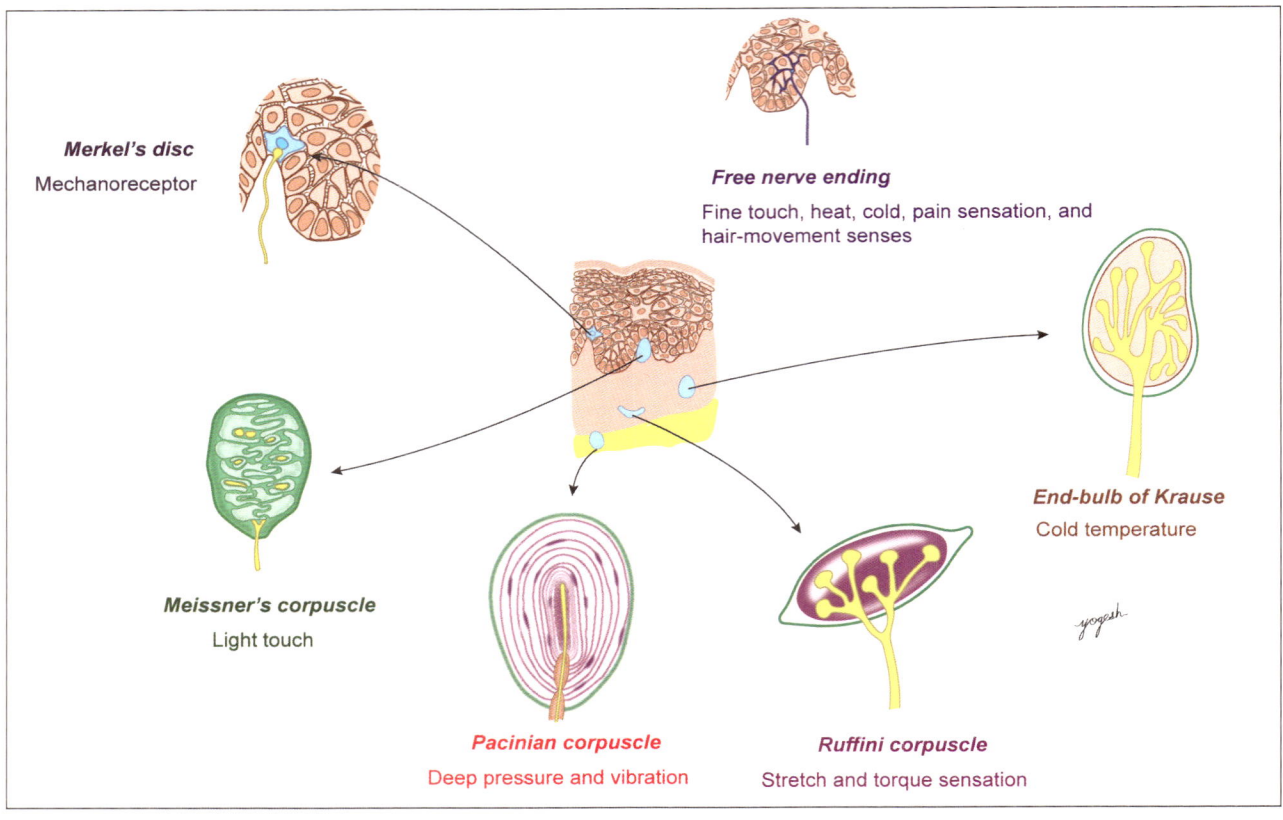

Fig. 14.9: Receptors in the skin.

endings and each one terminates as a small knob-like bulb. Ruffini corpuscles carry skin stretch and torque sensation.

- **End-bulb of Krause (Bulboid corpuscle):** End-bulbs of Krause are thermoreceptors, sensing cold temperatures. They are minute cylindrical or oval bodies with expansion of a medullated nerve fiber. They are located in conjunctiva of eye, in mucous membrane of lips and tongue, and epineurium of nerve trunks, penis and clitoris (called genital corpuscles), and in synovial membranes of certain joints. [Wilhelm Krause, 1833-1910, German anatomist].
- **Merkel discs:** Merkel discs/nerve endings are mechanoreceptors, a type of sensory receptor, that are found in basal epidermis and hair follicles.

APPENDAGES OF SKIN

- Epidermis gives rise to appendages of skin that support skin.
- Appendages of skin include hair follicles, hair, nail, sebaceous glands, eccrine sweat glands, and apocrine sweat glands.

HAIRS

- Hairs cover entire body except the following sites: Palm, sole, sides of hand and feet, lips, ventral surfaces and sides of digits, and part of genitalia.
- Hair growth and texture is influenced by hormones.

Some Interesting Facts
- With advancing age, because of lack of estrogen and estrogen-like hormones, hairline recedes in both male and female.
- Fine hairs and less number of hairs are adaptations in humans as compared to lower animals. It helps to enhance more sensory aspects of skin.
- In humans, subcutaneous fat helps in conservation of heat (Hairs perform same function in lower animals).

Skin and its Appendages

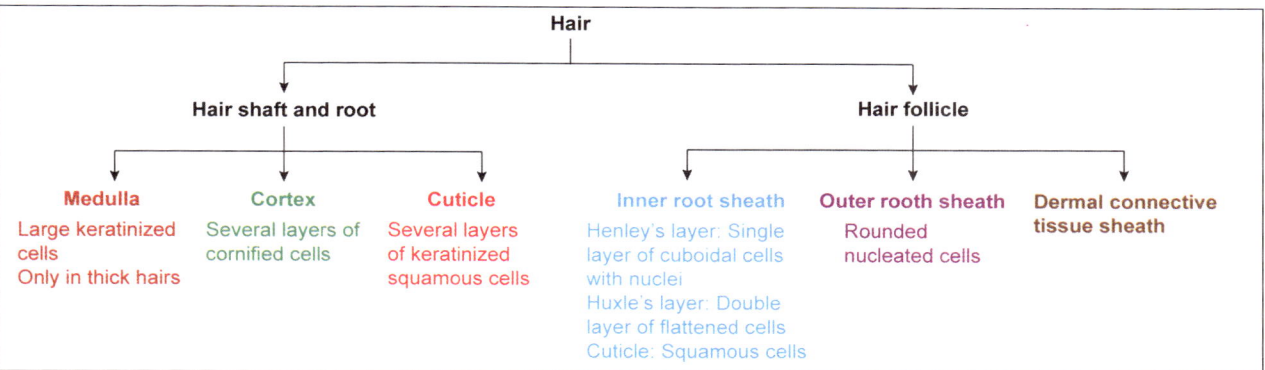

Flowchart 14.2: Histological structure of hair^{Viva}

Parts of Hair

Hair has the following parts (Flowchart 14.2):
1. *Shaft:* It is a visible part of hair that projects above surface of skin.
2. *Root*: It is a part of hair that is embedded in skin and enclosed by hair follicle.
3. *Bulb*: It is lower expanded end of root of hair.
4. *Hair papilla:* It is a part of the dermis that invaginates base of hair bulb.
5. *Hari follicle:* It is dermo-epidermal sheath that covers root of the hair.

Hair Shaft and Root

- Hair shaft and root consist of keratinized cells. Hence, hair is considered a modified part of stratum corneum of epidermis.
- Hair has three parts: Cuticle, cortex, and medulla.
- *Medulla:* It is a central part of hair. It consists of large keratinized cells. Medulla is a part of thick hairs, whereas it is absent in thin hairs.
- *Cortex:* It surrounds medulla. Hair mostly consists of cortex (80%). Cortex is made up of cornified cells containing hard keratin filaments and melanin pigments.
- *Cuticle:* It covers surface of hair. It consists of several layers of keratinized squamous cells. These cells are semitransparent, having distinct boundaries and resembles scales of fish.

Hair Follicle (Figs 14.10 and 14.11)

- Dermoepidermal covering of hair root forms a knob-like structure called hair follicle.
- Hair follicle produces hair.
- Each hair follicle has the following parts:
  1. *Infundibulum* extends from surface opening of follicle up to opening of sebaceous glands.

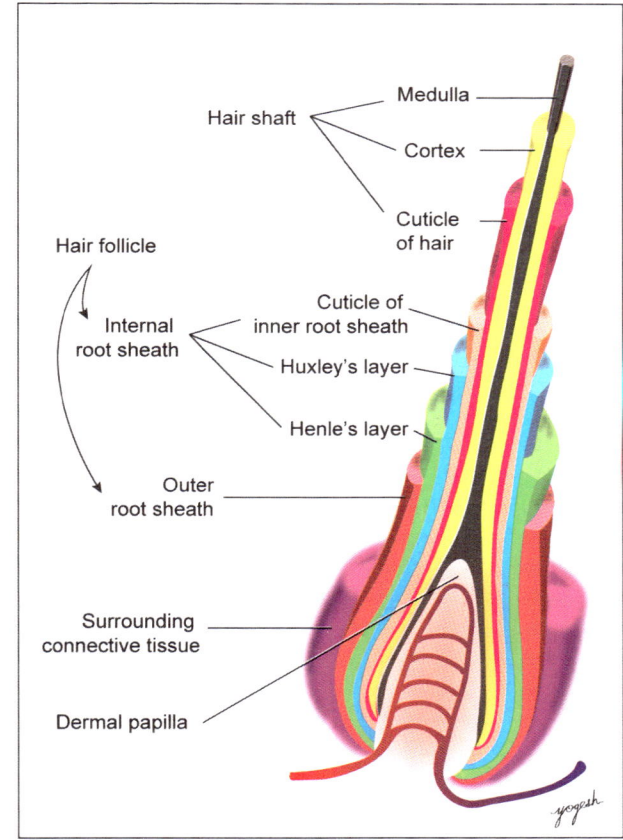

Fig. 14.10: Structure of hair.

  2. *Isthmus* extends from opening of sebaceous gland up to insertion of arrector pili/pilorum muscle.^{Viva}
  3. *Follicular bulge:* It contains epidermal stem cells and lies near insertion of arrector pili muscle.
  4. *Bulb and dermal papilla:* Bulb is lower expanded end of hair follicle. Dermal papilla invaginates base of hair bulb.
- Wall of hair follicle consists of 3 layers:
  1. Inner root sheath

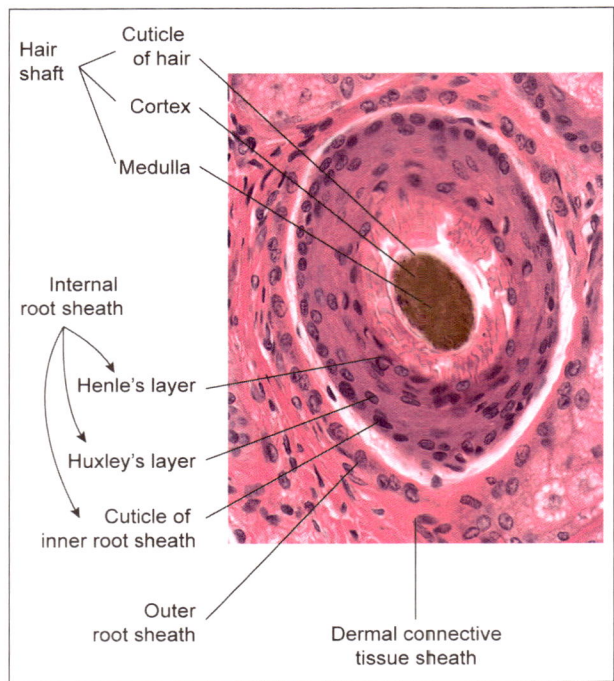

Fig. 14.11: Photomicrograph. Hair follicle (high magnification, H&E stain).

2. Outer root sheath (continuous with stratum spinosum)
3. Dermal connective tissue sheath

Inner root sheath
- Inner root sheath is a multilayered cellular coat that covers deep part of hair. It consists of the following three layers from outside inwards:
  1. *Henle's layer:* It consists of single layer of cuboidal cells with flattened nuclei. It is also called *stratum epitheliale pallidum.*[Neet] [Friedrich Henle, 1809–1885, German physician, anatomist].
  2. *Huxley's layer:* It consists of double layer of flattened cells that contain large eosinophilic trichohyalin granule.[Neet]
  3. *Cuticle:* Cuticle consists of squamous cells that cover outer free surface of hair shaft.

Outer root sheath
- It is continuous with stratum spinosum of epidermis.
- It consists of round nucleated cells.
- Outer root sheath is separated from dermal connective tissue sheath by a thick glassy membrane or basal lamina.

Matrix cells/hair matrix
- These are cells that surround bulb and dermal papilla.
- These cells are derived from follicular bulge.
- Matrix cells divide and provide continuous supply of cells for hair growth.
- Melanocytes are scattered among matrix cells. These melanocytes transfer melanin to developing hair cells.

Clinical Correlation
- Phases of hair growth:
  - *Anagen:* It is a time of new hair development.
  - *Catagen:* It is a period when hair growth stops.
  - *Telogen:* It is a period of hair loss because of follicular atrophy.
- Hair may be:
  - *Terminal hairs:* These are long and coarse hairs.
  - *Vellus hairs:* These are short and fine hairs. More than 80% of hairs of scalp are present in anagen phase. Most of the scalp hairs have very long anagen phase and short telogen phase.
- *Alopecia areata* (spot baldness): In this condition, hairs are lost in a small area of body. Area of alopecia areata does not show any scar, scale, or redness. At periphery of alopecia zone, *exclamation mark* hairs are present. It is characteristic of alopecia areata.[Neet]

Box 14.4: Arrector pili muscle

- Arrector pili muscle are small smooth muscles bundles attached at one end to dermis and another end to connective tissue sheath of a hair follicle.
- These muscles are attached to hair follicle that forms an obtuse angle with skin surface.
- Nerve supply: Sympathetic nerves.

Actions
- Hair stands on end/*goose-flesh appearance:* Contraction of muscle, on sympathetic innervation, produces hair-stand on end with slight depression at the dermal attachment of muscle. It gives goose flesh appearance.
- *Ejection of sebum:* As sebaceous glands lie between arrector pili muscle and skin, during contraction of muscle, sebaceous glands get squeezed. It results in release of sebum.

SEBACEOUS GLANDS

- Sebaceous gland is a *holocrine*, simple saccular gland present in dermis (Figs 14.12 and 14.13).[Neet, Viva]
- Usually, sebaceous gland opens into *pilosebaceous canal* at infundibulum of hair follicle by short duct.
- Hair-independent sebaceous glands are found in lips, areolae of nipple (Montgomery's tubercles), labia minora, and inner surface of prepuce.[Neet]

Skin and its Appendages

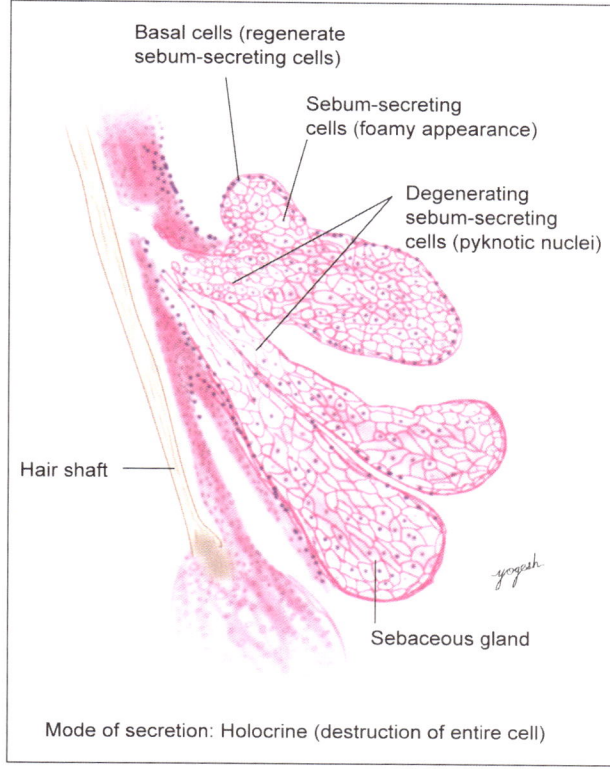

Fig. 14.12: Sebaceous gland.

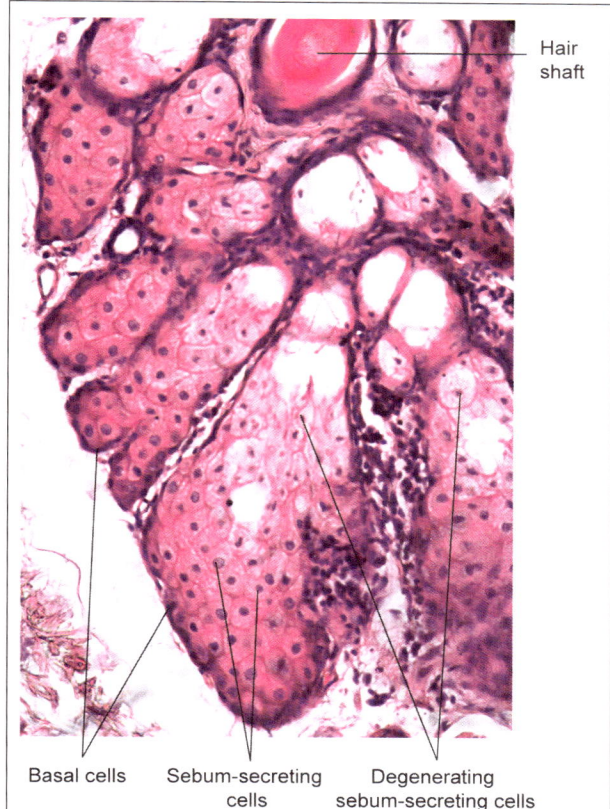

Fig. 14.13: Photomicrograph. Sebaceous gland (high magnification, H&E stain).

- Each sebaceous gland has two portions:
  1. Secretory portion (alveoli)
  2. Broad, short duct (lined by stratified squamous epithelium)^{Neet}
- Each alveolus consists of mass of polyhedral cells. Usually, alveolus does not have lumen.
- Each alveolus is lined by *basal cells and secretory cells*.
- *Basal cells* are outermost cells that rest on basement membrane. Basal cells divide mitotically to form inner secretory cells.
- *Secretory cells* resemble multilocular adipocytes. These cells are large polygonal cells with big, rounded nuclei. Cytoplasm of secretory cell is filled with lipid droplets.
- *H&E staining:* During preparation, lipid droplets get washed out; hence, the cytoplasm is stained lightly with eosin and cells show foamy appearance.
- *Secretion*
  Secretory cells synthesize and accumulate sebum. During this process, these cells undergo apoptosis. In the end, entire dead cell debris and lipids get secreted into duct as sebum (oily). This mode of secretion is called *holocrine secretion*.^{Neet}
- Sebaceous gland produces cathelicidin and β-defensin that improve water barrier function of skin.

> **Clinical Correlation**
> - *Seborrhea* or oily skin: It refers to overactive sebaceous glands that produce excess sebum.
> - *Acne vulgaris:* It occurs during adolescence in both sexes. In acne vulgaris, hair follicles get clogged with dead cell debris and sebum. It occurs as white head (closed by skin), back head (open, black because of oxidized melanin), pimple (trapped sebum under skin), or even scarring.
> - In 80% of cases, acne is genetically based. Increased hormonal levels during puberty enhance acne. *Comedo* is a clogged hair follicle.

SWEAT GLANDS

- Sweat glands produce sweat or perspiration.
- There are two types of sweat glands (Figs 14.14 and 14.15):
  1. *Eccrine* (typical or merocrine) sweat glands: These are distributed all over body **except** lips and external genitalia.
  2. *Apocrine* (atypical) sweat glands: These are present only in axilla, areola, nipple of mammary gland, skin around the anal opening, and external genitalia.^{Neet}

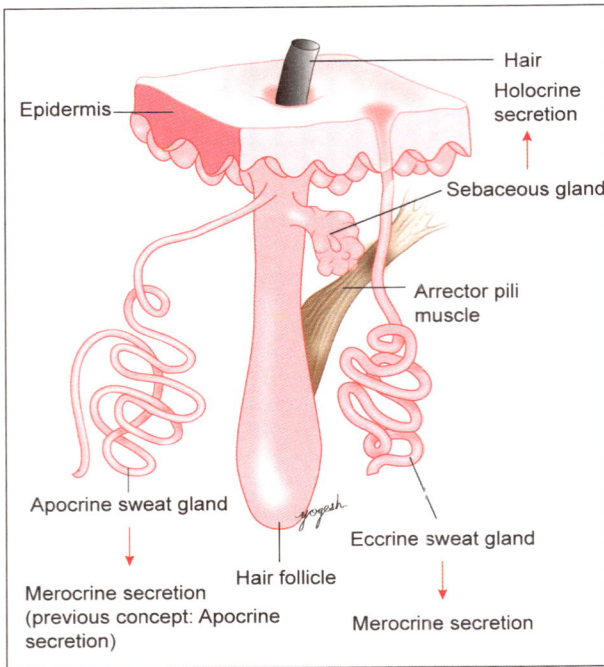

Fig. 14.14: Glands related to skin include apocrine and eccrine sweat gland, and sebaceous glands.

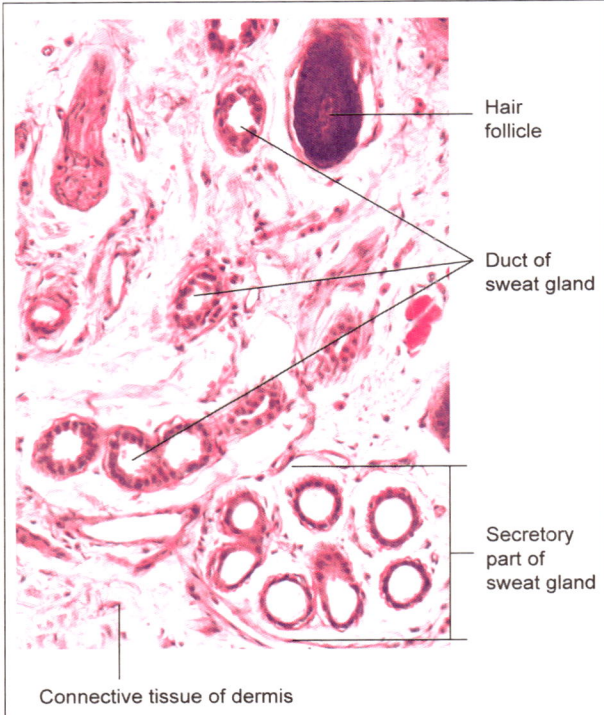

Fig. 14.15: Photomicrograph. Sweat gland (section of thin skin, H&E stain, high magnification).

- *Note:* Apocrine glands include glands of Moll in eyelids and ceruminous glands of the external acoustic meatus.^{MCQ}

Eccrine Sweat Glands
- Eccrine sweat glands are simple coiled tubular glands.^{Neet, Viva}
- These are distributed all over body except lips and external genitalia.
- These glands are most numerous in palms and soles, forehead, scalp, and axillae.
- They play a major role in regulation of body temperature.

Structure
- Eccrine sweat gland has two parts: 1. Duct and 2. Body or fundus.

1. Duct
- Gland has a long duct that runs through dermis. It opens on surface of epidermis through a funnel-shaped orifice.
- Duct is lined by two or more layers of cuboidal cells (stratified cuboidal epithelium).^{Neet}
- Duct ends on joining the epidermis and terminal part of excretory duct. It is lined by epithelial cells of epidermis.
- Ducts have smaller diameter than secretory portion (body) of gland, and ducts do not have myoepithelial cells.^{Identification feature}

2. Secretory part/body
- Secretory part of eccrine sweat gland consists of highly coiled terminal part of tube.
- Secretory part consists of inner lining epithelium, its basal lamina, and surrounding connective tissue of dermis.
- Secretory part is lined by a *single layer of cuboidal epithelium*.
- Lining epithelium consists of three types of cells:
  - *Clear cells:* These cells are separated from each other by intercellular canaliculi. These cells rest on basal lamina. Function: Secretion of water and electrolytes.
  - *Dark cells:* These cells stain dark on *H&E staining* because of abundant rough endoplasmic reticulum. These cells rest on apical surface of basal clear cells. Dark cells secrete proteins (defensins, cathelicidin). Note: Dark cell secretes their secretion by exocytosis (merocrine).^{MCQ}
  - *Myoepithelial cells:* These are contractile cells located between secretory cells and basal lamina. On *H&E staining*, myoepithelial cells are dark eosinophilic because of presence contractile filaments in cytoplasm. Myoepithelial cells help in ejection of secretions.

Apocrine/Atypical Sweat Glands

- Apocrine sweat glands are located in axilla, circumanal region, and mons pubis.
- Ducts of apocrine sweat glands open into hair follicle, just above levels of sebaceous ducts.^{MCQ}
- These are *simple, coiled tubular glands* (occasionally branched).
- Each gland has duct (excretory part) and body (secretory part).
- Secretory part of apocrine gland is located deep in dermis or may be in hypodermis.
- Lumen of apocrine glands are very wide and these lumen stores glandular secretions.
- *Previous concept:* During secretion, a part of cell is pinched off (apocrine secretion).
- *New concept:* Transmission electron microscopy showed that cells of apocrine sweat gland follow only *merocrine secretion* (exocytosis).^{Neet}
- Secretory portion is lined by simple cuboidal epithelium, myoepithelial cells, and basal lamina.
- *Modified apocrine sweat glands:* Ceruminous glands of external acoustic meatus and ciliary glands of eyelids.
- *Functions:* Production of protein-rich secretion including *pheromones*.

Clinical Correlation

- *Cystic fibrosis:* Cystic fibrosis is a genetic disorder caused by defect in cystic fibrosis gene of chromosome 7. It results in defective Cl^- transport because of defective CFTR protein channels [cystic fibrosis transmembrane conductance regulator].
- In cystic fibrosis, Cl^- concentration in sweat increases because of decreased reabsorption of sodium chloride from lumen of ducts of sweat glands.
- Apocrine glands become functional with puberty. Apocrine glands secrete pheromones (androstenol and androstenone in male and copulins in female).
- Eccrine sweat glands are stimulated by heat and stress. Apocrine sweat glands are stimulated by emotional and sensory stimuli.

NAILS

- Nails provide support to fingertips to carry out many movements.
- Nails are modified zones of epidermis.
- Nails consist of a tough protein called alpha keratin.

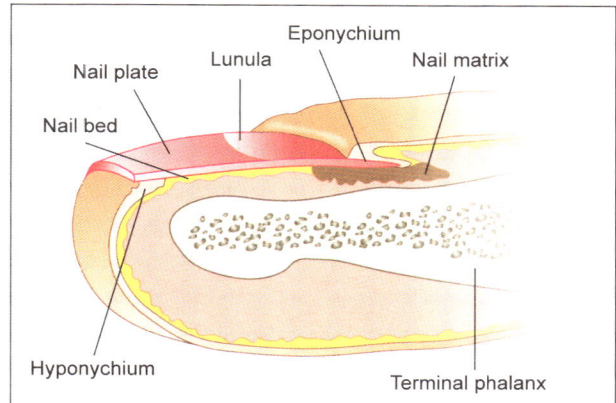

Fig. 14.16: Parts of nail (Source: Textbook of Human Embryology, Yogesh Sontakke, 1st Edn.)

Structure of Nail

Nail shows the following parts (Fig. 14.16):

1. *Nail plate* (body) consists of keratinized cells. Nail plate shows a free distal end and an embedded proximal end (root or radix). Nail plate is continuation of stratum lucidum and corneum of epidermis.^{MCQ}
2. *Nail bed* is a highly vascular connective tissue layer that lies deep to nail plate. Nail bed is a continuation of stratum basale and stratum spinosum of epidermis.
3. *Germinal matrix* is the thickened germinative zone at root of nail plate. These cells form nail plate.
4. *Proximal nail fold* is the fold of epidermis that covers nail root.
5. *Lunula* is proximal soft, half-moon-shaped white part of nail plate that overlies germinal matrix.
6. *Sterile matrix* is part of nail bed that lies under nail plate in continuation of germinal matrix but does not contribute to growth of nail plate. Sterile matrix does not have dermal papillae. It shows several parallel, and longitudinal ridges.
7. *Lateral nail folds* (nail wall) are epidermal folds that overlap sides of nail.
8. *Lateral nail grooves* are the grooves between lateral margin of nail plate and lateral nail folds.
9. *Eponychium* is an extension of base of nail plate or stratum corneum deep to proximal nail fold.
10. *Hyponychium* is part of stratum corneum (epidermis) that lies under the free edge of nail plate (*onyx* = nail in Greek).
11. *Cuticle* is skin that overlies the base of nail at the matrix.
12. *Perionychium* includes nail wall and cuticle area.

Some Interesting Facts

- Nail plate consists of hard keratin that does not desquamate.
- High sulfur content of keratin is responsible for hardness of nail plate.
- Corneocytes are nonnucleated cornified cells that form nail plate.
- Growth of nails:
  - Proliferation of cells of nail matrix produces continuous nail growth.
  - Growth of fingernails is faster than toe nails.

Clinical Correlation

1. *Onychia* is inflammation of nail folds that result in pus formation and shedding of nail.
2. *Onycholysis* (ingrown nails/unguis incarnates) is painful condition that involves injury of nail bed by ingrowing nail plate.
3. *Onychodystrophy* is deformation of nail.
4. *Onychogryposis/ ram's horn nail* is a hypertrophy of nail that produces ram's horn.
5. *Paronychia* is bacterial or fungal infection of nail base.
6. *Koilonychia*/spoon-shaped nails are caused by iron deficiency or vitamin B12 deficiency.

Box 14.5: Nail clubbing

- Nail clubbing involves bulbous swelling of nail bed that results in convex curved nails and increase in the angle between cuticle and nail plate.
- Nail clubbing is a deformity of nails associated with number of diseases.

Causes

- Reduction in amount of circulating oxygen (hypoxia) causes proliferation of nail bed and result in clubbing.
- Any disorder causing prolonged hypoxia can result in clubbing. For example, lung diseases, heart diseases, and so on.
- *Schamroth's window test* [Leo Schamroth, South African cardiologist, 1924–1988]:

  On opposing distal phalanges of corresponding fingers of opposite hands, a small diamond-shaped window is usually apparent between nail plates.
  If this window is obliterated, Schamroth test is considered as positive for clubbing.

SECTION 3

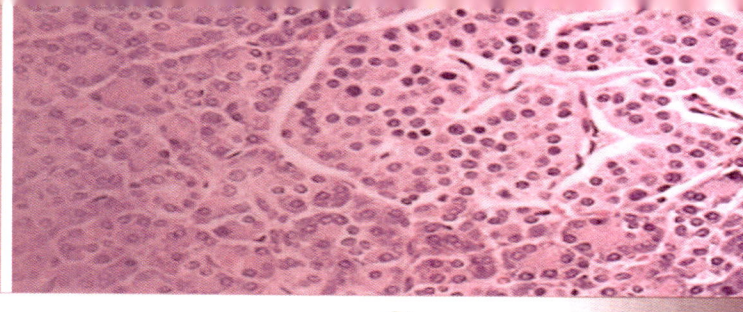

Systemic Histology

15. Respiratory System
16. Digestive System I: Oral Cavity and Associated Structures
17. Digestive System II: Esophagus and Stomach
18. Digestive System III: Small and Large Intestine
19. Liver, Gallbladder and Pancreas
20. Urinary System
21. Male Reproductive System I: Testis, Epididymis, Ductus Deferens
22. Male Reproductive System II: Accessory Sex Glands and Penis
23. Female Reproductive System I: Ovary, Uterus, and Vagina
24. Female Reproductive System II: Mammary Gland, Placenta, and Umbilical Cord
25. Endocrine System
26. Nervous System
27. Special Senses I: Eye
28. Special Senses II: Ear

CHAPTER 15

Respiratory System

Chapter Outline
- Nasal cavities
- Pharynx
- Larynx
- Epiglottis
- Trachea
- Bronchi
- Lungs

Competency achievement: The student should be able to:
AN25.1 Identify, draw and label a slide of trachea and lung.
AN43.2 Identify, describe and draw the microanatomy of epiglottis.

INTRODUCTION

- Respiratory system is primarily meant for oxygenation of blood. It involves transport of gases to lungs.
- Respiratory system consists of a *conducting portion* and a *respiratory portion*.
- Conducting portion transports air but does not participate in gaseous exchange. It consists of nasal cavities, pharynx, larynx, trachea, and bronchi up to respiratory bronchiole (Figs 15.1 and 15.2).

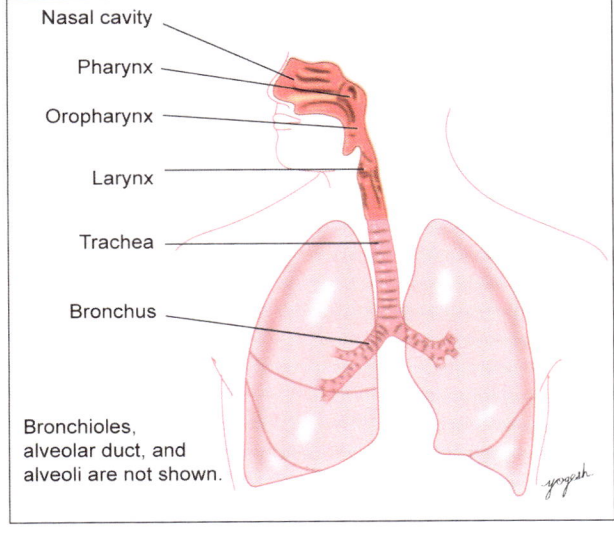

Fig. 15.1: Parts of respiratory passage.

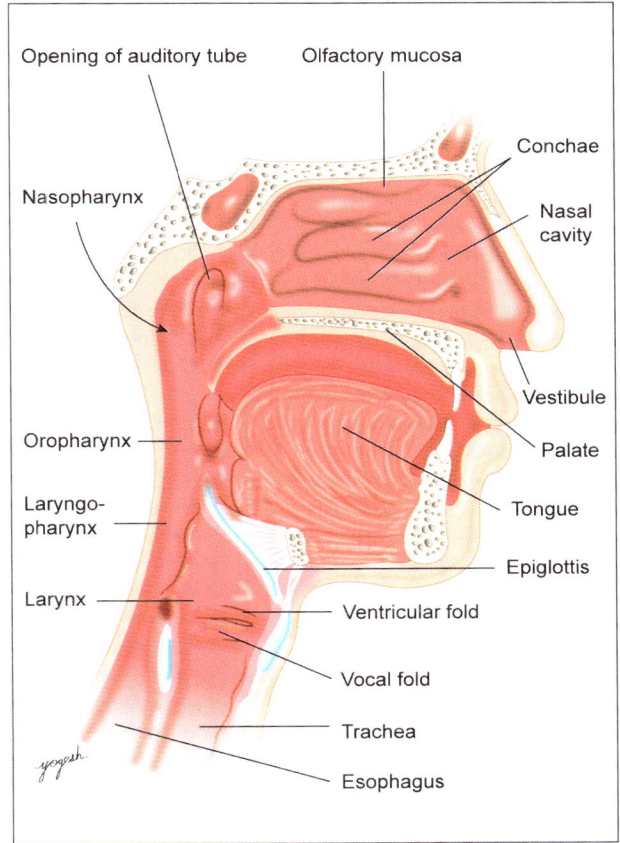

Fig. 15.2: Parts of respiratory tract showing nasal cavity, pharynx, larynx, and trachea.

167

- Respiratory portion is involved in gas exchange. It consists of respiratory bronchioles, alveolar ducts, alveolar sacs, and alveoli.
- Anatomically, upper respiratory tract consists of nasal cavity, paranasal air sinuses, and nasopharynx. Lower respiratory tract consists of larynx, trachea and lungs.
- Conditioning of air: During passage of air in respiratory tract, air undergoes conditioning that involves warming, moistening, and filtration.
- Respiratory tract shows *goblet cells* that secrete mucus. This mucus covers inner aspects of respiratory passage and traps particulate matter to keep passage moist.

NASAL CAVITIES

- Nasal cavities are paired chambers separated by a *nasal septum*.
- Extent: Nasal cavities extend from nostrils to the posterior nares.
- Nasal cavity anteriorly communicates with exterior and posteriorly with nasopharynx (Fig. 15.2).
- Mucosa of nasal cavity is grouped into three zones: Vestibule, respiratory zone, and olfactory zone (Flowchart 15.1).

Vestibule of Nasal Cavity

- Vestibule is anterior dilated part of nasal cavities.
- It is lined by stratified squamous epithelium.
- *Vibrissae:* Vestibule has *stiff hairs* called vibrissae. These hairs trap big particulate matter.^{Viva}
- Anterior part of vestibule is continuous with nasal cavity and it shows transition zone from stratified squamous epithelium to pseudostratified columnar epithelium.

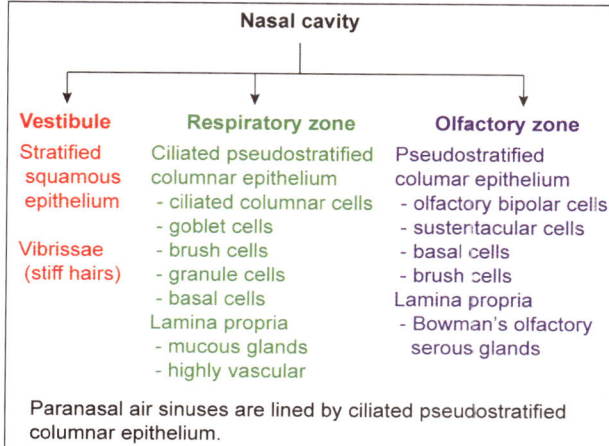

Flowchart 15.1: Histology of nasal cavity

Respiratory Zone of Nasal Cavity

- Respiratory zone of nasal cavities is lined by
  - *Ciliated pseudostratified columnar epithelium.*
  - Lamina propria is firmly adherent with deeper bones and cartilages.
- Respiratory zone on medial side shows nasal septum and on lateral side shows three shelf-like bony projections called *turbinate* or *conchae*.
- Lining epithelium of respiratory zone shows the following five types of cells:
  1. *Ciliated cells* are columnar cells with cilia that project into mucus covering of epithelium.
  2. *Goblet cells* are flask-shaped cells scattered in epithelium and secrete mucus.^{Viva}
  3. Nonciliated columnar cells (**brush cells**) are few. They have microvilli on free surface and secrete serous fluid.
  4. *Small granule cells* lie in basal layer and contain secretory granules.
  5. *Basal cells* lie along basal lamina and act as stem cells.
- Lamina propria of respiratory segment is highly vascular and helps in warming of inhaled air.
- In viral infections (common cold), lamina propria becomes edematous and blocks air passage. It creates difficulty in breathing.$^{Clinical\ fact}$
- Lamina propria contains numerous small *mucous acini* and some *serous demilunes*. It produces mucus to keep air passage moist.
- Lamina propria contains eosinophils, lymphocytes, and other immune cells. In allergic rhinitis, eosinophils increase in number.^{Viva}

Olfactory Zone of Nasal Cavity

- Olfactory segment is located in upper part of nasal cavity in a small area (10 cm^2) (Figs 15.2 and 15.3).
- Olfactory mucosa is yellowish in color, whereas respiratory mucosa is pink in color (highly vascular).
- Olfactory epithelium
  - It is a pseudostratified columnar epithelium (nonciliated, without goblet cells).^{Neet}
  - It has the following cell types:
    1. *Olfactory cells* (bipolar neurons): These are modified neurons that act as olfactory receptors.
    2. *Sustentacular (supporting) cells:* These are columnar cells that provide mechanical support to olfactory cells.
    3. *Basal cells:* These cells act like germinal cells for supporting cells.

Respiratory System

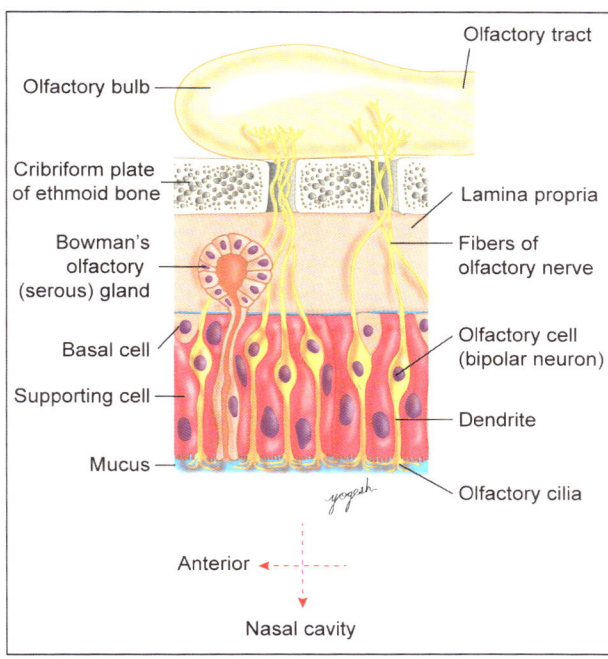

Fig. 15.3: Olfactory mucosa.

4. *Brush cells:* These are secretory cells with microvilli.
- Olfactory cells
  - These are bipolar neurons.
  - Apical surface of these cells shows dilatation called *olfactory vesicle.*
  - From olfactory vesicle, a number of nonmotile cilia arise. These cilia have odorant-binding proteins. These proteins bind with incoming odorant (dissolved in mucus) and generate an action potential.
  - This action potential (signal) is conveyed by axons of olfactory cells to brain through *olfactory nerve* (formed by axons of olfactory cells).
  - Note: Olfactory cells/neurons and some autonomic neurons are the only neurons that get regenerated in body throughout life.*Neet, Viva*
- Supporting cells
  - These are tall columnar cells with numerous microvilli.
  - Their nuclei are oval and occupy the apical portion.
  - These cells contain *lipofuscin* (yellow pigment) in cytoplasm.
  - Sustentacular cells provide physical and metabolic support to olfactory cells.

- Brush cells
  - These are few in number and have blunt microvilli.
  - These cells have synaptic contact with trigeminal nerve fibers and convey general sensation from mucosa to trigeminal nerve.*MCQ*
- Bowman's gland (olfactory glands)*Neet*
  - These are branched tubuloalveolar *serous glands.*
  - Their secretions get poured on epithelial surface and help in removing (washing) odorants.
  - Lipofuscin pigments of olfactory glands and supporting cells impart yellowing color to olfactory mucosa. [Sir William Bowman (1816–1892) was a British surgeon and anatomist discovered Bowman's capsule of nephron, Bowman's anterior limiting membrane of cornea and Bowman's olfactory glands.]
- Paranasal air sinuses are lined by respiratory mucosa, that is, thin ciliated pseudostratified columnar epithelium with numerous goblet cells.

PHARYNX

- Pharynx connects nasal cavity with larynx for communication of air.
- Simultaneously, it acts as a passage for food from oral cavity to esophagus.
- Pharynx is divided into nasopharynx, oropharynx, and laryngopharynx.
- Pharynx is a *fibromuscular tube.*

Layers of Pharynx

- Epithelium
  - Nasopharynx: Ciliated columnar or pseudostratified ciliated columnar epithelium.
  - Oropharynx and laryngopharynx: Stratified squamous epithelium.
- Lamina propria
  - Lamina propria shows diffuse lymphocytes.
  - Two lymphatics aggregation as follows:
  Tubal tonsil: Just underneath the epithelium, lymphatic follicles are aggregated around opening of Eustachian tube. These aggregations form *tubal tonsil.*
  Palatine tonsil: It lies in oropharynx (For details refer Chapter 11).
- Submucosa: Numerous mucous glands are present in submucosa.
- Muscle layer: It consists of skeletal muscle fibers of pharyngeal constrictors, palatopharyngeus, stylopharyngeus, and salpingopharyngeus.

> **Clinical Correlation**
>
> - *Ludwig's angina*
>   - It is a condition causing cellulitis and edema of the floor of mouth, tongue, and pharynx.
>   - This condition may cause airway obstruction, food passage obstruction.
>   - It is mostly caused by bacterial infection. [Wilhelm Fredrick van Ludwig, German physician 1790–1865].
> - *Diphtheria*
>   - It is caused by Corynebacterium diphtheria.
>   - It is a communicable disease (can spread from one person to another).
>   - It may cause airway obstruction as it involves pharynx, larynx, and trachea.

LARYNX

- Larynx is an airway passage that conducts air from laryngopharynx to trachea.
- It is a permanent (noncollapsible) passage consisting of mucous membrane that is supported by cartilages and muscles.
- Larynx also serves as an organ of phonation (speech).

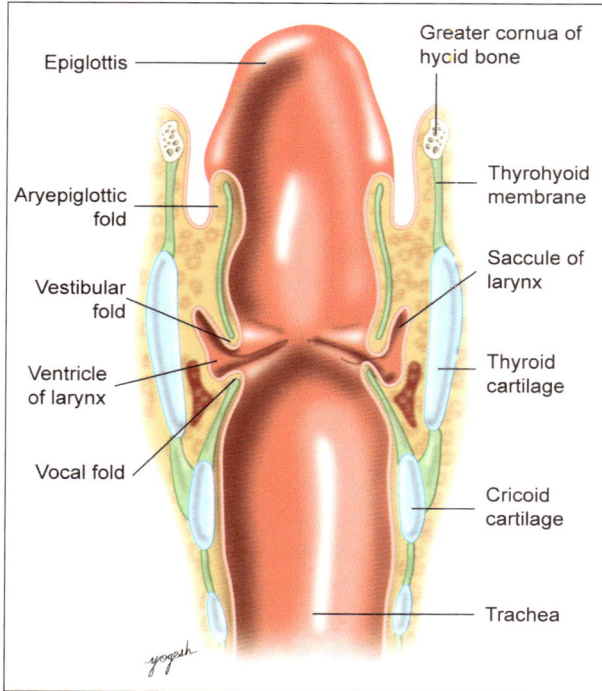

Fig. 15.4: Interior of larynx.

Cartilages of Larynx

- Larynx is supported by the following cartilages
  - Hyaline cartilages
    Thyroid (unpaired)
    Cricoid (unpaired)
    Arytenoid (paired)
  - Elastic cartilages
    Epiglottis (unpaired)
    Cuneiform (paired)
    Corniculate (paired)
- For further details on the structure of hyaline and elastic cartilages, refer Chapter 8.

Mucous Membrane of Larynx

- Mucous membrane of larynx shows two folds in the lumen of larynx as *superior vestibular folds* and *inferior vocal folds* (vocal cords) (Fig. 15.4).
- Space located above the vocal folds is called *ventricle of larynx*.
- Space between right and left vestibular folds is *rima vestibuli* and the space between vocal folds is *rima glottdis*.
- Division of cavity of larynx
  - *Vestibule of larynx:* Part of above vestibular folds
  - *Sinus or ventricle:* Dilated part between vestibular and vocal folds
  - *Infraglottic part:* Part below the vocal folds.
- *Sinus of Morgagni* may be prolonged upward as a diverticulum between vestibular fold and lamina of thyroid cartilage. This extension is known as *saccule of larynx*.

Features of Mucous Membrane of Larynx

- Anterior surface and upper part of posterior surface of epiglottis and upper part of aryepiglottic folds are lined by *stratified squamous epithelium*. This part of larynx comes in contact with food.
- Interior of larynx is lined by *ciliated pseudostratified columnar epithelium* except for *vocal folds that are lined by stratified squamous epithelium.*^MCQ This modification of epithelium may be because of continuous vibrations of vocal folds.
- Mucous membrane is loosely attached to cartilages except over vocal ligaments and over posterior surface of epiglottis. At these sites, it is firmly adherent.
- Mucous glands are numerous over epiglottis, lower part of aryepiglottic folds and saccule glands in saccule. They provide lubrication to vocal folds by means of secretions.

Respiratory System

- Lining cells of vocal folds show microvilli and microplicae (ridge-like folding of plasma membrane). These modifications help in **the maintenance** of moisture of vocal folds by retention of fluids.

> **Clinical Correlation**
> - Laryngitis: It is an inflammation of laryngeal mucosa. It may be acute or chronic.
> - **Singer nodules or teacher's nodules:** Misuse of vocal cords may produce singer's or teacher's nodules at the junction of anterior one-third and posterior two-thirds of vocal cord.

EPIGLOTTIS

Q. Write a short note on histology of epiglottis.

- Epiglottis is a flap-like structure that diverts food from oral cavity to esophagus and closes laryngeal inlet at the time of food passage.
- It consists of a central core of elastic cartilage covered by a mucous membrane.
- It has anterior and posterior surfaces and a free superior border.
- It develops from fourth pharyngeal arch.

Histology of Epiglottis

- Epiglottis shows mucosa covering core of elastic cartilage (Figs 15.5, 15.6 and Flowchart 15.2).

Mucosa

- The lining epithelium of epiglottis[Viva]
  - Nonkeratinized stratified squamous epithelium on its anterior/lingual surface, free border, and upper part of posterior surface.[Neet]

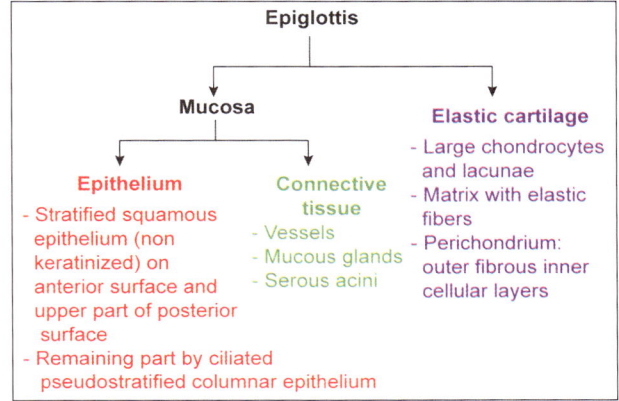

Flowchart 15.2: Histology of epiglottis

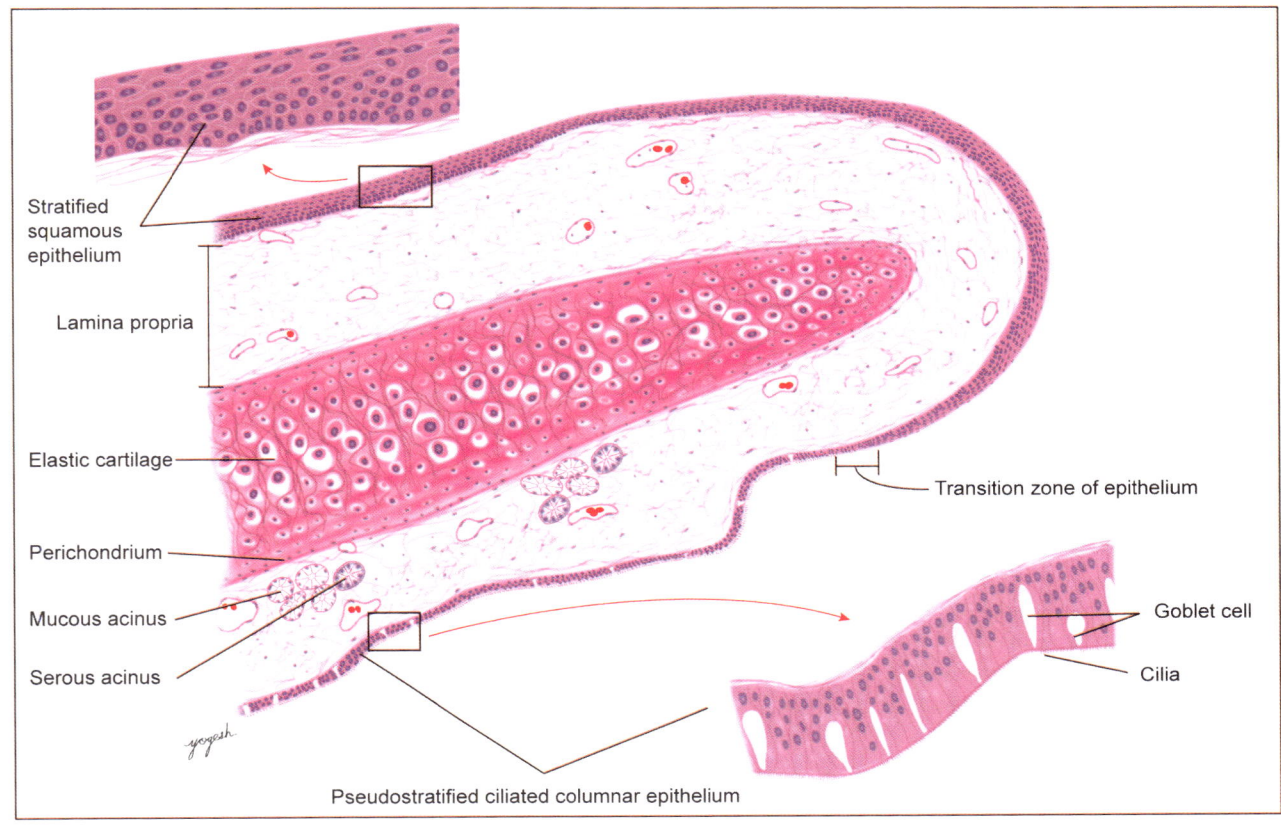

Fig. 15.5: Histology of epiglottis (practice figure).

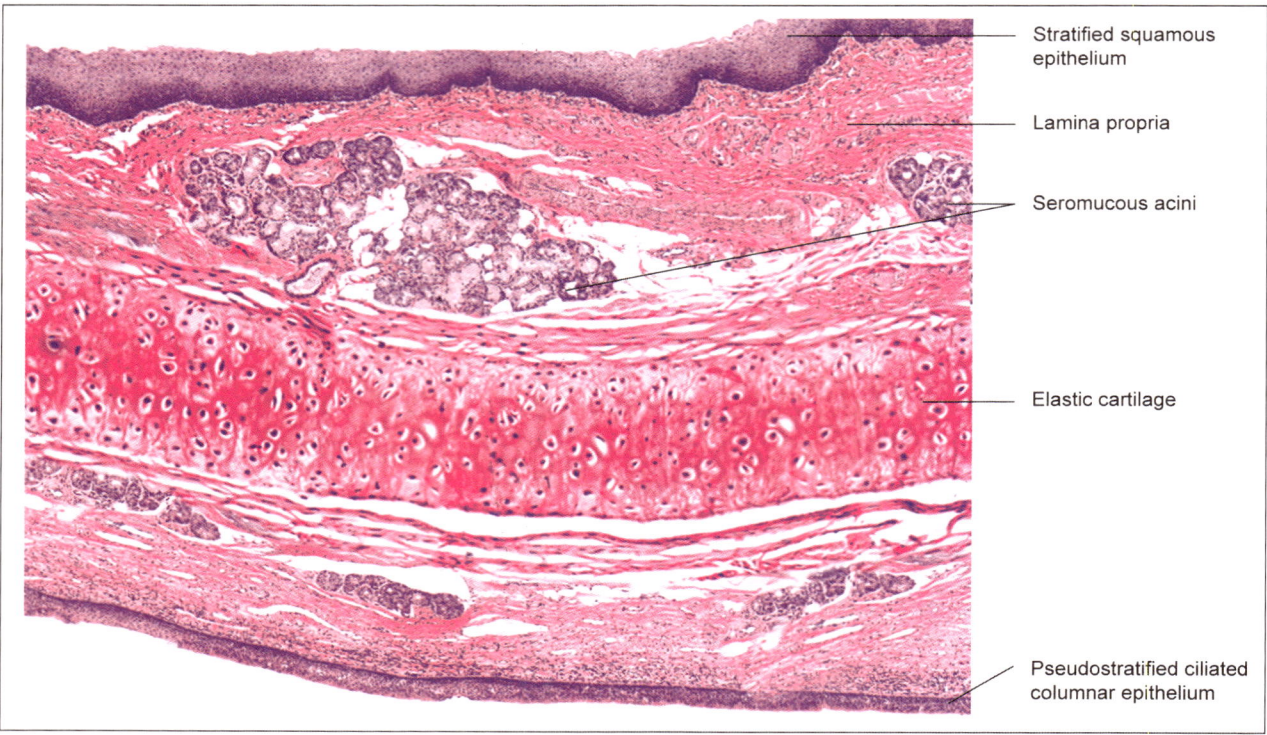

Fig. 15.6: Photomicrograph. Histology of epiglottis (low magnification, H&E stain).

- Ciliated pseudostratified columnar epithelium on rest of posterior surface.
- Goblet cells are seen in ciliated pseudostratified columnar epithelium.
- Few taste buds are present on posterior surface of epiglottis.
- Connective tissue/lamina propria
  - Mucosal lining is separated from elastic cartilage by a loose, vascular connective tissue.
  - *Mucous glands* are located in lamina propria, specifically on posterior surface of epiglottis. In addition to the mucous glands, some serous acini are also present.

Elastic Cartilage*Viva*

- Core of epiglottis is made up of typical yellow elastic cartilage.
- Elastic cartilage is characterized by presence of chondrocytes that lie within the lacuna and surrounded by elastic fibers containing matrix.
- Cartilage shows outer fibrous and inner cellular layers of perichondrium.

> **Summary (Examination Guide)**
> - Epiglottis has a core of elastic cartilage covered by mucous membrane.
> - Lining epithelium: Epiglottis is lined by ciliated pseudostratified columnar epithelium except at anterior surface and upper part of posterior surface where it is lined by stratified squamous epithelium (nonkeratinized).
> - Connective tissue is vascular and shows mucous and serous glands.
> - Elastic cartilage shows large chondrocytes and lacunae, a matrix with elastic fibers and perichondrium with outer fibrous and inner cellular layers.

TRACHEA

Q. Write a short note on histology of trachea.

- Trachea is a cartilaginous tube that acts as air passage from larynx to lungs.
- Length: about 10 cm.
- Diameter: about 2.5 cm outer and 1.5–2 cm inner diameter.

Respiratory System

- Trachea divides into main (primary) bronchi.
- Lumen of trachea is noncollapsible (remains open because of cartilages).*Viva*
- Unique feature of trachea: Presence of C-shaped hyaline cartilages.

Histology of Trachea

Wall of trachea shows (Figs 15.7 to 15.9 and Flowchart 15.3):
1. Mucosa
2. Submucosa
3. Cartilage–muscular layer
4. Adventitia

Mucosa

- Trachea is lined by *ciliated pseudostratified columnar* epithelium.*Neet, Identification feature*
- Cells of tracheal epithelium: Tracheal epithelium shows the following cells:
  - *Ciliated columnar cells:* These cells extend to full thickness of epithelium. Cilia appear as short hair-like projections (~250 cilia per cell). Cilia (mucociliary escalator) propel mucus and trapped particles toward pharynx and protect lungs.
  - *Mucous cells:* These are mucus-secreting cells and occupy full thickness of epithelium. On *H&E* staining, mucus is washed out and cells show clear cytoplasm with basally placed nucleus. These cells do not have cilia.
  - *Brush cells:* These are columnar cells with blunt microvilli. These cells form synapse with sensory nerve endings and function as receptor cells.*MCQ, Viva*

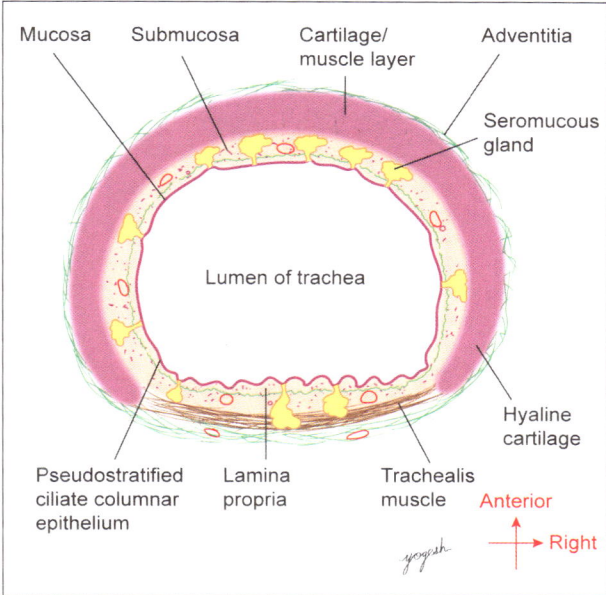

Fig. 15.7: Layers of trachea.

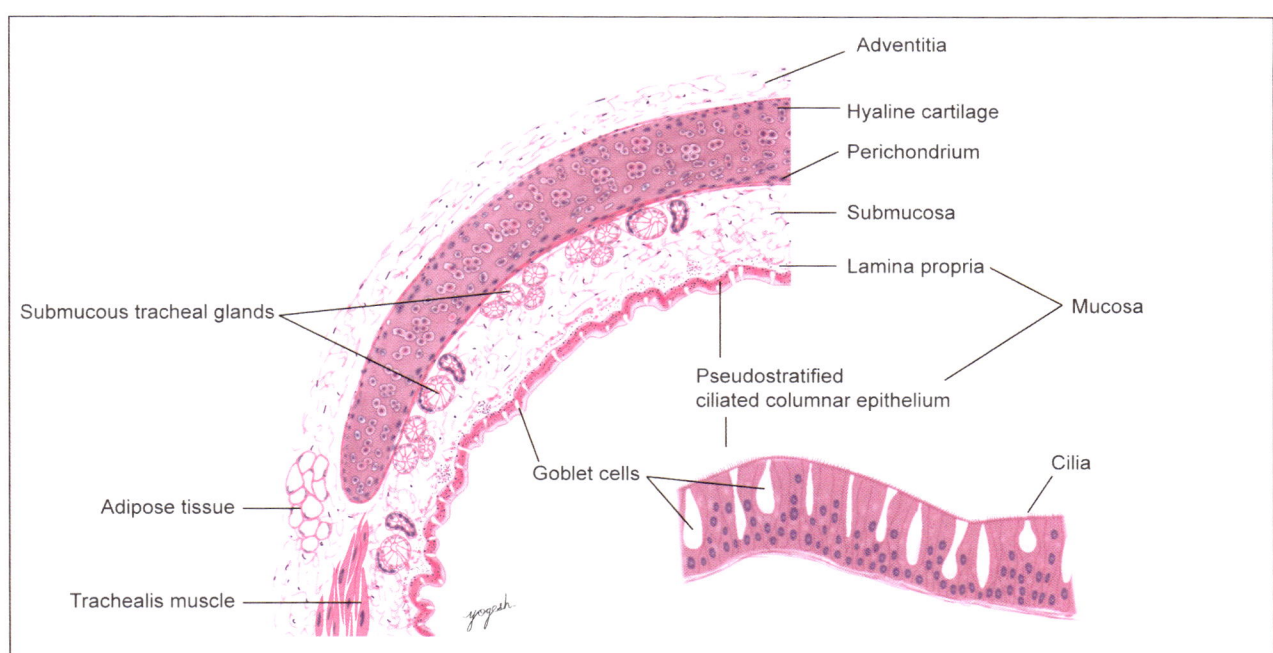

Fig. 15.8: Histology of trachea. Note: Elastic membrane (not distinguishable on *H&E* staining) separates lamina propria and submucosa (practice figure).

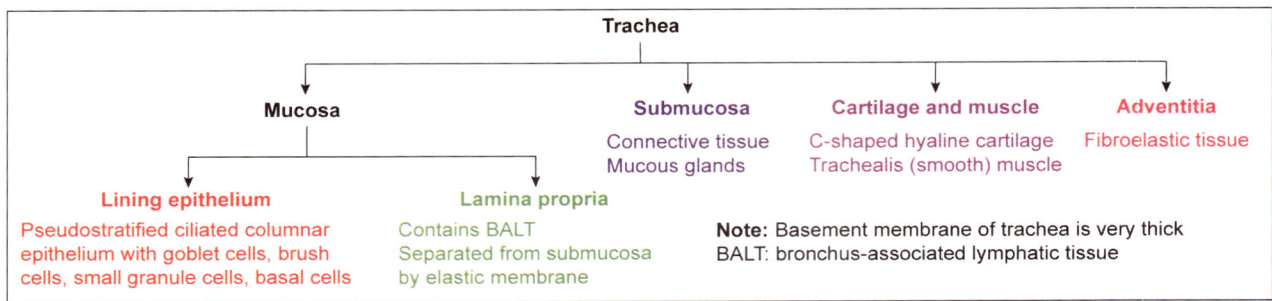

Flowchart 15.3: Histology of trachea.

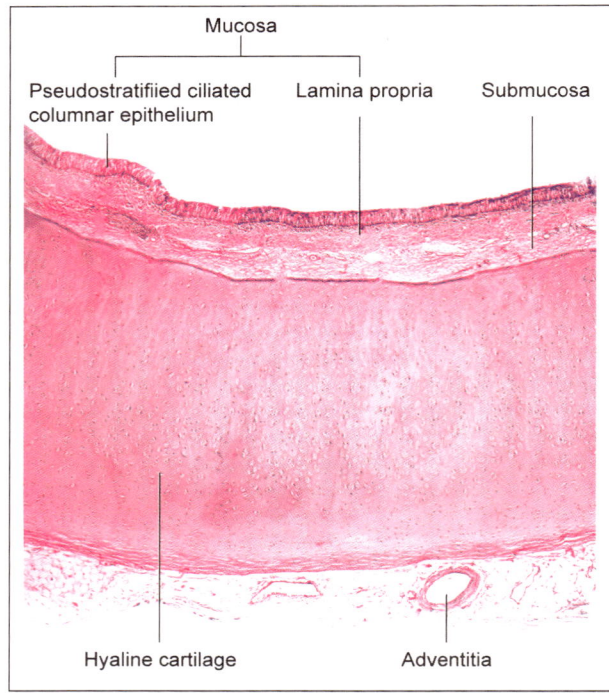

Fig. 15.9: Photomicrograph. Histology of trachea (low magnification, H&E stain).

- *Small granule cells/ Kulchitsky cell/K-cells:* These cells can be stained with silver for its identification. They function similar to enteroendocrine cells of gut and shows granules (secretory vesicles) containing catecholamines.^{Viva} [Nikolai Konstantinovich Kulchitsky, 1856–1925, Russian anatomist and histologist].
- *Basal cells:* These cells act as germinal cells for all other cells of tracheal epithelium. Their nuclei form a row adjacent to basal lamina.
- Basement membrane
  - Thick basement membrane is a characteristic feature of trachea.^{Viva}
  - *H&E staining:* Basement membrane is present as a glassy or homogeneous eosinophilic (pink) layer.
- Lamina propria
  - It consists of loose connective tissue.
  - It may show diffuse lymphocytes and lymphatic follicles in the form of bronchus-associated lymphatic tissue (BALT).
  - Lamina propria also contains numerous elastic fibers. Specifically, at the junction of lamina propria with submucosa, elastic fibers are more in number and they form an *elastic membrane*. This membrane is visible with orcein stain and not with H&E staining.

Submucosa

- On *H&E* staining, it is difficult to distinguish demarcation between lamina propria and submucosa.
- Submucosa contains mucous acini with serous demilunes and ducts of these glands (lined by cuboidal epithelium).
- Submucosa also contains lymphatic follicles, blood vessels, and lymphatics.

Tracheal Cartilage and Trachealis Muscle

- Trachea contains 16–20 C-shaped hyaline cartilage rings.^{Identification feature}
- Gap of C-shaped cartilage is bridged by fibroelastic tissue and trachealis muscle (smooth muscle).^{MCQ}
- With advancing age, hyaline cartilage may get calcified.
- *Hyaline cartilage:* It consists of chondrocytes lying in lacunae, surrounding homogenous matrix, and perichondrium (outer fibrous, inner cellular layer).

Adventitia

- It is a fibroelastic connective tissue layer that contains blood vessels and nerves.

Respiratory System

Summary (Examination Guide)

- Trachea has four layers: Mucosa, submucosa, cartilage–muscle layer and adventitia.
- Mucosa has pseudostratified ciliated columnar epithelium that has ciliated columnar cells, goblet cells (mucous secreting), brush cells (sensory), small granule cells (enteroendocrine-like), and basal cells (germinal cells).
- Epithelium rest on thick basement membrane and lamina propria that has bronchus-associated lymphatic tissue (BALT).
- Trachea has 16–20 C-shaped hyaline cartilages. Gaps of tracheal rings are filled by fibroelastic tissue and trachealis (smooth) muscle.
- Trachea is externally covered by fibroelastic tissue of adventitia.

Box 15.1: Bronchial tree

- Trachea divides into two principal (primary/main) bronchi (right and left) (Fig. 15.10 and Flowchart 15.4).
- Right bronchus is wider and shorter than left bronchus.
- Right bronchus divides into three secondary (lobar) bronchi, whereas left bronchus divides into two secondary bronchi.
- *Secondary bronchi* supply lobes of lungs.
- Secondary bronchi divide into 10 segmental (tertiary bronchi) that supply bronchopulmonary segments of lungs.
- *Tertiary bronchus* divides into numerous bronchioles.
- The smallest bronchioles are called *terminal bronchioles*.
- Terminal bronchioles divide to give rise to *respiratory bronchiole* and finally *alveolar duct* and *alveoli*.[Neet]
- Up to terminal bronchiole, as there is no gaseous exchange, this part of respiratory tract is called *conducting part*.
- Terminal bronchiole and distal to it, there occurs gaseous exchange; hence, this part of respiratory tract is called *respiratory part* (Fig. 15.11).

LUNG

Q. Write a short note on histology of lung.

- Lungs are a pair of organs that are principal site of gaseous exchange.
- Lungs consist of pleural covering, connective tissue septa, and lung parenchyma with airway passage.
- Principal bronchus divides into lobar bronchus that enter lung to form *intrapulmonary bronchi*.
- Lung parenchyma consists of bronchioles and alveoli.

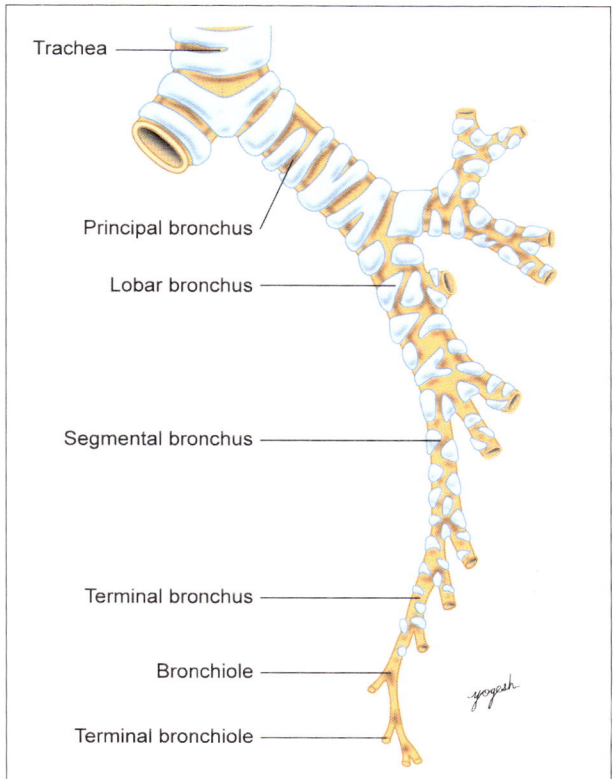

Fig. 15.10: Structures in conducting part of respiratory tract (no gaseous exchange).

Flowchart 15.4: Tracheobronchial tree.

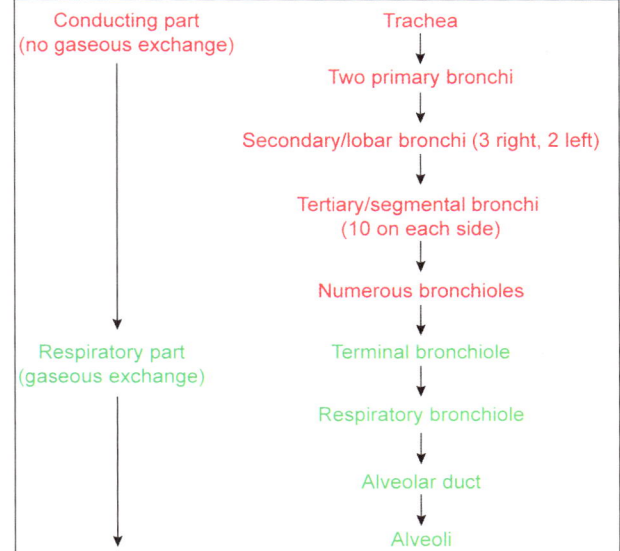

Note: Histological features of trachea and principal bronchi are same.

Intrapulmonary Bronchi

- Intrapulmonary bronchi include secondary (lobar) bronchi and tertiary or segmental bronchi.

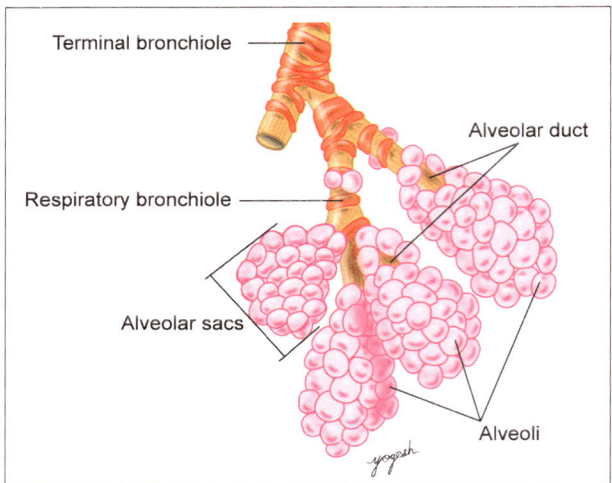

Fig. 15.11: Structures in respiratory part (zone of gaseous exchange) of respiratory tract.

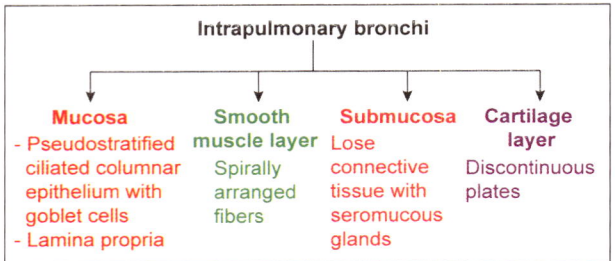

- Segmental bronchi divide into many small bronchi that finally form bronchiole (diameter ≤1 mm and no cartilage in their wall).

Histology of Intrapulmonary Bronchi

- Intrapulmonary bronchi have the following layers (Figs 15.12 to 15.15 and Flowchart 15.5):
  1. Mucosa
  2. Muscular layer
  3. Submucosa
  4. Cartilage
  5. Adventitia

Mucosa

- It consists of *pseudostratified ciliated columnar epithelium* with goblet cells.
- Height of epithelium decreases as the size of bronchus decreases.
- Lamina propria contains many elastic fibers and seromucous glands.

Muscular layer

- Smooth muscle layer forms a complete circumferential layer around the epithelium in intrapulmonary bronchi.
- Smooth muscle fibers are arranged spirally and help to maintain proper diameter of airway passage.

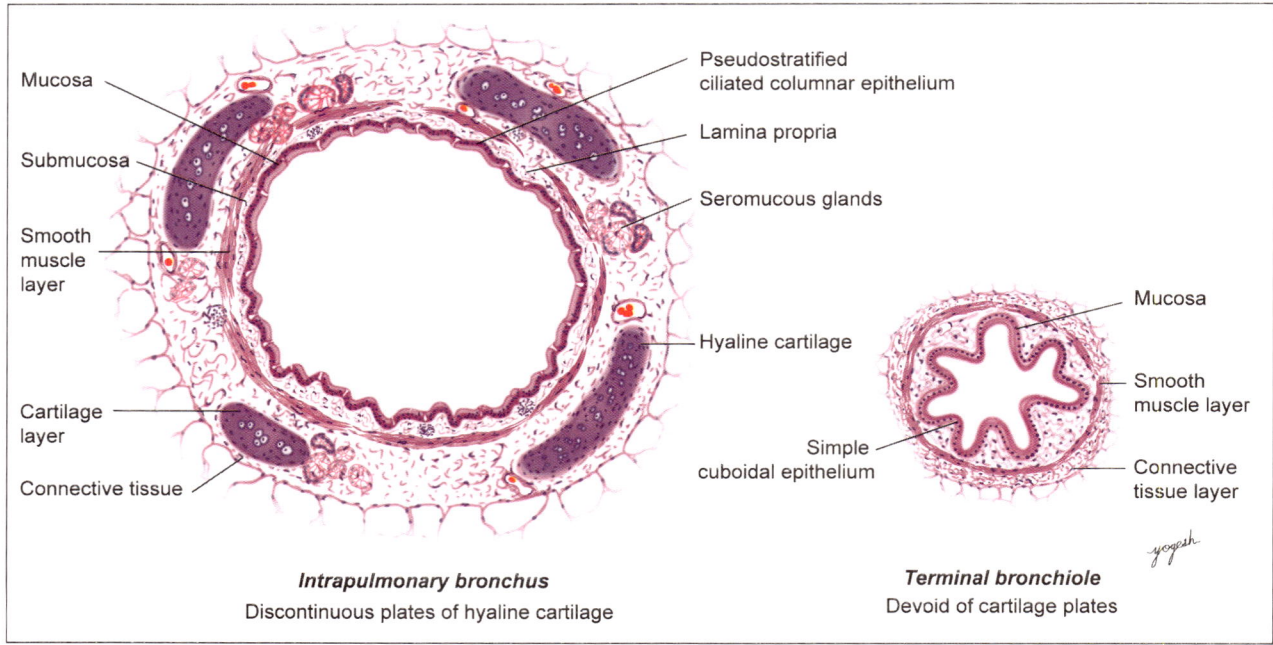

Fig. 15.12: Intrapulmonary bronchus and terminal bronchiole (practice figure).

Respiratory System

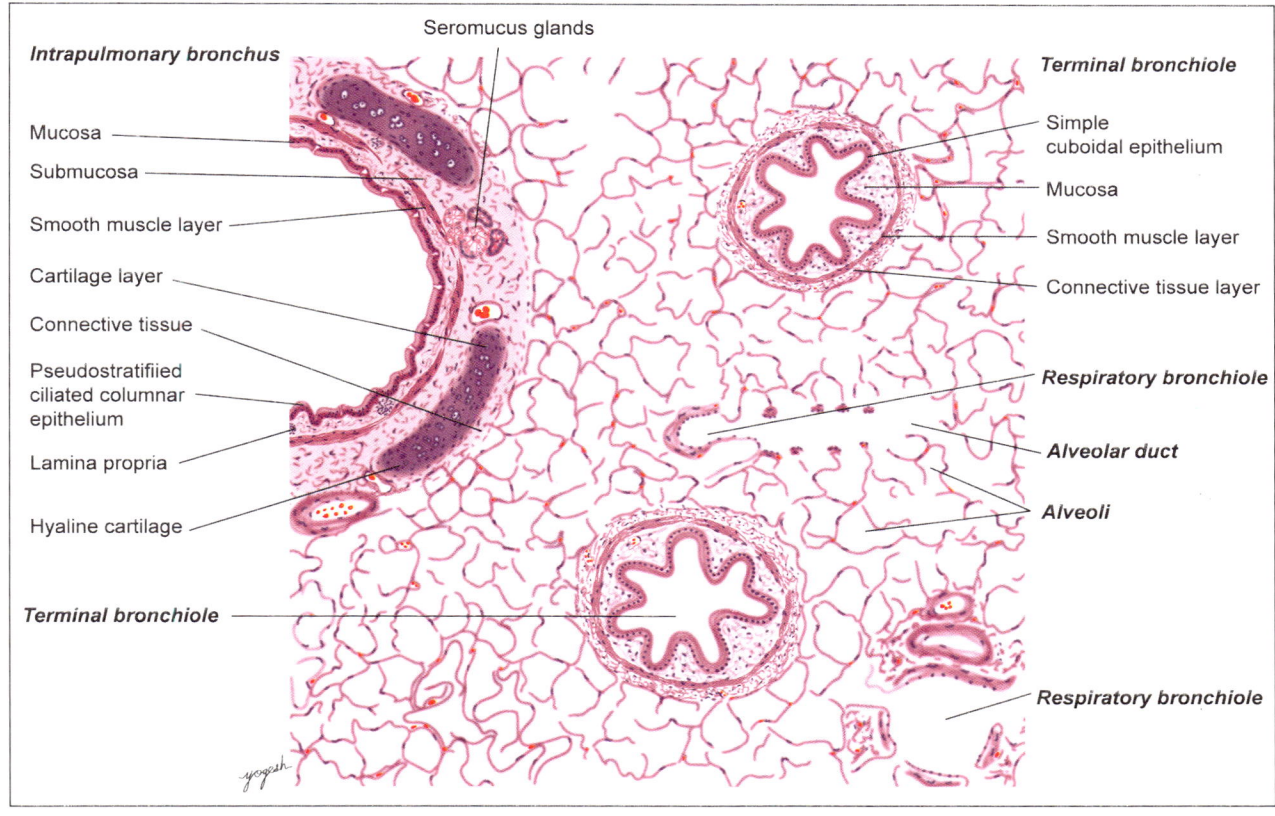

Fig. 15.13: Histology of lung (practice figure).

Submucosa
- It consists of loose connective tissue with seromucous glands.

Cartilage layer
- Intrapulmonary bronchiole shows presence of *discontinuous cartilage plates*.^{Identification feature}
- Note: Trachea and principal bronchus shows C-shaped single cartilage ring in a section and muscle layer that does not cover entire circumference.^{Identification feature}
- Cartilaginous plates help to keep bronchi open.

Adventitia
- Cartilaginous plates are externally surrounded by a connective tissue layer containing blood vessels and lung parenchyma.

Bronchioles
- Bronchioles are airway tubules that are^{Viva}
  1. Less than 1 mm in diameter
  2. Their wall does *not have cartilage* and submucosal glands^{Neet}
- *Pulmonary lobule:* It is a small part of bronchopulmonary segment that is supplied by a single bronchiole.
- Bronchiole further divides to give rise to *terminal bronchioles*.
- *Pulmonary acinus:* It is a small part of lung that is supplied by a terminal bronchiole.
- Terminal bronchiole further divides into *respiratory bronchiole* and *alveoli*.
- Respiratory bronchiolar unit: It is functional unit of lung and consists of a single respiratory bronchiole and alveoli supplied by it.
  Segmental bronchus → larger bronchiole → terminal bronchiole → respiratory bronchiole → alveolar duct → alveoli.^{Viva}

Structure of Bronchiole
- Bronchiole consists of the following layers (Figs 15.12, 15.14, 15.15 and Flowchart 15.6):
  Mucosa
  Smooth muscle layer
  Connective tissue layer
- Note: there is *no cartilage* layer.

Mucosa
- Lining epithelium varies according to site of the bronchiole as follows:
  1. Larger bronchioles: Ciliated pseudostratified columnar epithelium with goblet cells.

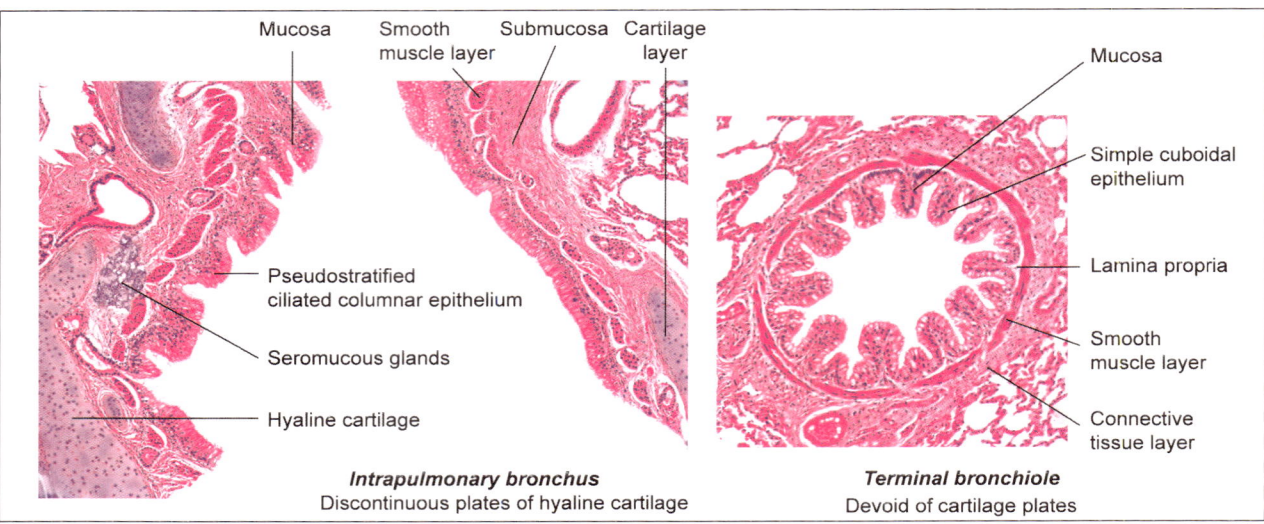

Fig. 15.14: Photomicrograph. Intrapulmonary bronchus (longitudinal section) and terminal bronchiole (transverse section) (high magnification, *H&E* stain).

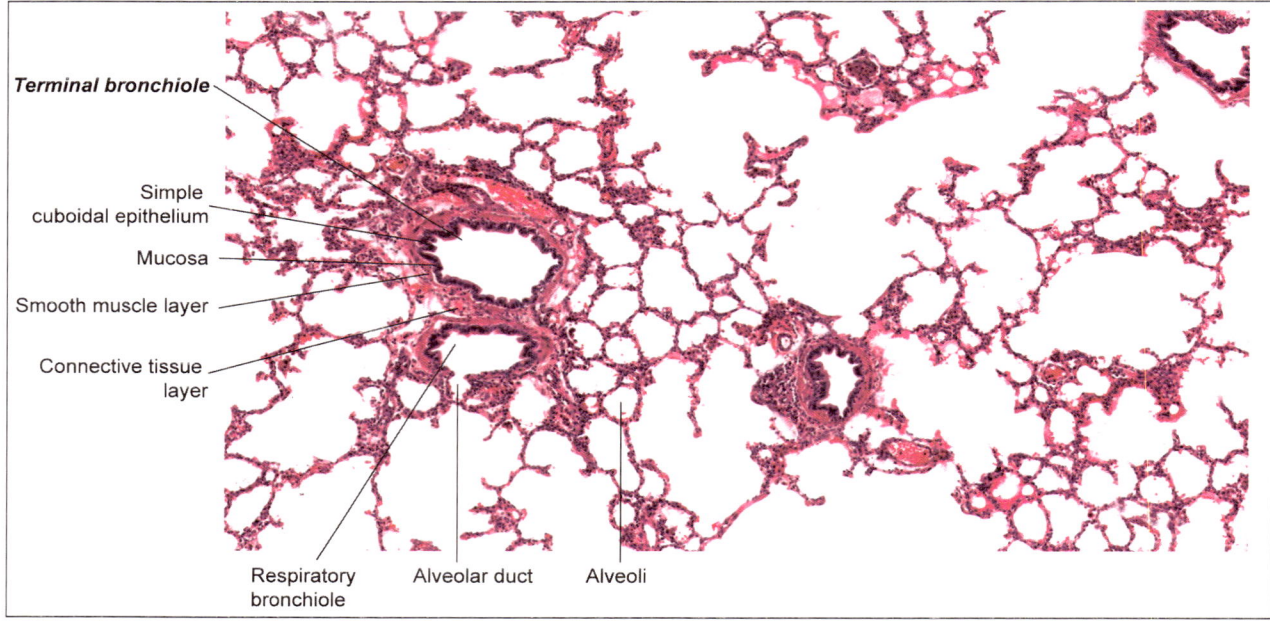

Fig. 15.15: Photomicrograph. Histology of lung (low magnification, *H&E* stain).

2. Medium bronchioles: Simple ciliated columnar epithelium with few goblet cells.
3. Smaller/terminal bronchioles: Simple cuboidal epithelium with Clara cells without goblet cells.

- What is absent in bronchioles? *Viva, identification feature*
  1. Bronchioles do not have cartilages in their wall.
  2. Bronchioles do not have seromucous glands in lamina propria.
  3. Terminal bronchioles do not have goblet cells.

- Clara cells:[Neet]
  - are nonciliated cells [Max Clara, 1899–1966, German anatomist].
  - are present *predominantly in terminal bronchioles*.[Neet]
  - replace goblet cells in terminal bronchioles.
  - have many microvilli on apical surface.
  - secrete
    Surface active protein (agent)
    Clara cell secretory protein (CC16)

Flowchart 15.6: Histology of bronchioles^{Viva}

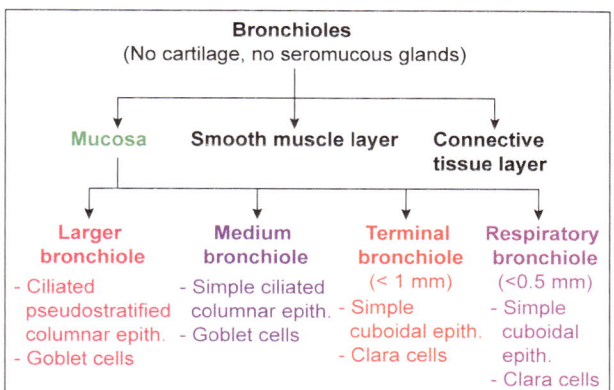

- *Surface-active agent* reduces surface tension and reduces collapsing tendency of airway passage.^{Neet}
- Clara cell protein is used as a marker for lung injury. It is present in bronchoalveolar lavage fluid and serum.
- Clara cell provides protection against inhaled harmful chemicals, protect alveoli (prevent emphysema), and work as stem cell.

Smooth muscle layer
- It is a predominant layer of the wall of bronchioles.
- It is under control of autonomic nervous system and regulates the passage of air through bronchioles.

Connective tissue layer
- Bronchioles are surrounded by small amount of connective tissue that separates bronchioles from adjacent structures.
- Connective tissue is rich in elastic fibers. These elastic fibers are responsible for recoiling of lungs.^{Viva}

Respiratory Bronchiolar Unit (Fig. 15.16)
- Respiratory bronchiolar unit is the smallest functional unit of lung.

Box 15.2: Asthma

- Asthma is an acute, episodic airway disease characterized by airway obstruction (difficulty in breathing).
- Pathophysiology: Asthma occurs because of spasm of smooth muscles of airway passage (bronchi and bronchioles). There is excessive mucus secretion and inflammation (swelling) of mucosa.
- Causes: There are many causes asthma that induce exposure to allergens (pollen grains, dust), exposure to cold air, and so on.
- Treatment: (1) Avoid allergen exposure, (2) Use bronchodilator drugs (salbutamol, ipratropium bromide) in acute cases.

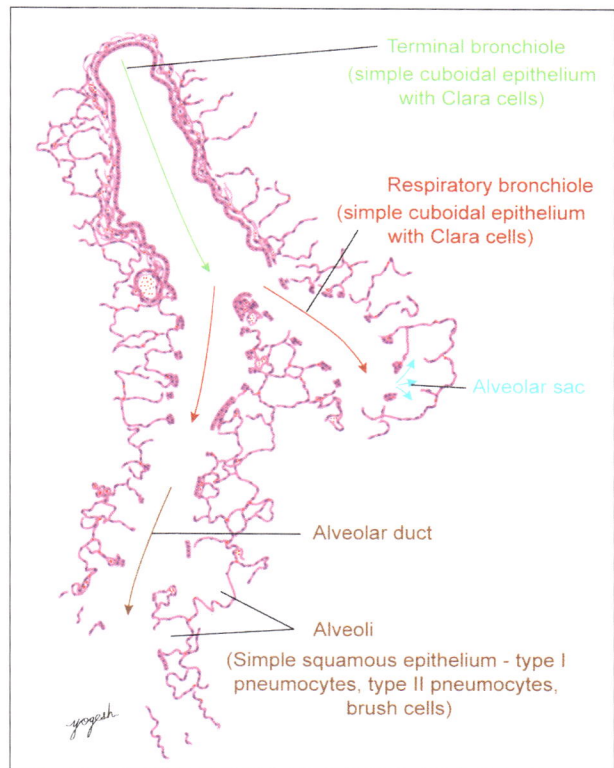

Fig. 15.16: Part of respiratory passage distal to terminal bronchiole.

- It consists of a single respiratory bronchiole and alveoli.

Respiratory Bronchiole
- It usually measures less than 0.5 mm in diameter
- It participates in gaseous exchange, hence called respiratory bronchiole.

Layers
1. Simple cuboidal epithelium: These cells gradually lose cilia as moves toward distal side of bronchiole.
2. Smooth muscle cells surround the epithelium.
3. A layer of delicate connective tissue separates respiratory bronchiole from adjacent structures.
- Epithelium also shows Clara cells.
- Respiratory bronchiole shows few alveolar outpouchings.

Alveolar ducts and alveolar sacs
- Each respiratory bronchiole gives rise to 2–3 alveolar ducts.
- Each alveolar duct gives rise to space called *alveolar sac* that is surrounded by clusters of alveoli. The surrounding alveoli open into the alveolar sac.

Respiratory bronchiole → Alveolar duct → Alveolar sac → Alveoli

The differences between bronchus and bronchioles are listed in Table 15.1.

Alveoli

- Alveoli are thin-walled polyhedral, sac-like terminal air spaces of respiratory system that constitute the actual site for air exchange.
- Each lung contains 150–250 million alveoli.
- Total surface area of alveoli is 75 m^2 (equal to the approximate surface area of a tennis court).
- Size of each alveolus is about 200 μm in diameter.
- *Alveolar septum*
  - Adjacent alveoli are separated from each other by a thin layer of connective tissue containing blood capillaries. This alveolar septum also contains fibroblasts and macrophages.
  - Alveoli are lined by simple *squamous epithelium* along with some other cells.
  - *Interalveolar pores/pores of Kohn:* These are the opening of alveolar septa that help in the communication of air between adjacent alveoli. [Hans Kohn, 1866-1935, German physician].*Viva*

Cells of Alveolar Epithelium (Fig. 15.17 and Flowchart 15.7)

- Alveolar wall is lined by type I pneumocytes, type II pneumocytes, and occasional brush cells.*Viva*

Type I Pneumocytes (95%)

- These are simple squamous cells connected with each other by occluding junctions.
- Type I pneumocyte cannot undergo cell division.

Flowchart 15.7: Different types of cells in respiratory epithelium (Fig. 15.16).*Neet*

Q. List the cells lining respiratory passage.

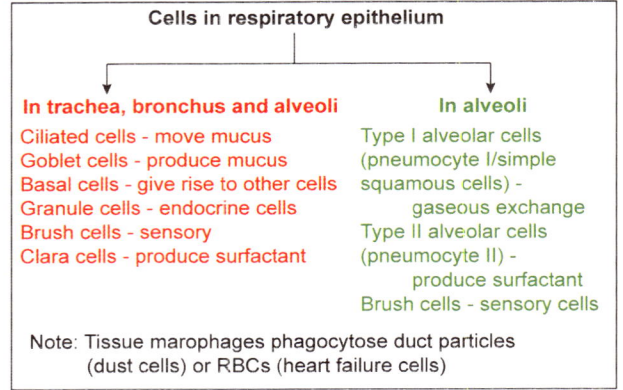

Q. List the microscopic differences between bronchus and bronchiole.

Table 15.1: Differences between bronchus and bronchiole

Characteristics	Bronchus	Bronchiole
Diameter	More than 1 mm	Less than 1 mm
Epithelium	Pseudostratified ciliated columnar epithelium with goblet cells	Large bronchioles: Simple columnar cells with few cilia and few goblet cells
		Small bronchioles: Simple columnar or simple cuboidal cells without cilia and without goblet cells
Smooth muscle layer	Present between mucosa and cartilage layer	Present between mucosa and adventitia
Cartilages	Irregular plates of cartilage present	Cartilages absent
Seromucous glands	Seromucous glands are present in submucosa	Glands are absent

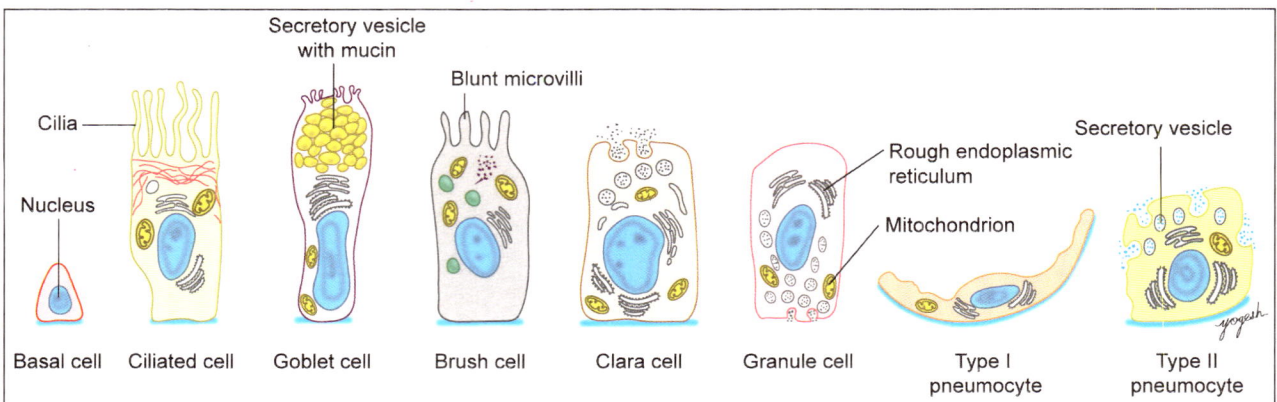

Fig. 15.17: Cells of respiratory passage.

Type II Pneumocytes (5%)

- These are also called septal cells or great alveolar cells or type II alveolar cells.
- These cells are cuboidal (rounded) in shape and abundant cytoplasm is present.
- These cells produce surfactant, dipalmitoylphosphatidylcholine (DPPC). This surfactant helps to reduce surface tension and keeps the alveoli open.*Viva*
- Transmission electron microscopy (TEM)
  On TEM, type II pneumocytes show presence of *lamellar bodies:* stacks of membrane-bound granules in apical zone of cells.*Viva*
- Function
  1. Type II pneumocyte act as progenitor of type I cells.
  2. Production of surfactant (Note: Clara cells also produce surfactant).

Brush Cells

- Few brush cells are also present in alveolar epithelium.
- These cells act as receptors to monitor quality of air entering in alveoli.

Box 15.3: Alveolar macrophages

- Alveolar macrophages are present in connective tissue as well as in alveolar lumen.
- Alveolar macrophages are the first-line defense against lung infection.
- The main function of these cells is phagocytosis and they perform the following actions:
  1. Removal of dust particles (hence, also called *dust cells*).*Neet, Viva*
  2. Removal of carbon and tar in smokers.
  3. Removal of pollen grains.
  4. Removal of red blood cells in heart failure patients. In heart failure, red blood cells enter in alveoli from adjacent capillaries. These cells are phagocytosed by alveolar macrophages and cytoplasm of macrophage becomes brick-red colored because of hemosiderin. These cells are also called *heart failure cells.*ced*Viva*
- *Mycobacterium tuberculosis* bacteria cannot be killed by alveolar macrophages. These bacteria get accumulated in macrophages and form multinucleated giant macrophage.

Box 15.4: Blood–air barrier*Viva*

Q. Write a short note on blood–air barrier.

- Gaseous exchange between alveolar air and blood occurs through blood–air barrier (Fig. 15.14).
- The thinnest blood–air barrier consists of the following components:
  1. Thin layer of surfactant
  2. Simple squamous epithelium of lung alveoli
  3,4. Fused basal lamina of alveolar epithelium and capillary endothelium
  5. Continuous (non-fenestrated) capillary endothelium

Clinical Correlation

- *Pneumonia:* It is the inflammation of lung alveoli. It may be caused by microorganisms, allergens, drugs, and so on.
- *Lung cancer:* Toxic elements in cigarette smoke converts pseudostratified ciliated columnar epithelium of respiratory tract to stratified squamous epithelium. Later, this change may lead to squamous cell carcinoma (lung cancer).
- *Metaplasia:* It is alteration of one kind of epithelium to another type.

  Pseudostratified ciliated columnar epithelium $\xrightarrow{\text{Cigarette smoke}}$ Stratified squamous epithelium

- *Acute respiratory distress syndrome (ARDS)* or *hyaline membrane diseases:* It is a rapid respiratory failure due to inflammation of lung epithelium. It may be either neonatal ARDS or adult ARDS. Neonatal ARDS occurs because of insufficient surfactant.
- *Bronchitis* is an inflammation of bronchi and it may be acute or chronic.
- *Immotile cilia syndrome (Kartagener's syndrome)* is characterized by immotile cilia. It is also called primary ciliary dyskinesia. It is an autosomal recessive disorder. It affects respiratory tract, fallopian tube (infertility), and sperms (immotile sperms). Failure of ciliary movements in respiratory epithelium results in repeated infections.
- *Emphysema:* It is an abnormal permanent *dilatation* of airway distal to terminal bronchiole; cigarette smoking and air pollution are common causative agents.

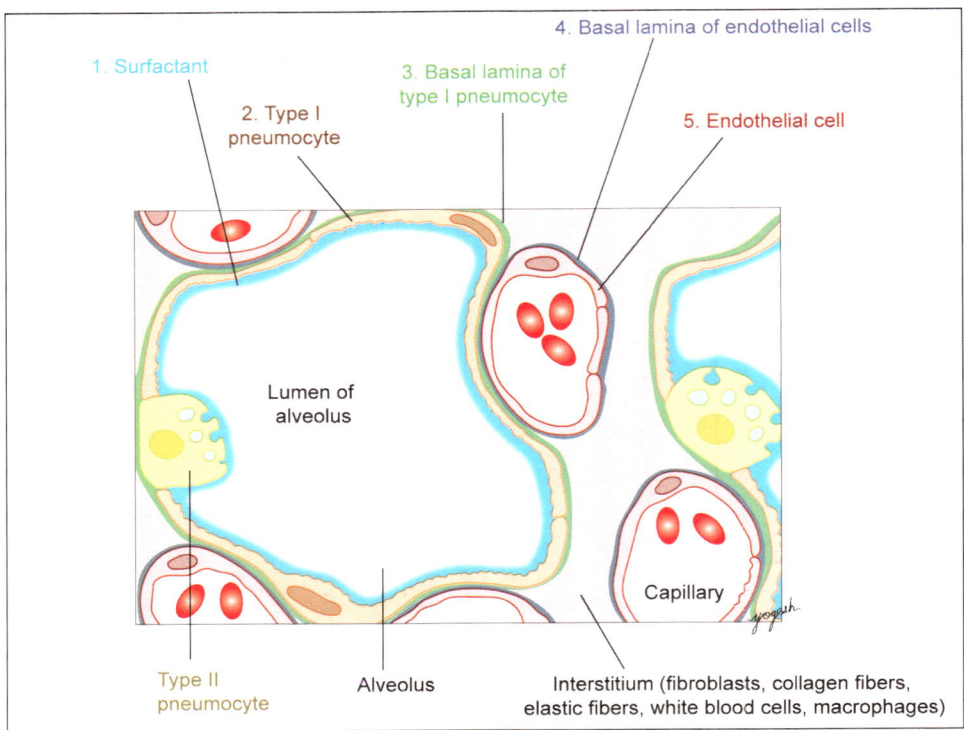

Fig. 15.18: Blood–air barrier.

Summary (Examination Guide) (Fig. 15.18)

- Lung is covered by mesothelium of visceral pleura and connective tissue layer.
- Lung consists of intrapulmonary bronchi, bronchioles, and alveoli.

Intrapulmonary bronchi
- These include lobar bronchus, segmental bronchus, and terminal bronchus.
- Intrapulmonary bronchi are lined by pseudostratified ciliated columnar epithelium with goblet cells and lamina propria (contains seromucous glands). There is a complete circumferential smooth muscle layer. Submucosa is supported by discontinuous cartilaginous plates.

Bronchioles
- Bronchioles are < 1 mm in diameter and do not have cartilage plates.
- Bronchioles show transition from ciliated pseudostratified columnar epithelium to ciliated columnar and finally simple cuboidal epithelium. In terminal bronchioles, Clara cells replace goblet cells.
- Bronchioles show smooth muscle layer covered by a connective tissue layer.
- Respiratory bronchiole is lined by simple cuboidal epithelium and is surrounded by smooth muscles.

Alveoli
- These are thin-walled polyhedral sacs lined by simple squamous epithelium (type I pneumocytes) with few type II pneumocytes (produces surfactant).
- Interalveolar spaces contain a small amount of connective tissue and non-fenestrated (continuous) capillaries.
Trachea → principal bronchi → lobar bronchi → segmental bronchi → large bronchioles → terminal bronchioles → respiratory bronchioles → alveolar ducts → alveolar sacs → alveoli.

CHAPTER 16

Digestive System I: Oral Cavity and Associated Structures (Lip, Tooth, Tongue, Salivary Glands)

Chapter Outline
- Oral cavity
  - Lip
  - Tooth
- Tongue
- Salivary glands

Competency achievement: The student should be able to:
AN43.2 Identify, describe and draw the microanatomy of tongue, salivary glands

INTRODUCTION

- Digestive system performs functions of ingestion, digestion, and absorption of food and water.
- Digestive system consists of (Fig. 16.1):
  - Oral cavity and associated structures such as lips, teeth, tongue, and salivary glands
  - Gastrointestinal tract that includes esophagus, stomach, small and large intestines
  - Associated glands such as liver, gallbladder, and pancreas
- Oral cavity helps in ingestion of food and water with the help of saliva.
- Oral cavity is lined by nonkeratinized stratified squamous epithelium. This epithelium is supported by lamina propria.
- Lamina propria consists of loose areolar tissue.
- Part of oral cavity is lined by parakeratinized epithelium. This epithelium has superficial cells with nuclei. These cells get exfoliated.
- Lamina propria has few mucous and serous glands.
- Oral cavity is surrounded by salivary glands such as parotid, submandibular, and sublingual glands.
- Oral cavity also performs immunological functions with the help of palatine tonsil, lingual tonsil and other diffuse mucosa-associated lymphatic tissue.

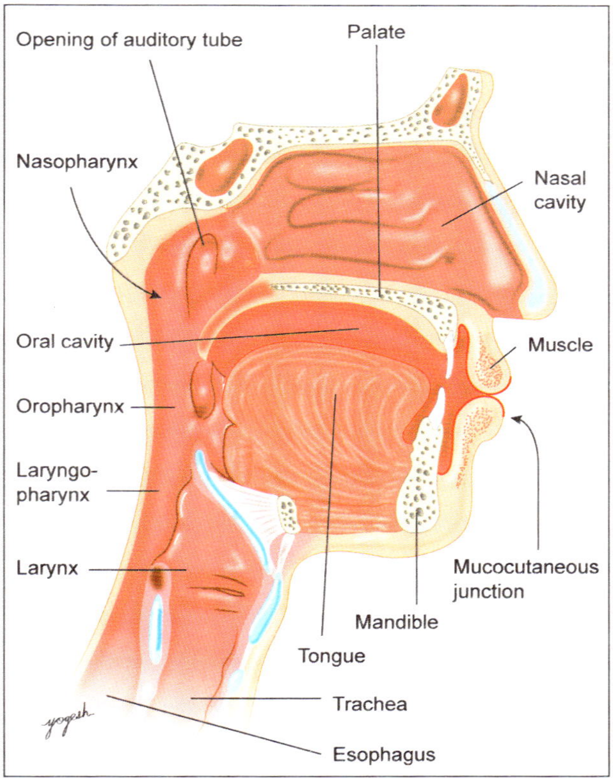

LIP

- Lip is a mucomuscular fold having core made of skeletal muscles (Fig. 16.2).

Fig.16.1: Upper part of oral cavity and pharynx.

- Lip is externally lined by skin and internally by mucous membrane.
- Free margin of lip shows mucocutaneous junction.

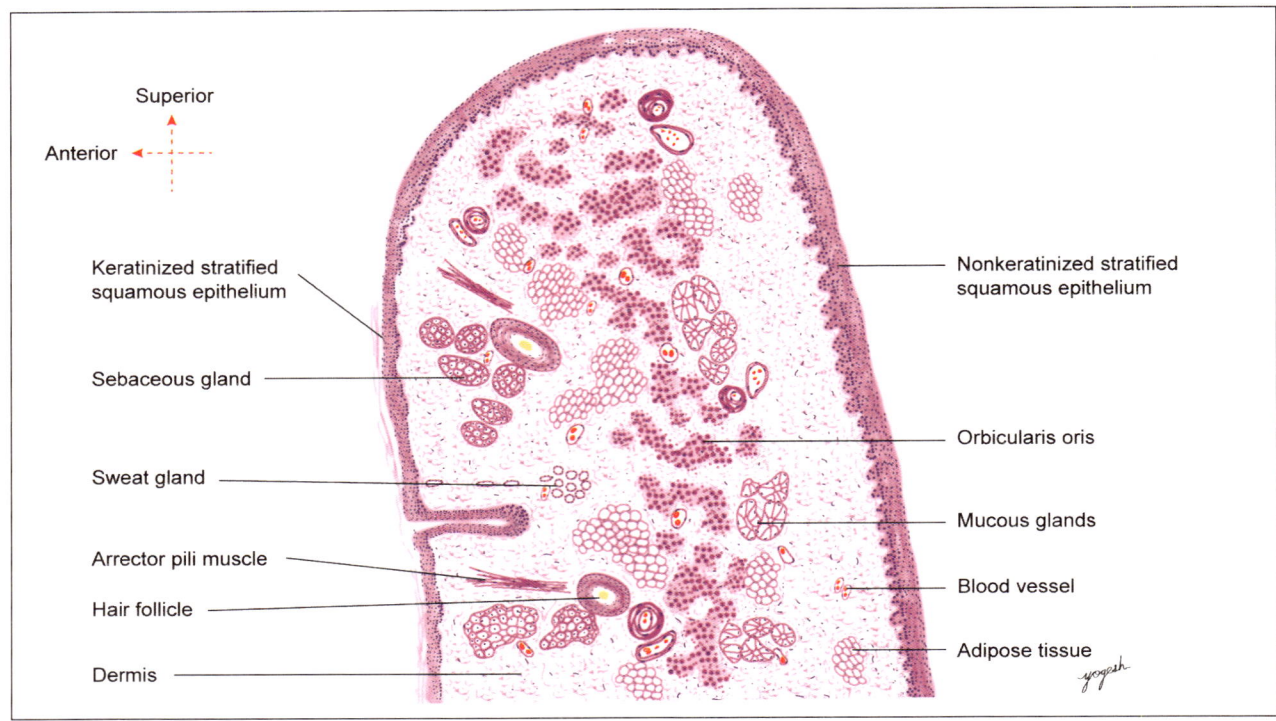

Fig. 16.2: Histology of lower lip (sagittal section) (practice figure).

- Mucocutaneous junction is also called *vermilion*/red margin.
- Large number of blood vessels that are present beneath epithelium give red color to the lip.
- Skin covering the lip is lined by stratified squamous epithelium (epidermis), hair follicles, sweat glands, and sebaceous glands.
- Mucous membrane of lip is lined by nonkeratinized stratified squamous epithelium. This epithelium is thick and has prominent *rete ridges*.
- Rete ridges are finger-like extensions of epithelium that projects into the underlying connective tissue.
- Long rete ridges help to withstand frictions.
- Parakeratinization: Mucosa of lip shows parakeratinization.
- Red margin is highly sensitive to the touch because of presence of more sensory receptors, such as Meissner's corpuscles.

TEETH

- Teeth are located in the alveolar sockets of maxilla and mandible.
- In children there are 10 deciduous milk teeth in each jaw (2 incisors, 1 canine, and 2 molar teeth on each side of jaw), whereas in adults, there are 16 permanent teeth in each jaw (2 incisors, 1 canine, 2 premolar, and 3 molar teeth on each side of the jaw).
- Alveolar processes of mandible and maxilla, and part of teeth are covered by gum.

Histology of Tooth

- Tooth has three parts (Figs 16.3, 16.4 and Flowchart 16.1):
  1. Crown: It lies superficial to gum and visible in oral cavity.
  2. Root: It is covered by gum and bony alveolar process.

Clinical Correlation

- *Fordyce' spots/granuloma:* These are visible sebaceous glands seen in oral mucosa, lips, face, and genitals. These are physiologically seen in 70–80% people [John Fordyce, 1858–1925, American dermatologist].
- *Peutz-Jeghers syndrome* is an autosomal dominant disorder that involves formation of polyps (abnormal growths) in intestine and dark spots on lips and oral mucosa.
- *Cheilitis* is an inflammation of lips. Cheilitis most commonly involves angles of mouth. It results in red, cracked, and scaly lips.

Digestive System I: Oral Cavity and Associated Structures (Lip, Tooth, Tongue, Salivary Glands)

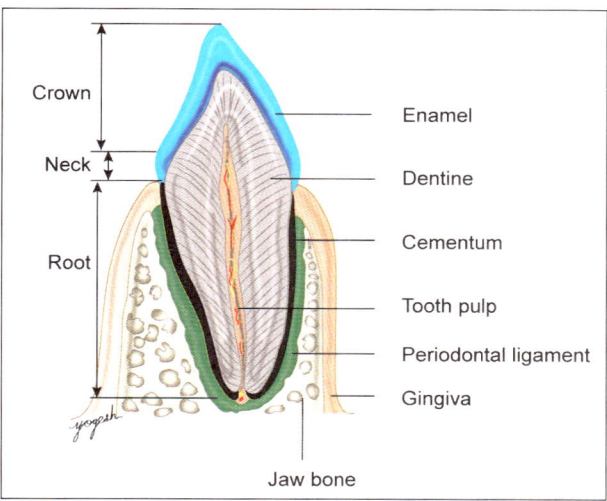

Fig. 16.3: Parts of tooth (schematic diagram).

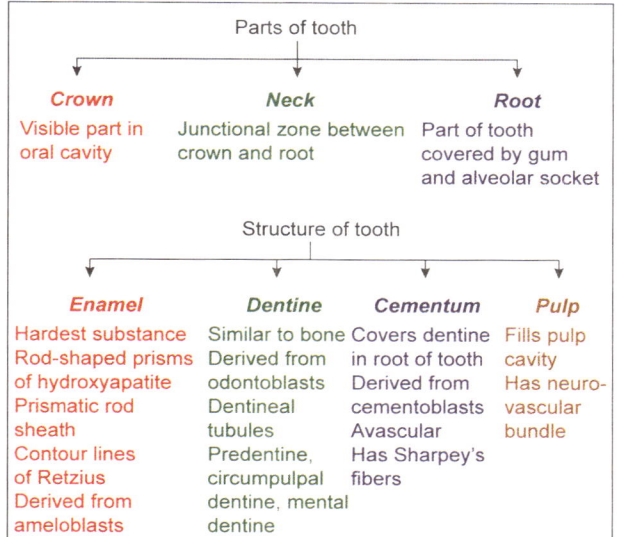

Flowchart 16.1: Structure and histology of tooth

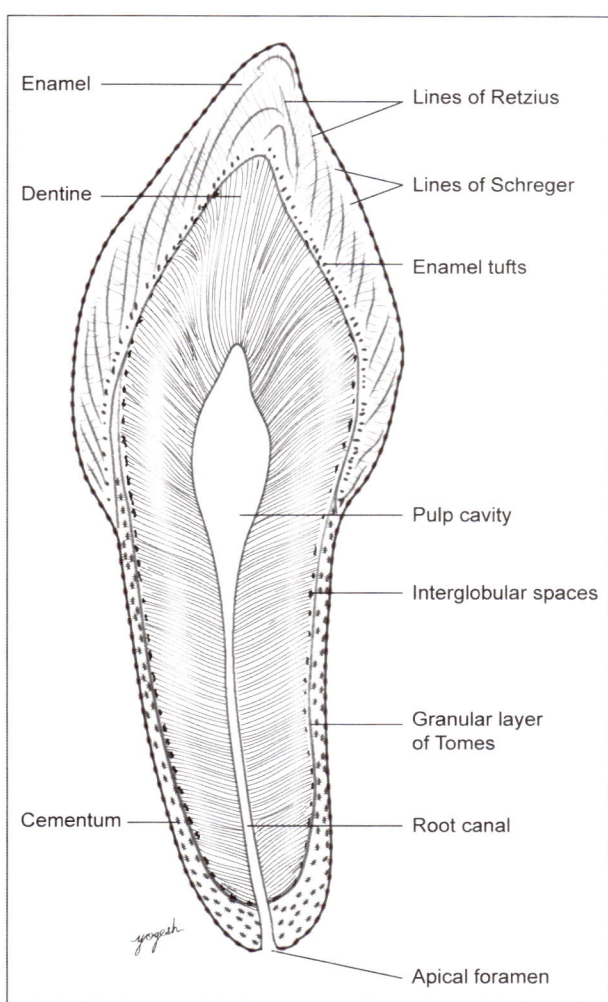

Fig. 16.4: Longitudinal section of dry tooth (practice figure). Note: Draw this figure using HB pencil.

3. Neck: It is a small part that lies at the junction of crown and neck.
- Tooth is made up of four specialized zones/coats as follows:
  1. Enamel: It is the hardest substance of body. It covers crown of tooth.
  2. Dentine: It forms a major portion of tooth. It lies deep to the enamel in crown and cementum in root.
  3. Cementum: It is a bone-like calcified tissue. It is present in root of tooth and covers dentine.
  4. Pulp cavity: Dentine encloses a cavity called pulp cavity. This cavity is filled with pulp that consists of connective tissue, blood vessels, and nerves. Pulp cavity continues as root canal in alveolar process.
- Periodontal ligament anchors cementum to alveolar socket.

Enamel

- It is the hardest substance in the body
- It is made up of calcium hydroxyapatite (96–98%).
- *Clinical crown* is a part of enamel that is visible in the oral cavity.
- Enamel consists of rod-shaped prism of crystals of hydroxyapatite. Prisms radiate from dentinoenamel junction to enamel surface.
- *Prismatic rod sheath:* It is a thin layer of organic matrix that covers prism.
- *Ameloblasts:* These cells form enamel. On eruption of tooth, ameloblasts are lost and there is no further deposition of enamel.

- *Contour lines of Retzius:* Enamel is deposited in waves by ameloblasts. This results in growth lines at right angle to the direction of enamel rods. These lies are called contour lines/striae of Retzius [Anders Adolph Retzius, 1796–1860, Swedish anatomist].
- *Lines of Schreger:* Alternating light and dark lines seen in enamel of the tooth that begin at the dentoenamel junction and end before they reach the enamel surface; they may represent areas of enamel rods cut in cross-sections dispersed between areas of rods cut longitudinally [John Hunter, 1728–1793, Scottish surgeon, anatomist].
- *Neonatal line:* It is an incremental growth line that represents the junction of enamel formed before and after birth.
- *Enamel tufts:* These are projections entering the enamel from dentoenamel junction.
- *Enamel lamellae:* These are projections entering from free surface of enamel.
- *Enamel spindles:* Dentineal tubules that extend into enamel form enamel spindles.

Dentine

- Dentine forms the wall of pulp cavity.
- It consists of 80% of inorganic salts and 20% organic material.
- Hardness of dentine is similar to the bone.
- Dentine contains hydroxyapatite salts that provide hardness.
- *Odontoblasts:* These are columnar cells that form dentine.
- *Dentineal tubules:* Dentineal tubules radiate outward form pulp cavity to the outer wall of tooth.
- Dentineal tubules are occupied by processes of odontoblasts in living state. These tubules lie parallel to each other.
- *Fibers of Tomes:* Protoplasmic processes of odontoblasts that occupy the dentineal tubule are called fibers of Tomes.
- *Predentine:* Newly formed layer of dentine by odontoblast is called predentine. In later stage, predentine gets mineralized.
- *Incremental lines of von Ebner:* These are less mineralized lines that separate layers of dentine. These lines indicate rhythmic growth pattern of dentine.
- *Granular layer of Tomes:* It is a thin layer of dentine adjacent to cementum. This layer appears granular on histological section [Sir John Tomes, 1815-1895, English dentist and anatomist].
- *Mantle dentine:* It is less mineralized zone of dentine near dentoenamel junction.
- *Circumpulpal dentine:* It forms the major part of dentine and lies between predentine and mantle dentine.

Cementum

- Cementum covers dentine in the root of tooth.
- It is a thin layer of bone-like material
- *Cementoblasts:* These are large cuboidal cells that form cementum.
- *Periodontal ligament:* It anchors cementum to the bony alveolar socket.
- *Cementocytes:* These are mature cementoblasts.
- Cementocytes are similar to osteocytes of bone and get trapped in lacunae of mineralized matrix of cementum. Processes of cementocytes are connected with that of adjacent cementocytes through canaliculi.
- *Sharpey's fibers:* Collagen fibers of periodontal ligament extend into cementum as Sharpey's fibers.

Pulp

- Pulp cavity of the tooth contains pulp.
- It consists of fibroblasts, macrophages, mast cells, collagen fibers, and ground substance.
- Pulp receives neurovascular bundle through *apical foramen* of tooth.
- Pulp cavity is lined by odontoblasts.
- Neurovascular bundle forms network deep to the odontoblast layer

---

Clinical Correlation

Dental caries/tooth decay
- It is the breakdown of tooth.
- Dental caries occurs in the form of pits or fissures.
- It occurs because of lack of proper oral hygiene.
- If the dental caries reaches up to pulp cavity, it becomes painful (because of sensory nerve endings).

TONGUE

Q. Draw a well-labelled diagram of histology of tongue.

Q. Draw a well-labelled diagram of histology of circumvallate papilla.

- Tongue is a mucomuscular organ having core of skeletal muscles covered with mucous membrane.
- Tongue helps for taste, speech, mastication, and deglutination.

Gross Features of Tongue

- Tongue is a conical-shaped organ having root, tip, and body (Fig. 16.5).
- Root of tongue is attached to mandible and hyoid bone.
- Tip of tongue is free and comes in contact with central incisors.

Digestive System I: Oral Cavity and Associated Structures (Lip, Tooth, Tongue, Salivary Glands)

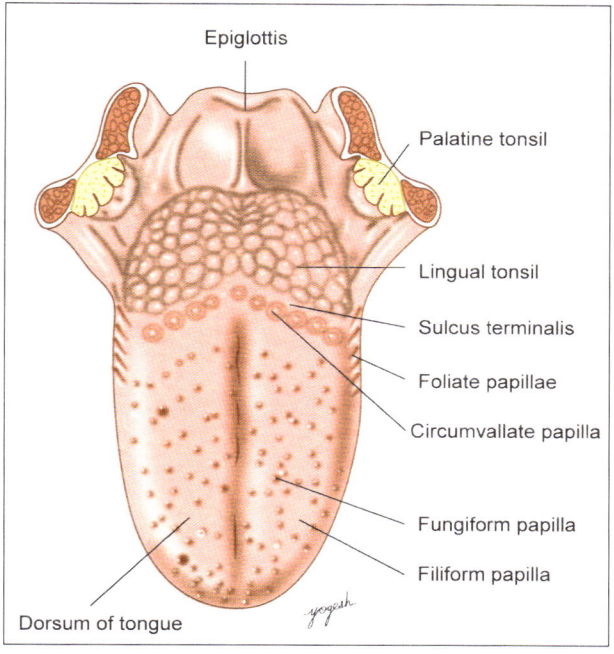

Fig. 16.5: Features of dorsal surface of tongue.

- Body has dorsal and ventral surfaces.
- Dorsal surface is divided into anterior two-third or oral part and posterior one-third or dorsal part by V-shaped *sulcus terminalis.*
- Apex of the sulcus terminalis shows a small depression called *foramen cecum* (point of embryonic thyroglossal duct).
- Dorsal surface of oral part is rough because of number of surface elevations called *papillae.*
- Pharyngeal part shows elevation of *lingual tonsils* (aggregation of lymphatic follicles covered by mucosa).

Papillae of Tongue

- Dorsal surface of the body of tongue shows projections called *lingual papillae* (Fig. 16.6).
- Lingual papillae are projections of lamina propria covered by mucous membrane.
- There are four types of lingual papillae as follows:
  1. Filiform papillae: These are most numerous and smallest papillae. They are minute conical projections that are covered by keratinized stratified squamous epithelium. They do not contain taste buds (Fig. 16.7).
  2. Fungiform papillae: These are mushroom-shaped projections projecting above filiform papillae. They are present mostly near the tip and can be easily identified as small pink spots. They have taste buds in their epithelium (Fig. 16.7).
  3. Circumvallate papillae: They are large, dome-shaped, 8–12 papillae. They are located just anterior to the sulcus terminalis. Each papilla is surrounded by a circular sulcus/trench. Base of the trench has openings of ducts of serous glands of von Ebner (Fig. 16.8).
     Secretions of these glands rinse the sulcus. Wall of sulcus (moat-like invagination) has taste buds. Core of the circumvallate papillae consists of connective tissue, vessels, and nerves.
  4. Foliate papillae: They consist of parallel rows of ridges near the margin of tongue in front of sulcus terminalis. Foliate papillae are rudimentary in humans (well developed in rabbits).

Box 16.1: Taste buds

- Taste buds are neurosensory epithelial structures (Fig. 16.9).
- Taste buds are present on fungiform and circumvallate papillae of tongue, oropharynx, soft palate, and epiglottis.

Structure

- Taste buds extend through the thickness of epithelium.
- *H&E* staining: Taste buds appear as onion-like, oval, pale staining epithelial structures.

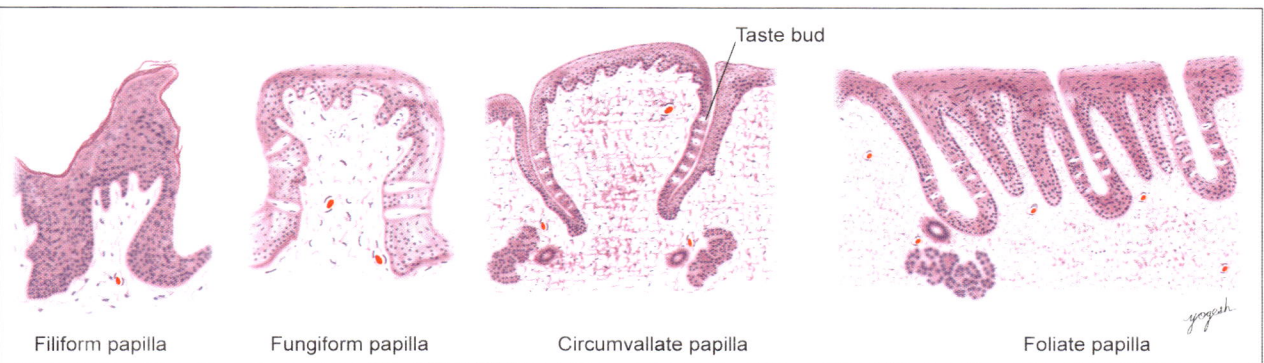

Fig. 16.6: Tongue papillae (practice figure).

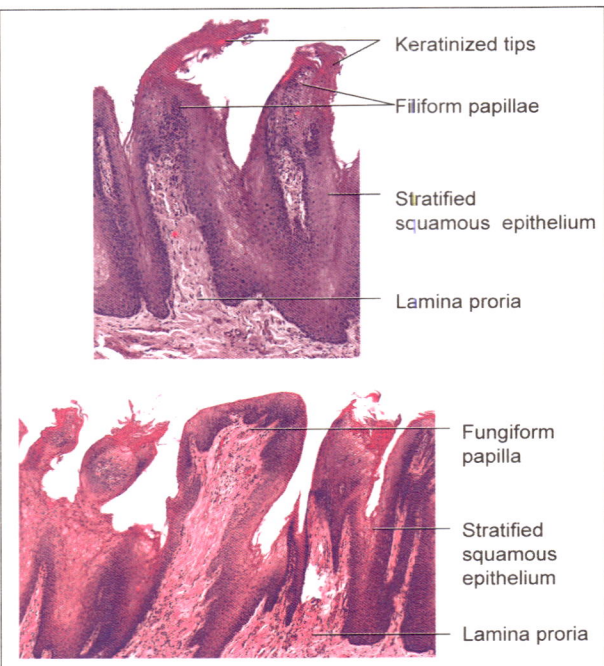

Fig. 16.7: Photomicrograph. Filiform and fungiform papillae high magnification, *H&E* stain).

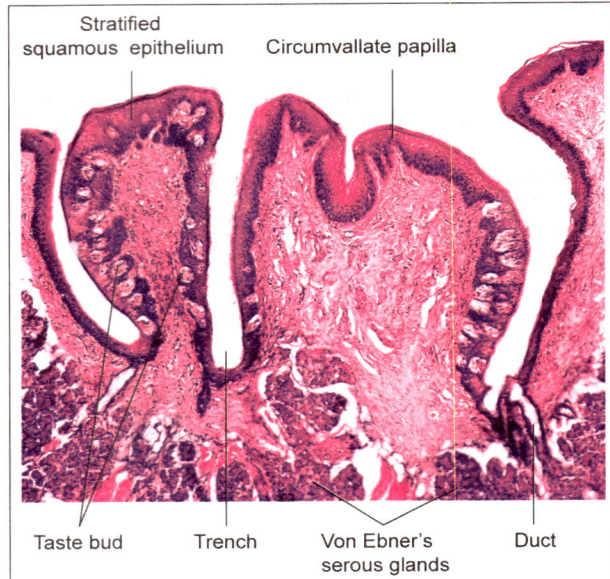

Fig. 16.8: Photomicrograph. Circumvallate papilla (high magnification, *H&E* stain).

Muscles of Tongue

- Core of tongue is formed by intrinsic and extrinsic striated muscles.
- Intrinsic muscles of tongue are arranged as longitudinal, transverse, and vertical bundles.
- Along with these, extrinsic muscles also enter the tongue and run in various directions.
- Muscle bundles are supported by loose connective tissue, adipose tissue, mucous lingual glands, von Ebner's serous glands, vessels, nerves, and lymphatics.

- Length: 50–80 μm, width: 30–50 μm
- Taste/gustatory pore: It is a small opening on the surface of taste bud.
- Histologically, taste bud consists of three cells.
- 1. *Neuroepithelial/sensory cell:* These are elongated cells that extend from basal lamina of epithelium to the taste pore. Their apical surface shows few microvilli. Basal portion of these cells synapse with afferent sensory processes of facial, glossopharyngeal, and vagus nerves. Life span of these cell is 10 days.
  2. *Supporting cells:* These are elongated cells that extend from basal lamina to the taste pore. They support receptor cells and secrete amorphous dense material at taste pore.
  3. *Basal/stem cells:* These are small dark cells situated near the basal lamina. They multiply and replace supporting and receptor cells.
- Mechanism
  - Chemicals (tastants) stimulate receptor cells and generate signals for sweet, sour, salty, bitter, and delicious tastes.
  - Bitter, sweet, and delicious tastants activate G-protein coupled taste receptors.
  - Sour and salty tastants activate ion channels.
- Tip of tongue detect sweet taste, posterolateral to tip detect salty atste, followed by sour taste.
- Circumvallate papillae detect bitter and delicious taste.

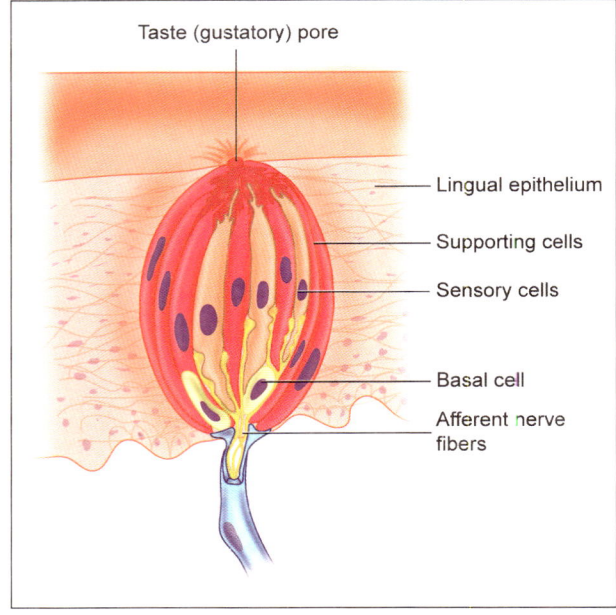

Fig. 16.9: Taste bud.

Digestive System I: Oral Cavity and Associated Structures (Lip, Tooth, Tongue, Salivary Glands)

> **Summary (Examination Guide)**
> - Tongue consists of mucous membrane that covers core of skeletal muscle fibers (Figs16.10, 16.11 and Flowchart 16.2).
> - Mucous membrane has:
>   – Lining epithelium – nonkeratinized stratified squamous epithelium *Identification feature*
>   – Lamina propria – loose connective tissue
> - Mucosa shows projecting papillae such as: *Identification feature*
>   1. Filiform: Small, conical projections with keratinized tips
>   2. Fungiform: Mushroom-shaped projections
>   3. Circumvallate: Dome-shaped papillae surrounded by circular sulcus
>   4. Foliate: Rudimentary papillae
> - Taste buds: Fungiform and circumvallate papillae have taste buds that open as taste pores. Taste buds have receptor, supporting, and basal cells.
> - Skeletal muscle fibers in tongue are arranged longitudinally, transversely, and vertically.
> - Tongue also shows mucous lingual salivary glands and von Ebner's serous salivary glands.

SALIVARY GLANDS

- Salivary glands secrete saliva in the oral cavity.
- Salivary glands include:
  – Major salivary glands such as parotid, submandibular, and sublingual glands. These glands open into oral cavity with the help of long ducts.

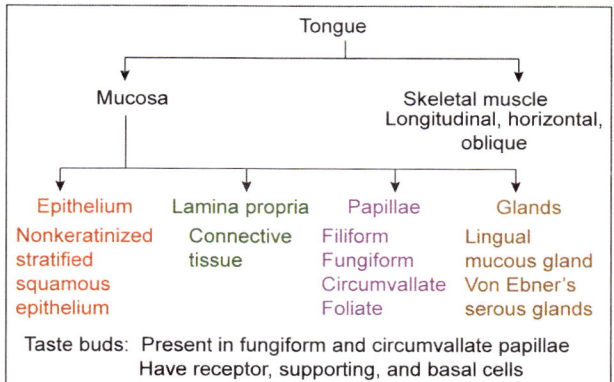

Flowchart 16.2: Histology of tongue

  – Minor salivary glands: These are small salivary glands located in lamina propria of lips, cheeks, soft palate, and tongue.
- Each salivary gland has duct and secretory unit/acini.

Histology of Salivary Gland

- Salivary gland consists of highly branched duct system and well-developed secretory acinar unit (Fig. 16.12 and Flowchart 16.3).
- Acini are made up of pyramidal cells.
- Based on the nature of secretory cells, acini are classified as serous acini, mucous acini, and mixed acini.
- Glandular tissue is surrounded by connective tissue capsule.

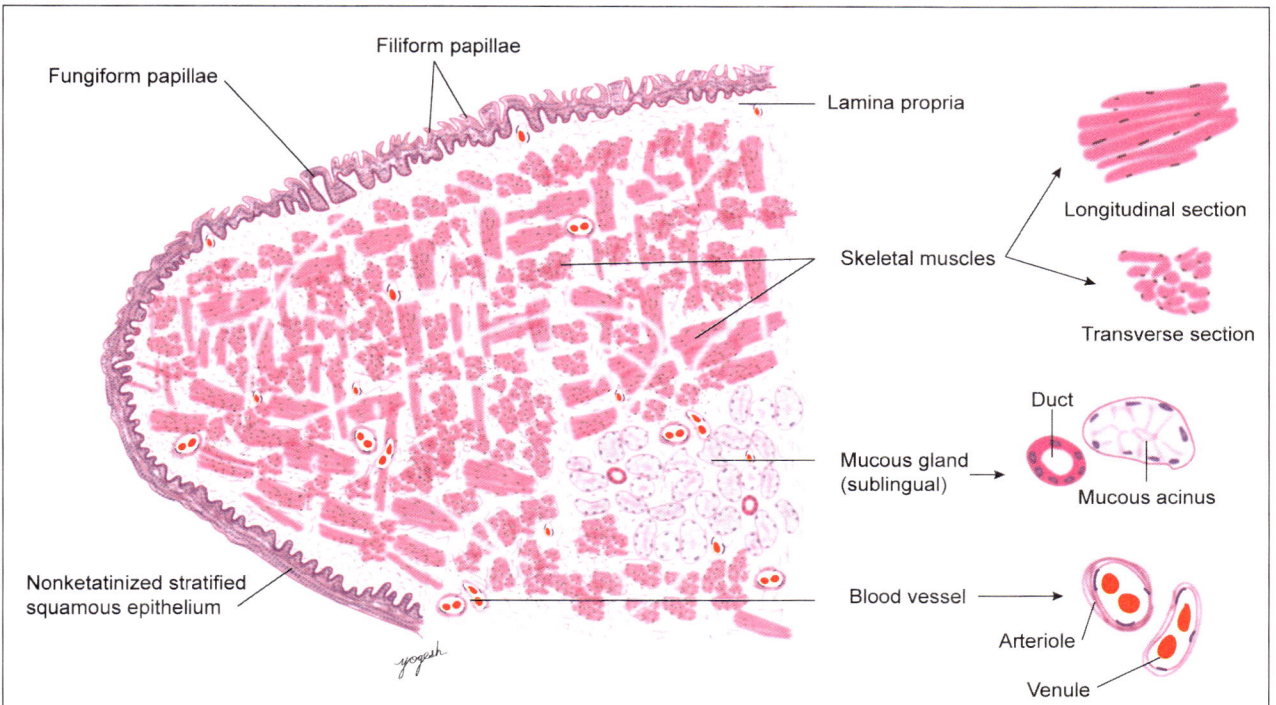

Fig. 16.10: Histology of anterior part of tongue (longitudinal section, practice figure).

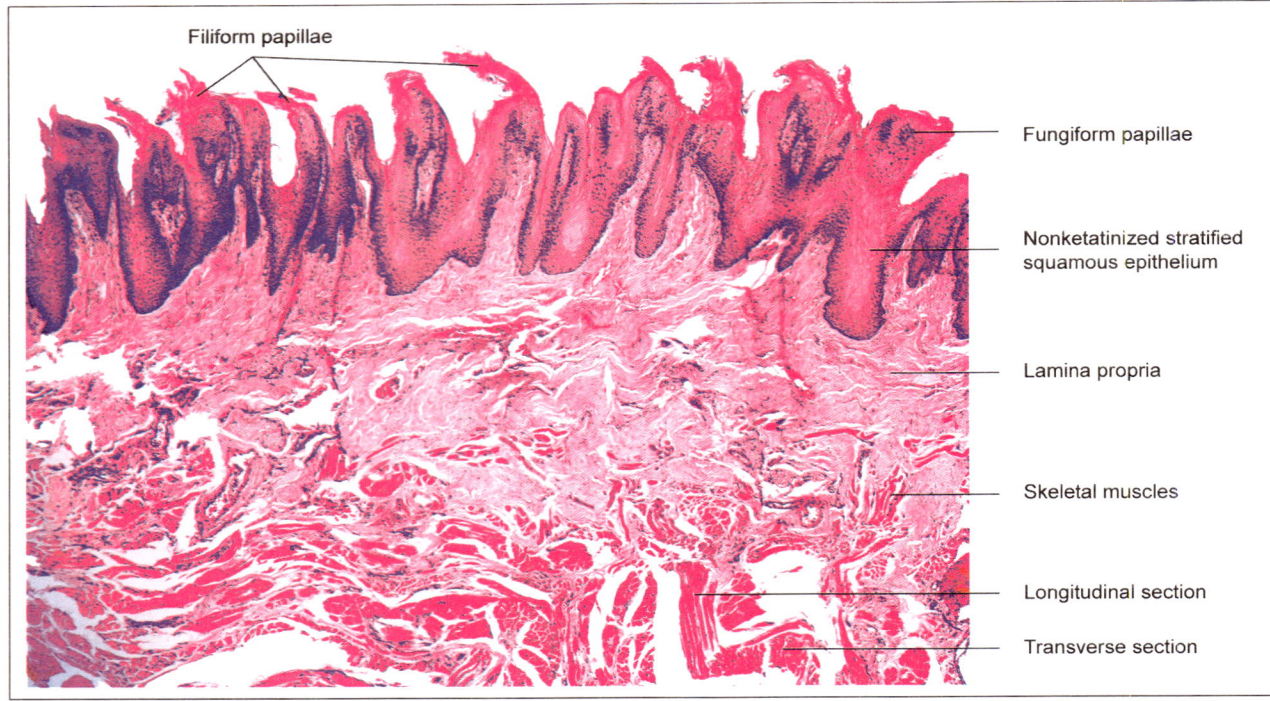

Fig. 16.11: Photomicrograph. Longitudinal section of anterior part of tongue (low magnification, *H&E* stain).

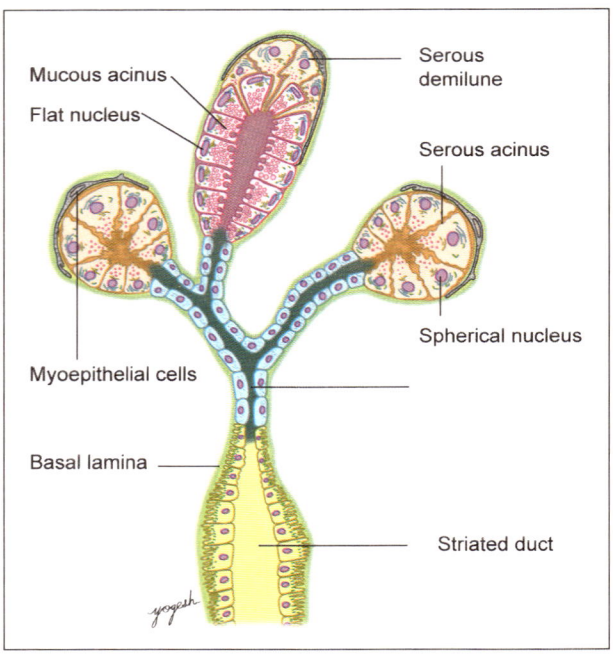

Fig. 16.12: Schematic representation of mixed salivary gland.

- Septa arising from capsule divide the gland into number of lobes and lobules.

Salivary Ducts

- Main salivary duct of the gland divides to form lobar, interlobular, and intralobular (striated and intercalated) ducts.

Intercalated duct

- These are lined by low cuboidal epithelium.
- These ducts connect secretory acini with larger ducts.
- These are predominant in serous glands.
- Functions: Absorption of Cl^- ions and secretion of HCO_3^- ions in saliva.

Striated ducts

- These ducts connect intercalated ducts with interlobular ducts (Fig. 16.13).
- These are lined by simple columnar epithelium.
- Basal portion of these epithelial cells shows numerous infoldings of plasma membrane. It helps in accommodation of numerous mitochondria and increasing surface area.
- On *H&E* staining, basal infoldings give striated appearance; hence, called striated duct.
- Striated ducts are predominantly present in serous glands.
- Functions: Resorption of Na^+ and secretion of K^+ and HCO_3^- in saliva.
- Striated ducts are absent in mucous glands.

Excretory ducts

- They include interlobular, lobar, and main excretory ducts.
- These duct shows gradual epithelial transformation from simple columnar to stratified cuboidal or columnar epithelium.
- Main excretory ducts open into the oral cavity.

Flowchart 16.3: Histology of salivary glands.

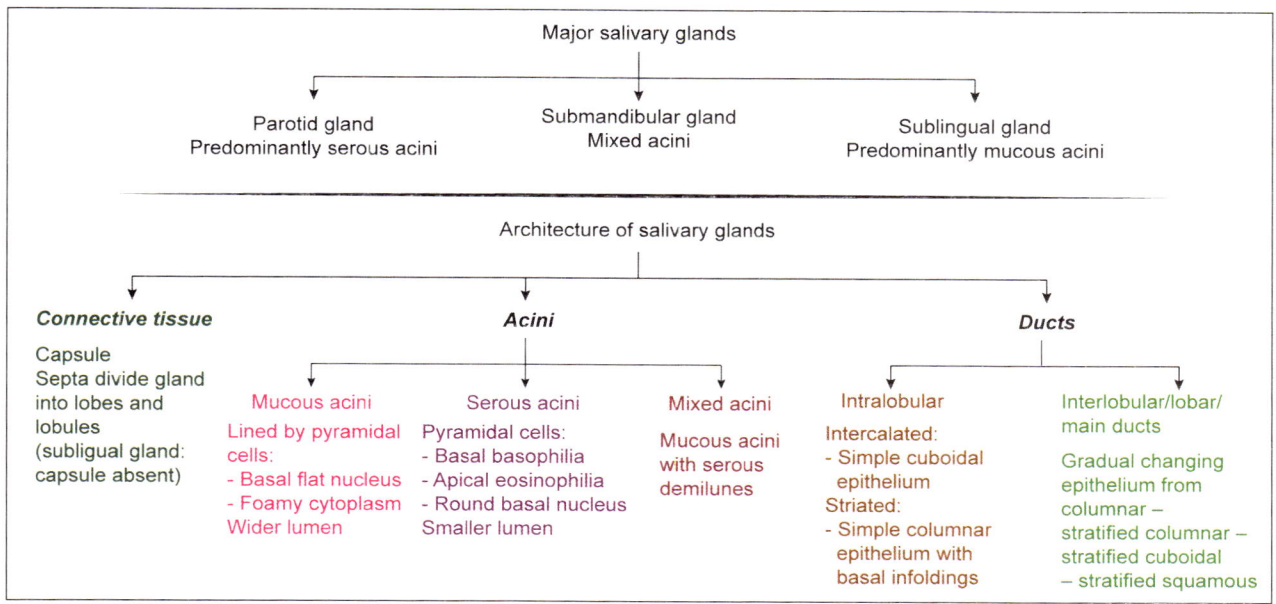

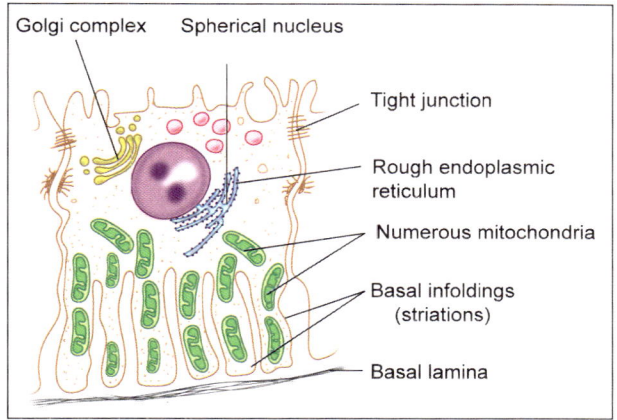

Fig. 16.13: Ultrastructure of a cell from striated duct.

Secretory Acini

- Salivary glands are tubuloalveolar glands salivary gland have serous, mucous, and mixed acini.

Serous acinus

- Serous acini secrete protein-rich, watery secretions.
- These acini are lined by pyramidal-shaped simple columnar epithelium.
- Serous cells have (Fig. 16.14):
  – Rounded basal nucleus
  – Large amount of rough endoplasmic reticulum that gives basal basophilia
  – Well-developed Golgi complex and secretory vesicles that gives apical eosinophilia

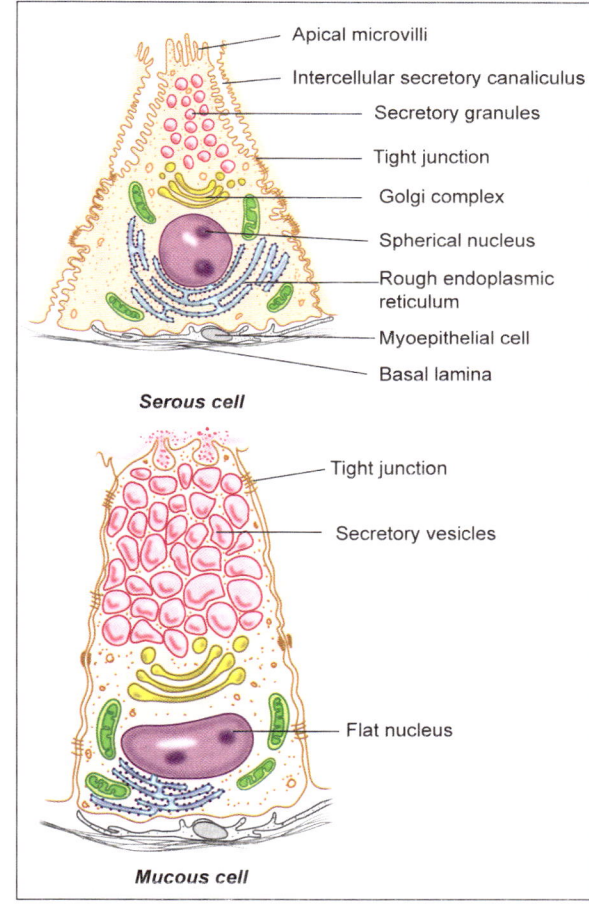

Fig. 16.14: Ultrastructure of serous and mucous cells.

Mucous acinus
- Mucous acini secrete thick mucoid secretions.
- These acini are lined by pyramidal-shaped simple columnar epithelium.
- Mucous cells have (Fig. 16.14):
  - Flat, elongated and basally placed nucleus
  - Foamy cytoplasm (mucus removed during tissue processing)
  - Mucous acini have wider lumen than serous acini

Mixed acini
- Mixed acini secrete both mucus and enzyme-rich watery secretions.
- Mixed gland has mucous acini with serous demilunes.
- Mixed acini are lined by mucous cells and these cells are capped by demilune of serous cells. All serous cells open into the lumen of acinus by fine canaliculi.
- *New concept:* Serous demilunes are preparation artifact that are formed during tissue processing because of swelling of mucous cells.
- These swollen cells push serous cells to produce serous demilune.

Myoepithelial cells
- These are also called basket cells or myoepithelium.
- These are star-shaped cells that are present between epithelium and basal lamina of acinus.
- They have actin filaments in their cytoplasm.
- Their contractions help the acini to expel the secretions.

Differences between serous and mucous cells are listed in Table 6.1. Differences between serous and mucous acini are listed in Table 6.2.

Parotid Gland
- Parotid gland is the largest salivary gland.
- It is covered by thick capsule and divided into number of lobes and lobules (Figs 16.15 and 16.16).
- Main secretory duct/Stenson's duct opens into the vestibule of mouth opposite to the upper second molar tooth.
- Acini: Parotid gland mainly consists of serous acini. These acini are surrounded by myoepithelial cells. *Identification feature*
- Ducts: Parotid gland has number of intralobular (intercalated and striated) ducts, and interlobular and lobar ducts. *Identification feature*
- Intercalated ducts are lined by low cuboidal epithelium.
- Striated ducts are lined by simple columnar epithelium with basal infoldings.
- Other ducts are lined by stratified cuboidal to stratified squamous epithelium.
- In between acini, adipose tissue is also present.

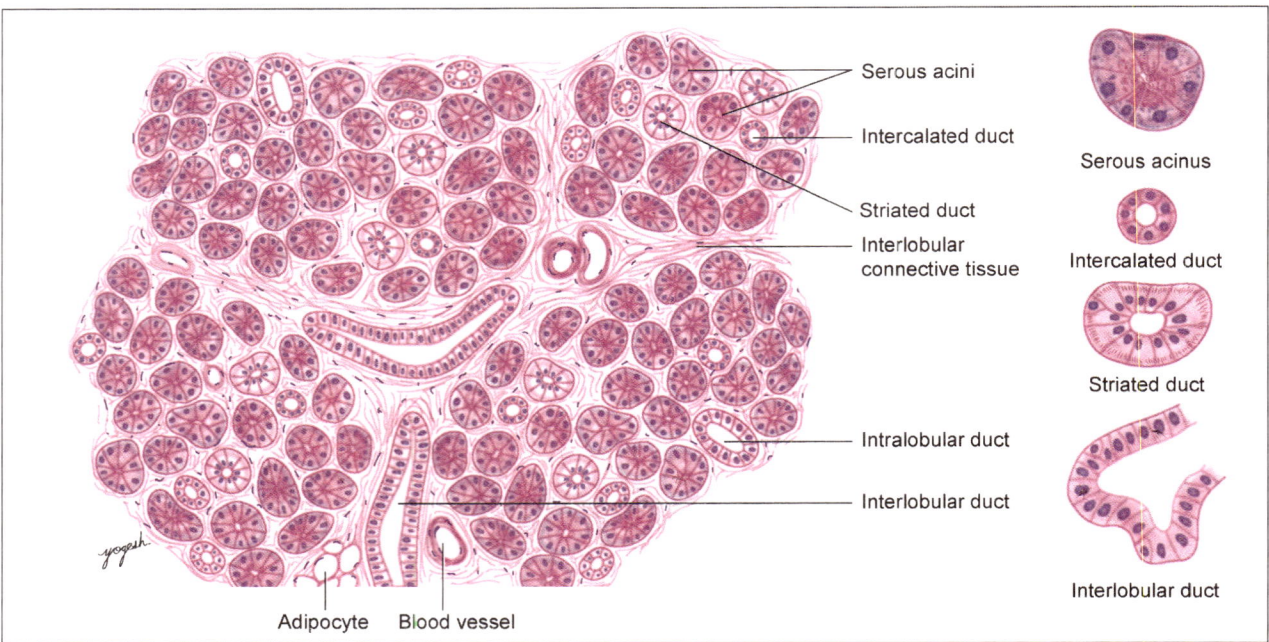

Fig. 16.15: Histology of parotid (serous) salivary gland (practice figure).

Digestive System I: Oral Cavity and Associated Structures (Lip, Tooth, Tongue, Salivary Glands)

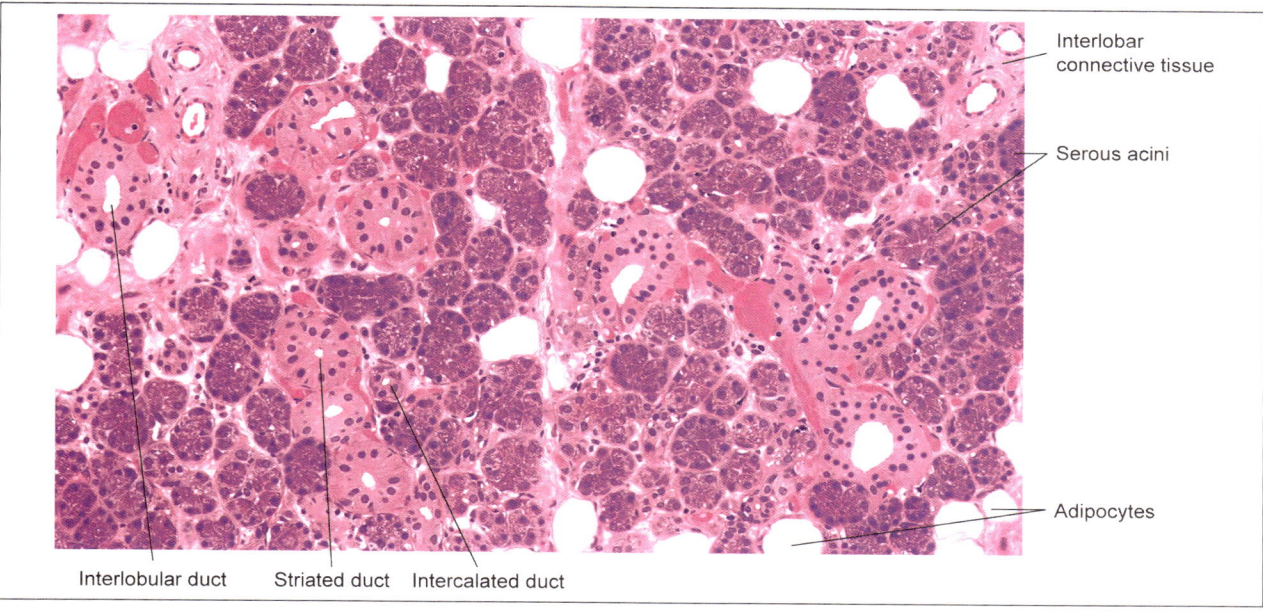

Fig. 16.16: Photomicrograph. Histology of parotid (serous) gland (low magnification, *H&E* stain).

Submandibular Gland

- Submandibular gland is mixed salivary gland.
- It has a well-defined capsule. Septa arising from capsule divide the gland into number of lobes and lobules (Figs 16.17 and 16.18).
- Acini: Gland shows presence of both serous and mucous acini. Few mucous acini also show serous demilunes. *Identification feature*
- Ducts: Gland has lobar, interlobular, and intralobular (striated and intercalated) ducts. *Identification feature*

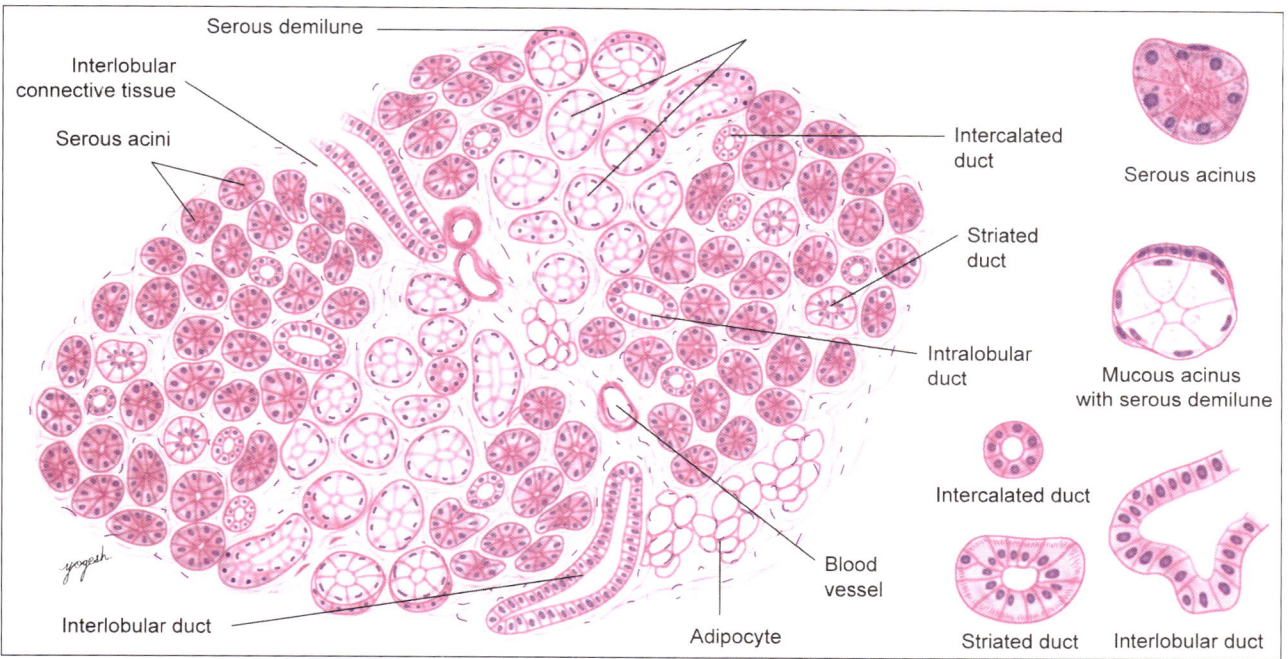

Fig. 16.17: Histology of submandibular (mixed) salivary gland (practice figure).

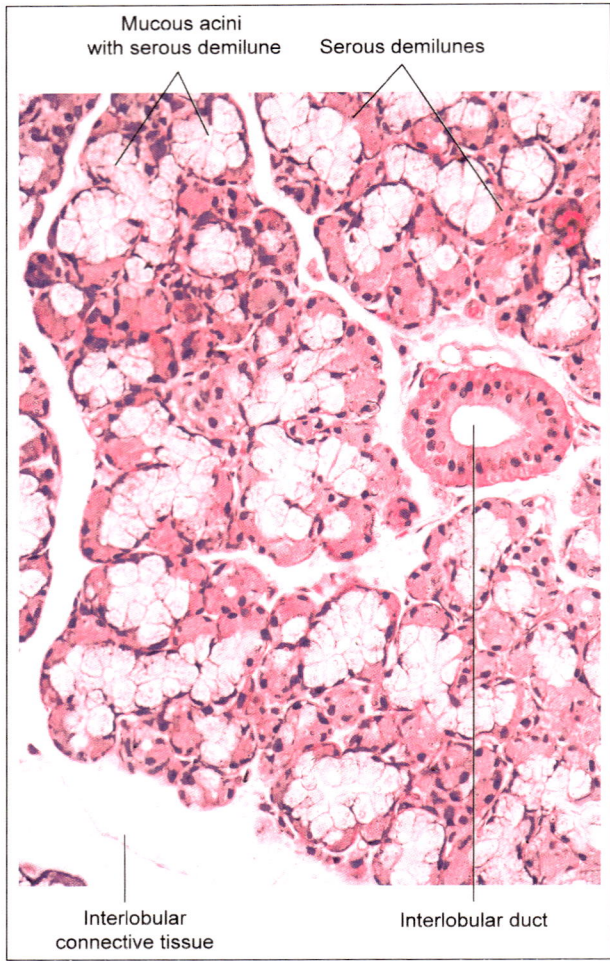

Fig. 16.18: Photomicrograph. Histology of submandibular (mixed) gland (low magnification, *H&E* stain).

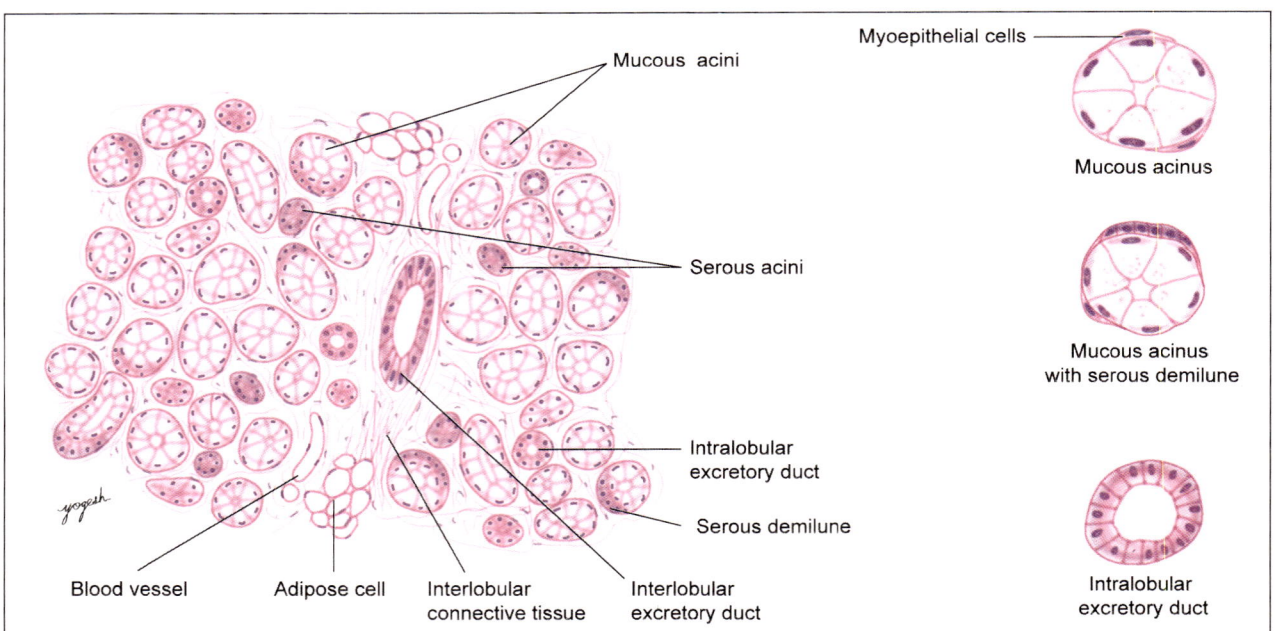

Fig. 16.19: Histology of sublingual (predominantly mucous) salivary gland (practice figure).

Digestive System I: Oral Cavity and Associated Structures (Lip, Tooth, Tongue, Salivary Glands)

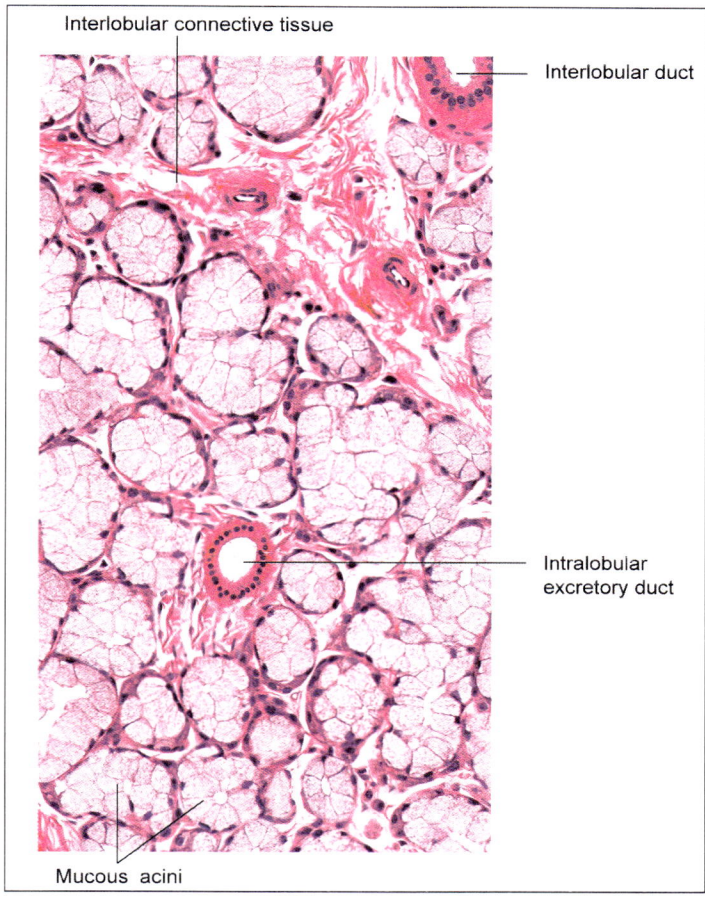

Fig. 16.20: Photomicrograph. Sublingual (predominantly mucous) salivary gland (low magnification, *H&E* stain.

- Intercalated ducts are less in number than in the parotid gland.

Sublingual Gland
- These are small masses of glandular tissue that lie in the substance of tongue.
- Sublingual gland is not surrounded by well-defined capsule (Figs 16.19 and 16.20).
- Acini: Sublingual gland predominantly has mucous acini. Few serous and seromucous acini are also present.
- Mucous secretory units are tubular (not purely acinar).
- Ducts: Sublingual glands do not have intercalated duct (rarely present) and striated ducts are also very few. Interlobular and lobar ducts are present.

CHAPTER 17

Digestive System II: Esophagus and Stomach

Chapter Outline
- General structure of GIT
- Esophagus
- Stomach
  - Internal structure
  - Cardiac region
  - Fundic or body region
  - Cells of fundic glands
  - Pyloric region

Competency achievement: The student should be able to:

AN52.1 Describe and identify the microanatomical features of gastrointestinal system: Oesophagus, fundus of stomach, pylorus of stomach

AN52.3 Describe and identify the microanatomical features of cardiooesophageal junction

- Gastrointestinal tract (GIT) is a long muco-muscular tube that extends from proximal part of esophagus to distal part of anal canal.
- GIT includes esophagus, stomach, duodenum, ileum, jejunum, colon, vermiform appendix, and anal canal.
- GIT shares common structural features that are essential for digestion, absorption, and transport of food material.

GENERAL STRUCTURE OF GIT

- GIT consists of four layers (from inside outward) (Fig. 17.1 and Flowchart 17.1):*Viva*
  1. *Mucosa:* It consists of lining epithelium, lamina propria, and muscularis mucosae.
  2. *Submucosa:* Consists of dense irregular connective tissue.
  3. *Muscularis externa* has inner circular and outer longitudinal smooth muscle layer.
  4. *Serosa* is a connective tissue layer covered by peritoneum. Adventitia is only connective tissue layer.

Mucosa

- Mucosa consists of three layers: Epithelium, lamina propria, and muscularis mucosae.*Viva*

Epithelium

- Lining of gut is *simple columnar epithelium* except at
  1. Esophagus (lined by stratified squamous epithelium)
  2. Terminal part of anal canal (lined by stratified squamous epithelium)
- The major functions of epithelium are protection, absorption, and secretion.
- Absorptive function of gut is supported by large surface area.
- To increase the surface area, intestine shows following modification (specifically in small intestine):*Viva, MCQ*

Flowchart 17.1: General structure of GIT

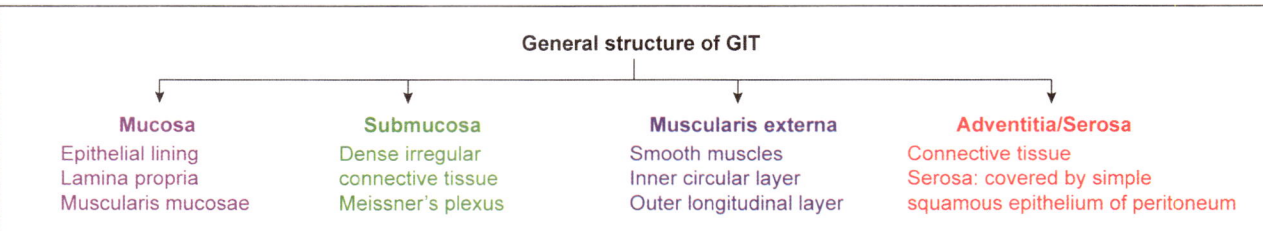

196

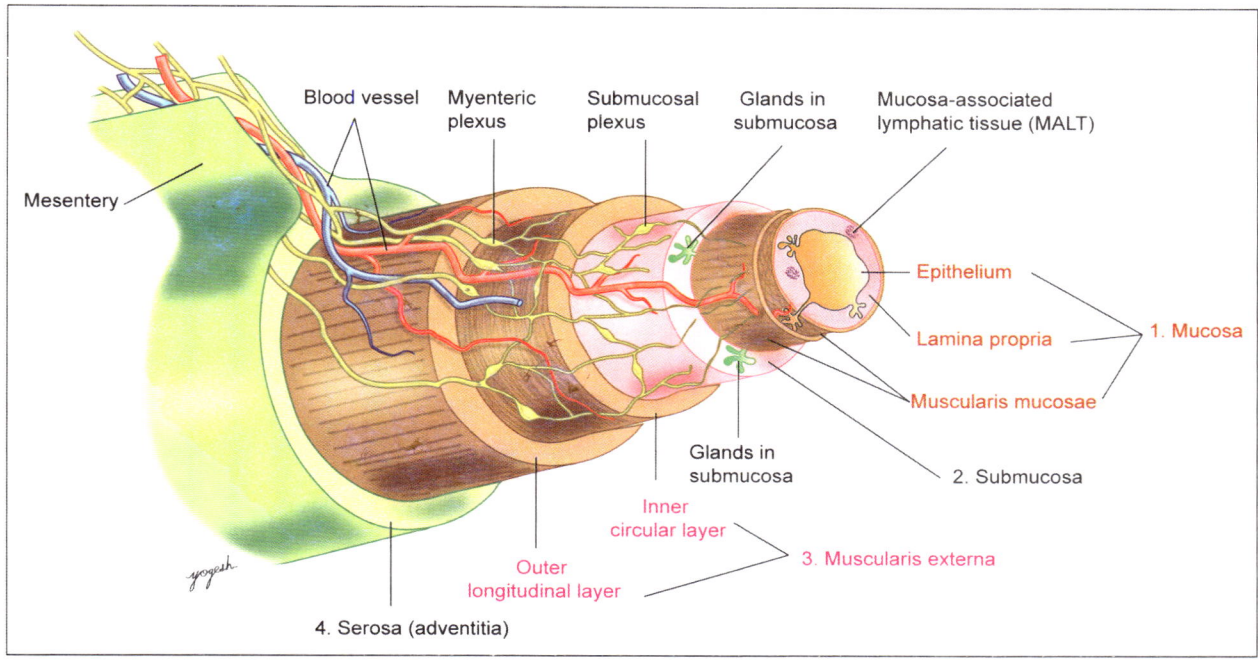

Fig. 17.1: Layers of intestine.

1. *Plicae circularis*: These are circumferential submucosal folds.
2. *Villi*: These are finger-like mucosal projection.
3. *Microvilli*: These are cell-surface projections.
4. Other than these three modifications, the length of intestine and crypts (depressions of epithelium in lamina propria) also increase absorptive power of intestine.

- Intestine also performs secretory function that provides lubrication factors, digestive enzymes, and even antibodies.
- Secretory function of intestine is supported by
  1. *Unicellular secretory cells* of epithelium.
  2. *Simple tubular glands*: These arise from lining epithelium and extend into lamina propria. These are also called as *crypts*.
  3. *Submucosal glands* are compound tubuloalveolar mucous secreting glands that lie in submucosa. These are present in esophagus and duodenum.
4. *Extramural glands:* These are supportive glands that pour their secretion into lumen of gut through ducts. These include liver (bile) and pancreas (pancreatic juice). Embryologically, these glands are derived from endoderm of gut.

Lamina Propria

- Lamina propria is a layer of loose connective tissue that supports epithelium.
- It consists of blood vessels and lymphatic vessels. These vessels help in transport of absorbed nutrients.
- Lamina propria has *gut-associated lymphatic tissue* (GALT) in the form of diffuse lymphatic tissue and lymphatic nodules. GALT plays major role in protection, phagocytosis, and antibody secretion. In ileum, lymphatic nodules occupy lamina propria and submucosa to form *Peyer's patches*.[Neet]
- Lamina propria also provide space for mucosal depressions that form *mucosal glands*. For examples, gastric glands in stomach and crypts of Lieberkühn in intestine.

Muscularis Mucosae

- Muscularis mucosae is the *smooth muscle cell* layer that separates mucosa from submucosa.
- Muscle cells are arranged in *two layers* as an inner circular and outer longitudinal layer.
- Contractions of muscularis mucosae can change shape of mucosa and it facilitates absorption and secretion.
- Muscularis mucosae extend into mucosal folds but not into villi.

Submucosa

- Submucosa is a *dense irregular connective tissue* layer.[MCQ]
- It contains numerous blood vessels, lymphatics, and occasional glands (in esophagus and duodenum).

- Submucosa also shows few unmyelinated nerve fibers and ganglionic cells that form submucosal Meissner's plexus.*Neet, Viva*
- Submucosa allows movement of mucosa over muscularis externa.

Mucularis Externa

- Muscularis externa consists of smooth muscles arranged in *two layers:* inner circular and outer longitudinal (ICOL).
- Exceptions for this arrangement are
  - Upper third of esophagus has striated muscles, middle third of esophagus has both striated and smooth muscles.
  - Stomach has inner oblique, middle circular, and outer most longitudinal muscle layer.
  - In large intestine/colon, longitudinal fibers form prominent bundles called *taenia coli*.
- In some part, circular muscle layer forms a thick band that works as *sphincter* or *valves*. For example, pharyngoesophageal sphincter (part of cricopharyngeus), lower esophageal sphincter, pyloric sphincter, ileocecal valve, and internal anal sphincter.
- Between inner circular and outer longitudinal layers, Auerbach's plexus (myenteric plexus) is present.*Neet, Viva*
- *Function:* Contractions of muscularis externa propel content of intestinal lumen. These movements are called peristalsis. Autonomic (enteric) nervous system controls movements of the muscularis externa.

Serosa/Adventitia

- It is an outer most connective tissue covering of intestine.
- If intestine is covered by a layer of peritoneum (mesothelium – simple squamous epithelium), the covering layer is called *serosa*.
- If the intestine is covered only by connective tissue, the covering layer is *adventitia*.
- Large blood vessels, lymphatics, and nerves traverse through serosa.

ESOPHAGUS

- Esophagus is a mucomuscular tube that conveys food and liquid from pharynx to stomach.
- Esophagus lies in the neck and thoracic region. It is fixed and separated from adjacent structures by connective tissue.
- Length: 25 cm.
- Lumen of esophagus remains normally collapsed and opens only during passage of a food substance.
- Lumen of esophagus has longitudinal folds.
- Esophagus has constrictions at the following sites:*Viva, MCQ*
  1. At the beginning of esophagus due to cricopharyngeus muscle (pharyngoesophageal sphincter)
  2. At crossing of arch of aorta
  3. At crossing of left main bronchus
  4. At the level of entry through diaphragm.

Histology of Esophagus

- Histologically, esophagus has four layers: Mucosa, submucosa, muscularis externa, and adventitia (Figs 17.2 to 17.4 and Flowchart 17.2).

Mucosa

- Mucosa consists of the following layers:
  1. Epithelium: Esophagus is lined by *nonkeratinized stratified squamous epithelium*.*Identification feature*
  2. *Lamina propria:* It consist of loose areolar tissue and few lymphatic nodules.
  3. *Muscularis mucosae:* It consist of only longitudinal smooth muscle fibers. It is thicker as compared to other parts of gut.*Identification feature, Neet, Viva*

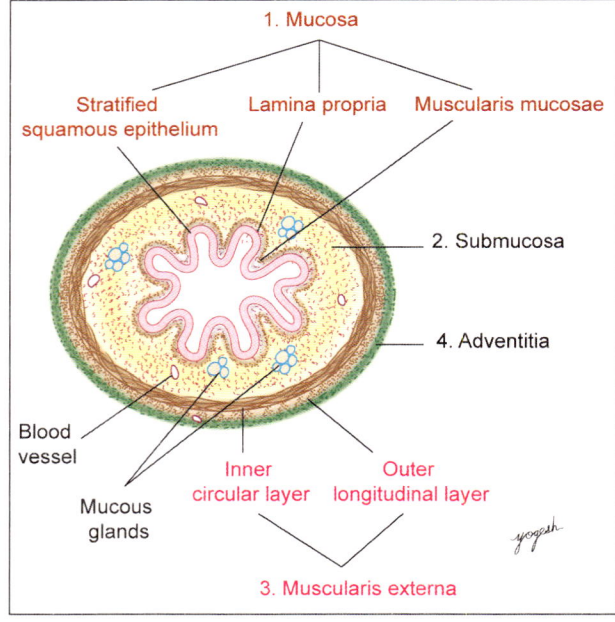

Fig. 17.2: Transverse section of esophagus. It consists of four layers and has star-shaped lumen.

Digestive System II: Esophagus and Stomach

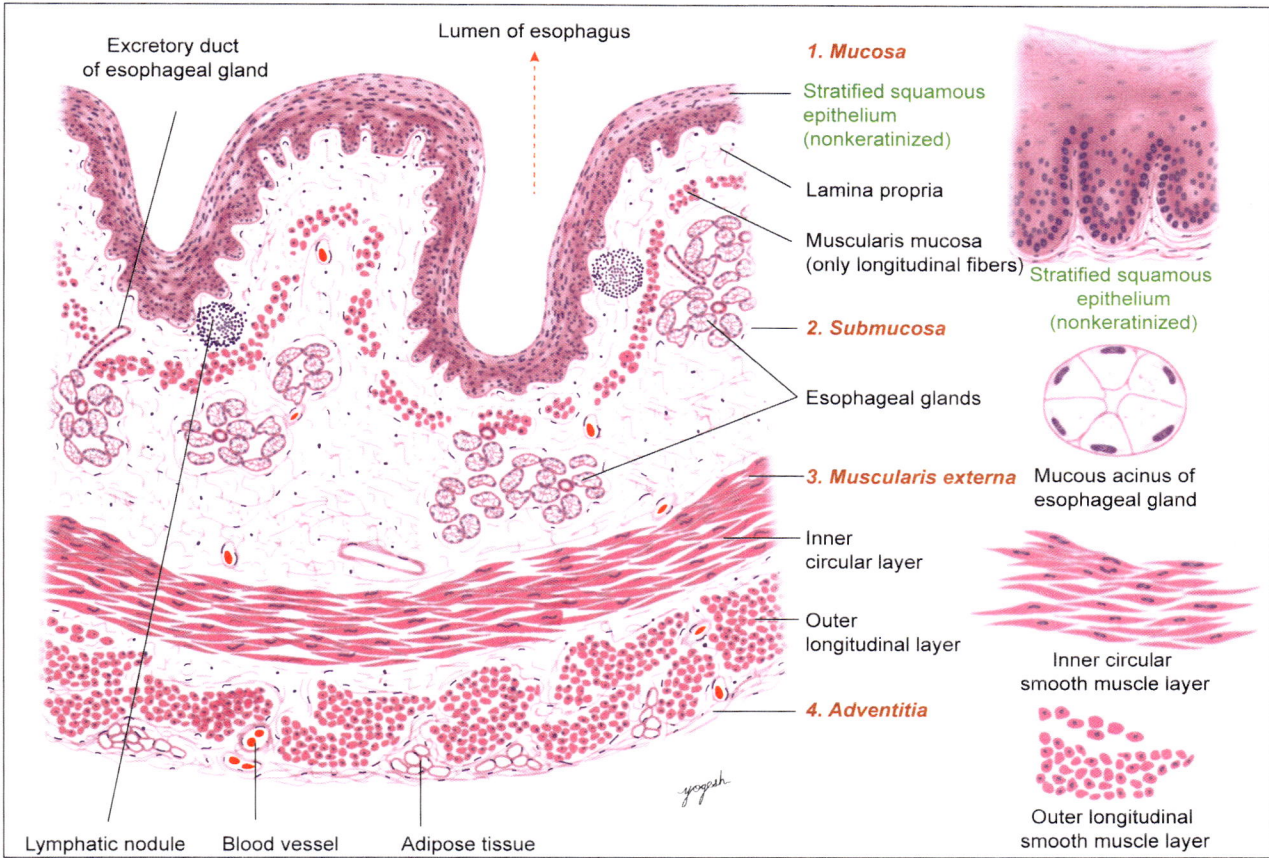

Fig. 17.3: Histology of lower part of esophagus (practice figure). Note: In upper one-third, wall of esophagus shows skeletal muscles in muscularis externa; in middle third, both skeletal and smooth muscles; whereas in lower-third only smooth muscles are present.

Flowchart 17.2: Histology of esophagus

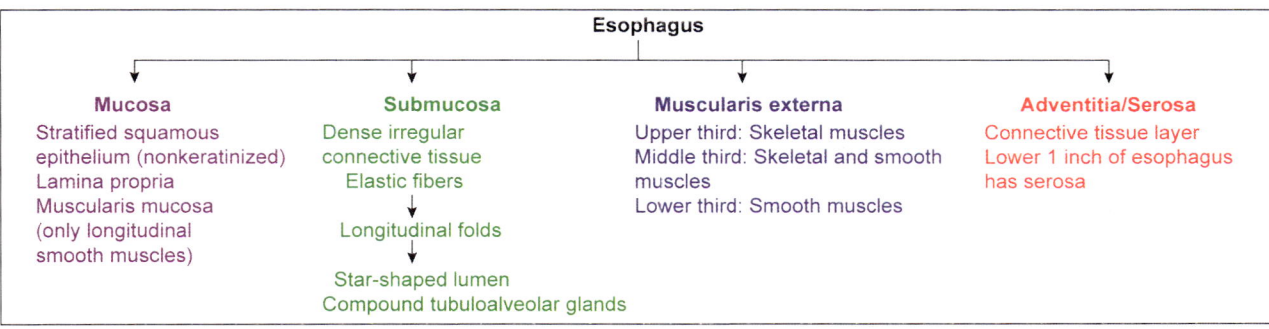

- Mucosa of esophagus shows longitudinal folds that disappear on distention of esophagus.
- Lamina propria gives finger-like projections into the epithelium. These projections prevent separation of epithelium from underlying connective tissue.

Submucosa

- It has *dense irregular connective tissue* that consists of bundles of collagen fibers, elastic fibers, large blood vessels, and nerves.
- Because of presence of elastic fibers, submucosa is folded, and lumen of esophagus is irregular (star-shaped). *Viva*
- *Branched tubuloalveolar mucous glands* are present in submucosa. Ducts of these glands pass through lamina propria and open into lumen of esophagus. *Viva*
- Glands are predominantly seen in lower part of esophagus.

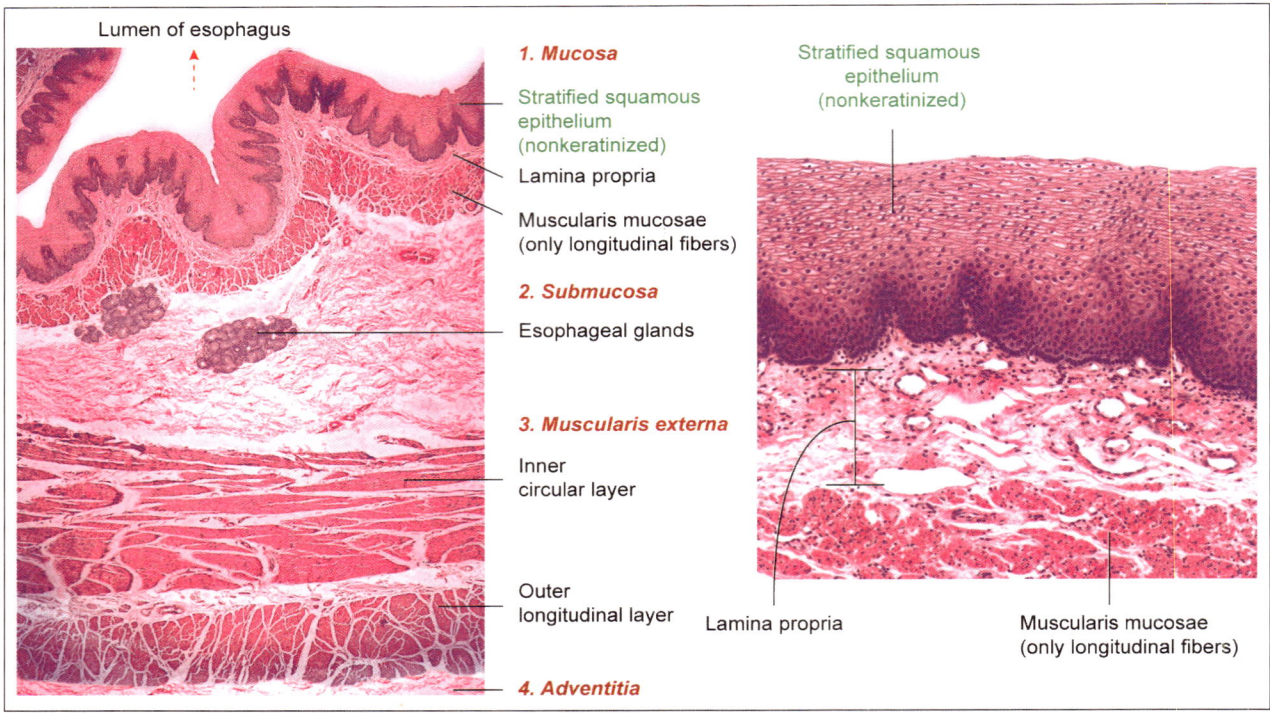

Fig. 17.4: Photomicrograph. Histology of lower part of esophagus.

Muscularis Externa

- Muscularis externa of esophagus shows the following composition:^{MCQ}
  1. Upper third of esophagus: Skeletal muscle
  2. Middle third of esophagus: Both smooth and skeletal muscles
  3. Lower third of esophagus: Smooth muscles only
- Muscles are arranged as inner circular and outer longitudinal layer.
- Between two layers, myenteric plexus (Auerbach's plexus) is present.
- Muscularis externa is toughest layer of esophagus.^{Neet}

Adventitia/Serosa

- Esophagus is surrounded by dense fibrous tissue (adventitia).
- Serosa: Lower 1 inch of esophagus is covered by peritoneum (serosa).

Functions of Esophagus

1. Transport of food and liquid from pharynx to stomach.
2. Esophageal glands secrete mucus that protects esophagus from acidic contents of stomach.
3. No absorption, no digestion.

Some Interesting Facts

- *Cardiac glands:* These are mucous glands in the lamina propria of the lower end of esophagus. It protects esophagus from exposure to acidic contents of the stomach.
- *Lower esophageal sphincter (LES):* It is present at the junction of esophagus with stomach. LES is only a physiological sphincter as it does not exist anatomically.

Summary (Examination Guide)

Esophagus has the following layers:

- *Mucosae:* It consists of stratified squamous epithelium (nonkeratinized), lamina propria, and muscularis mucosa (thick, longitudinal smooth muscles).
- *Submucosa:* It consists of dense irregular connective tissue with elastic fibers and compound tubuloalveolar glands.
- *Muscularis externa:* In upper third of esophagus, it has skeletal muscle fibers; in middle third, both skeletal and smooth muscle fibers; whereas in lower third, only smooth muscle fibers.
- *Adventitia:* Esophagus is surrounded by connective tissue. Only lowest 1 inch, it is surrounded by serosa (peritoneum).

Digestive System II: Esophagus and Stomach

Clinical Correlation
- *Achalasia cardia:* It is also called cardiospasm. In achalasia cardia, because of neuromuscular dysfunctions, lower esophageal sphincter (cardiac sphincter) fails to relax. It results in *megaesophagus* (dilatation of esophagus) and patient complaints of dysphagia (difficulty in swallowing) and in severe cases there may be a regurgitation of undigested food in respiratory tract.
- *Gastroesophageal reflux disease* (GERD): In GERD, because of failure of lower esophageal sphincter mechanism, the acidic contents of stomach enter in the lower part of esophagus. It causes heart burn (chest pain) and inflammation of esophagus.
- *Barrett's esophagus:* In Barrett's esophagus, lining epithelium of esophagus changes from stratified squamous to simple columnar epithelium with goblet cells. The main cause of Barrett's esophagus is GERD. This is a precancerous condition.

STOMACH

- Stomach is a hollow muscular organ that lies between esophagus and duodenum.
- Anatomically, stomach has fundus, body, and pylorus parts, and cardiac and pyloric ends.
- Histologically, stomach shows three regions: cardiac, fundic, and pyloric regions (Fig. 17.5).
  1. *Cardiac region:* It is a small part of stomach that lies at cardiac end (at gastroesophageal junction).
  2. *Fundic (body) region:* It includes fundus and body of stomach. Histological features of fundus and body parts are similar.
  3. *Pyloric region:* It connects stomach with duodenum.
- Histologically, stomach shows usual four layers of gut, that is, mucosa, submucosa, muscularis externa, and serosa. Gastric mucosa shows presence of gastric glands (Fig. 17.6).

Internal Structure of Stomach

- *Rugae:* Inner surface of stomach shows longitudinal mucosal folds/ridges called *rugae*. These rugae allow stomach to distend when filled and rugae disappear on stomach distention.*Viva*
- *Gastric pits:* Mucosal surface of stomach shows numerous depressions called *gastric pits*. These are openings of simple tubular gastric glands.*Viva*
- *Gastric canals:* Mucosal folds lie longitudinally along lesser curvature of stomach. These are called *gastric canals*.
- *Mucus coating/visible mucus:* Surface epithelial cells of stomach secrete thick, gel-like mucus that covers the internal surface of stomach, and protects stomach from acidic contents.

Some Interesting Facts
- Prostaglandins (PGE2) enhance mucus and bicarbonate secretion, and thus protect gastric mucosa from acidic damage.
- Nonsteroidal antiinflammatory drugs (NSAIDS), such as, aspirin suppress production of prostaglandins and make gastric mucosa prone to damage → gastric ulcers.

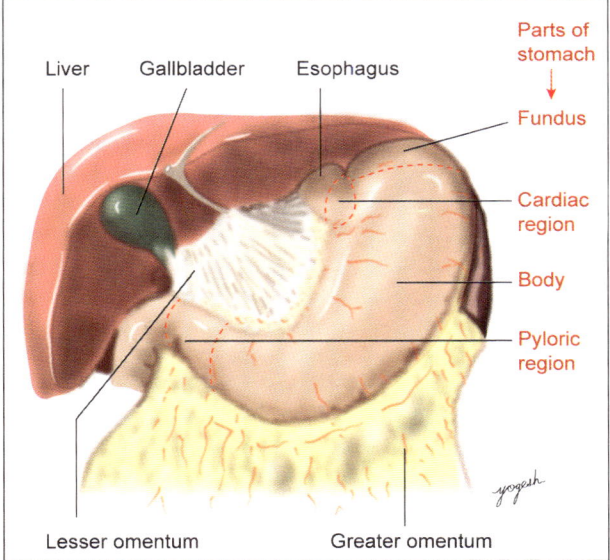

Fig. 17.5: Regions of stomach for histological description.

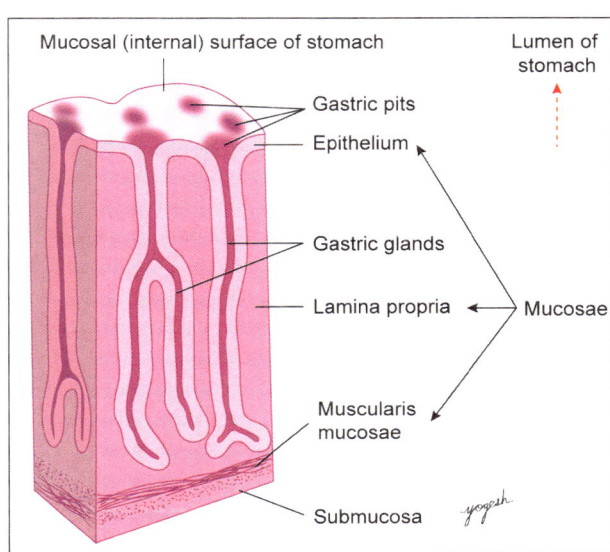

Fig. 17.6: Location of gastric glands in lamina propria.

CARDIAC REGION OF STOMACH

Q. Write a short note on histology of cardiac region of stomach.

- A section of stomach in cardiac region shows four layers: Mucosa, submucosa, muscularis externa, and serosa (Figs 17.7, 17.8 and Flowchart 17.3).

Mucosa

- Mucosa of cardiac region shows three layers: Epithelium, lamina propria, and muscularis mucosae.
- *Epithelium:* Simple columnar epithelium with basal oval nuclei. Epithelial cells secrete mucus and hence also called *mucous surface cells.* These cells show vacuolated cytoplasm as mucus is washed during the slide preparation. *Viva*
- Note: There are *no goblet cells and microvilli* in stomach (microvilli and goblet cells are present in small intestine). *Viva*
- *Lamina propria:* Lamina propria contains *mucous secreting, simple tubular cardiac glands.* These glands are lined by simple columnar epithelium with flattened basal nuclei. Apical cytoplasm of these cells is filled with mucin granules (may show vacuolated appearance on *H&E staining*). Ducts of cardiac glands open as the *gastric pits.*
- *Muscularis mucosae* consists of smooth muscle cells that are arranged as inner circular and outer longitudinal layers.

Submucosa

- Submucosa consists of dense irregular connective tissue. It has blood vessels, nerve fibers, and Meissner's (submucosal) plexus.

Flowchart 17.3: Histology of cardiac part of stomach

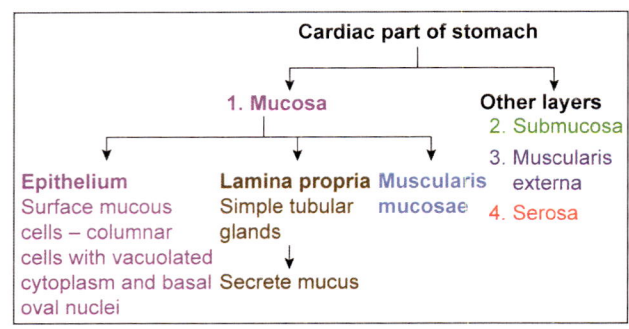

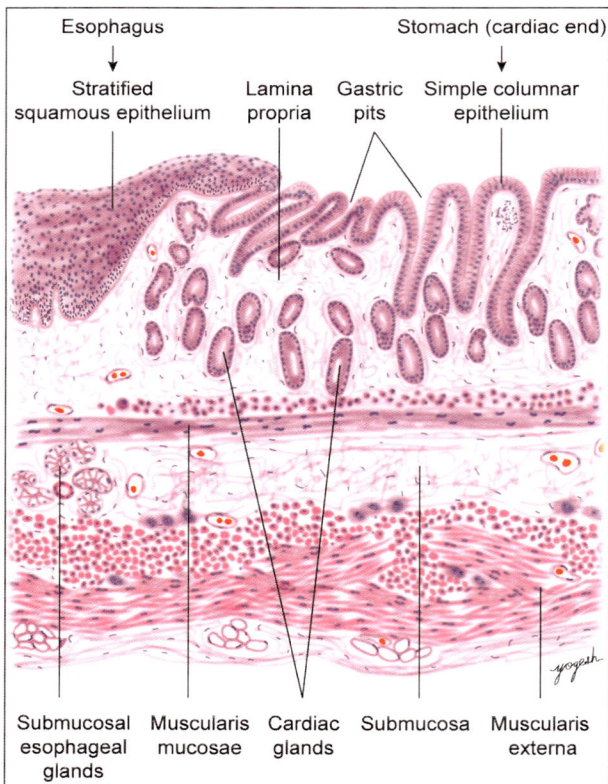

Fig. 17.7: Histology of gastroesophageal junction (longitudinal section, practice figure).

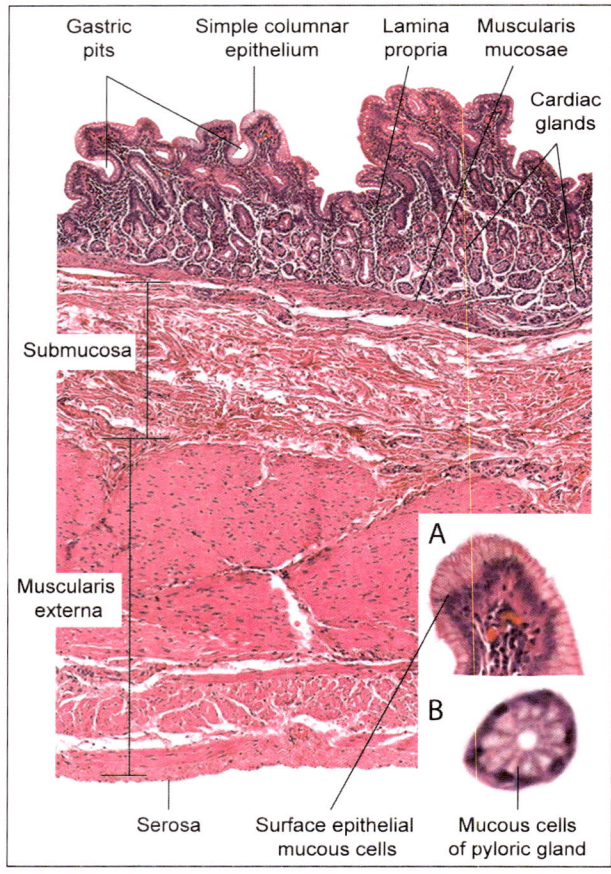

Fig. 17.8: Photomicrograph. Histology of cardiac part of stomach (low magnification).

Muscularis Externa

- *Previous concept:* Smooth muscles of stomach are arranged as an outer longitudinal, middle circular, and inner oblique layer.
- *New concept:* Histologically distinct layers of muscularis externa cannot be differentiated. Smooth muscles of muscularis externa are oriented randomly. *Viva*
- Myenteric or Auerbach's plexus is present between bundles of smooth muscle fibers.

Serosa

- Stomach is covered by a connective tissue layer with mesothelial lining of visceral peritoneum.
- Along lesser and greater curvatures, peritoneum continues as lesser and greater omentum, gastrosplenic and gastrophrenic ligaments.

FUNDIC OR BODY REGION OF STOMACH

Q. Write a short note on the histology of fundic or body region of the stomach.

- A section of stomach in fundic or body region shows four layers: Mucosa, submucosa, muscularis externa, and serosa (Figs 17.9, 17.10 and Flowchart 17.4).

Mucosa

- Mucosa of fundic (body) region shows three layers: Epithelium, lamina propria, and muscularis mucosae.

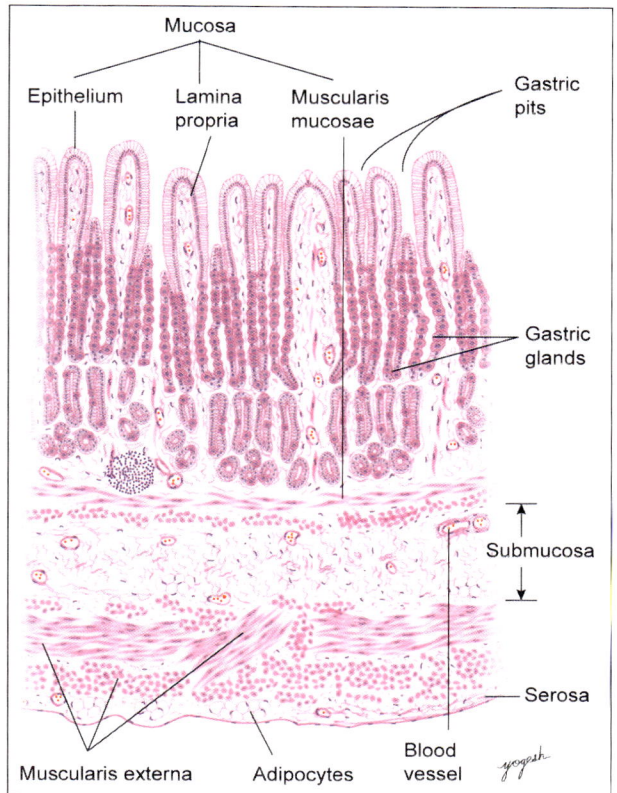

Fig. 17.9: Histology of body/fundus of stomach at low magnification (practice figure).

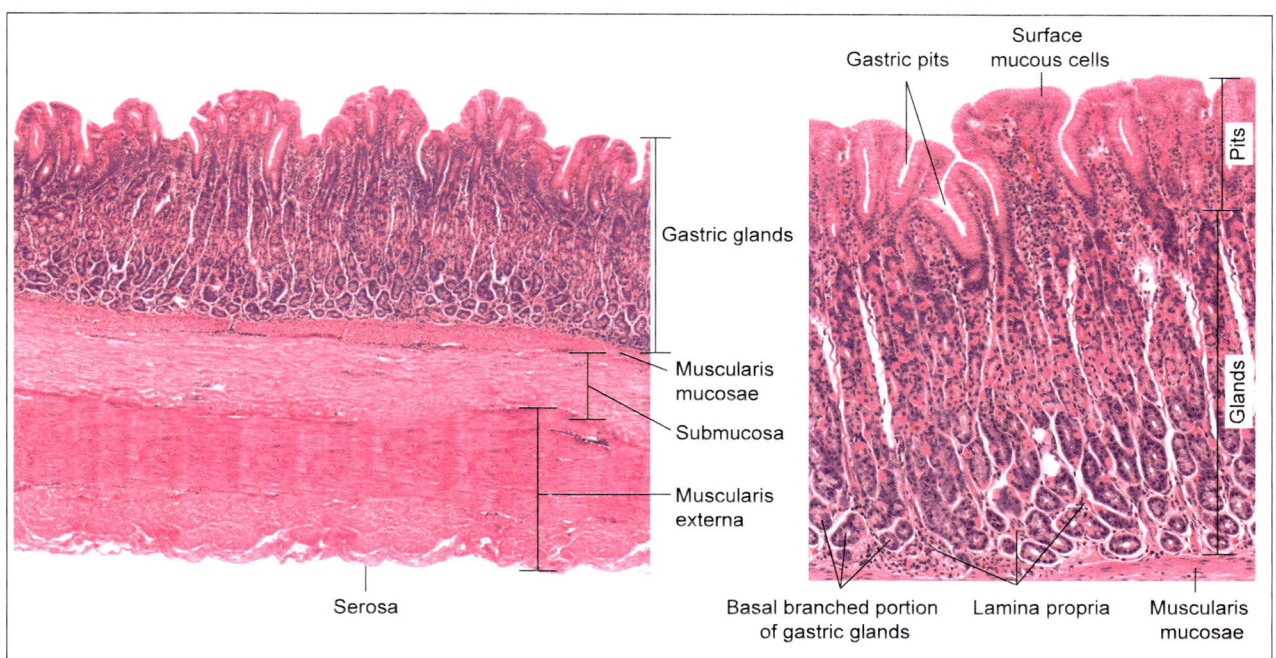

Fig. 17.10: Photomicrograph. Fundus/body region of stomach. (entire stomach wall on left, X40 and low magnification of gastric mucosa on right, X100; *H&E* stain).

Flowchart 17.4: Histology of fundic (body) region of stomach

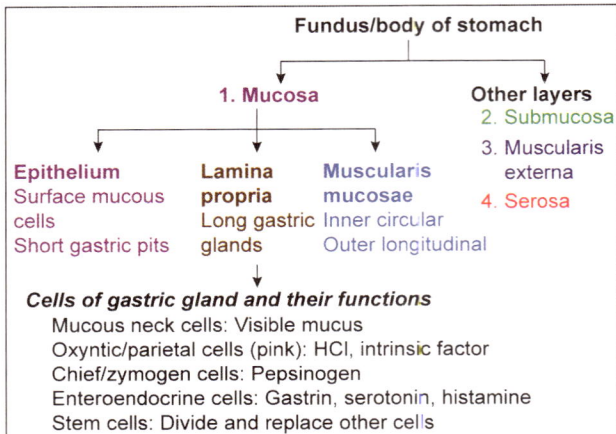

- *Epithelium:* Stomach is lined by simple columnar *surface mucous cells.* These cells show presence of mucinogen granules in apical part and basal oval nucleus.
- *H&E staining:* Surface mucous cells show vacuolated apical cytoplasm as mucus is removed during slide preparation.
- *Periodic acid–Schiff (PAS) staining:* Mucus takes deep magenta stain.
- *Toluidine blue staining:* Blue-colored glycoproteins of mucus is seen.
- *Lamina propria* shows presence of simple branched tubular glands called *gastric or fundic glands.* These glands extend from bottom of gastric pit (surface epithelium) to muscularis mucosae. Each gastric gland is connected with gastric pit by a small narrow segment called isthmus.
- Isthmus of gastric gland has stem cells that divide and migrate toward gastric pit and toward gastric glands.
- Each gastric gland has
  - Neck segment – It lies adjacent to isthmus. It is a narrow and long segment.
  - Fundic segment/base – It is a short and wide segment. Fundic segment usually divides into two or three branches.
- Gastric glands are lined by mucous neck cells, chief cells, parietal/oxyntic cells, enteroendocrine cells, and some undifferentiated cells.

Muscularis Mucosae, Submucosa, Muscle Layer, Serosa

- Structures of muscularis mucosae, submucosa, muscle layer, and serosa in fundic or body region of stomach are same as that of cardiac region of stomach.

CELLS OF FUNDIC GLANDS OF STOMACH

Q. List the cells of fundic glands of stomach.

- Fundus or body of stomach has branched tubular glands that have mucous neck cells, chief cells, parietal (oxyntic) cells, enteroendocrine cells, and some undifferentiated stem cells (Figs 17.11 to 17.13 and Flowchart 17.5). *Viva*

Mucous Neck Cells

- These are located in the neck region of fundic glands, just beneath gastric pits. *Neet*
- These are columnar cell with basal oval nucleus.
- Cytoplasm shows apical mucinogen granules (foamy appearance on H&E staining). *Neet*
- These cells produce soluble mucus (*Note:* Surface mucous cells produce insoluble/cloudy mucus). *Neet*

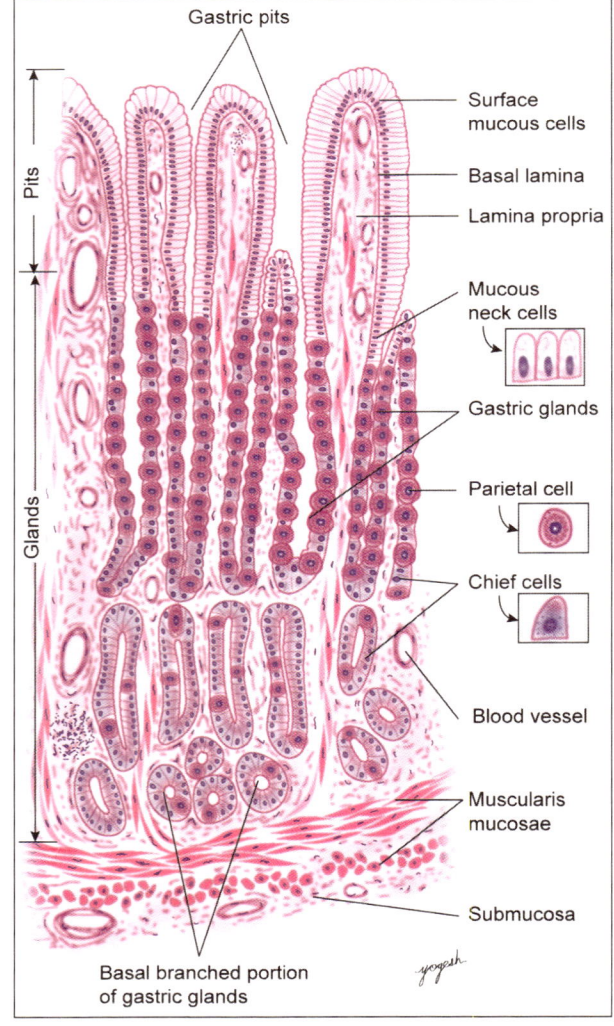

Fig. 17.11: Gastric mucosa at high magnification showing gastric glands (practice figure).

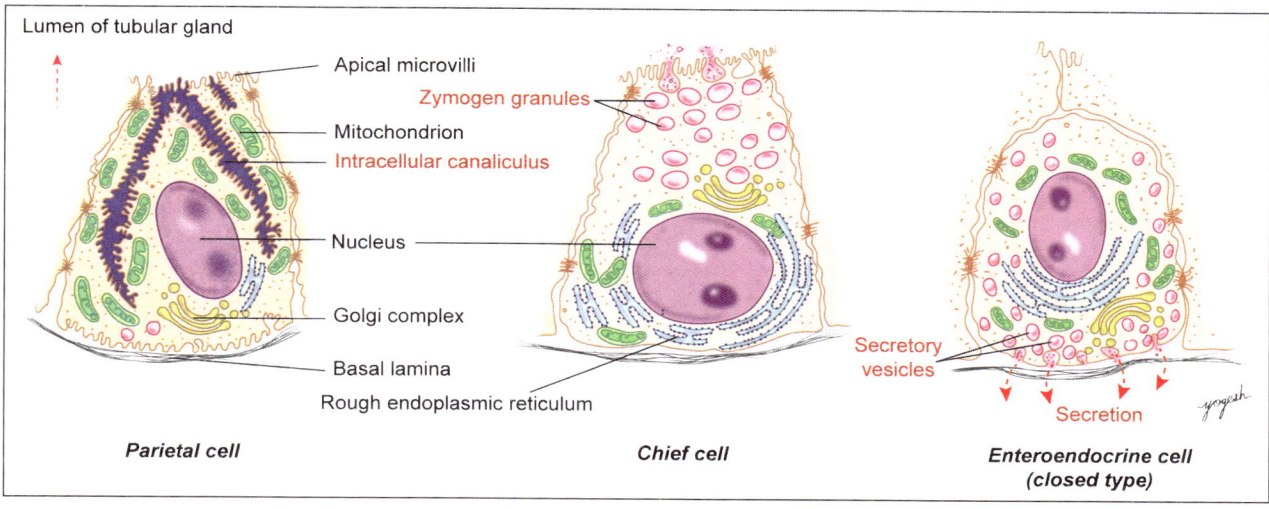

Fig. 17.12: Cells in glands of stomach.

Flowchart 17.5: Cells of gastric glands

	Mucous neck cells	Chief/zymogen cells	Parietal/oxyntic cells	Enteroendocrine cells	Adult stem cells
Location	Neck of gland	Lower third of gland	Upper part of gland	Lower part of gland	Neck region of gland
Identification feature	Columnar cell with oval nucleus	Dark basophilic cytoplasm	Dark acidophilic cytoplasm	Silver staining: Argyrohilic cells	Can be identified by immunohistochemistry
Function	Soluble mucus	Pepsinogen	HCl, intrinsic factor	Gastrin, serotonin, histamine	Divide and migrate upward and downward
Lifespan	6 days	150–200 days	60–90 days	4–6 days	–

Note: Surface mucous cell: Life span is 3–5 days.

- Some mucous neck cells give rise to stem cells in the neck region of gland that later replace surface mucous cells.
- Mucous cells are replaced every 5–7 days.

Chief or Zymogenic Cells

- These are blue in color on *H&E* staining and also called peptic cells.
- These are located in deeper/basal part (lower one-third) of the gastric glands in fundic and body part of stomach.
- These cells synthesize proteins (pepsinogen); hence their cytoplasm contains a large quantity of rough endoplasmic reticulum (rER). This rER takes basophilic (blue/hematoxylin) stain in basal part of cell (*basal basophilia*).
- Apical portion of the cell has secretory zymogen granules that impart slight *apical eosinophilia*.
- *Function:* Secretion of *pepsinogen* – a precursor of proteolytic enzyme pepsin.
- *Electron microscopy:* Cell shows abundant rER in basal part and secretory granules (Golgi apparatus) in apical part. Luminal surface of cells shows numerous small microvilli.

Parietal (Oxyntic) Cells

- These are mostly found in upper part and neck region of gastric glands in fundus and body part of the stomach.
- These are large triangular cells with a spherical nucleus. Apex of cell is directed toward lumen of gland and base toward basal lamina.

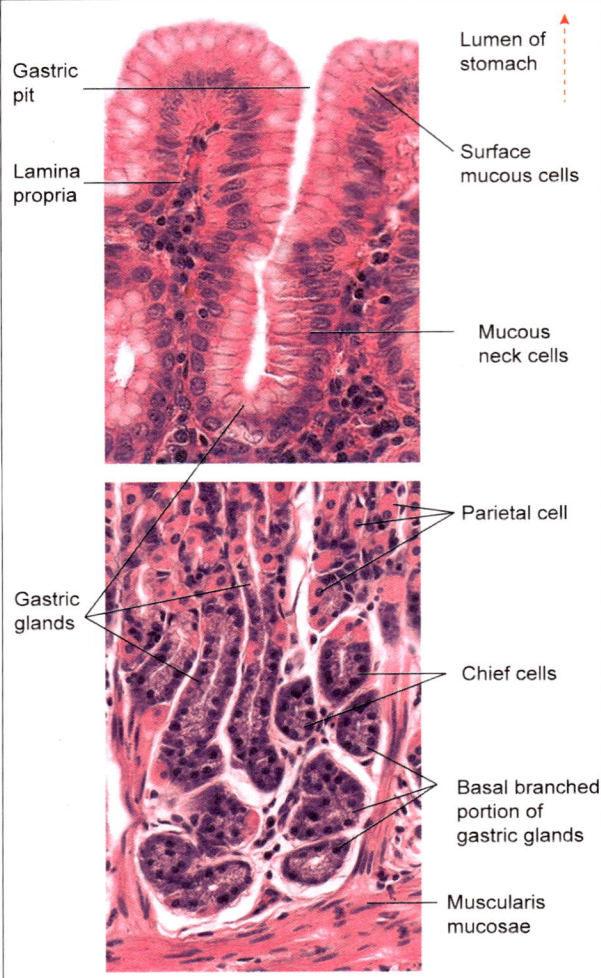

Fig. 17.13: Photomicrograph. Gastric mucosa at high magnification showing gastric glands (at high magnification only a portion of gland can be seen, hence in this photomicrograph, two separate views of gastric gland are shown, upper image shows superficial part and lower image shows deeper part of the gland).

- *H&E staining:* These cells take dark acidic (pink) stain. As these cells stain strongly with eosin, they are called *oxyntic cells.*
- *Electron microscopy:* Parietal cells have an intracellular canalicular system and tubulovesicular membrane system. Apical cell membrane shows several invaginations that form intracellular canaliculi.
- Wall of canaliculi shows a number of small microvilli. Cytoplasm contains numerous mitochondria.
- *Immunohistochemistry:* Wall of canaliculi contains a number of proton (H^+) pumps and Cl^- pumps. These pumps help in secretion of HCl.
- *Function:* Parietal cells secrete *HCl and intrinsic factor.*^Neet
- *Note:* Intrinsic factor binds with vitamin B_{12} and helps in its absorption. Deficiency of intrinsic factor leads to vitamin B_{12} deficiency and pernicious anemia.

- Lifespan of parietal cell is 150–200 days.^Neet
- Parietal cells have gastrin receptors, histamine (H2) receptors, and acetylcholine receptors.

Enteroendocrine Cells

- These cells are mostly present in lower portion of gastric glands.
- **Types of enteroendocrine cells**
  1. *Closed type:* These cells rest on basal lamina and do not reach lumen of gland.
  2. *Open type:* These cells have microvilli that reach lumen of glands.
- *H&E staining:* These cells remain unstained on *H&E* staining; hence, difficult to identify.
- *Silver staining:* These cells are argentaffin or argyrophilic cells (stained by silver salts).
- *Functions:* Secretion of gastrin, serotonin, and histamine directly into the blood vessels.

Stem Cells

- Some undifferentiated stem cells are present in neck region of gastric glands.
- These cells divide and move upward and downward to replace other cells.

PYLORIC REGION OF STOMACH

Q. Write a short note on histology of pyloric region of stomach.

A section of stomach in pyloric region shows four layers: Mucosa, submucosa, muscularis externa, and serosa (Figs 17.14, 17.15 and Flowchart 17.6).

Mucosa

- Mucosa of pyloric region shows three layers: Epithelium, lamina propria, and muscularis mucosae.
- *Surface epithelium* is lined by tall columnar surface mucous cells.
- *Lamina propria* shows presence of pyloric glands.

Flowchart 17.6: Histology of pyloric part of stomach

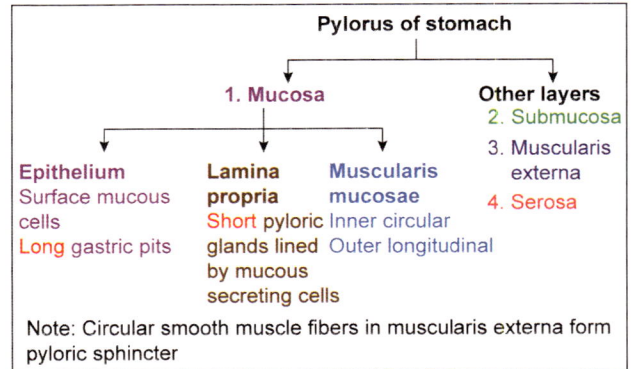

Digestive System II: Esophagus and Stomach

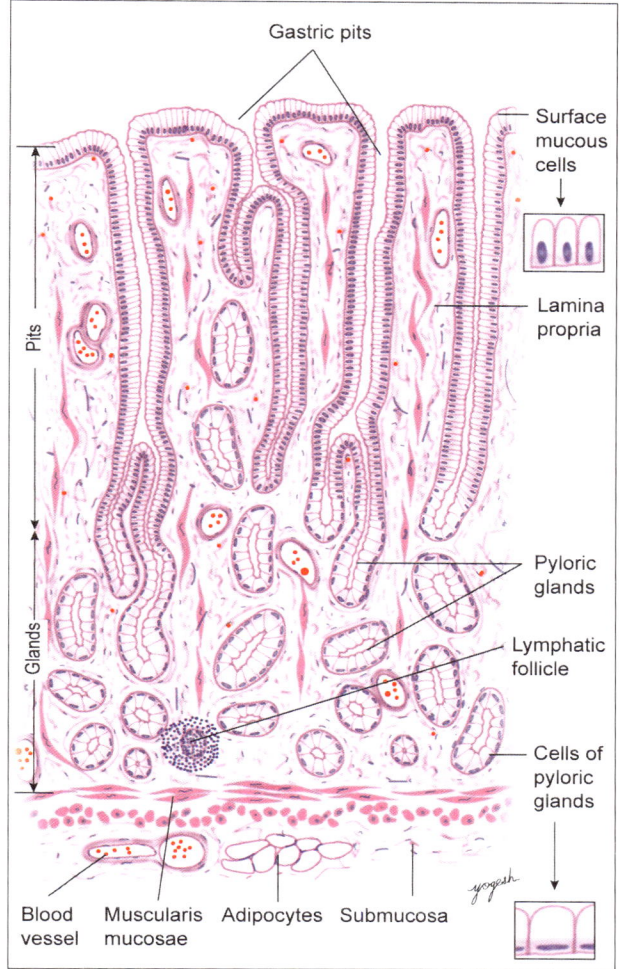

Fig. 17.14: Histology of pyloric part of stomach showing only mucosa and part of submucosa. Note: Muscularis externa and serosa are not shown in this figure (practice figure).

- *Gastric pits* of pyloric glands are deep and occupy about the two-third thickness of mucosa.^{Identification feature}
- Pyloric glands are shorter than fundic glands.^{Identification feature} Glands occupy only lower half or third of the mucosa.
- Pyloric glands are coiled branched tubular glands with wider lumen than fundic glands.
- Pyloric glands are lined by only one type of cell that are similar to the neck mucous cells.^{Identification feature}
- These cells produce mucus.
- Occasional enteroendocrine cells are also present.
- *G cells* are present in the deeper part of pyloric glands and in duodenum. These cells secrete gastrin.^{Viva}

Muscularis Mucosae, Lamina Propria, and Submucosa

- The structure of muscularis mucosae, lamina propria, and submucosa in the pyloric region of stomach are same as that of the cardiac region of stomach.

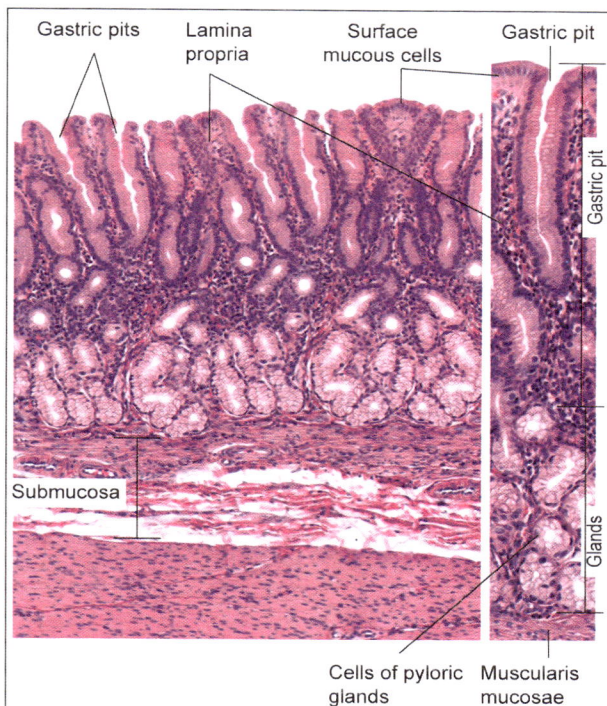

Fig. 17.15: Photomicrograph. Histology of pyloric part of stomach (low magnification on left, High magnification on right, H&E stain).

Muscularis Externa

- It has thicker circular smooth muscle coat that forms *pyloric sphincter*.^{Identification feature}

Serosa

- Stomach is covered by a connective tissue layer with mesothelial lining of visceral peritoneum.

The differences between histology of fundic (body) and pyloric region of stomach are listed in Table 17.1.

Clinical Correlation
• *Gastritis* is inflammation of lining epithelium of stomach. The most common symptoms of gastritis are upper abdominal discomfort (pain), heartburn, nausea, and vomiting.
• *Gastric ulcer* is a discontinuity of epithelial lining of stomach. These ulcers produce abdominal pain that improves with eating. Common causes of gastric ulcers are *Helicobacter pylori* bacterial infection, nonsteroidal antiinflammatory drugs, tobacco, smoking, and stress.
• *Pernicious anemia:* Failure of parietal cells to produce intrinsic factor results in deficiency of vitamin B_{12}. Intrinsic factor is essential for absorption of vitamin B_{12} in the small intestine. Deficiency of vitamin B_{12} produces pernicious anemia. Treatment: Injection of vitamin B_{12} (cobalamin).

Q. List the differences between histology of fundic (body) and pyloric part of stomach.^{Viva}

Table 17.1: Differences between histology of fundic (body) and pyloric region of stomach

Feature	Fundus or body of stomach	Pyloric region of stomach
Gastric pit	Shallow, occupy upper third thickness of mucosa	Deeper, occupy about two-third thickness of mucosa
Glands	Occupy lower 2/3rd thickness of mucosa	Occupy lower 1/3rd thickness of mucosa
– Coiling at base	Less coiled	More coiled
– Lumen	Narrow	Wider
– Cells	Parietal cells, chief cells, mucous neck cells	Mostly one type; Mucus-secreting cells (chief cells are absent)

Summary (Examination Guide)

- A section of stomach shows four layers: Mucosa, submucosa, muscularis externa, and serosa.
- *Mucosa:* It is lined by surface mucous cells. These are simple columnar cells with basal oval nuclei and secrete visible mucus.
- Mucosa shows gastric pits (openings of glands).
  - Fundus/body: Short gastric pits
  - Pylorus: Long gastric pits
- Glands: Branched tubular glands.
  - Cardiac: Cardiac glands shows mucus-secreting cells.
  - Fundus/body: Long gastric glands that show pink oxyntic cells (HCl, intrinsic factor), neck mucous cells (mucus), blue colored deeper chief cells (pepsinogen), enteroendocrine cells (histamine, gastrin).
  - Pylorus: Pyloric glands are short and mostly lined by mucus-secreting cells.
- *Muscularis mucosae* shows inner circular and outer longitudinal smooth muscles.
- Submucosa: It consists of dense irregular connective tissue and has blood vessels, nerve fibers, and Meissner's (submucosal) plexus.
- *Muscularis externa:* Randomly oriented smooth muscle cells: Inner oblique, middle circular, and outer longitudinal layers. In pylorus, thick circular fibers form pyloric sphincter.
- *Serosa:* Stomach is covered by a connective tissue layer with mesothelial lining of visceral peritoneum.

CHAPTER 18

Digestive System III: Small and Large Intestine

Chapter Outline

- Small intestine
  - General features
  - Cells of small intestine
  - Duodenum
  - Jejunum
  - Ileum
- Peyer's patches
- Large intestine
  - Colon
  - Vermiform appendix
  - Anal canal

Competency achievement: The student should be able to:

AN52.1 Describe and identify the microanatomical features of gastrointestinal system: Duodenum, jejunum, ileum, large intestine, appendix

SMALL INTESTINE

- Small intestine is a 6 m long mucomuscular tube.
- Small intestine has three parts:
  1. Duodenum: First 25 cm part that extends from stomach to duodenojejunal junction
  2. Jejunum: Middle 2.5 m long part
  3. Ileum: Distal 3.5 m long part that continues with large intestine at ileocecal junction

GENERAL FEATURES OF SMALL INTESTINE

- Small intestine is the site of digestion and absorption of nutrients.
- For sufficient digestion and absorption, small intestine has the following modification that increases surface area:
1. *Plicae circularis* (circular folds) or valves of Kerckring (Fig. 18.1)
   These are permanent circular folds that contain core of submucosa. These folds are predominantly seen in duodenum (except in first 5–6 cm) and jejunum. Plicae circularis are absent in terminal part of ileum. These folds decrease the speed of passage of intestinal contents and increase intestinal surface area.
2. *Villi* (Fig. 18.2)
   These are finger-like and leaf-like projections of lamina propria.

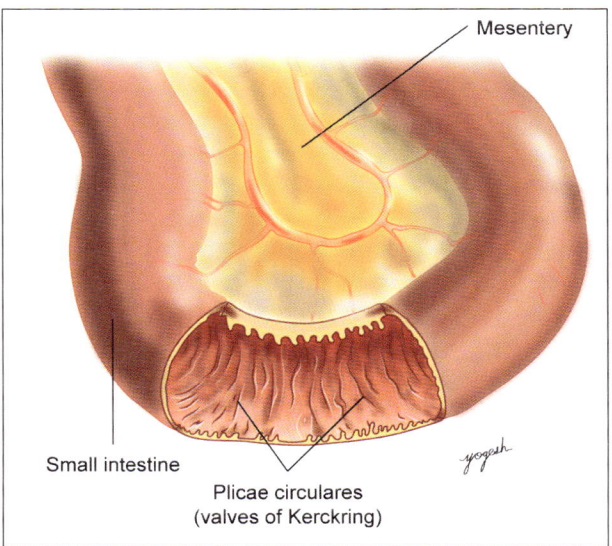

Fig. 18.1: Segment of small intestine showing plicae circulares.

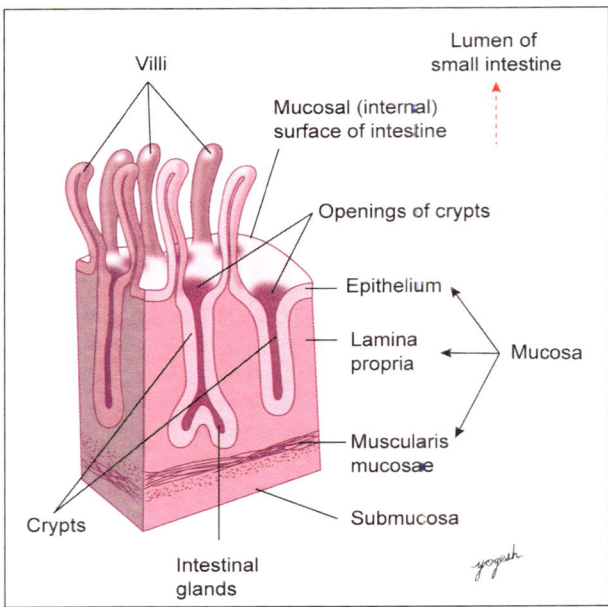

Fig. 18.2: Villi of small intestine.

Core of villus contains blood vessels and lacteal (lymphatic vessels).

Villi give a velvety appearance to intestinal surface on gross examination.

3. *Microvilli*

Epithelial lining of intestine shows numerous microvilli (striated border) along its luminal surface.

4. *Crypts of Lieberkühn*

These are simple tubular intestinal glands that extend in the lamina propria up to muscularis mucosa. These glands are lined by tall columnar epithelium that is continuous with epithelial lining of villi.

CELLS OF SMALL INTESTINE

- Intestine is lined by simple columnar epithelium. This lining epithelium consists of five types of cells: Enterocytes, goblet cells, Paneth cells, enteroendocrine cells and M cells (Fig. 18.3, Table 18.1).

Enterocytes/Absorptive Columnar Cells

- Enterocytes are the main absorptive cells of small intestine.
- These are tall columnar cells with basal oval nucleus.
- Apical (luminal) surface of these cells has a *striated border* formed by *regularly arranged microvilli.* ^{Viva}
- Each microvillus has a core of vertical microfilaments covered by plasma membrane. These vertical microfilaments insert on a network of terminal web (horizontally arranged microfilaments in apical part of the cell).
- Lateral surface of enterocyte shows flattened cytoplasmic processes that interdigitate with similar processes of adjacent cells.
- Luminal sides of adjacent enterocytes have tight junctions that establish a barrier between intestinal lumen and intercellular fluid.
- *Function:* Enterocyte absorbs nutrients and secretes enzymes required for terminal digestion.

Goblet Cells

- Goblet cells are unicellular glands that secrete mucus.
- Number of goblet cells increases gradually from duodenum toward terminal part of ileum.
- *Shape:* Goblet cell has a shape similar to a drinking glass–broad above and narrow stem toward basement membrane.

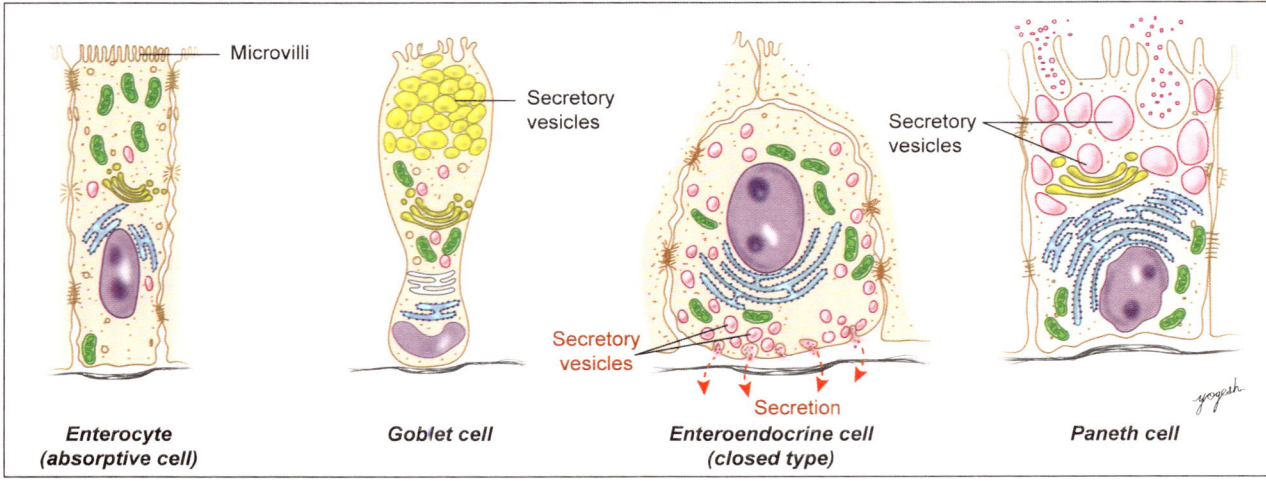

Fig 18.3: Cells of small intestine.

Q. List the cells of small intestine with their functions.

Table 18.1: Cells of small intestine^Viva

Cell	Identification	Function
Enterocyte	Tall columnar cell with basal oval nucleus and striated border	Absorption Secretion of terminal enzymes
Goblet cell	Vacuolated apical portion, basal-flat nucleus, glass-like cell, PAS – magenta color	Unicellular gland Mucus secretion
Paneth/Zymogen cell	Intensely acidophilic cytoplasm, oval basal nucleus, zymogen granules	Phagocytosis Secretion of lysozymes, α-defensins Maintenance of normal bacterial flora
Enteroendocrine cell	*Silver staining:* black color *Argentaffin cell*	Secretion of enkephalins, vasoactive inhibitory peptides
M cell	Present in epithelium overlying Peyer's patches	Antigen transporting cell Transfers intestinal bacterial antigens to lymphocyte, dendritic cells
Undifferentiated/stem cell	Columnar cell Short irregular microvilli	Divide to form other cells

- *H&E staining:* Apical portion of cell contains mucinogen granules. These granules are removed during H&E staining; hence, apical portion of goblet cells look empty. Nucleus is pushed toward base and becomes flattened.
- *Electron microscopy:* Cell shows wide apical and narrow basal portions. Cell shows abundant mucinogen granules in apical portion.
- *PAS staining:* Apical portion shows presence of bright magenta-colored mucinogen.

Paneth Cells (Zymogen Cells)^Neet

- Paneth cells are present in clusters at the bases of intestinal glands [Joseph Paneth, 1857–1890, Austrian physiologist].
- These cells have *intensely acidophilic* (pink/eosinophilic) refractile secretory vesicles/granules in apical portion (do not have foamy cytoplasm).^Neet
- Nucleus of Paneth cell is oval and basally placed.
- *Electron microscopy:* Apical portion shows supranuclear Golgi apparatus and small quantity of basal rough endoplasmic reticulum.
- *Functions:* Secretion of zymogen granules containing lysozymes, α-defensins, cryptidines, TNF-α, and zinc.^Neet
- *Note:* Lysozyme and α-defensins help Paneth cells to *control normal bacterial flora of small intestine* and thereby maintain innate immunity of crypts. Paneth cell can phagocytose bacteria.
- *Lifespan:* 30 days.
- *Special stains:* Phloxine–tartrazine gives a red color to Paneth cells.
- *Special character:* Paneth cells migrate toward base of intestinal crypts rather than migrating toward tip of villi.^Neet

Enteroendocrine/Argentaffin Cells

- These are few cells present among epithelium of intestine.
- These cells produce different peptide hormones such as enkephalins, vasoactive inhibitory peptide (VIP).
- *Silver staining:* These cells can be stained by silver salts; hence, called *argentaffin cells*.
- There are two types of enteroendocrine cells:^Neet
  - Closed type: These cells do not reach lumen of gland/crypt. These cell lies between basal lamina and other intestinal cells.
  - Open type: These cells reach lumen of gland. These cells secrete CCK, secretin, GIP, motilin, and gastrin hormones.

M Cells

- These are epithelium cells that overlie Peyer's patches and other intestinal lymphatic follicles.^Viva
- *Shape:* M-cell has deep pocket-like recess (space) that accommodate lymphocytes, macrophages, and dendritic cells.
- M-cell has few microfolds on its apical surface (no microvilli).
- M-cells have protein receptors that catch bacteria and transfer bacterial proteins to macrophages that reside in cell recesses.
- Thus, M-cell acts as *antigen-transporting cell*.^Neet, Viva

Intermediate Cells (Undifferentiated Cells)

- These cells behave similar to stem cells and give rise to other intestinal epithelial cells.
- Intestinal stem cells are present in lower half of intestinal gland or crypts of Lieberkühn.[Neet]
- These cells cannot be differentiated with *H&E staining*. These are columnar cells with short, irregular microvilli and some apical cytoplasm.

DUODENUM

Q. Write a short not on histology of duodenum.

- Duodenum is proximal part of small intestine.
- Length: 25 cm (10 inches).
- It receives food material from stomach. This material is highly acidic.
- Duodenum also receives secretions of liver (bile) and pancreas (pancreatic juice) in the second part through common bile duct and accessory pancreatic ducts. Pancreatic juice is alkaline and neutralizes acidic content of stomach in duodenum.
- Initial 2.5 cm of duodenum lies in peritoneum while rest of the duodenum is retroperitoneal.

Histology of Duodenum

- Wall of duodenum consists of four layers: Mucosa, submucosa, muscularis externa, and serosa or adventitia (Figs 18.4, 18.5 and Flowchart 18.1).

Mucosa

- Duodenum shows
  - *Plicae circularis:* These are permanent circular folds having a core of submucosa
  - *Villi:* These are finger-like mucosal projection having a core of lamina propria. Villi contain fenestrated capillaries, blind-end lacteals (lymphatics), and smooth muscle cells.
- *Epithelium:* Villi are lined by *simple columnar epithelium* with few goblet cells.
- *Microvilli:* Luminal surface of columnar epithelial cells shows striated border due to regularly placed microvilli.

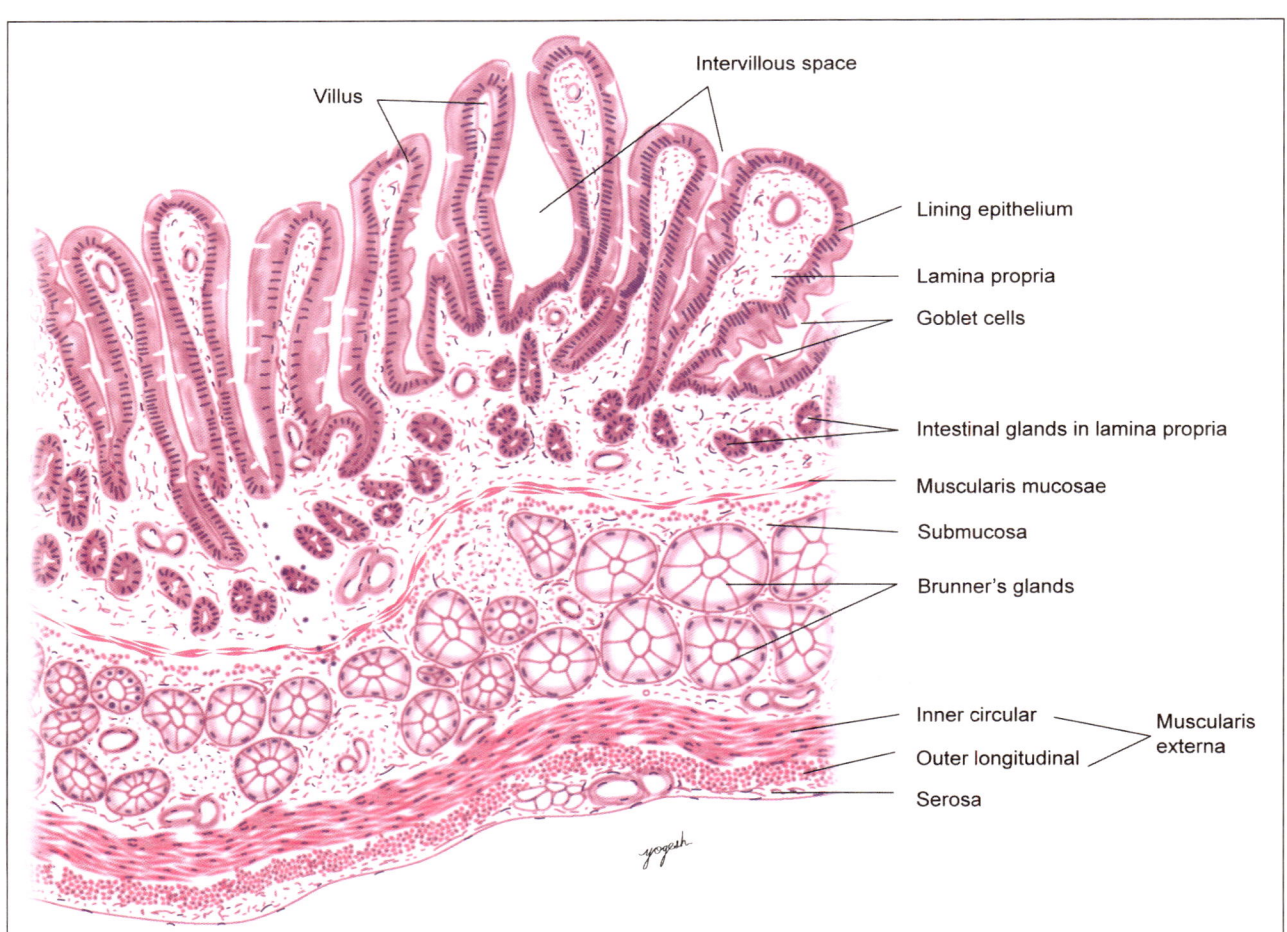

Fig. 18.4: Histology of duodenum. Low magnification (practice figure).

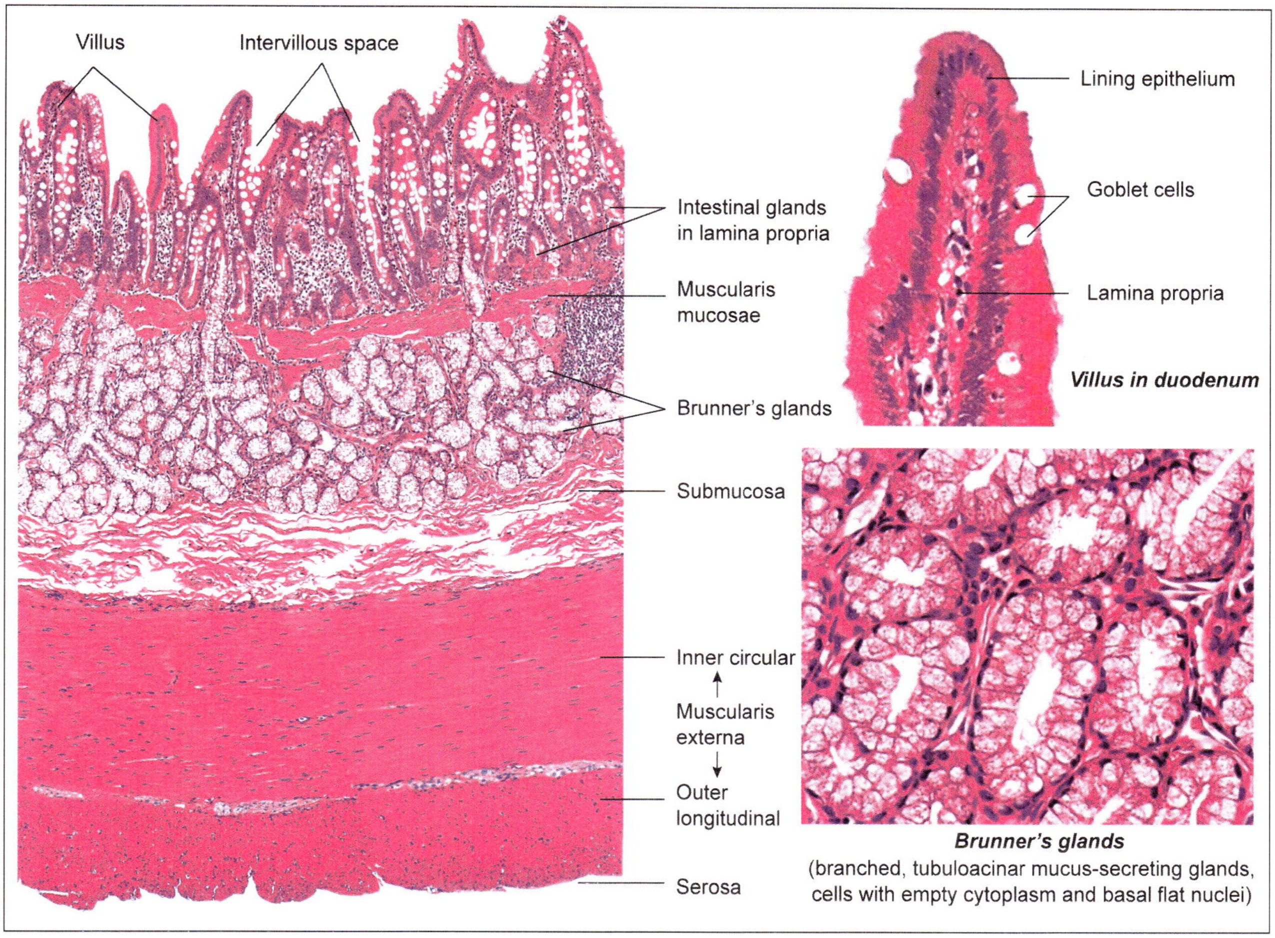

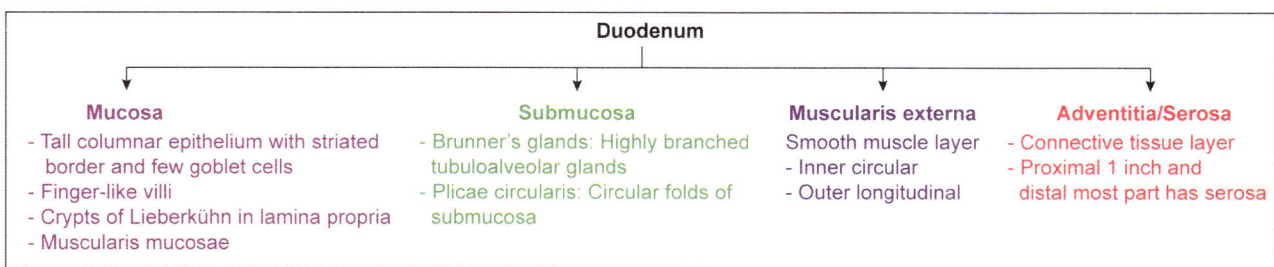

Fig. 18.5: Photomicrograph. Histology of duodenum (low magnification on left, high magnification of villus and Brunner's glands on right).

Flowchart 18.1: Histology of duodenum

```
                              Duodenum
        ┌─────────────┬──────────────┬────────────────┬──────────────┐
      Mucosa        Submucosa    Muscularis externa   Adventitia/Serosa
```

Mucosa	Submucosa	Muscularis externa	Adventitia/Serosa
- Tall columnar epithelium with striated border and few goblet cells - Finger-like villi - Crypts of Lieberkühn in lamina propria - Muscularis mucosae	- Brunner's glands: Highly branched tubuloalveolar glands - Plicae circularis: Circular folds of submucosa	Smooth muscle layer - Inner circular - Outer longitudinal	- Connective tissue layer - Proximal 1 inch and distal most part has serosa

- *Intestinal glands/crypts of Lieberkühn:* These are short tubular glands formed by invagination of bases of crypts in lamina propria. These glands are lined by columnar cells, goblet cells, Paneth cells, and enteroendocrine cells.
- *Muscularis mucosa* has inner circular and outer longitudinal layers of smooth muscle cells.
- Some smooth muscle fibers of muscularis mucosa enter the core of villi.

Submucosa

- *Brunner's glands:* These are highly branched, tubuleoacinar mucus-secreting glands in submucosa of duodenum. *Identification features, Viva, Neet*
- Ducts of these glands pass through muscularis mucosa and open into bases of villi.
- Brunner's glands (duodenal glands) have acini lined by simple cuboidal or low columnar pyramidal cells. These cells have an empty cytoplasm and basal flat nucleus (typical mucous cell). *Viva*

- *Function:* Secretion of mucus that protects duodenum from acidic content of stomach. Secretion of human epidermal growth factor that increases cell division of epidermal cells and inhibits secretion of HCl.
- Brunner's glands occupy most of the submucosa.

Muscle Layer

- It has inner circular and outer longitudinal smooth muscle coats.

Serosa/Adventitia

- Most of the duodenum is covered by connective tissue (adventitia) except a small part is covered by peritoneum (serosa).

> **Summary (Examination Guide)** (Fig. 18.4)
> - Duodenum has four layers: Mucosa, submucosa, muscularis externa, and serosa/adventitia.
> - Duodenum shows finger-like villi lined by simple columnar epithelium and few goblet cells. Epithelium cells show striated border because of microvilli.
> - Crypts of Lieberkühn/intestinal glands are present in lamina propria above muscularis mucosa.
> - Brunner's glands are highly branched, tubuloalveolar mucous glands that are located in submucosa. *Identification features*
> - Brunner's glands are present deep to muscularis mucosa.
> - Submucosal folds are circular folds called plicae circularis.
> - Muscularis externa has inner circular and outer longitudinal smooth muscle layers.
> - Most of the duodenum is covered by adventitia except a small portion is covered by peritoneum (serosa).

JEJUNUM

Q. Write a short note on histology of jejunum.

- Jejunum is the middle part of small intestine that lies between duodenum and ileum.
- Length: ~2.5 m.
- Wall of jejunum has four layers: Mucosa, submucosa, muscularis externa, and serosa (Figs 18.6, 18.7 and Flowchart 18.2).

Mucosa

- Mucosa of jejunum shows
  - *Plicae circularis:* These are permanent circular folds having a core of submucosae.
  - *Villi:* Villi in jejunum are tongue-shaped. These are mucosal projection having a core of lamina propria. *Identification feature*
- Epithelial lining, microvilli, intestinal glands, and muscularis mucosa: same description as that in duodenum.

Submucosa

- Submucosa of jejunum consists of connective tissue blood vessels, Meissner's plexus, and lymphatics.
- Note: Brunner's glands and Peyer's patches are absent. *Identification feature, Viva*

Muscularis Externa

- It has inner circular and outer longitudinal smooth muscle coats.

Serosa/Adventitia

- Jejunum is covered by a layer of peritoneum (serosa).

ILEUM

- Ileum is distal part of small intestine.
- It opens in cecum at ileocecal junction.
- Length: 3.5 m.
- Wall of ileum has four layers: Mucosa, submucosa, muscularis externa, and serosa (Figs 18.8 and 18.9).

Mucosa

Ileum shows

- *Plicae circularis:* These are permanent circular folds having core of submucosa. These are spares in ileum and even absent in terminal part of ileum.

Flowchart 18.2: Histology of jejunum

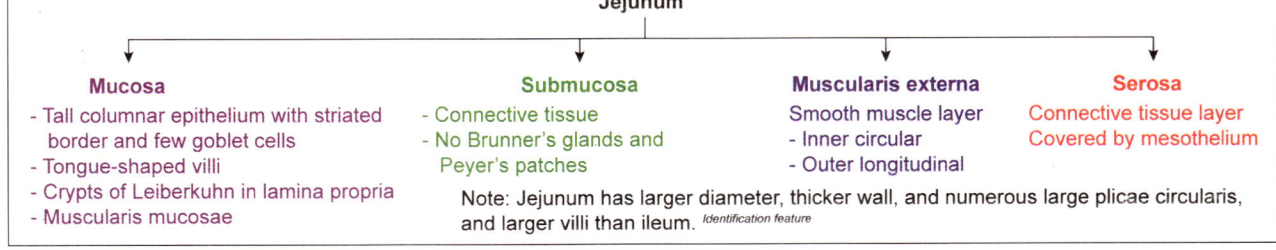

Digestive System III: Small and Large Intestine

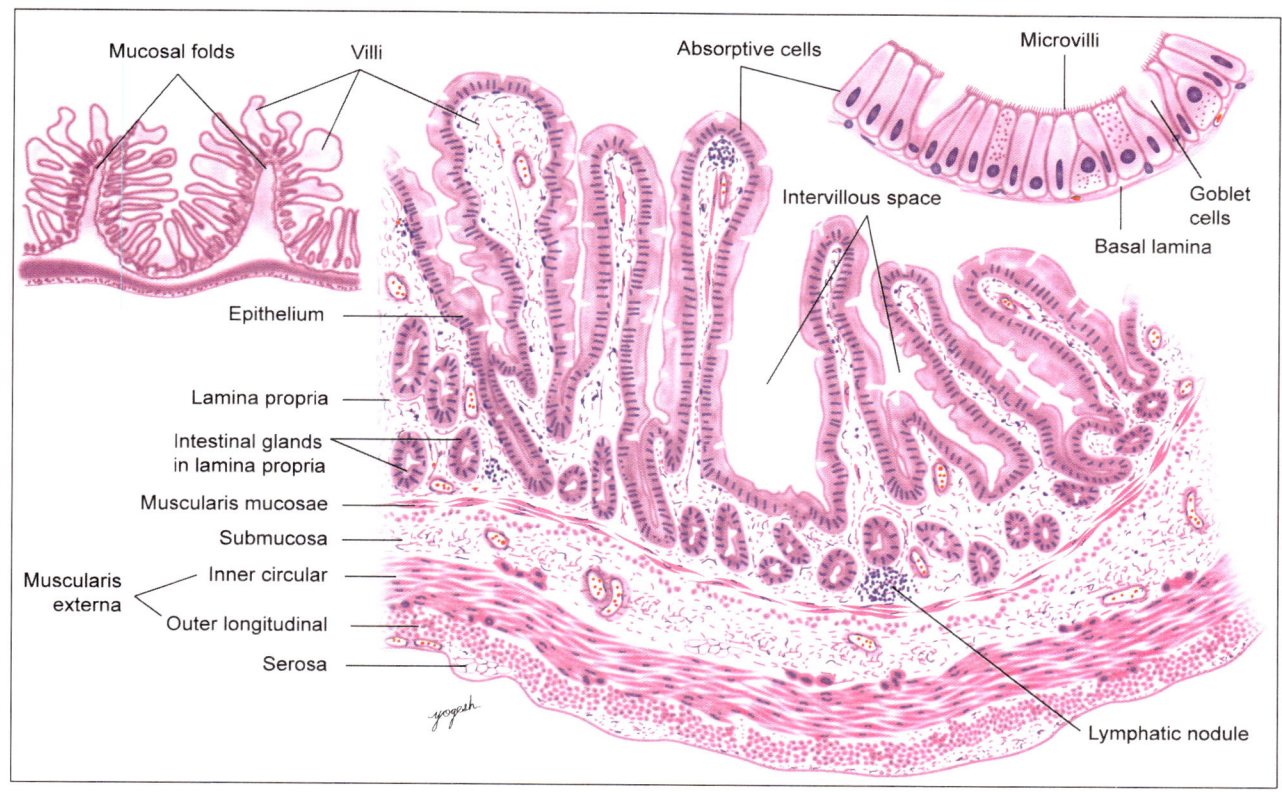

Fig. 18.6: Histology of jejunum (typical features of small intestine). Low magnification (practice figure).

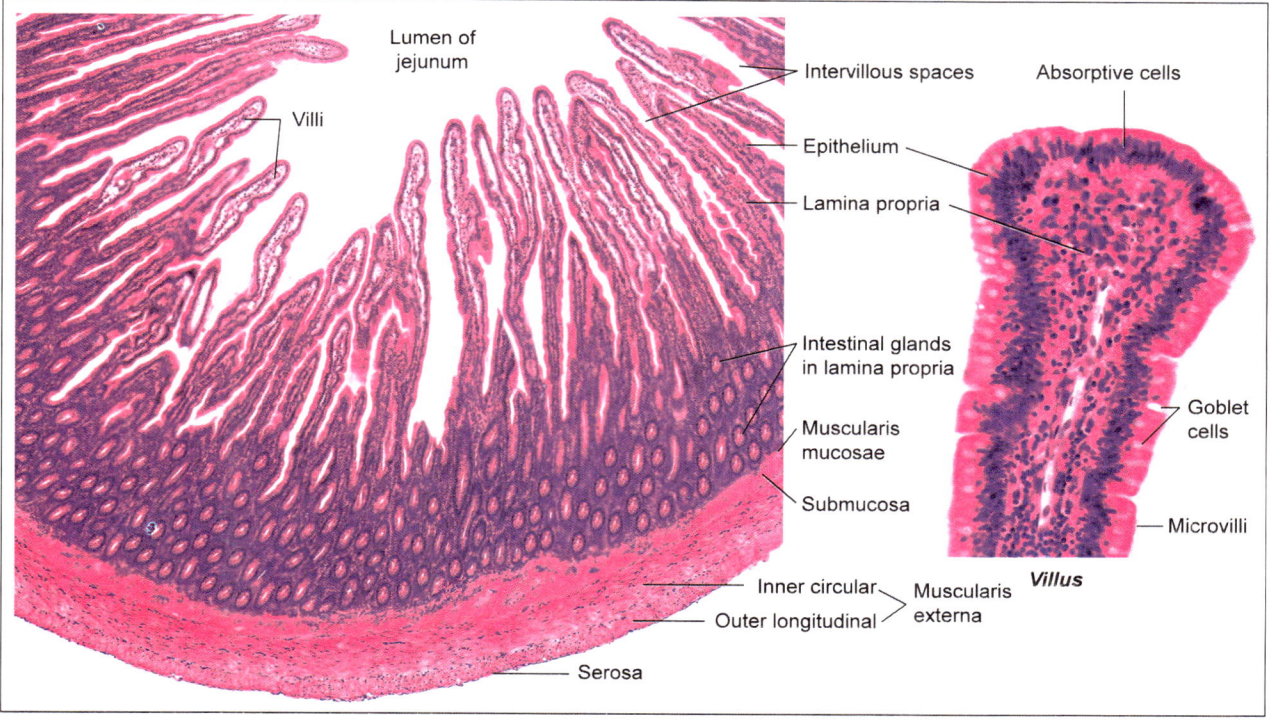

Fig. 18.7: Photomicrograph. Histology of jejunum (low magnification on left and villus at high magnification on right).

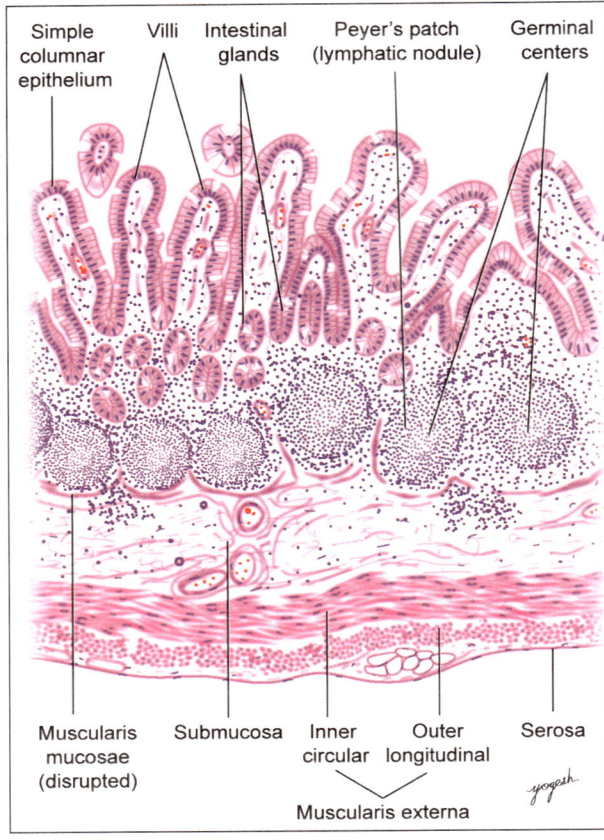

Fig. 18.8: Histology of ileum (practice figure).

- *Villi:* Only few, short, finger-like villi (mucosal projections with a core of lamina propria) are present.
- *Lining epithelium:* Simple columnar epithelium with striated border (microvilli) and goblet cells.
- *Lamina propria:* Lamina propria contains intestinal glands and Peyer's patches.*Neet, Identification feature*
- *Muscularis mucosa* is thin and even absent at the site of large Peyer's patches.

Submucosa, Muscularis Externa, Serosa

- Few authors mentioned that Peyer's patches are present in submucosa. But histologically Peyer's patches are present in lamina propria and may extend into submucosa.*Neet*

Some Interesting Facts

In ileum,
- Villi are thin, slender, finger-like.
- Lamina propria shows presence of lymphatic follicles.
- M cells are present in epithelium that overlie Peyer's patches.

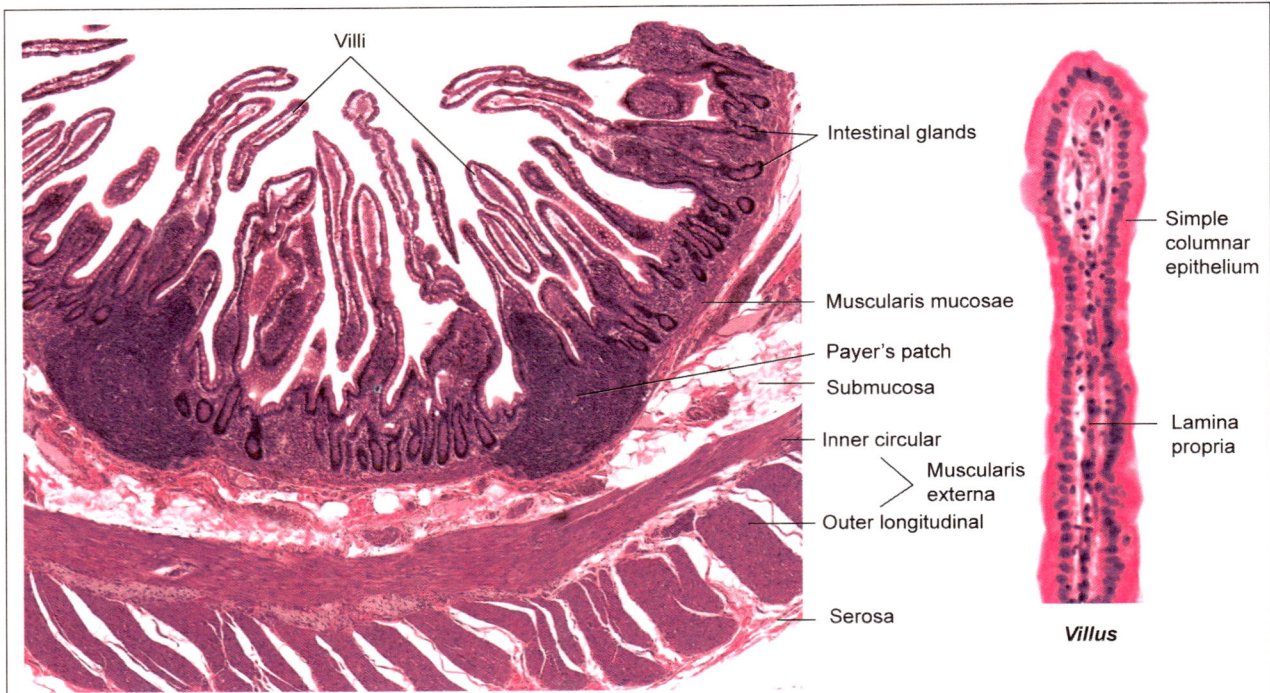

Fig. 18.9: Photomicrograph. Histology of ileum (low magnification on left, villus at high magnification on right, *H&E* stain).

> **Box 18.1:** Peyer's patches
>
> **Q. Write a short note on Peyer's patches.**
> - Peyer's patches are organized lymphatic nodules in lamina propria of terminal part of ileum.
> - These are elongated thickening of intestinal mucosa (few centimeters in length).
> - Number: About 100 Peyer's patches are present in ileum.
> - Peyer's patches are aggregation of lymphatic follicles.
> - At many places, Peyer's patches cross muscularis mucosa and extend into submucosa.
> - Peyer's patches form a part of gut-associated lymphatic tissue (GALT).
> - Peyer's patches are found in antimesenteric border of ileum.
> - *M-cell:* These are columnar epithelial cells that overlie Peyer's patches. These cells have recesses to accommodate lymphocytes and macrophages. M-cell presents bacterial antigens to immune cells.
> - *Function:* Peyer's patches help to maintain normal bacterial intestinal flora and prevent infections.

LARGE INTESTINE

- Large intestine consists of cecum, vermiform appendix, colon (ascending, transverse, descending, and sigmoid), rectum and anal canal.
- Gross anatomically, large intestine shows three cardinal features (Fig. 18.10):*Viva*
  1. *Taenia coli:* These are three narrow thickened bands longitudinal smooth muscle fibers of muscularis externa. Taenia are absent in appendix, rectum, and anal canal.*Viva*
  2. *Haustrations:* These are dilatations (sacculations) of colon.
  3. *Appendices epiploicae* (omental appendices): These are small pockets of fat on outer surface of large intestine.

COLON

- A section of colon shows four layers: Mucosa, submucosa, muscularis externa, and serosa (Figs 18.11 to 18.13 and Flowchart 18.3).

Mucosa

- Mucosa consists of lining epithelium, lamina propria, and muscularis mucosa.
- *Epithelium:* Colon is lined by *simple columnar epithelium* and number of *goblet cells.* Epithelial cells show microvilli (striated border) on absorptive cells.*Identification feature*
- In large intestine (colon), plicae circularis (mucosal folds) and villi are absent.*Identification feature* Hence, mucosa of large intestine has smooth surface.
- *Glands:* Lamina propria is occupied by short *simple tubular intestinal glands* or crypts of Lieberkühn.*Identification feature* These glands are lined with simple columnar cells and may goblet cells.

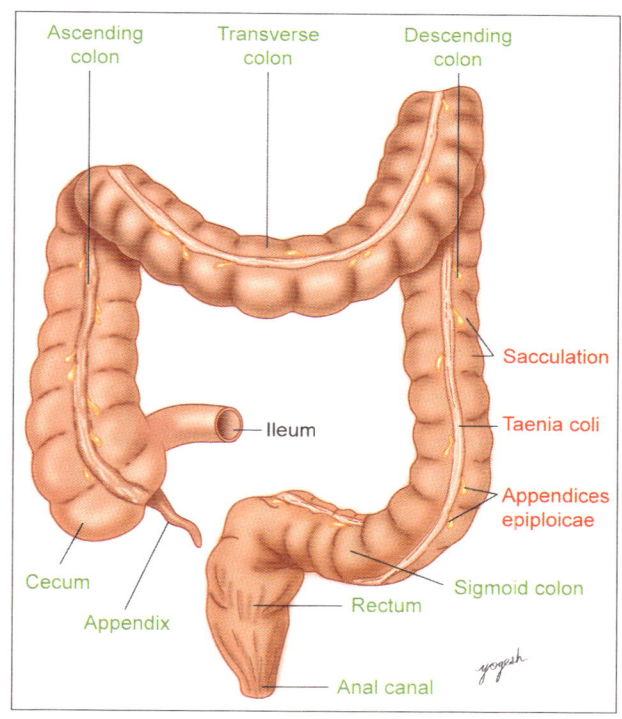

Fig. 18.10: Parts of large intestine and its features.

- Note: Paneth cells are absent in large intestine.*Neet*
- Some *caveolated tuft cells* are present in colon.
- *Stem cells* are located at the bottom of gland.
- Surface epithelial cells and goblet cells have a lifespan of 5–6 days.*MCQ*
- Lifespan of enteroendocrine cells is 4 weeks.*MCQ*
- Large intestine performs absorption of water and electrolytes and production of mucin that lubricates its contents.

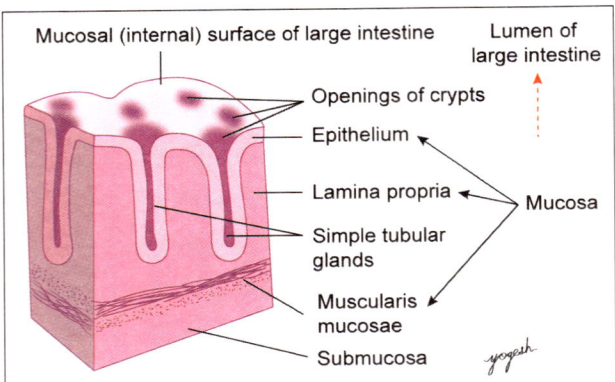

Fig. 18.11: Location of simple tubular glands in lamina propria of large intestine.

- Lamina propria shows collagen table (thick collagen fibers) between basal lamina and epithelium. Collagen table regulates transport of water and electrolytes.
- *New concept:* There is pericryptal fibroblast sheath in lamina propria of colon. These fibroblasts replicate and migrate toward luminal surface and may differentiate to form macrophages.
- Lamina propria shows discrete lymphatic nodules that are regularly spaced.

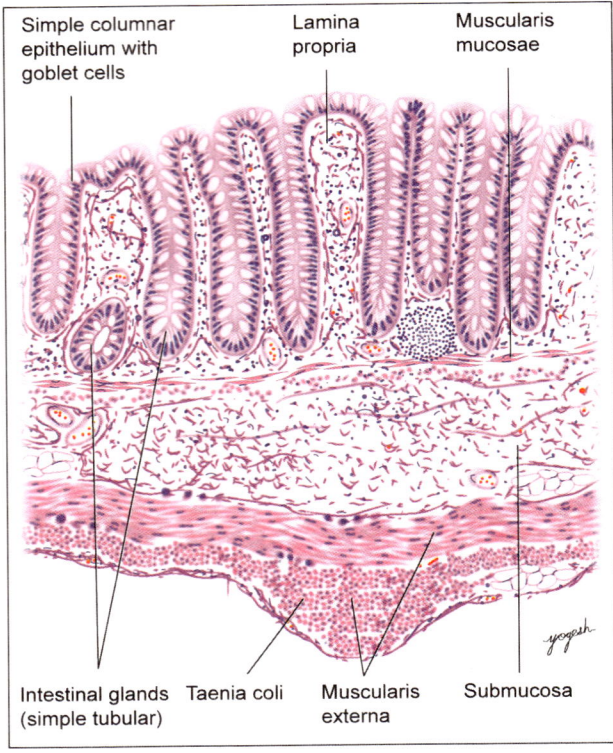

Fig. 18.12: Histology of large intestine (practice figure).

Flowchart 18.3: Histology of colon

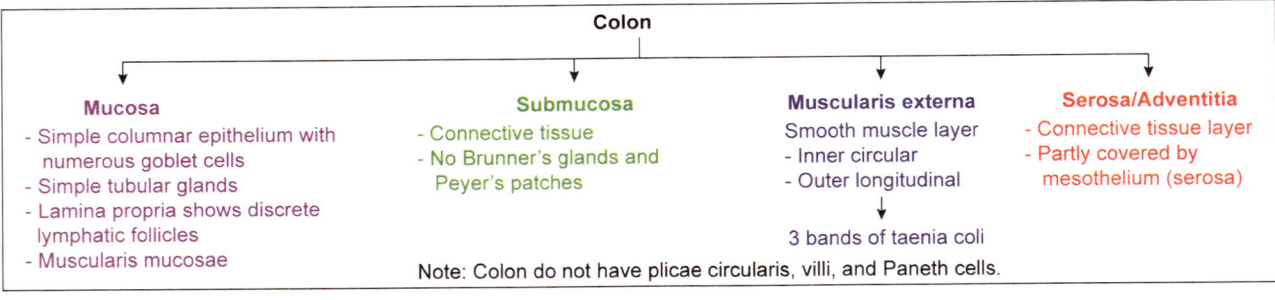

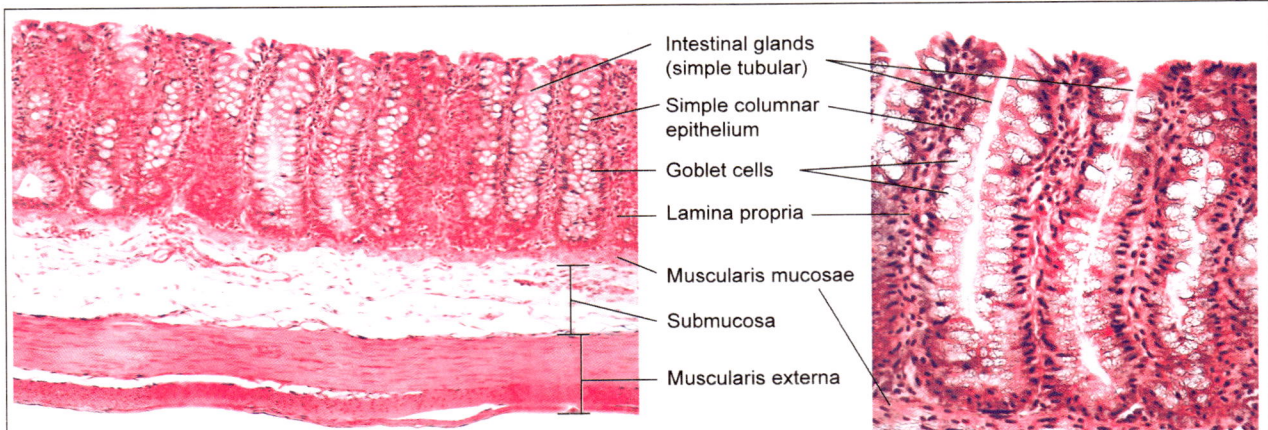

Fig. 18.13: Photomicrograph. Histology of colon/large intestine (low magnification on left, mucosa at high magnification on right, *H&E* staining).

- *New concept:* Lamina propria of large intestine shows presence of occasional lymphatics. (*Previous concept*: Large intestine do not have lymphatics in lamina propria).^Neet

Submucosa
- Submucosa consists of dense irregular connective tissue.

Muscularis Externa
- It consists of thin inner circular and outer longitudinal smooth muscle fibers.
- Longitudinal fibers form three thick bundles as tenia coli (even visible on gross examination).
- Because of shorter length of tenia coli than other layers, large intestine shows sacculations.

Serosa
- Colon is covered by connective tissue and peritoneum except at its retroperitoneal parts.
- Colon shows presence of pockets of fat called appendices epiploicae that are covered by peritoneum (mesothelium/simple squamous epithelium).

Summary (Examination Guide)
- Colon shows four layers: Mucosa, submucosa, muscularis externa, and serosa.
- *Mucosa* is lined by simple columnar absorptive cells with microvilli and goblet cells.
- *Lamina propria* is filled with intestinal glands (crypts of Lieberkühn). These glands are lined by number of goblet cells. Lamina propria shows discrete lymphatic follicles.
- *Submucosa* consists of dense irregular connective tissue.
- *Muscularis externa* has inner circular and outer longitudinal fibers. Longitudinal fibers form three bands of taenia coli.
- Externally colon is covered by *serosa/adventitia*.
- Colon does not have plicae cirularis, villi, and Paneth cells.

VERMIFORM APPENDIX

Q. Write a short note on histology of vermiform appendix.

- Appendix is a blind-ended tubular appendage extending from cecum.
- It is the narrowest part of intestine.
- Histologically, appendix shows four layers of gut: Mucosa, submucosa, muscularis externa, and serosa (Figs 18.14, 18.15 and Flowchart 18.4).

Mucosa
- Mucosa is lined by *simple columnar epithelium* with microvilli, *goblet cells*, and M cells.^Identification feature
- *Lamina propria* contains short *tubular intestinal glands* lined by simple squamous epithelium with goblet cells.
- Lamina propria is mostly occupied by large and small lymphatic follicles that even may cross muscularis mucosa and extend into submucosa.^Identification feature

Submucosa
- It consists of connective tissue.
- Many lymphatic follicles extend from lamina propria to submucosa.^Identification feature

Muscularis Externa
- It consists of inner circular and outer longitudinal muscle coat. Note: Though appendix is a part of large intestine, it does not have taenia coli.^Identification feature

Serosa
- Appendix is entirely covered by peritoneum (serosa).

Some Interesting Facts
- Because of enlarged follicles, lumen of appendix may be star-shaped or even obliterated.
- In adults, appendix may become fibrosed.
- Appendicitis is inflammation of appendix.
- Carcinoid is a tumor of enteroendocrine cells. Appendix is a common site for carcinoid.

Flowchart 18.4: Histology of appendix

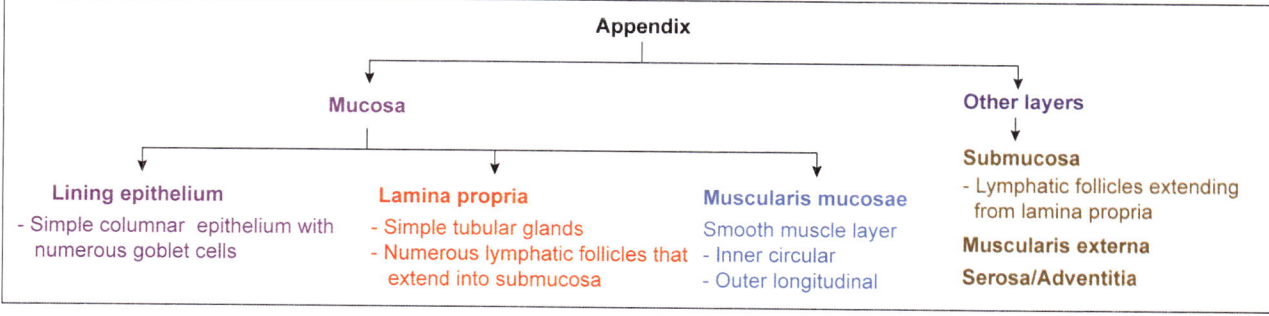

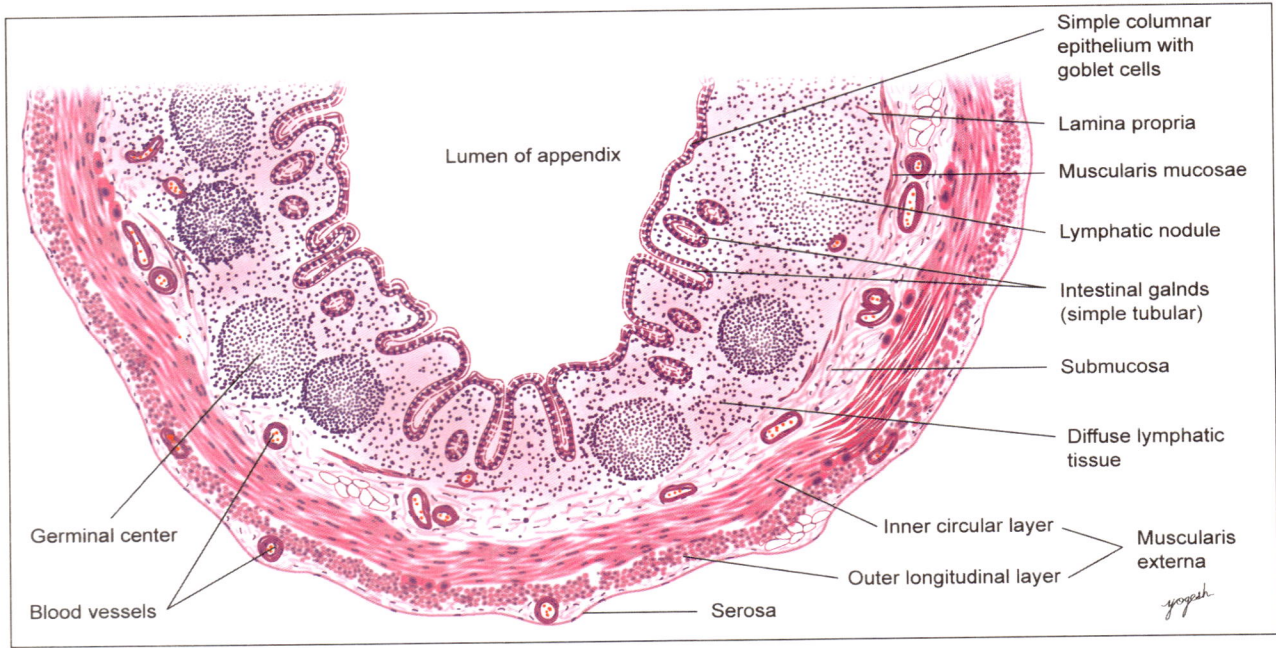

Fig. 18.14: Histology of appendix (practice figure).

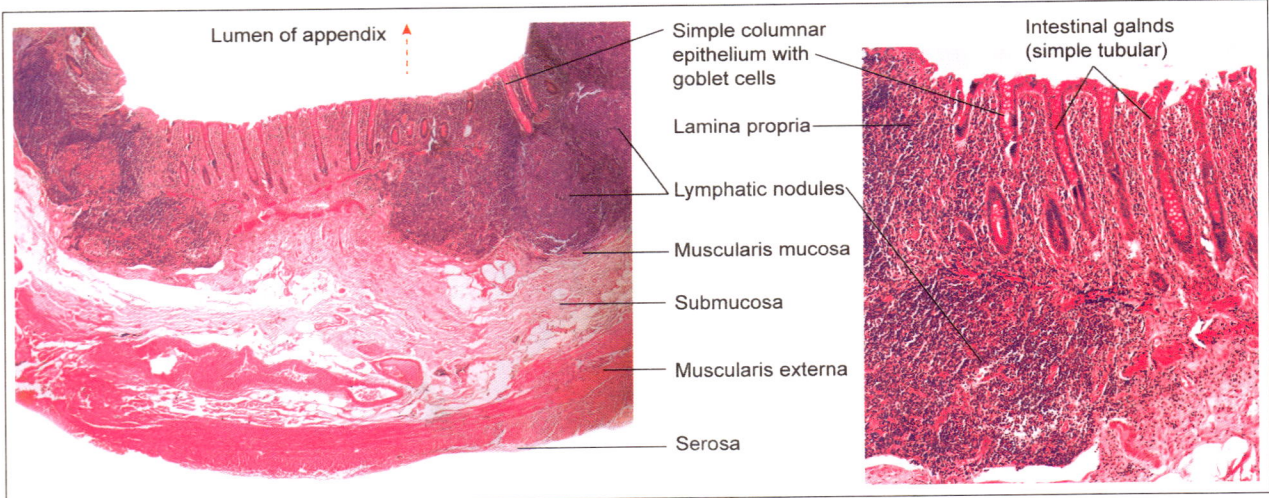

Fig. 18.15: Photomicrograph. Histology of appendix (low magnification on left, high magnification on right, H&E stain).

ANAL CANAL

- Anal canal is the terminal part of intestine.
- Length: 4 cm.
- Anal canal shows four layers: Mucosa, submucosa, muscularis externa, and adventitia (Fig. 18.16, Flowchart 18.5).

Mucosa

- Epithelial lining of anal canal shows transition from simple columnar epithelium to stratified squamous epithelium as follows:
  - Upper one-third of anal canal: Simple columnar epithelium.
  - Middle one-third of anal canal: Nonkeratinized stratified squamous epithelium.
  - Lower one-third of anal canal (below pectinate line): Keratinized stratified squamous epithelium (skin). *Neet*
- Mucus membrane of upper third show 6–12 longitudinal folds called *anal columns of Morgagni*. It also shows a few *short intestinal glands* [Giovanni Battista Morgagni, 1682–1771, Italian anatomist].

Digestive System III: Small and Large Intestine

Flowchart 18.5: Histology of anal canal

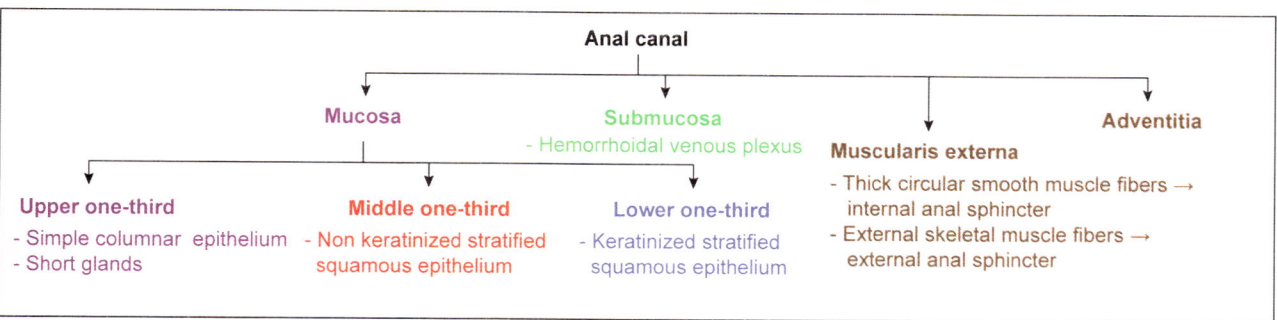

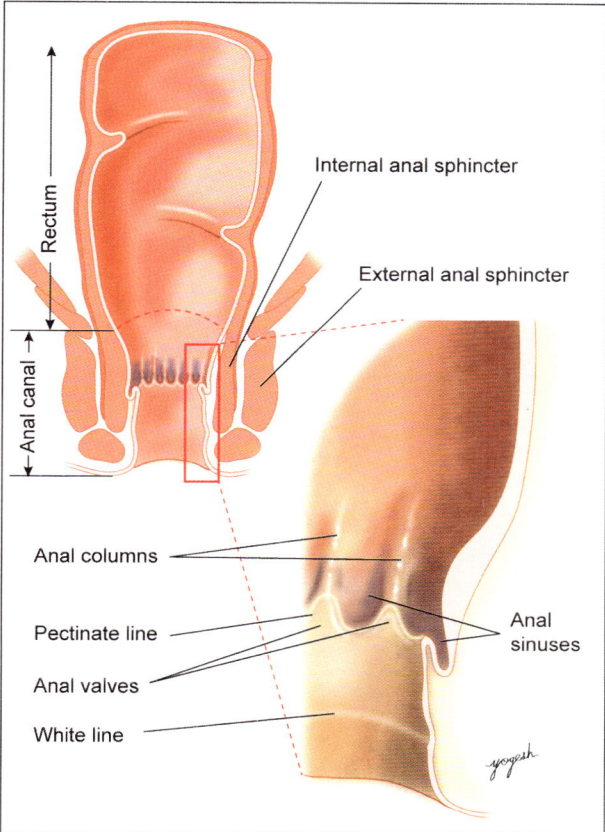

Fig. 18.16: Internal features of lower part of rectum and anal canal (coronal section).

- At the junction of upper and middle third of anal canal, anal columns fuse to form transverse folds called *anal valves*, along a line called pectinate line.
- Middle third of anal canal has bluish appearance due to presence of deeper dense venous plexus.
- Junction of middle and lower third is represented by a *white line of Hilton*. [John Hilton, 1805-1878, British surgeon].

- Above anal valves, there are depressions called *anal sinuses*. Apocrine sweat glands (circumanal glands) open into each sinus.

Submucosa

- Submucosa contains numerous venous plexuses called *hemorrhoidal plexuses* (internal hemorrhoidal plexus above pectinate line and external hemorrhoidal plexus below pectinate line).

Muscularis Externa

- Anal canal has inner circular and outer longitudinal smooth muscle fibers.
- Thick circular smooth muscle layer forms *internal anal sphincter*.
- Outside muscularis externa, a layer of skeletal muscle fibers is present. These fibers form *external anal sphincter*.

Adventitia

- Anal canal is surrounded by a connective tissue coat of adventitia.

Clinical Correlation

- *Fistulas:* These are false communications between anal canal and skin of perianal region.
- *Internal hemorrhoids:* This is enlargement and dilatation of hemorrhoidal veins. As submucosa in middle third of anal canal shows portacaval anastomosis, in portal hypertension, internal hemorrhoids are seen.
- *External hemorrhoids* are present in lower third of anal canal and covered by skin.
- *Adenocarcinoma of colon* is the second most common cancer of humans. Adenocarcinoma is a malignant (spreading) tumor of intestinal glands.

- *Ulcerative colitis* is an inflammation and ulceration of rectum and colon; it produces damage to mucosa and submucosa and causes bloody diarrhea.
- *Typhoid ulcer:* It is caused by infection of Salmonella typhi bacteria. It involves ileum. It causes swelling of lymphoid tissue and ulceration of mucosa covering these lymphoid tissues.
- *Celiac disease:* It is a gluten-sensitive enteropathy caused by gluten proteins of wheat. It involves damage to villi that results in malabsorption.

Some Interesting Facts

- Rectum: Histologically rectum is similar to that of colon except for the following:
  - Taenia coli are absent in rectum.
  - Appendices epiploicae are absent in rectum.
  - Only front and side of upper third and front of middle third of the rectum is covered by peritoneum (serosa), whereas rest is covered by adventitia.

CHAPTER 19

Liver, Gallbladder and Pancreas

Chapter Outline
- Liver
- Gallbladder
- Pancreas

Competency achievement: The student should be able to:
AN52.1 Describe and identify the microanatomical features of gastrointestinal system: Liver, gallbladder, pancreas

LIVER
- Liver is the largest gland of body (weight about 1,500 g).
- It is a modified exocrine gland with many other functions.

Gross Organization of Liver
- Liver is supplied by hepatic artery (oxygenated blood) and portal vein (blood from gut).
- Liver is drained by hepatic veins into the inferior vena cava.
- Secretions of liver (*bile*) are carried by bile canaliculi to extrahepatic biliary apparatus.
- Anatomically, liver is divided into right, left, quadrate, and quadrate lobes.
- Functional segmentation of liver corresponds to blood supply and bile drainage. It is surgically and clinically more important.

Structural Organization of Liver
- Liver shows the following functional components:
  - Capsule and connective tissue stroma
  - Parenchyma (hepatocytes)
  - Sinusoids and other blood vessels
  - Perisinusoidal space of Disse
  - Bile canaliculi

Connective Tissue Capsule
- Liver is enclosed by a connective tissue capsule (*Glisson's capsule*). [Francis Glisson, 1597–1677, British physician, anatomist].
- Connective tissue extends in the parenchyma of liver along with branches of portal veins (along with hepatic artery and bile canaliculi).
- *Reticular fibers* (type III collagen fibers): Finer reticular fibers form a network (reticulum) in liver to support liver parenchyma. Reticular fibers are *argentophilic* fibers because they can be stained with *silver* impregnation method (become black on silver staining).*Neet*

Hepatocytes (Liver Cells)
- Liver parenchyma consists of *liver cells* or *hepatocytes*.
- These are *large, polygonal cells* (20–30 μm size).*Visu*
- Nuclei: Hepatocytes show large, spherical nuclei that are present at the center of cells. Nuclei show huge *euchromatin* (open-phase nuclei) as these cells are metabolically active (synthesize proteins).
- Nuclei show 1–2 nucleoli. Many hepatocytes are *binucleated* (contains 4n amount of DNA).*Neet, Visu*
- Lifespan: 5 months.
- *Regeneration capability:* Liver has capability of regeneration after loss of liver tissue.
- Cytoplasm: Cytoplasm is slightly *acidophilic* (eosinophilic)
- Special stains:
  - Large number of mitochondria can be demonstrated by *vital staining.*
  - PAS staining for *glycogen* deposits.
  - Sudan staining for lipid droplets.
  - H&E staining/PAS staining for *brown lipofuscin pigment* within lysosomes.

Surfaces of Liver Cells

Liver cells show the following surfaces (Fig 19.1):

1. *Sinusoidal surface* faces adjoining sinusoids. This surface of hepatocyte shows microvilli that project into the *space of Disse*. Microvilli increase surface area of cells for transport of nutrients across hepatocytes.
2. *Canalicular surface* that forms wall of bile canaliculus (0.5 μm diameter) along with adjacent hepatocytes. *Bile canaliculi* are separated from remaining intercellular spaces by tight junctions.
3. *Intercellular surface* that face toward adjacent hepatocytes.

Blood Vessels of Liver

- Liver has dual blood supply through *hepatic portal vein* (75%) and *hepatic artery* (25%) (Flowchart 19.1).^{Viva}
- Portal veins carry the nutrients and toxic materials absorbed from the intestine, blood from spleen and pancreas.
- Liver produces bile that is drained by bile canaliculi → hepatic ducts and finally enter the extrahepatic biliary apparatus.
- *Portal triad:* In liver, a branch of *hepatic artery, portal vein*, and *bile ductule* run together in the form of portal triad.^{MCQ} Note: Central vein or hepatic vein do not form a part of portal triad (Fig. 19.2).^{Neet}
- The blood from the portal vein and hepatic artery enter into *hepatic sinusoids* (Figs 19.3 and 19.4).
- Hepatic sinusoids drain into central vein → sublobular vein → hepatic vein and finally into the inferior vena cava.
- *Note:* Hepatic veins do not have valves.^{Viva}

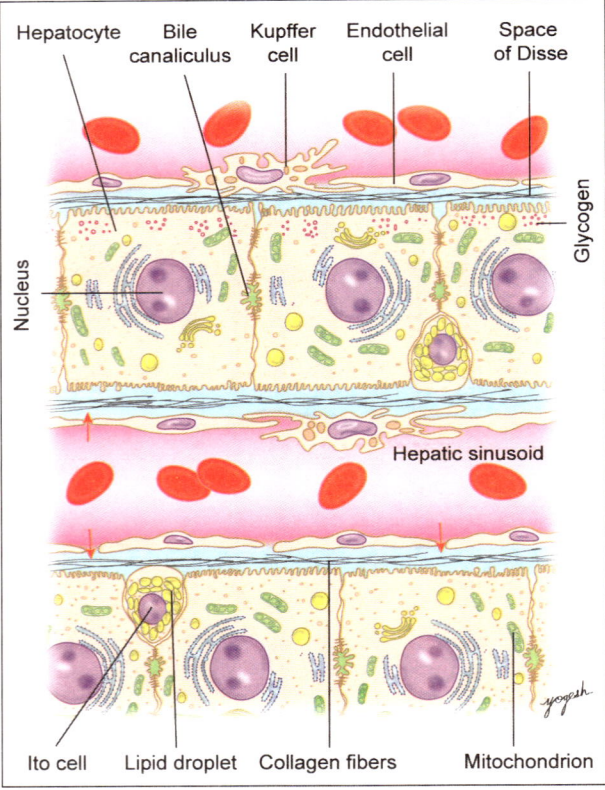

Fig. 19.1: Surfaces of hepatocytes, space of Disse, and Kupffer cell. Fenestrations are shown with red arrows.

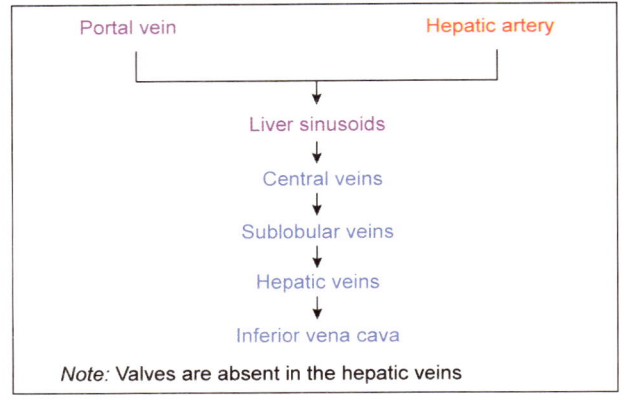

Flowchart 19.1: Blood supply of liver

Note: Valves are absent in the hepatic veins

Box 19.1: Concept of liver lobules

Q. Write a short note on liver lobules.

Q. Write a short note on classical hepatic lobule.

- The structural organization of liver form liver lobules.
- For descriptive purposes, researchers have described three different forms of liver lobules such as classical lobule, portal lobule, and liver acinus (Fig. 19.5, Flowchart 19.2).^{Viva}

Classical liver lobule

- It is a *hexagonal* mass with central vein (terminal hepatic venule) in the center and surrounded by *radiating anastomosing plates or cords of hepatocytes.*^{Neet}
- Adjacent plates of hepatocytes are separated by sinusoids.

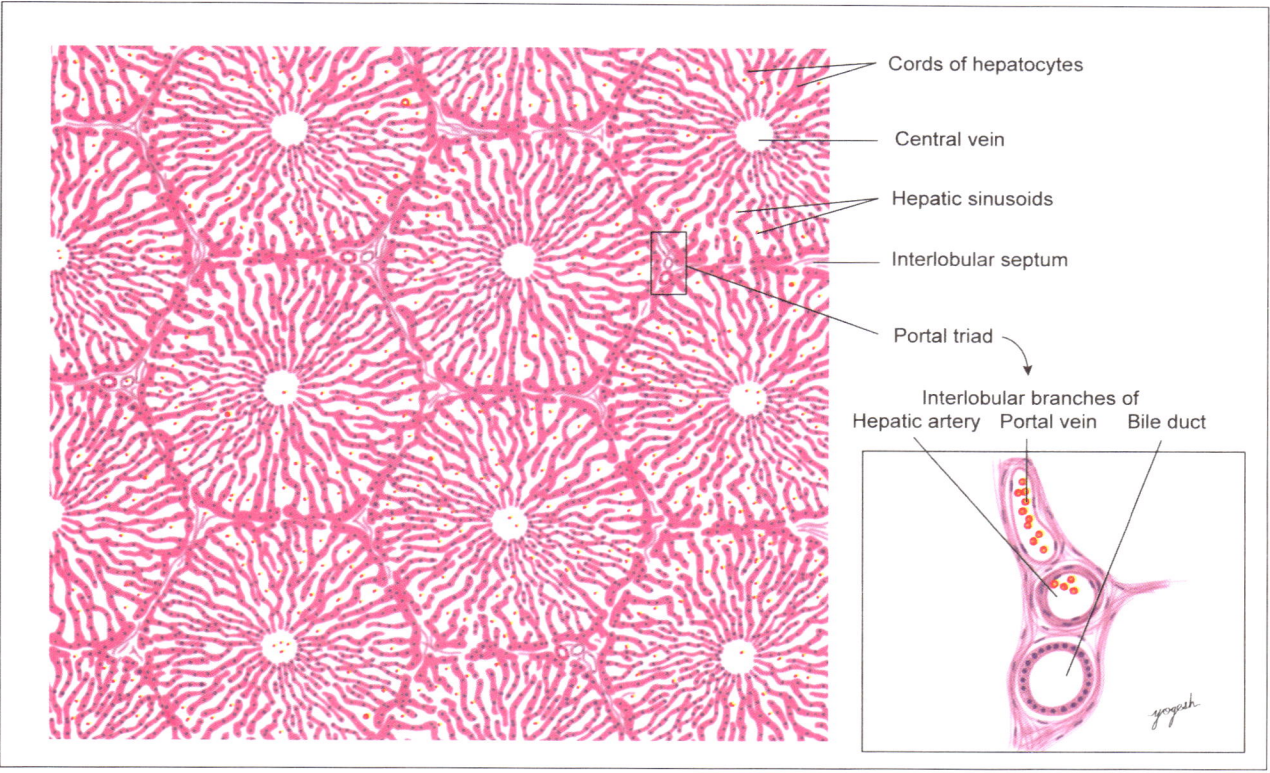

Fig. 19.2: Histology of liver (low magnification, practice figure).

- Between adjacent classical lobule, a small quantity of connective tissue with portal triad is present.
- At the angle of hexagon, portal triad runs in portal canals (connective tissue area).
- *Space of Mall:* It is a space between the connective tissue stroma of portal canals and outermost hepatocytes. It is also called *periportal space of Mall*. It is the site for lymph formation in liver.[Neet, Viva]
- In pigs, classical lobules are clearly seen because of thick connective tissue, but in humans, these lobules are not notably separated from each other.

Portal lobule
- It is a *triangular* area of liver parenchyma around each portal triad.[Viva]
- It is considered as the *functional lobule* as bile duct (in portal triad) lies at the center.
- Central veins lie at the corners of portal lobule.

Liver acinus
- It is the *structural and functional unit* of liver.
- It has two axes:
  Short axis: Between two closest portal triads.
  Long axis: Between two closest central veins.
- Liver acinus has 3 zones as follows:
  Zone 1: It is near to portal triads. It receives more oxygenated blood. It is exposed to more toxins.[Viva, Clinical fact, Neet]
  Zone 2: It lies between zone 1 and 3.
  Zone 3: It lies near to central veins. It receives less oxygenated blood; hence, more prone to hypoxic injuries.[Viva, Clinical fact, Neet]

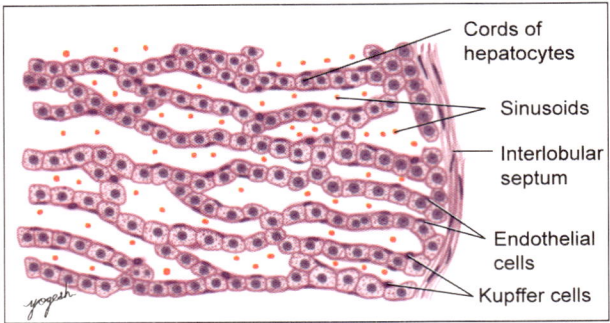

Fig. 19.3: Histology of liver (high magnification, practice figure).

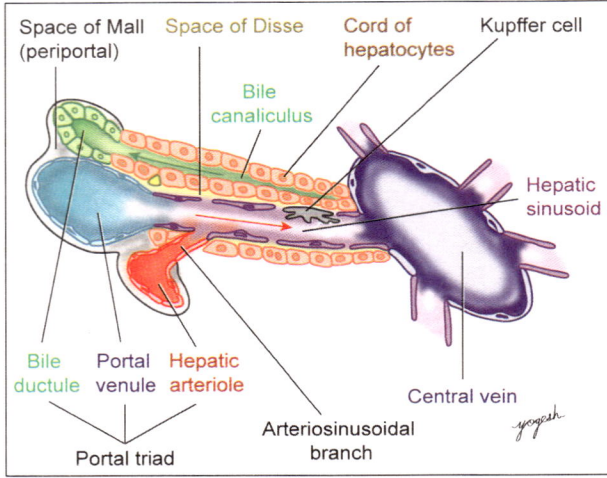

Fig. 19.4: Blood supply and bile drainage of liver cells. Note: The direction of bile flow (green arrow) is opposite to that of the direction of blood flow (red arrow).

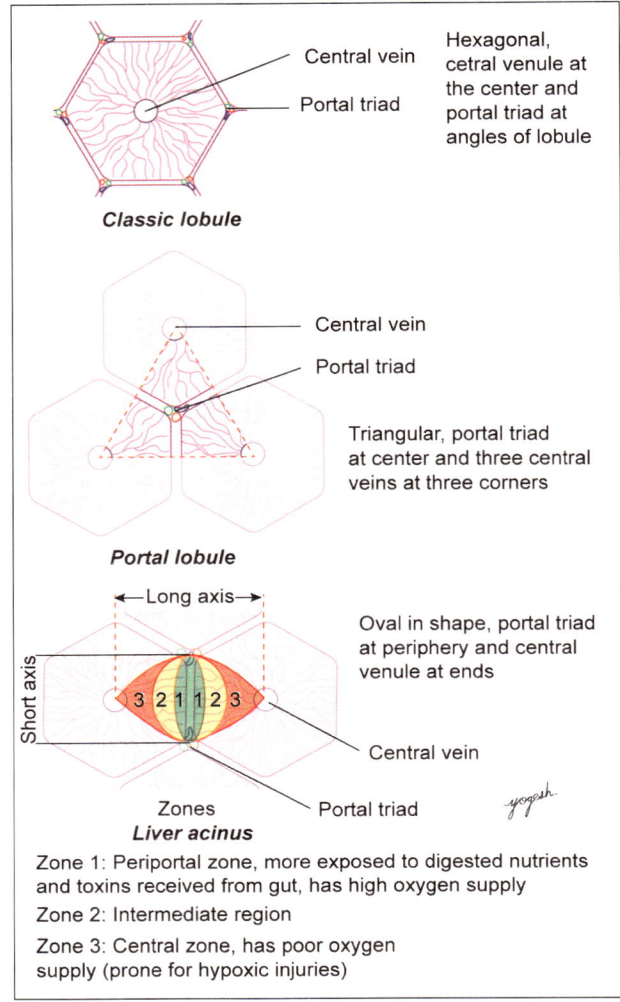

Fig. 19.5: Comparison of three models of liver architecture.

Box 19.2: Liver sinusoids

- Cords (plates) of hepatocytes are separated by liver/hepatic sinusoids.
- *Sinusoids* are lined by
  1. Discontinuous endothelium with discontinuous basal lamina.
  2. *Stellate sinusoidal macrophages (Kupffer cells):* This is the peculiarity of hepatic sinusoids. *Neet*
- *Space of Disse* (perisinusoidal space): Sinusoidal epithelium is separated from underlying hepatocytes by a small extracellular space, called space of Disse. Microvilli of hepatocytes project into the space of Disse. *Neet*
- *Note:* There is no significant barrier between blood and hepatocytes because of
  - Large gaps between adjacent endothelium cells
  - Discontinuous basal lamina of endothelium
- Space of Disse is the site for hematopoiesis in fetal life. *Neet*
- *Hepatic stellate cells (Ito cells)* are mesenchymal originated cells that lie in perisinusoidal space of Disse. Ito cells are involved in *storage of vitamin A* and lipids. *Neet*
- *Note:* In many liver disorders, Ito cells lose their storage function and get converted into myofibroblasts that ultimately results in liver fibrosis. *Clinical fact*

Flowchart 19.2: Liver lobules

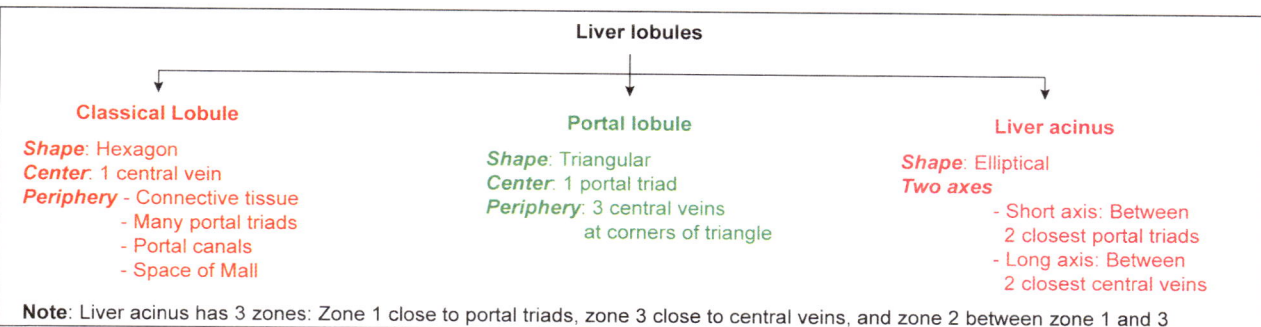

Liver lobules

Classical Lobule
- *Shape*: Hexagon
- *Center*: 1 central vein
- *Periphery* - Connective tissue
  - Many portal triads
  - Portal canals
  - Space of Mall

Portal lobule
- *Shape*: Triangular
- *Center*: 1 portal triad
- *Periphery*: 3 central veins at corners of triangle

Liver acinus
- *Shape*: Elliptical
- *Two axes*
  - Short axis: Between 2 closest portal triads
  - Long axis: Between 2 closest central veins

Note: Liver acinus has 3 zones: Zone 1 close to portal triads, zone 3 close to central veins, and zone 2 between zone 1 and 3

Some Interesting Facts

- Each hepatocyte contains 200–300 *peroxisomes*. These peroxisomes use oxygen to generate hydrogen peroxide (H_2O_2) and enzyme *catalase* to degrade this H_2O_2. Peroxisomes help in[Neet]
  1. Detoxification of drugs (for example, alcohol)
  2. Oxidation (breakdown) of fatty acids
  3. Gluconeogenesis
  4. Metabolism of purines
- Hepatocytes contain smooth endoplasmic reticulum that help in
  1. Detoxification of toxins and drugs
  2. Cholesterol synthesis[MCQ]
- Hepatocytes contain large *Golgi apparatus*.
- Hepatocytes contain number of *lysosomes* near bile canaliculus. These lysosomes may show lipofuscin (pigment granules).
- Details of various liver cells are given in Table 19.1.

Table 19.1: Cells of liver

Cell	Location	Major Functions
Hepatocytes	Cords or plates	Production of bile Detoxification of toxic chemicals Storage of glycogen
Kupffer cells[Neet]	Lining of sinusoids	Modified macrophages; hence, phagocytosis[Neet]
Ito cells/Hepatic stellate cells	Perisinusoidal space of Disse	Storage of vitamin A and lipids[Neet] Become myofibroblasts in liver diseases → liver fibrosis[Clinical fact]
Sinusoidal endothelium	Lining of sinusoids	Gap between endothelial cells facilitate transport
Hemopoietic cells (only in fetal life)	Perosinusoidal space of Disse	Hematopoiesis

Box 19.3: Intrahepatic biliary tree

- Intrahepatic biliary tree drains exocrine liver (secreted bile) and conveys it to extrahepatic biliary tree through right and left hepatic ducts.

Intrahepatic biliary tree consists of the following (Flowchart 19.3):

- *Bile canaliculus:* Formed between adjacent surface of hepatocytes.
- *Intralobular (Intrahepatic) ductules or canals of Hering:* Bile canaliculi drain the bile into intralobular ductules. These are lined by simple cuboidal epithelium. [Karl Ewald Konstantin Hering, 1834–1918].
- *Interlobular ducts:* Intralobular ducts drain into interlobular ducts that run through the interlobular connective tissue septa. These ducts are lined by simple cuboidal to columnar epithelium and form a part of portal triad.[Neet]
- *Right and left hepatic ducts:* Interlobular ducts join to form right and left hepatic ducts that later join to form common hepatic ducts outside the liver.
- *Note:* Bile flows centripetally opposite to the flow of blood in the sinusoids. Bile flows away from central vein, toward the portal triad.[Viva]
- *Duct of Luschka/accessory bile duct:* It is a small bile duct that drains either in to gallbladder or in to right hepatic duct. It lies between the inferior surface of liver and superior surface of gallbladder.[MCQ] [Hubert von Luschka, 1820–1875, German anatomist].

Note:

- Liver secretes about 1 liter of bile per day.
- Extrahepatic biliary apparatus is composed of common hepatic ducts, cystic duct, gallbladder, and common bile duct.
- Common bile duct opens into the second part of duodenum along with the main pancreatic duct at *ampulla of Vater*. This opening is guarded by *sphincter of Oddi* [Abraham Vater, 1684–1751, German anatomist; Ruggero Oddi, 1864–1913, Italian physiologist and anatomist]

Flowchart 19.3: Intrahepatic biliary tree

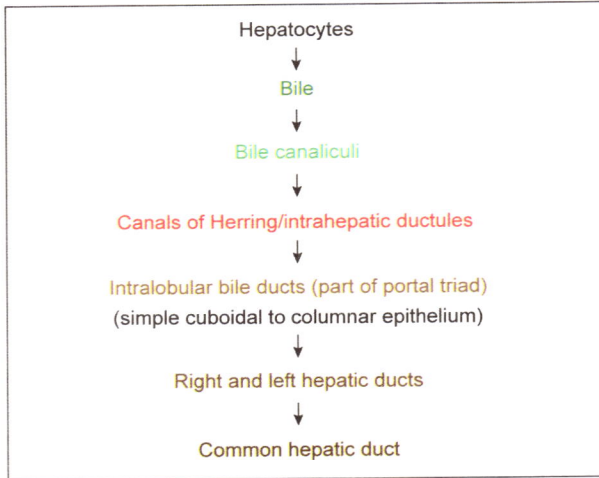

Clinical Correlation

- *Hepatitis:* It is inflammation of liver.^{Viva} Hepatitis may be caused by viruses (hepatitis A virus, hepatitis B virus, and so on), or bacteria or drugs.
- *Cirrhosis of liver:* In this condition, hepatocytes undergo necrosis (death) and get replaced by *fibrous tissue*.^{Viva} It is produced by alcohol, drugs, chemical, viruses, and autoimmune liver diseases.
- *Portal hypertension:* It is an increased resistance to the flow of portal blood through the liver causing increased blood pressure in portal vein. Cirrhosis or many other diseases produce portal hypertension. In portal hypertension, the portacaval anastomotic channels (veins) dilate.
- *Wilson disease:* It is an autosomal recessive disease of *copper metabolism.* Cause: Deficiency of copper transport protein due to a mutation in ATP7B gene.^{Neet} Results: Deposition of copper in liver, cornea, and brain causing cirrhosis of liver and *neurological malfunctions*.
- *Hepatic coma and liver failure:* In cases of large destruction of liver cells (liver failure), liver cannot detoxify material; hence, waste products get accumulated in blood. It causes hepatic coma (unconsciousness) and even death.

Summary (Examination Guide) (Flowchart 19.4)

Q. Write a short note on histology of liver.

- Liver is covered by a thin connective tissue Glisson's capsule.
- Liver shows classical hepatic lobules (hexagonal in shape).
- Central vein lies in the form of space at the center of lobule.
- Cords of hepatocytes: Arranged radially, radiating away from central vein.
- Portal triad: It consists of *identification feature, Neet, Viva*
  - Branch of portal vein (irregular lumen, simple squamous epithelium)
  - Branch of hepatic artery (circular lumen, simple squamous epithelium)
  - Interlobular bile duct (circular lumen, simple cuboidal to columnar epithelium.)
- *Liver sinusoids:* They separate cords of hepatocytes and are lined by discontinuous endothelium, Kupffer cells, and discontinuous basal lamina.
- *Hepatocytes* are large polygonal cells with large central nucleus and granular eosinophilic (pink) cytoplasm.
- Adjacent lobules are separated by thin connective tissue septa.

Flowchart 19.4: Histology of liver

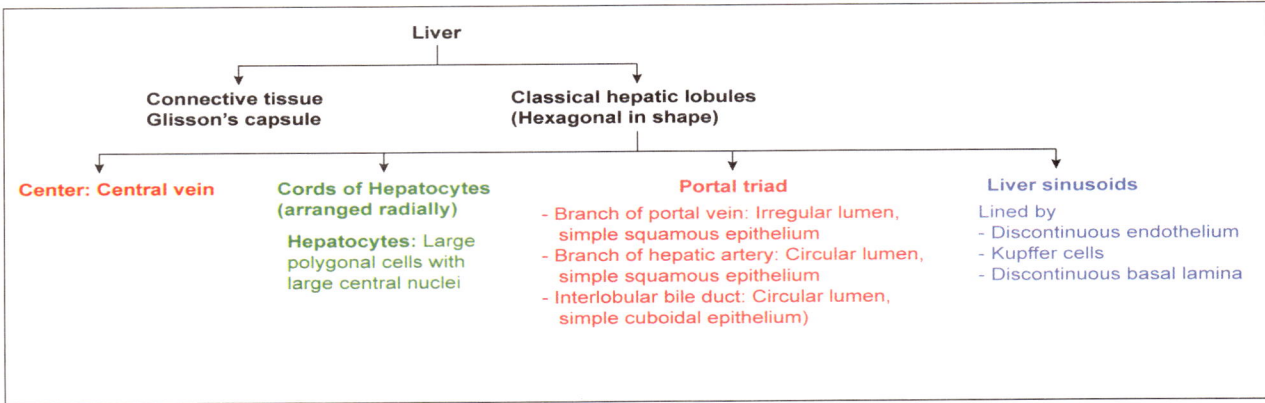

Liver, Gallbladder and Pancreas

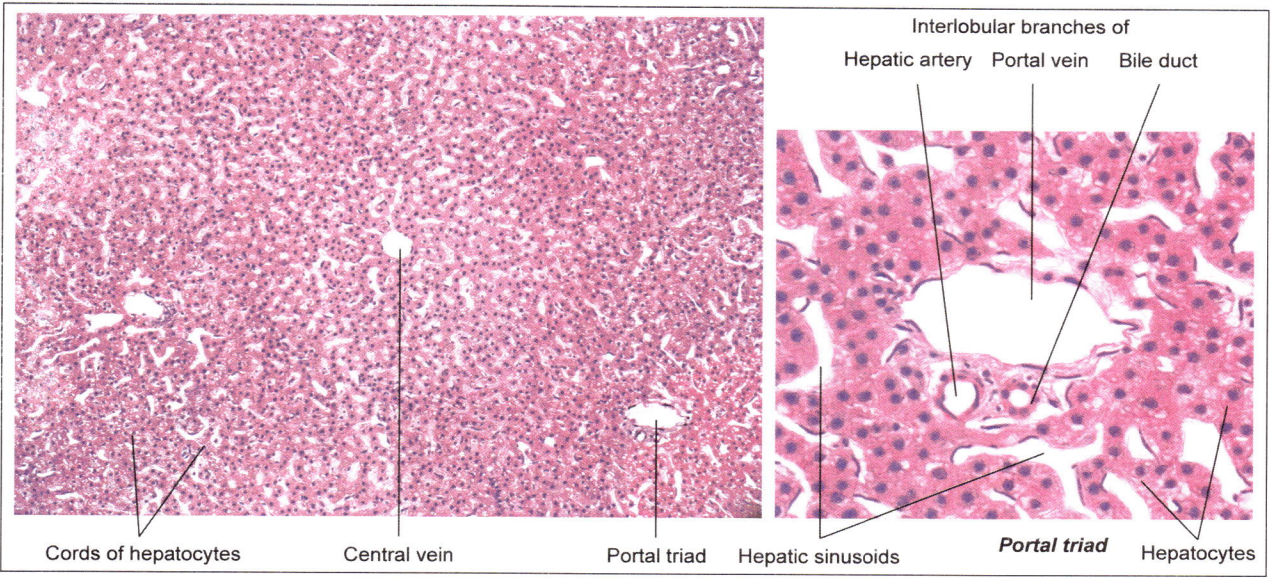

19.6: Photomicrograph. Histology of liver (low magnification on left, portal triad at high magnification on right, *H&E* stain).

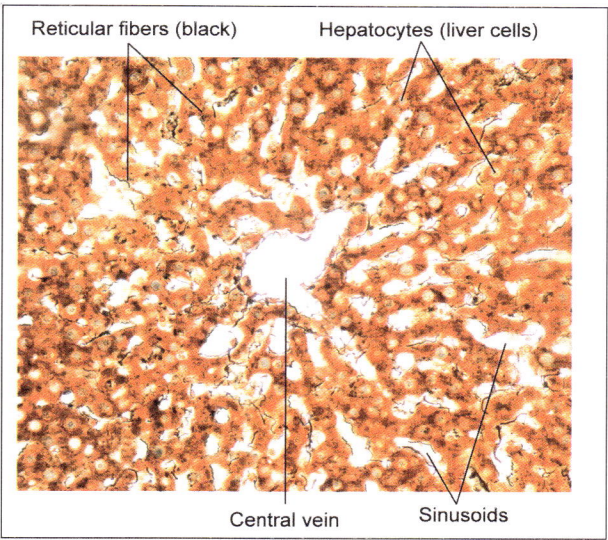

Fig. 19.7: Photomicrograph. Liver showing reticular fiber (high magnification, Gomori's silver impregnation staining technique).

GALLBLADDER

- Gallbladder is a pear-shaped *mucomuscular sac* that concentrates and temporarily stores the bile.
- Capacity: 30–50 ml.
- Location: It is situated in the fossa for gallbladder on the inferior surface of liver.
- It receives bile from liver through a cystic duct.

Histology of Gallbladder

- Gallbladder has following three layers (Fig. 19.8, and 19.9):
  - Mucosa
  - Fibromuscular coat
  - Serosa/adventitia
- Note: There is no submucosa and muscularis mucosae in gallbladder.

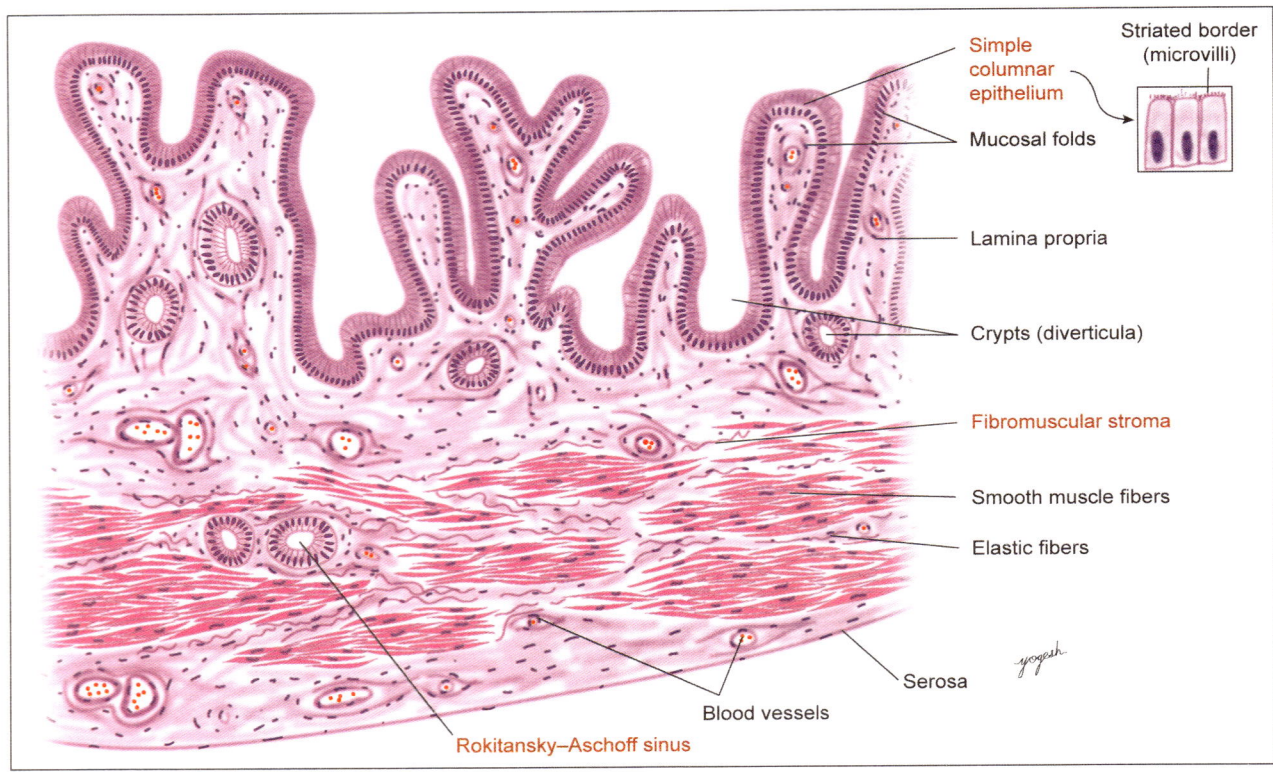

Fig. 19.8: Histology of gallbladder (practice figure).

Mucosa

- Interior of gallbladder shows numerous muscular folds.
- Lining epithelium:
  Simple columnar epithelium with basally placed ovoid nucleus and faint eosinophilic cytoplasm.[Neet]
  Epithelial cells show numerous apical *microvilli* to increase the surface area for absorption.[Neet]
- Epithelium shows apical *striated border* (*some authors described it as brush border*) because of the presence of microvilli.[Neet]
- *Lamina propria:* It consists of connective tissue and number of fenestrated capillaries. Lamina propria of gallbladder does not have lymphatic vessels.[MCQ]
- There is *no muscularis mucosae and submucosa* in wall of gallbladder.
- Lamina propria may show presence of crypts because of mucosal folding.
- Lamina propria near the neck of gallbladder may show presence of mucous glands.

Fibromuscular Coat/muscularis Externa

- It consists of bundles of *smooth muscle cells* with interspaced collagen and elastic fibers.
- Smooth muscle cells are *not organized* like gut. They run in different directions.
- Few deep diverticula of mucosa extend into the muscularis externa. These are called *Rokitansky-Aschoff sinuses*. They look like glands, but they are just extensions of mucosa. [Carl Freiherr von Rokitansky, 1804–1878, pathologist; Ludwig Aschoff, 1866–1942, German pathologist].
- Note: Fibromuscular coat is seen in gallbladder, biliary tree, and ureter.[Neet]

Serosa/Adventitia

- It consists of *thick layer of dense connective tissue*, blood vessels, lymphatics, autonomic nerves, and elastic fibers.
- Surface of gallbladder that is not related to liver is covered by serosa – a layer of visceral peritoneum with a mesothelium (simple squamous epithelium).

Clinical Correlation

- *Cholecystitis* is an *inflammation* of gallbladder.
- *Cholelithiasis* is formation of *stones* in gallbladder (gall stones).

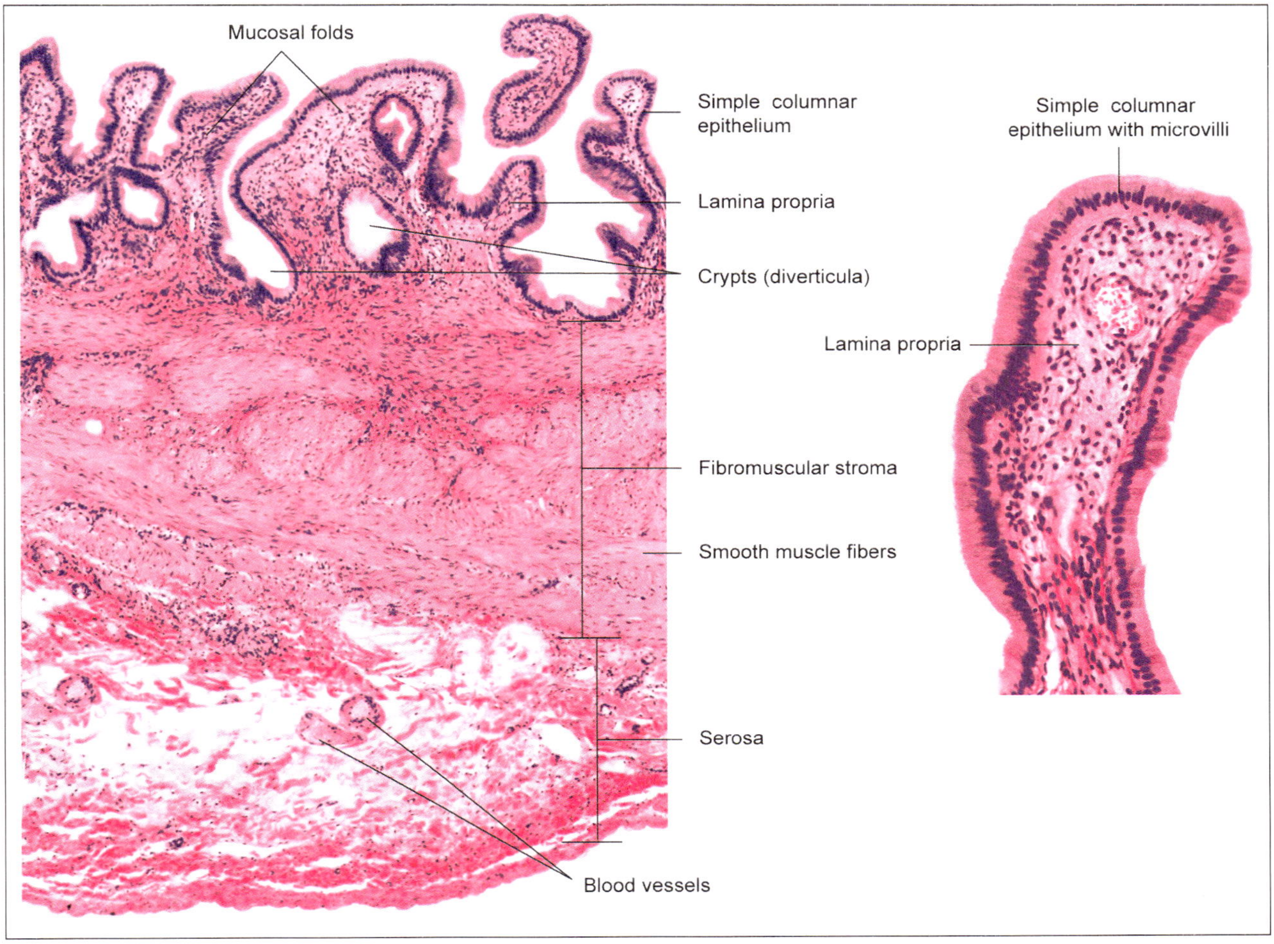

Fig. 19.9: Photomicrograph. Histology of gallbladder (low magnification on left, epithelium at high magnification on right, *H&E* stain).

Summary (Examination Guide) (Flowchart 19.5)

Gallbladder shows three layers as follows:
- Mucosa: It is lined by tall columnar cells with striated border because of the presence of microvilli. Nuclei are elongated and basally placed. Cytoplasm is light eosinophilic (pink color). Lamina propria consists of connective tissue.
- Fibromuscular coat: It consists of bundle of smooth muscle fibers with interspaced collagen and elastic fibers.
- Serosa/adventitia: Other than inferior surface (covered by peritoneum), gallbladder is covered by adventitia.
- Gallbladder shows absence of four structures: *Neet, Identification feature*
- Following features differentiate gallbladder from intestine:
  1. Villi
  2. Goblet cells
  3. Submucosa
  4. Properly organized muscularis externa.

Flowchart 19.5: Histology of gallbladder.

Gallbladder
- **Mucosa**
  - Simple columnar cells with striated border (microvilli)
  - Lamina propria: Connective tissue
- **Fibromuscular coat**
  - Bundle of smooth muscle fibers with interspaced collagen and elastic fibers
- **Serosa/adventitia**
  - Other than inferior surface (covered by peritoneum) gallbladder is covered by connective tissue adventitia

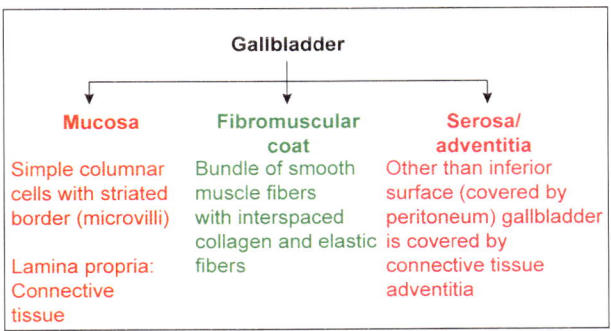

PANCREAS

- Pancreas is located retroperitoneally, extending from concavity of duodenum to hilum of spleen.
- Pancreas shows head, neck, body, and tail.

Pancreatic Ducts

Exocrine part of pancreas is drained by (Fig. 19.10):
1. *Pancreatic duct of Wirsung* that extends through the entire length of pancreas. It opens in to the second part of duodenum at hepatopancreatic ampulla of Vater along with common bile duct. This opening is guarded by sphincter of Oddi that prevents entry of bile and intestinal contents in to pancreas and also regulates flow of bile.
2. *Accessory pancreatic duct of Santorini* drains a small part of pancreas at minor duodenal papilla. [Giovanni Domenico Santorini, 1681–1737]

Histology of Pancreas

Capsule

- A thin layer of loose connective tissue forms a capsule of pancreas.
- Septa extend from capsule in the substance of gland and divide gland into ill-defined lobules.

> **Box 19.4:** Santorini
>
> - He was an Italian anatomist (1681–1737).
> - Following are some of his inventions:
>   1. Santorini's cartilage: Corniculate cartilage of larynx
>   2. Santorini's concha: Superior nasal concha
>   3. Duct of Santorini: Accessory pancreatic duct
>   4. Santorini's muscle (Albinus muscle): Muscle that draws the angle of mouth laterally
>   5. Santorini's vein: It passes through the parietal foramen.
>   6. Santorini's plexus of veins: Located in retropubic space or cave of Retzius, lie between pubis symphysis and urinary bladder [Anders Adolph Retzius, 1796–1860, Swedish anatomist]

Exocrine and Endocrine Pancreas

- Parenchyma of pancreas is divided into two components according to its functions:
  A. *Exocrine pancreas:* It produces enzymes and bicarbonates that get secreted into second part of duodenum through pancreatic *ducts.*
  B. *Endocrine pancreas* (Islets of Langerhans): It secretes glucagon and insulin *into the blood.*

Exocrine Pancreas (Serous Gland)

- Exocrine pancreas is a compound *tubuloalveolar/ tubuloacinar serous gland.*
- **Pancreatic acini** (Fig. 19.11):
  - Pancreatic acini are *serous acini* (round or oval in cross sections) with small lumen.
  - *Epithelial lining:* Simple columnar cells having narrow luminal and broad basal surface. Nuclei are spherical and basally placed.
  - *H&E staining:* Secretory cells show *basal basophilia and apical eosinophilia.* Basal basophilia is because of rough endoplasmic reticulum, whereas apical eosinophilia is because of numerous secretory vesicles, zymogen granules, and Golgi apparatus.
  - *Zymogen granules:* These are secretory granules contain digestive enzymes (proteases, amylases, lipases, and nucleases). Zymogen granules increase in fasting.^(MCQ, Viva) Zymogen granules are released by exocytosis.
  - *Centroacinar cells:* These are located at the center of acini. They represent the beginning of intercalated ducts that invaginate acini.^(Neet, Viva) Centroacinar cells show *pale staining cytoplasm* with centrally placed *flattened nucleus* (like squamous cells).^(Viva) Centroacinar cells secrete bicarbonate ions in pancreatic juice.
  - Concept: Acinus is a balloon with straw of centroacinar cells.

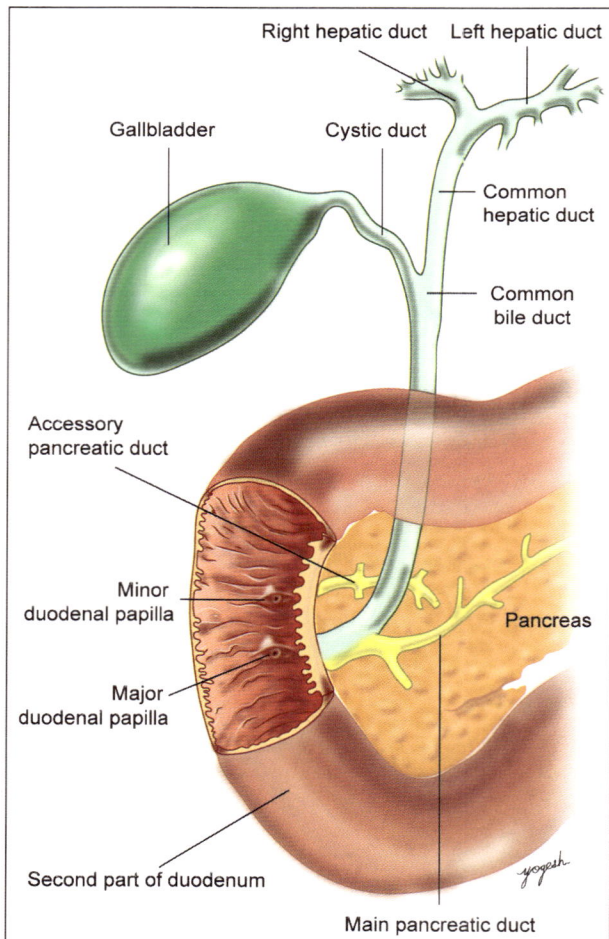

Fig. 19.10: Relationship of hepatic, pancreatic, and cystic ducts and openings of ducts in second part of duodenum.

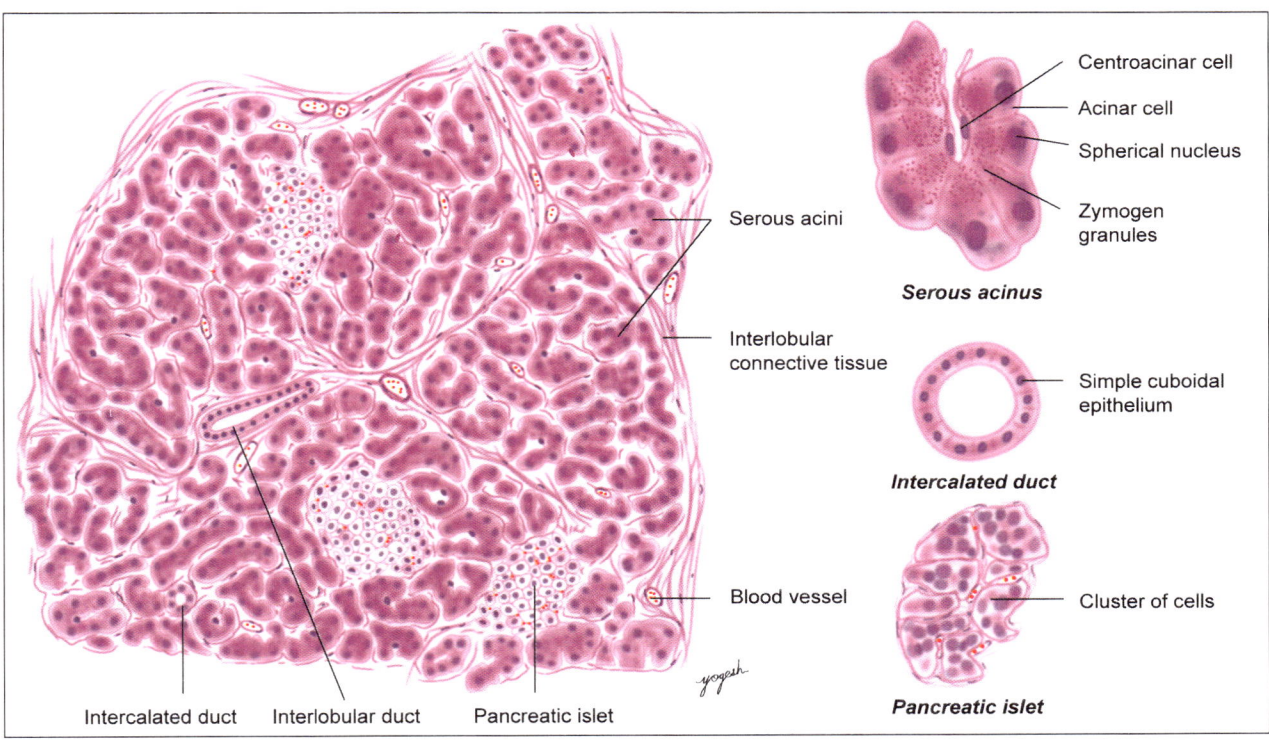

Fig. 19.11: Histology of pancreas (low magnification, practice figure).

- **Duct system of pancreas** (Table 19.2 and Fig. 19.12)
  - Histologically, exocrine pancreas shows following ducts:
    Intercalated (intralobular) ducts → interlobular ducts → main and accessory pancreatic ducts.
  - *Intercalated duct:* These are intralobular ducts that begin as centroacinar cells. They are lined by *simple squamous* to *very low simple cuboidal epithelium*.
  - *Note:* There are *no striated ducts* in pancreas. Striated ducts are present in parotid gland.^{Neet}
  - Intercalated ducts open into *interlobular ducts* that are lined by *cuboidal to low columnar* epithelium.
  - *Main and accessory pancreatic ducts* are lined by *simple columnar* epithelium.

Table 19.2: Exocrine pancreas

Component	Epithelium
Acini	Simple columnar cells (basal basophilia, apical eosinophilia)
Centroacinar cells	Simple squamous to low cuboidal epithelium
Intercalated duct	Low cuboidal epithelium
Interlobular duct	Cuboidal to low columnar cells
No striated duct	
Main and accessory ducts	Simple columnar epithelium

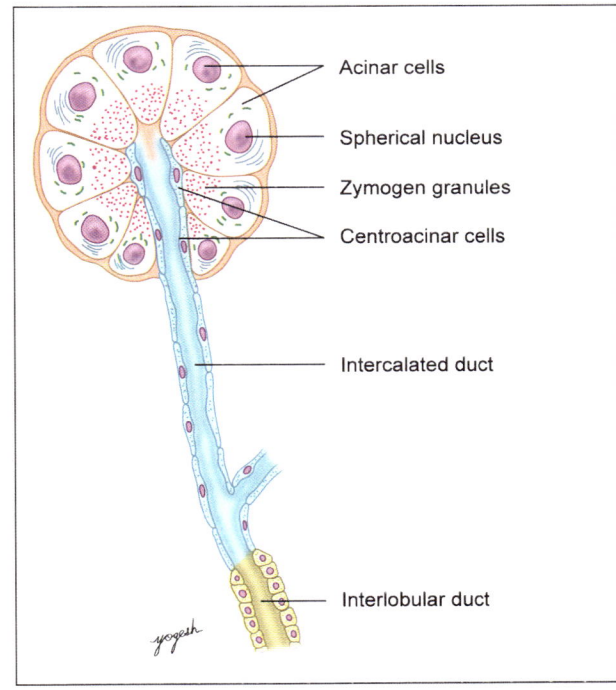

Fig. 19.12: Pancreatic duct system.

- Intercalated ducts add bicarbonates and water in pancreatic secretions.

- Exocrine pancreatic secretions are under the control of *secretin* and *cholecystokinin* (CCK) hormones as well as autonomic nerves.

Endocrine Pancreas

- Endocrine pancreas consists of numerous small *clusters* (group of cells) or *islands* that are scattered in the parenchyma of pancreas. These cluster of cells are called Islets of Langerhans (Fig. 19.13).^Viva
- Human pancreas contains about 1 million islets (about 1–2% of volume of pancreas).
- *H&E staining:* Islets of Langerhans consists of *clusters of pale staining polygonal cells* with numerous capillaries. These islets are surrounded by serous pancreatic acini (dark staining).^Viva
- Note: On *H&E* staining, cells of islets of Langerhans cannot be differentiated.

- *Mallory-Azan staining with Zenker's formal fixation:* It reveals three types of cells:
  1. Red A or alpha cells
  2. Brownish orange B or beta cells
  3. Blue D or delta cells
- *Immunohistochemical staining method:* In addition to alpha, beta, and delta cells, islets of Langerhans show few other cells such as F cells or PP cell, D 1 cell, and enterochromaffin cells.
- For details of various cells of islets of Langerhans, refer Table 19.3.

> **Some Interesting Facts**
> - **Insulin** decreases blood glucose level and its absence results in *diabetes mellitus.*
> - Insulin is essential for normal cell growth and function.
> - *Glucagon* enhances blood glucose level (opposite to insulin).
> - *Somatostatin* (secreted by D cells) inhibits secretion of both insulin and glucagon.
> - Blood glucose level above 70 mg/dL stimulates the beta cells for insulin secretion, whereas blood glucose level below 70 mg/dL stimulates glucagon secretion.
> - Islets of Langerhans are supplied by fenestrated capillaries that easily allow entry of hormone in circulation.
> - Note: Difference between pancreas and parotid (salivary) gland: Though both show serous acini, there are three basic differences^Viva
>   1. Pancreatic islets of Langerhans
>   2. Pancreatic centroacinar cells
>   3. No striated ducts in pancreas (few intralobular ducts)

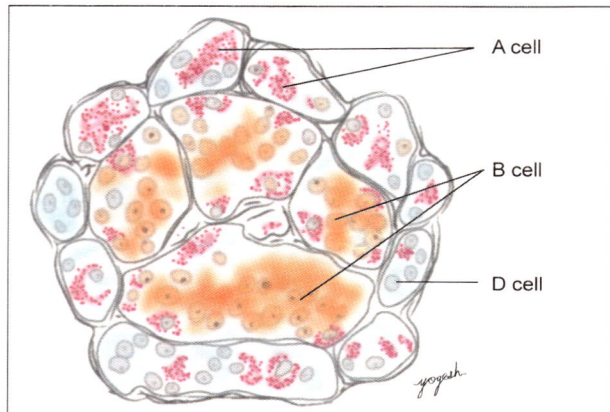

Fig. 19.13: Islets of Langerhans. Mallory-Azan staining showing red A or alpha cells, brownish-orange B or beta cells, and blue D or delta cells.

Table 19.3: Cells of islets of Langerhans

Cell	Function	Remarks
Alpha/A cells/A2 cells	Glucagon	Constitute about 15–20% of cells of islets Arranged toward periphery of islets Stain brightly with acid fuchsin
Beta/B cells	Insulin	Constitute about 60–70% of cells of islets Arranged at the center of islets Stain with aldehyde fuchsin
Delta/D cells/Type III cells/ A1 cells	Somatostatin	Constitutes about 5–10% of cells of islets Peripherally placed These are argyrophilic cells (stains with silver) Stain with acid fuchsin
PP cells/F cells	Pancreatic polypeptide	
D1 cells	Vasoactive intestinal peptide (VIP)	
EC cells	Serotonin, motilin, substance P	

Summary (Examination Guide) (Flowchart 19.6, Fig. 19.14 and 19.15)

- Pancreatic parenchyma shows exocrine as well as endocrine components.

Exocrine pancreas (serous compound tubuloalveolar part):
- It secretes bicarbonates and digestive enzymes.
- It consists of
  Serous acini are lined by tall columnar cells that show basal basophilia (because of SER) apical eosinophilia (because of SER) and spherical basal nuclei.
  Centroacinar cells (simple squamous cells) line intercalated ducts.
- Interlobular ducts are lined by simple cuboidal to low columnar epithelium.
- Main and accessory pancreatic ducts are lined by simple columnar epithelium.

Endocrine pancreas (Islets of Langerhans)
- These are lightly stained *clusters of polygonal cells.*
- Mallory–Azan staining and immunohistochemistry shows
  – Alpha cells (A cells): Secrete glucagon
  – Beta cells (B cells): Secrete insulin
  – Delta cells (D cells): Secrete somatostatin
- Few other cells (PP, D-1, enterochromaffin cells) are also seen in islets of Langerhans.
- Endocrine pancreas is supplied by fenestrated capillaries.

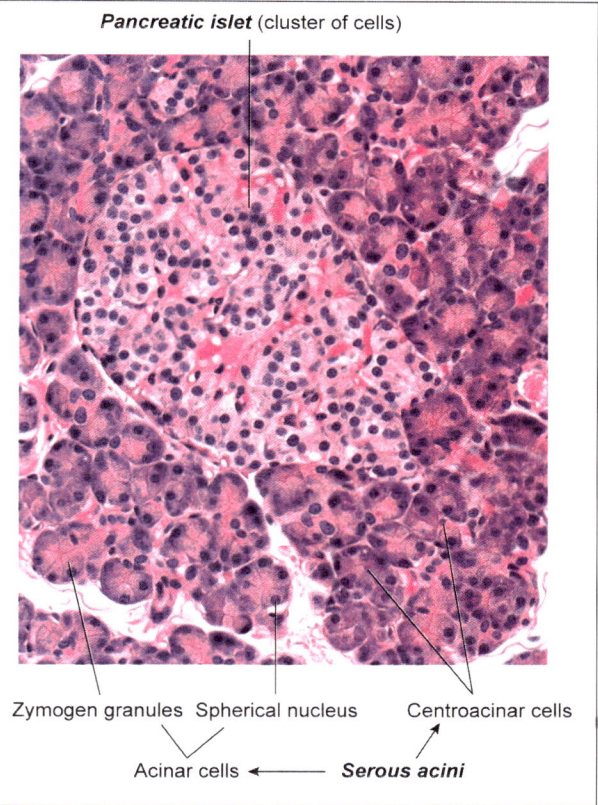

Fig. 19.15: Photomicrograph. Histology of pancreas (High magnification, *H&E* stain).

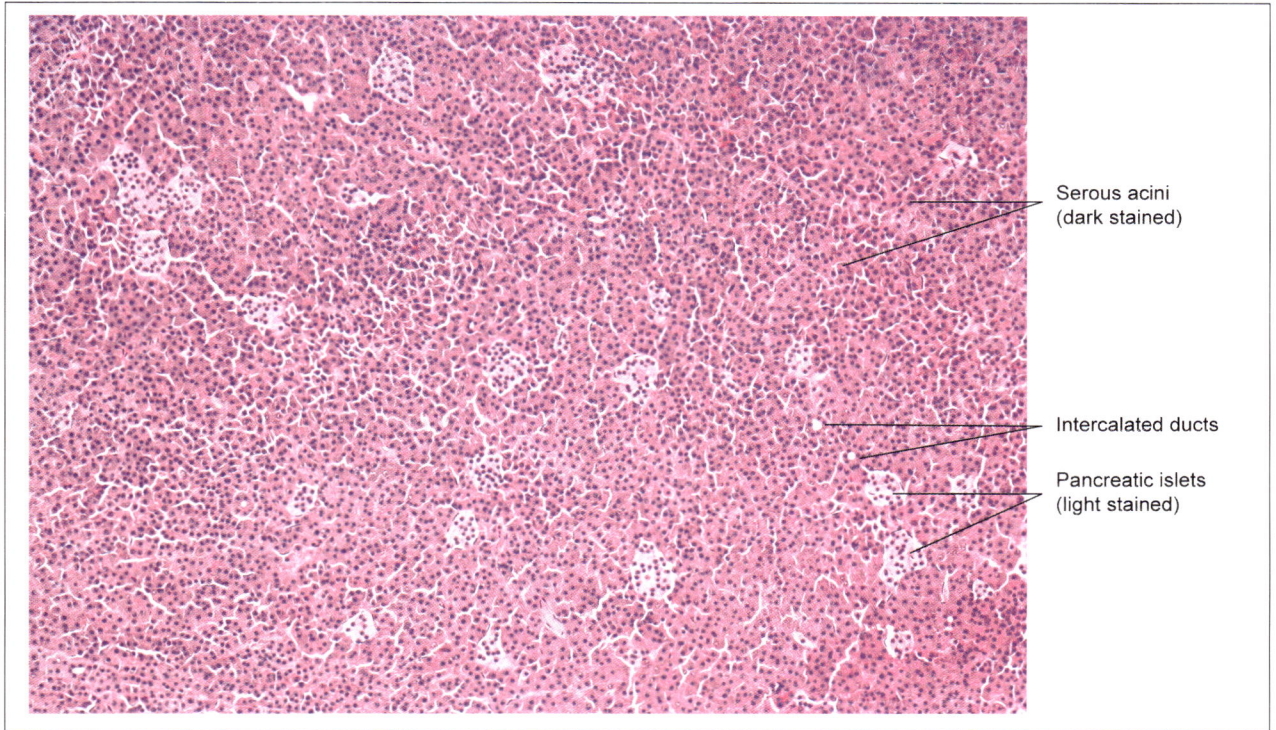

Fig. 19.14: Photomicrograph. Histology of pancreas (low magnification, *H&E* stain).

Flowchart 19.6: Histology of pancreas

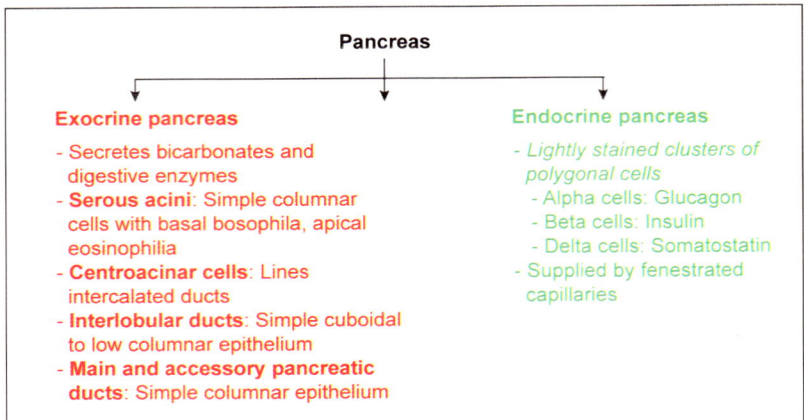

Clinical Correlation

- *Acute pancreatitis:* It is an acute inflammation of pancreas that has severe complications and high mortality (death) rate. It occurs because of abnormal activation of proteolytic pancreatic enzymes in the pancreas (usually these enzymes get activated in the intestine). Activated enzymes cause inflammation, edema, and cellular death.
- *Chronic pancreatitis:* It is long-standing inflammation of pancreas (repeated attacks of mild acute pancreatitis).
- Serum *amylase* and serum *lipase* levels get elevated in both acute and chronic pancreatitis.[Neet]
- *Diabetes mellitus:* Failure of beta cells to produce insulin results in diabetes mellitus (high blood sugar levels). Note: *Type I* diabetes mellitus occurs because of pancreatic failure, whereas type II diabetes mellitus result because of insulin resistance (failure of cells to respond to insulin).

CHAPTER 20

Urinary System

Chapter Outline
- Kidney
- Ureter
- Urinary bladder
- Urethra

Competency achievement: The student should be able to:

AN52.2 Describe and identify the microanatomical features of urinary system: Kidney, ureter and urinary bladder

INTRODUCTION

- Urinary system consists of the following:
  - A pair of kidneys
  - A pair of ureters
  - Urinary bladder
  - Urethra

Main Functions of Kidney

- Kidney helps in the ***purification*** of blood by ultrafiltration and removal of metabolic waste products.
- Kidneys conserve body fluid and electrolytes and maintain their balance.
- Kidneys also function as an *endocrine* organ by production of:
  1. *Erythropoietin:* It helps in the formation of red blood cells. Erythropoietin production depends on blood oxygen levels.
  2. *Renin:* Renin converts angiotensinogen to angiotensin I that helps in blood pressure regulation.
  3. *Vitamin D3:* Kidney enzyme 1-hydroxylase converts 25-hydroxy vitamin D3 (produced in liver) to active 1,25 dihydroxy vitamin D3.

KIDNEY

Gross Structure of Kidney

- Each kidney is a bean-shaped organ covered by a capsule.
- Medial border of kidney has *hilum* through which vessels and nerves enter the kidney. At hilum, *renal pelvis* (space) continues as ureter (Fig. 20.1).
- Space that occupies vessels, nerves, and renal pelvis at hilum of kidney is called *renal sinus.*
- Renal pelvis is divided into *two major calyces* (upper and lower). Each major calyx is divided into a number of cup-shaped *minor calyces* that show conical projections of kidney called *papillae.*
- On examination with naked-eye, kidney shows the following structures (Fig. 20.1 and Flowchart 20.1):
  - Outer reddish-brown *cortex*
  - Inner pale *medulla*
- Cortex receives 90–95% of kidney's blood supply; hence, it is reddish-brown.
- *Capsule:* Capsule of kidney is composed of two layers:
  - Outer layer of fibroblast and collagen fibers
  - Inner layer of myofibroblasts (their clear function is not known)
- *Renal pyramids* are triangular projections of renal medulla. Apical portion of renal pyramid faces renal pelvis and base faces cortex.

Flowchart 20.1: Structure of kidney.

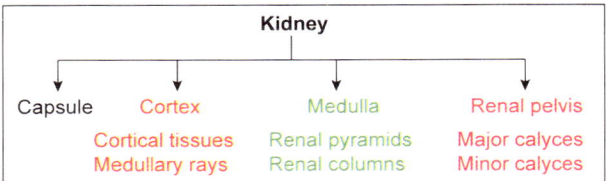

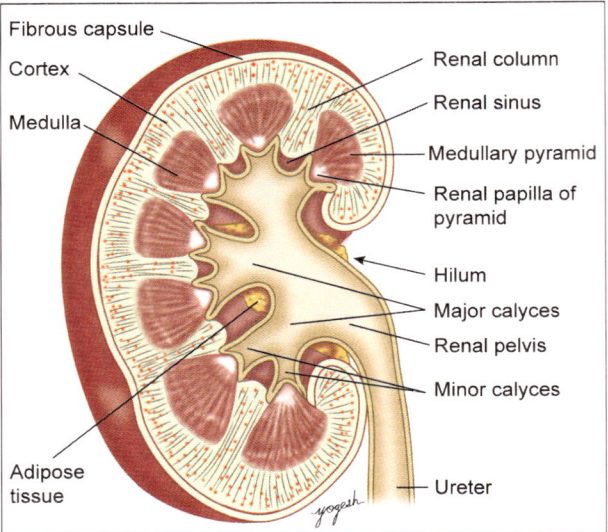

Fig. 20.1: Coronal section of kidney.

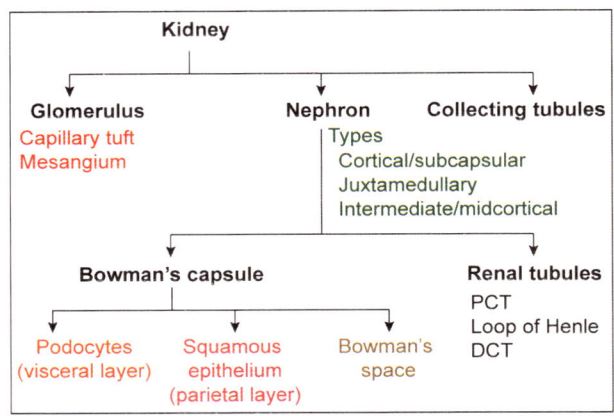

- Renal cortex shows *striations*. Light lines (400–500 in number) are extensions of medulla into the cortex and these are called *medullary rays of Ferrein*.^{MCQ} Medullary rays contain straight tubules of nephron and collecting ducts.
- *Cortical labyrinths* are regions of cortex between adjacent medullary rays.
- *Renal columns of Bertin* represents cortical tissue that is extended between adjacent renal pyramids.
- *Papilla* is the apical portion of each pyramid. Papilla projects into minor calyx.^{Neet}
- *Area cribrosa* is perforated area at the tip of renal papilla because of collecting ducts openings.
- *Kidney lobe:* Each pyramid with the surrounding cortical tissue forms a lobe of the kidney. Each kidney contains 8–18 lobes (multilobed kidney). Lobulation is a prominent feature of fetal kidney but in adult kidney lobes are indistinct.^{Viva}
- *Kidney lobule:* Similar to secretory unit of exocrine glands, collecting ducts of medullary ray and surrounding cortical tissues constitutes kidney lobule.^{Viva}

Microscopic Structure of Kidney (Figs 20.2 to 20.9 and Flowchart 20.2)

Nephron

- Nephron is the structural and functional unit of kidney.^{Viva}
- Each kidney contains approximately 2 million nephrons.^{Viva}
- Each nephron consists of renal corpuscle and long renal tubule. Renal tubule is made up of proximal convoluted tubule, loop of Henle, and distal convoluted tubule (Fig. 20.4).
- Distal convoluted tubule connects collecting tubule.

> **Box 20.1:** Types of nephrons^{Viva}
>
> Based on location of renal corpuscles, nephrons are classified as:
> 1. **Cortical or subcapsular nephrons:** Their renal corpuscles lie in outer cortex. They have short loops of Henle that extend only into the outer part of medulla.
> 2. **Juxtamedullary nephrons:** Their renal corpuscles lie at the junction of cortex and medulla. They have long loops of Henle and ascending thin segments. They help in maintenance of urine concentration.^{MCQ}
> 3. **Intermediate or mid-cortical nephrons:** Their renal corpuscles lie in mid-region of cortex. They have average length loop of Henle.

Renal Corpuscle/Malpighian Corpuscle

- Renal corpuscle is a spherical structure
- It consists of the following parts:
  - *Glomerulus:* A tuft of blood capillaries.
  - *Bowman's (renal/glomerular) capsule:* A cup-like double-layered covering of glomerulus.
  - *Urinary/Bowman's space:* It is a space between two layers of Bowman's capsule (urinary space).

Glomerulus

- It is a spherical ball of tuft of blood capillaries.
- It receives blood through *afferent arteriole* and drains into *efferent arteriole*. Diameter of efferent arteriole is less than that of afferent arteriole.
- *Vascular pole:* Site of entry-exit of afferent-efferent arterioles in the glomerulus is referred as *vascular pole*.
- *Urinary pole:* Opposite to the vascular pole, Bowman's capsule continues as proximal convoluted tubule. This pole is called *urinary pole*.

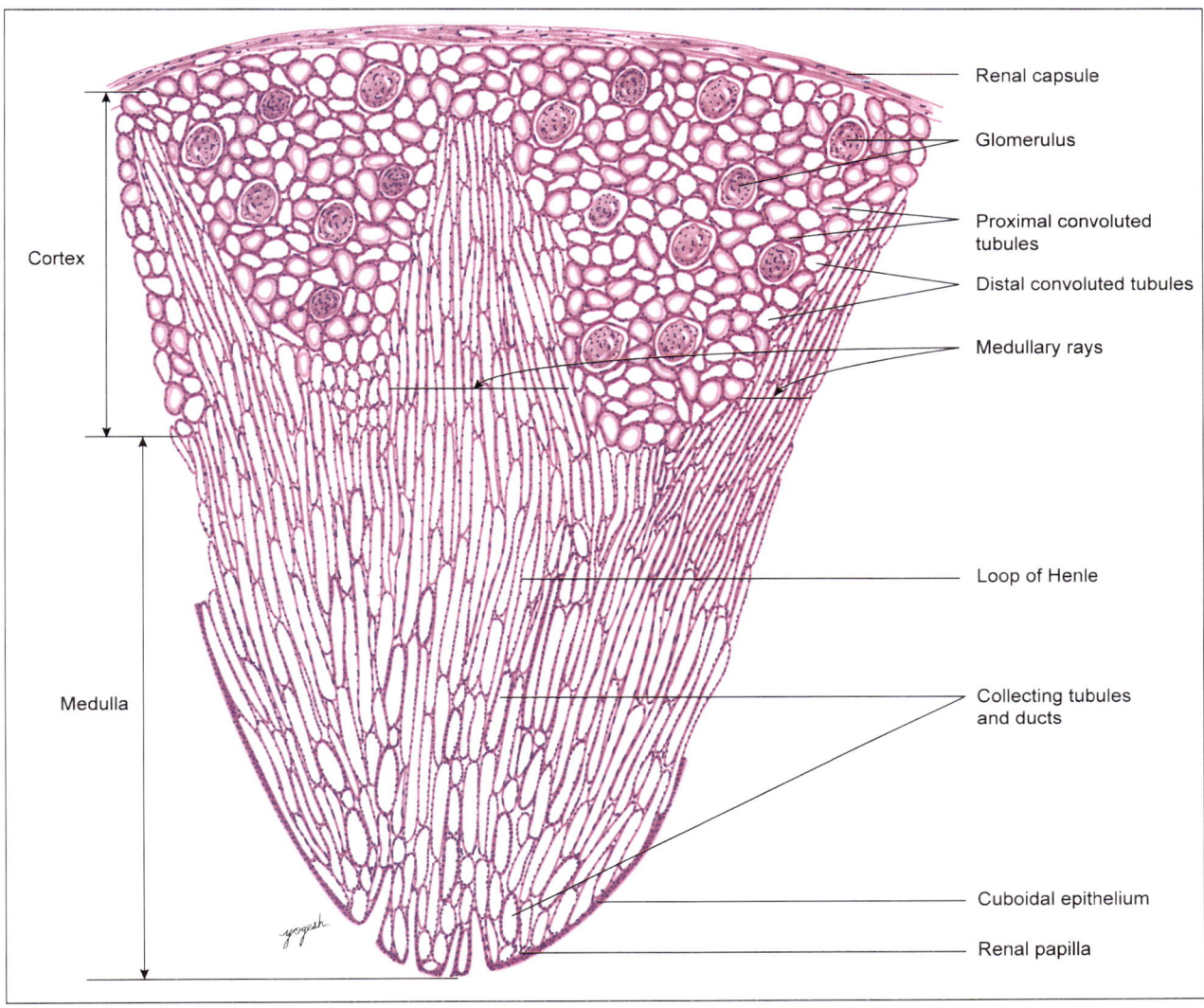

Fig. 20.2: Histology of kidney (low magnification, practice figure).

Box 20.2: Filtration apparatus of kidney^{Viva}

Q. Write a short note on glomerular filtration barrier.

- Filtration barrier or apparatus consists of three components (Fig. 20.5):
  1. **Endothelium of glomerular capillaries**
     Endothelium of glomerular capillaries is fenestrated that has large pores (70–90 nm).
  2. **Glomerular basement membrane (GBM)**
     It consists of fused lamina of endothelium and podocytes of Bowman's capsule. It forms principal component of filtration barrier and prevents filtration of plasma proteins.
  3. **Visceral layer of Bowman's capsule/podocytes**
     The Bowman's capsule has two layers:
     (a) Outer *parietal layer* of squamous cells, (b) Inner *visceral layer* of podocytes
- *Podocytes* have processes called pedicels or *foot processes* that extend toward glomerular capillaries.
- *Filtration slits:* Elongated spaces (25 nm wide) between interdigitating foot processes are called filtration slits. It helps in ultrafiltration.
- *Filtration slit membrane* or *slit diaphragm:* It spans slits between adjacent foot process.
- Glomerular filtration apparatus is a semipermeable-barrier that has discontinuous endothelium and epithelium, but continuous basement membrane.

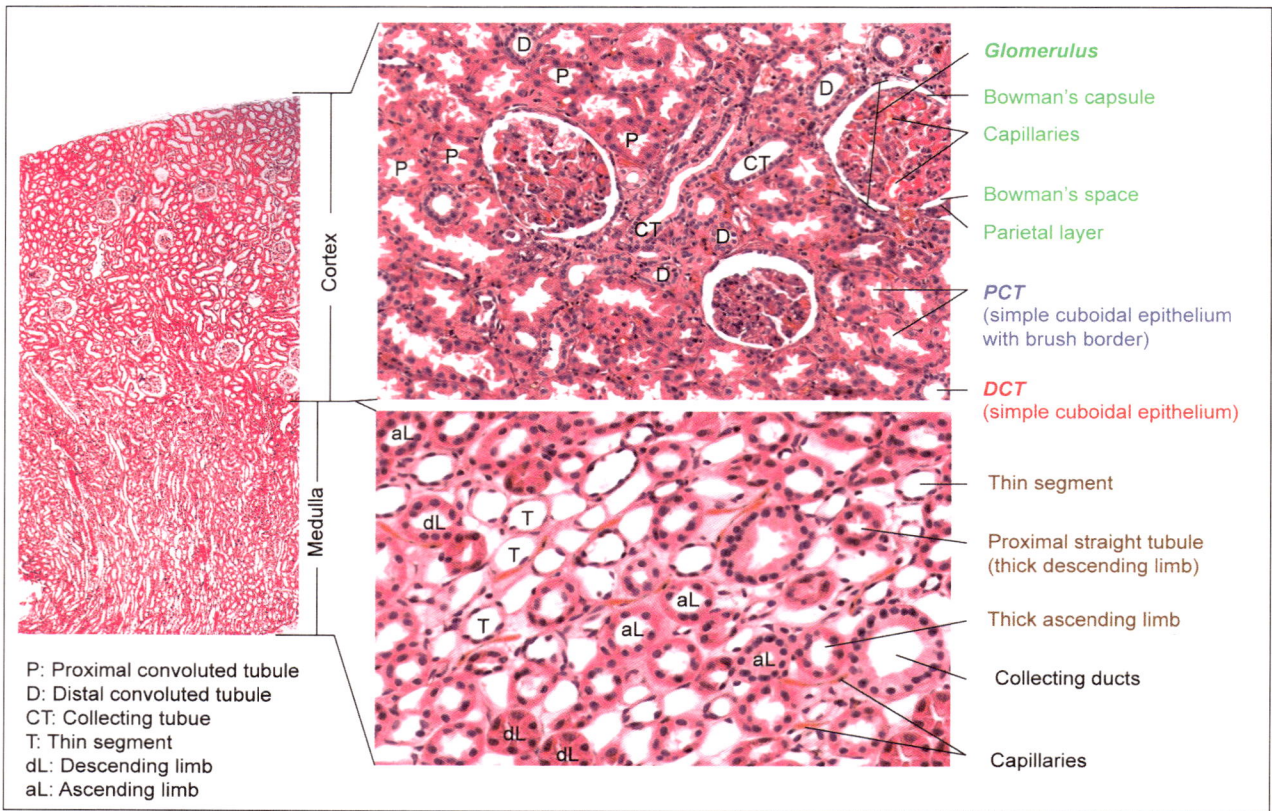

Fig. 20.3: Photomicrograph. Histology of kidney (low magnification on left, cortex and medulla at high magnification on right, H&E stain)

Box 20.3: Mesangium

- Glomerular capillaries are held together by mesangial cells and their extracellular matrix.
- These mesangial cells along with associated extracellular matrix are called *mesangium.*
- Mesangial cells work similar to pericytes of capillaries and are embedded in basal lamina of capillaries.
- *Lacis cells:* These are mesangial cells along the vascular pole and these cells form part of juxtaglomerular apparatus.

Functions of mesangial cells
1. Phagocytosis of aggregated proteins from glomerular basement membrane (cleaning of glomerular basement membrane)
2. Support podocytes
3. Secretion of interleukin-1 (IL-1) and platelet-derived growth factor (PDGF)[Neet]
- Note: Unlike other phagocytic cells (monocyte-derived), mesangial cells are derived from smooth muscle cell precursors.[Neet]
- Mesangial cells have *angiotensin II receptors* and these cells help in regulation of blood flow through glomerulus.

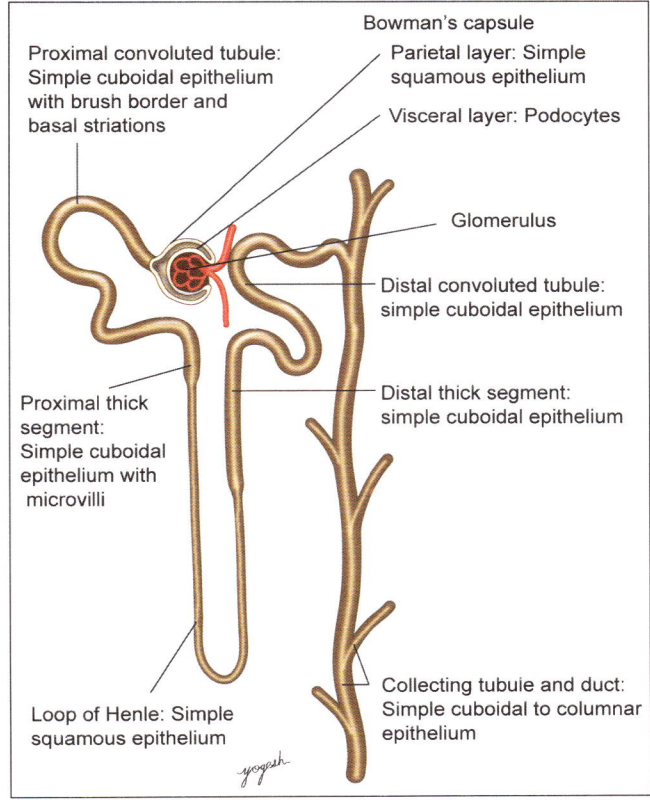

Fig. 20.4: Parts of nephron and corresponding lining epithelia.[Neet]

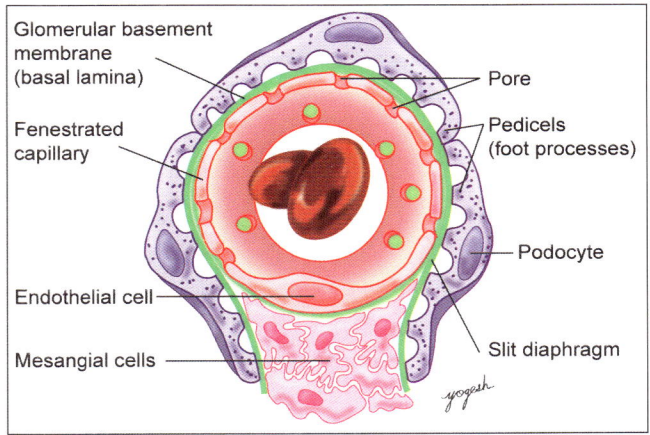

Fig. 20.5: Filtration apparatus of kidney.

Some Interesting Facts
- Basis for maintenance of blood pressure is formed by renin–angiotensin–aldosterone system.
- ACE inhibitors (enalapril, captopril) are useful in the treatment of hypertension.
- Proteins and RBCs cannot cross glomerular ultrafiltration barrier.
- In glomerulonephritis (inflammation of glomeruli), proteins and RBCs cross the filtration barrier and enter in urine.
- Proteinuria is the presence of proteins in urine.
- Hematuria is presence of RBCs in urine.

Box 20.4: Juxtaglomerular apparatus

Q. Write a short note on juxtaglomerular apparatus.

- Juxtaglomerular apparatus is a group of specialized cells near the vascular pole of renal corpuscle (Figs 20.6, 20.7 and Flowchart 20.3).
- It consists of juxtaglomerular cells, macula densa and extraglomerular mesangial cells (Lacis cells).

Juxtaglomerular cells (Flowchart 20.4)
- These are modified *smooth muscle cells* of wall of *afferent arteriole*.[Neet]
- Function: Secretion of *renin*.[Neet]

Macula densa
- These are specialized cells of *distal convoluted tubule* that lie adjacent to afferent and efferent arteriole.
- Macula densa cells are narrow, *columnar* and crowded cells (other cells of DCT are cuboidal).[Neet]
- *Nuclei* of these cells are *crowded* and overlapping; hence, these cells are called macula densa.

Lacis cells or extraglomerular mesangial cells
- Mesangial cells near the juxtaglomerular cells modify to form Lacis cells.
- These cells have *lace-like network forming processes*.
- These cells show receptors for angiotensin II and probably regulate glomerular filtration rate.

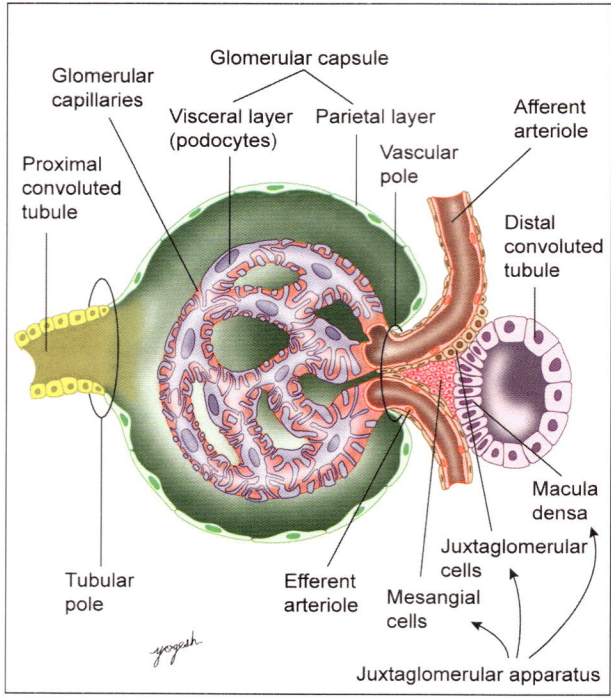

Fig. 20.6: Structure of renal corpuscle and JG apparatus.

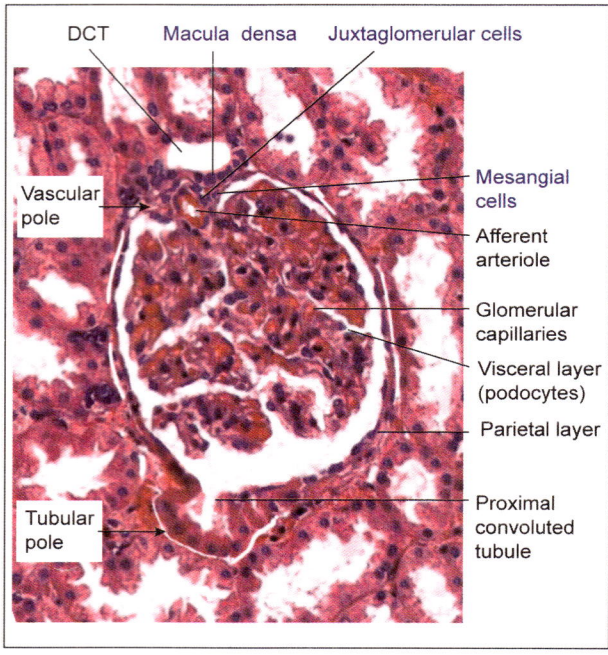

Fig. 20.7: Photomicrograph. Structure of renal corpuscle.

Flowchart 20.3: Juxtaglomerular apparatus

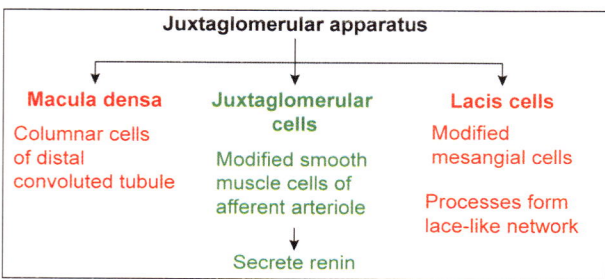

Flowchart 20.4: Role of JG cells

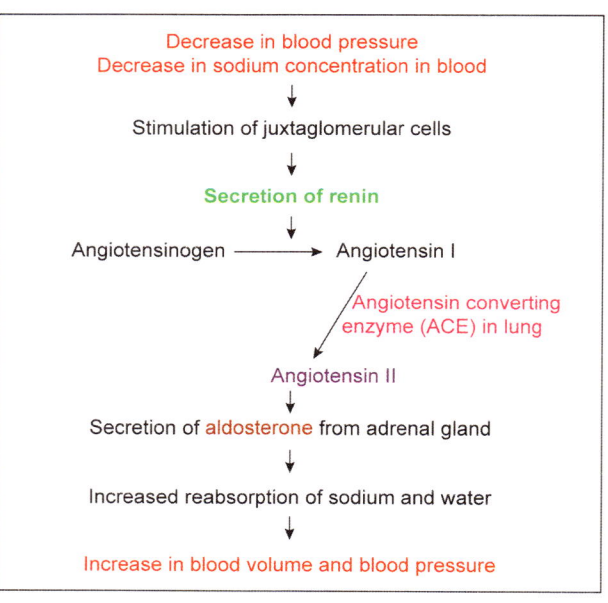

Renal Tubule

- Renal tubule consists of proximal convoluted tubule (PCT), proximal straight tubule, loop of Henle, distal straight tubule, and distal convoluted tubule (DCT) (Figs 20.4 and 20.8).
- Renal tubule receives glomerular filtrate from Bowman's capsule at PCT and continues at DCT with collecting tubules.
- Renal tubule is lined with simple (single-layered) epithelium.

Proximal convoluted tubule (40–60 μm in diameter)

- It receives ultrafiltrate from urinary pole of Bowman's capsule.
- It is lined by *simple cuboidal epithelium with brush border*, central spherical nucleus, and pink (eosinophilic) cytoplasm.
- Electron microscopy: Following are the features of cells of PCT:[Neet]
  - *Brush border:* These are long, closely packed straight *microvilli.*
  - *Tight junctions:* They are present on apical portion of cells.
  - *Basal striations:* Longitudinally oriented mitochondria give basal striated appearance.

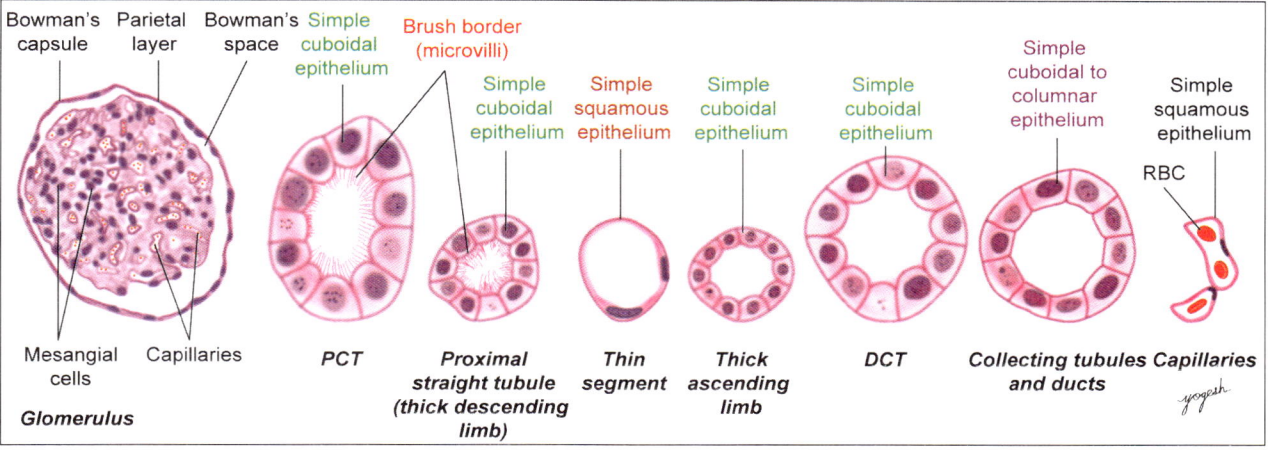

Fig. 20.8: Different components of nephron (practice figure). PCT, proximal convoluted tubule; DCT, distal convoluted tubules; RBC, red blood cell.[Neet]

- Note: Brush border and basal striations increase the surface area of cells.
- *Functions:* Reabsorption of 80% of ultrafiltrate (about 150 L per day)
- In PCT, Na^+/K^+-ATPase pump and aquaporin (AQP 1) proteins are mainly responsible for reabsorption of water.
- PCT also reabsorbs amino acids, glucose, and polypeptides

Proximal straight tubule (thick descending limb of loop of Henle)
- It connects PCT and loop of Henle.
- Some authors consider proximal straight tubule as part of PCT and some as thick descending limb of loop of Henle.
- Cells of proximal straight tubule are shorter than that of PCT. These cells have less developed brush border, basal and lateral foldings and fewer mitochondria than PCT.

Thin segment of loop of Henle (ansa nephoni)
- Length of thin segment of loop of Henle is variable according to nephron. It is longest in juxtamedullary nephrons, whereas shortest in cortical nephrons.
- *H&E staining:* Thin segment of loop of Henle is lined by simple squamous (even low cuboidal) epithelium with few microvilli, pale staining cytoplasm, and bulging elongated nucleus (Note: It resembles a venule in cross section).

Distal straight tubule (thick ascending limb)
- It is the part of ascending limb of loop of Henle.
- It is lined by large cuboidal cells with light pink (eosinophilic) cytoplasm and apically located nuclei.

Distal convoluted tubule (DCT)
- DCT is about one third long as that of PCT.
- DCT is lined by simple cuboidal epithelium with centrally placed spherical nuclei (without brush border).[Neet]
- Functions: Its main function is reabsorption of Na^+, secretion of K^+, and reabsorption of bicarbonate ions (that makes urine acidic). DCT works under the control of aldosterone in increasing the absorption of Na^+ ions.

Some Interesting Facts
- The differences between PCT and DCT are listed in Table 20.1.
- Thin segment of loop of Henle shows four types (I to IV) of epithelial cells but their specific functions are not yet clear.
- Thin ascending limb of loop of Henle is impermeable to water.[MCQ]

Collecting Tubules and Ducts
- Collecting tubules (40–50 μm in diameter) begin in cortex as a continuation of DCT and proceed to medullary rays.
- In the medullary ray, collecting tubules join to form collecting ducts.
- These collecting ducts run toward the apex of pyramid. They join to form *papillary duct of Bellini* (200 μm).[Neet] [Lorenzo Bellini, 1643–1704, Italian physician and anatomist]. Duct of Bellini opens on the free surface of papilla.
- *H&E staining:* Circular crosssection of collecting tubules and ducts show clear outline of cells. This

Q. List the differences PCT and DCT.

Table 20.1: Differences between proximal convoluted tubule and distal convoluted tubule (Fig. 20.9)^Viva

Characteristics	PCT	DCT
Length	Longer	Shorter (one third of PCT)
Diameter	Wide (60 μm)	Narrow (15–30 μm)
Epithelium	Simple cuboidal or low columnar	Simple cuboidal
H&E staining of cytoplasm	Dark pink stained than DCT	Light pink stained
Nuclei in each cross-section of tube	Fewer	More, equally spaced
Lumen of tubule	Star-shaped, irregular	Circular or oval, regular
Brush border	Present	Absent^Neet

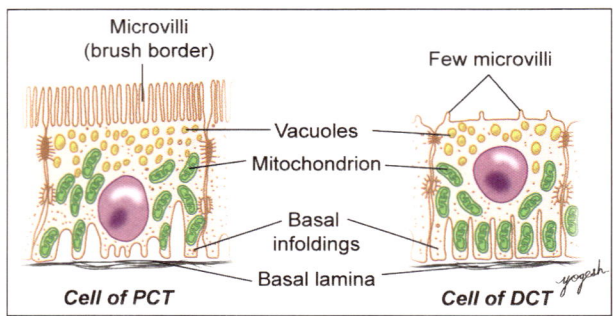

Fig. 20.9: Ultrastructural differences between cells of proximal and distal convoluted tubules.

distinguishes them from convoluted tubules (irregular sections and indistinct cell outlines).^Viva, MCQ

- Collecting tubules are lined by *simple cuboidal* epithelium without brush border but it becomes *columnar* as the size of duct increases.
- Cell types: Collecting tubules and ducts are lined by
  - *Light (clear) cells:* These are called CD cells (collecting duct cells). These cells have single cilium and few short microvilli.^MCQ Theses cells have ADH-regulated water reabsorption aquaporin-2 (AQP-2) channels. Defective *AQP 2 gene* causes *diabetes insipidus.*^Neet These cells show basal infoldings.
  - *Dark cells (intercalated cells):* These are few. These cells do not show basal infoldings.

Renal Microvasculature

- Each kidney is supplied by *renal artery* (Fig. 20.10 and Flowchart 20.5).
- Renal artery divides to form *lobar* and then *interlobar* arteries.

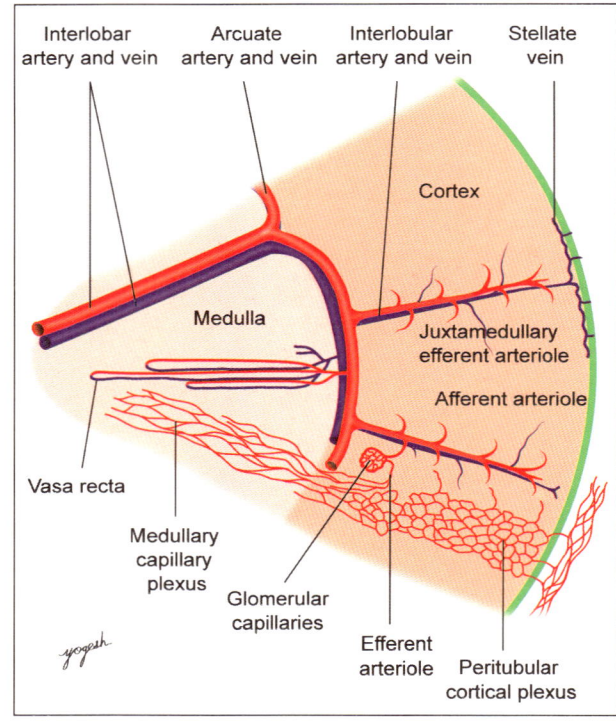

Fig. 20.10: Blood supply of kidney.

- Interlobar artery dive to form *arcuate artery* along the base of pyramids.
- Arcuate arteries form *interlobular arteries* that traverse cortex toward capsule.
- Interlobular arteries give *afferent arterioles*.
- Afferent arterioles give rise to a network of *glomerular capillaries* that unite to form *efferent arteriole*.
- Efferent arterioles form second set of capillaries called *peritubular capillaries*.
- Efferent arterioles form the juxtamedullary glomeruli that form *vasa recta* and help in *countercurrent exchange system*.

Flowchart 20.5: Blood supply of kidney

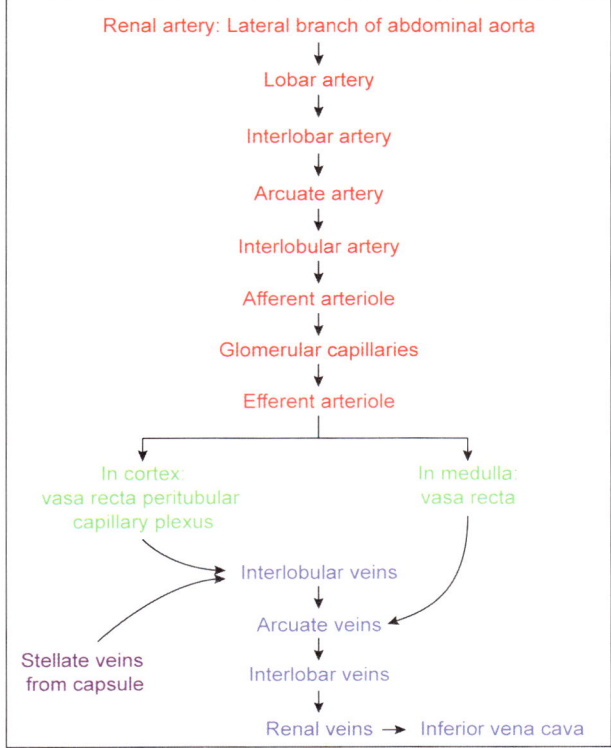

- Peritubular capillaries in cortex drain into *interlobular vein*, and later into *arcuate vein, interlobar veins* and finally *renal veins*.
- Capsule drains into *stellate veins* and finally into *interlobar veins*.

Summary (Examination Guide) (Figs 20.2 and 20.8)
- Kidney is covered by a connective tissue capsule.
- Kidney has outer cortex and inner medulla.
- Kidney shows presence of renal corpuscles and renal tubules.

Renal corpuscle consists of the following:
- Glomerulus: tuft of capillaries
- Bowman's capsule: It has outer *parietal layer* (simple squamous epithelium) and inner *visceral layer* (made up of podocytes). *Bowman's space* lies between visceral and parietal layers (urinary space).

Renal tubules consist of the following:
- *Proximal convoluted tubules:* They have star-shaped indistinct lumen lined with *simple cuboidal epithelium* with prominent *brush border*.
- *Proximal straight tubule:* It is lined with *simple cuboidal epithelium* and has less developed microvilli.

- *Loop of Henle:*
  - Thin segment of loop of Henle is lined with *simple squamous epithelium.*
  - Thick segment of loop of Henle is lined with *cuboidal epithelium.*
- *Distal convoluted tubules:* They have regular oval/round lumen lined by *simple cuboidal epithelium* (no brush border).
- *Collecting tubules and ducts:* DCT continues as collecting tubules and later as ducts that finally open on the surface of renal pyramids.
- Collecting tubules and ducts are lined by *simple cuboidal to columnar epithelium.*
- Cortex and medulla show numerous sections of blood vessels.

URETERS

- Ureter is a *mucomuscular tube* that carries urine from renal pelvis to urinary bladder.
- Length: 25–35 cm.
- Lumen: star-shaped.
- Wall of ureter has the following layers (Figs 20.11, 20.12 and Flowchart 20.6):
  - Inner mucous membrane layer
  - Middle smooth muscle layer
  - Outer adventitial (fibrous coat) layer

Mucous Membrane

Mucous membrane consists of the following layers:
- *Epithelial lining* is transitional epithelium (4–5 cell thick).
- *Lamina propria:* Connective tissue layer.
- Mucosa shows numerous longitudinal folds; hence, the lumen has a *star-shaped* appearance.

Smooth Muscle Coat

- Smooth muscles are arranged in three layers: inner longitudinal, middle circular and outer longitudinal. These layers are not distinctly marked from each other.
- Outer longitudinal muscle layer is present only in lower two-thirds of ureter.

Flowchart 20.6: Histology of ureter

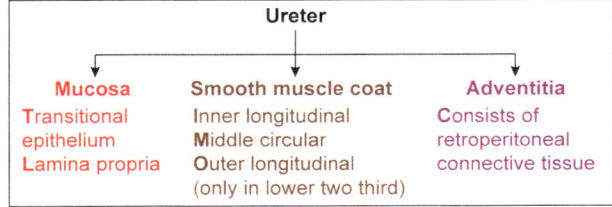

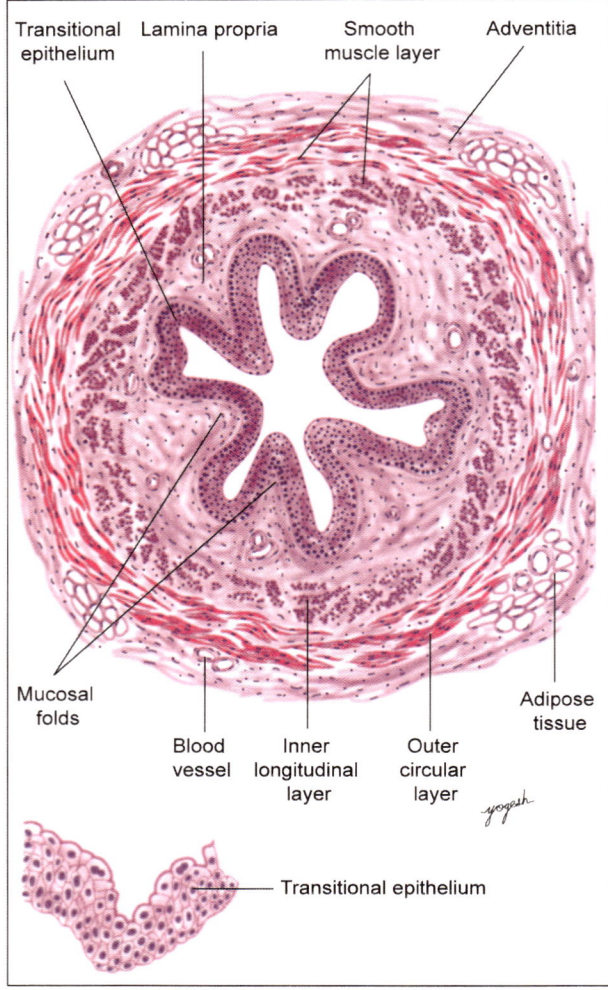

Fig. 20.11: Histology of transverse section of ureter (practice figure).

Adventitia

- Ureter is embedded in retroperitoneal connective tissue that forms a layer of adventitia.
- Adventitia contains adipose tissue, blood vessels, nerves, and lymphatics.

Summary (Examination Guide)

- Ureter is mucomuscular tube with star-shaped lumen.
- It has three layers
  1. Inner mucous membrane: It is lined by transitional epithelium and lamina propria (shows longitudinal folding).*Viva*
  2. Middle smooth muscle layer having inner longitudinal, middle circular, and outer longitudinal layers.
  3. Outer adventitia: Connective tissue coat having blood vessels, nerves, and lymphatics.

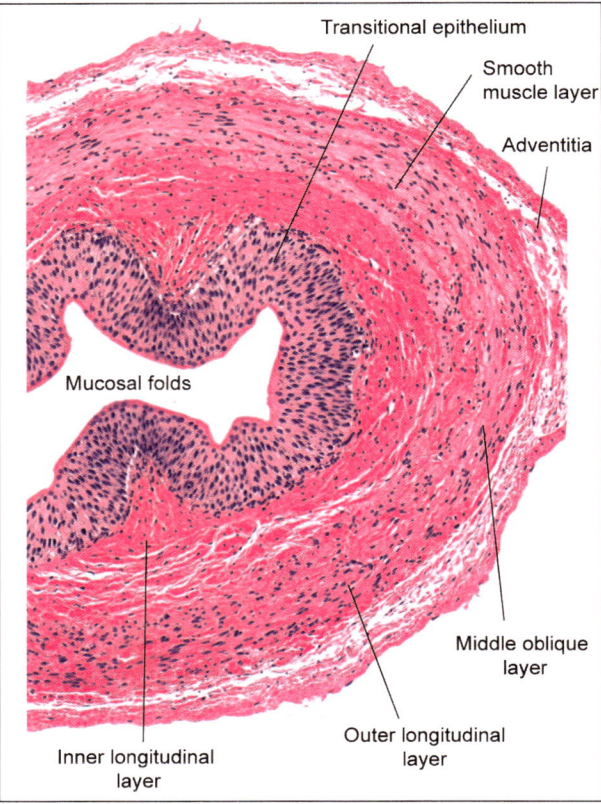

Fig. 20.12: Photomicrograph. Histology of transverse section of lower part of ureter (high magnification, H&E stain).

Some Interesting Facts

- Arrangement of muscle in gut is inner circular and outer longitudinal and reverse in ureter.*Viva*
- In longitudinal section of smooth muscles, nuclei look round, whereas in transverse section, nuclei look elongated or spindle-shaped.
- Apical layer of transitional cells may have two nuclei (binucleate).*MCQ*
- Ureter passes obliquely through bladder wall; hence, on bladder contraction during micturition, ureteric openings get compressed and it prevents reflux of urine in ureters.

URINARY BLADDER

- It is a mucomuscular bag that functions as a reservoir of urine.
- It receives urine from two ureteric openings and expels the urine into urethra.
- The wall of urinary bladder has three layers (Figs 20.13, 20.14 and Flowchart 20.7):
  – Inner mucous layer

Urinary System

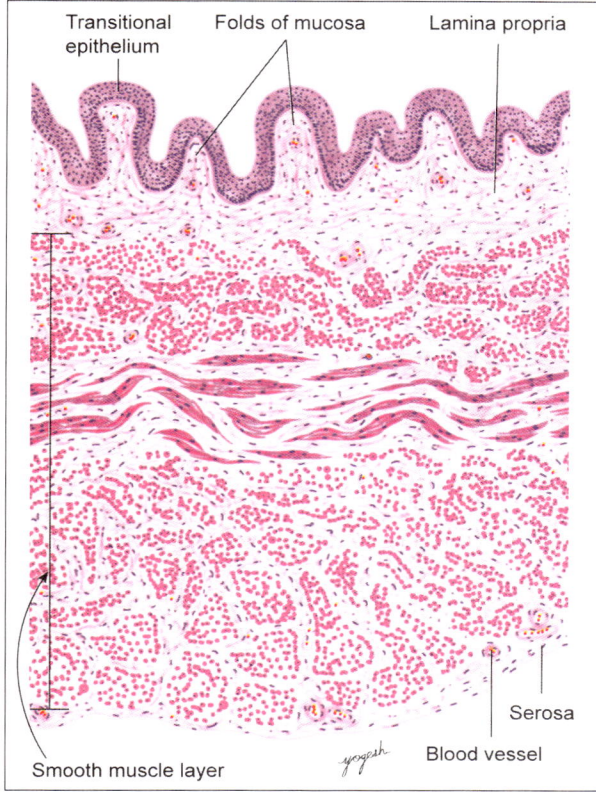

Fig. 20.13: Histology of transverse section of urinary bladder (practice figure).

Flowchart 20.7: Histology of urinary bladder

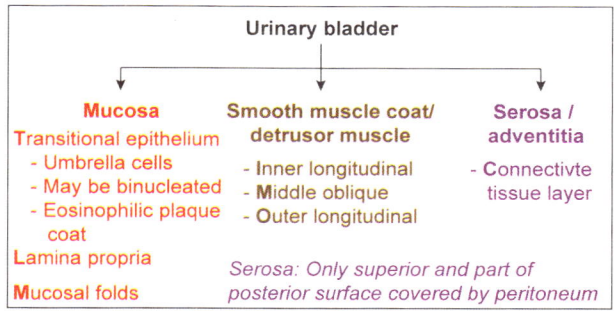

- Middle thick smooth muscle coat
- Outer serous layer

Mucous Membrane

- Interior of urinary bladder is lined by *transitional epithelium.*[MCQ] It shows apical dome-shaped (umbrella) cells on luminal surface. Some of these cells may be binucleated. In empty bladder, the cells of transitional epithelium are cuboidal in shape and bulge into the lumen.
- *Transmission electron microscopy:* Superficial cells are covered by thick plaques (modified area of apical plasma membrane). Plaque takes dark eosinophilic stains.[Viva]

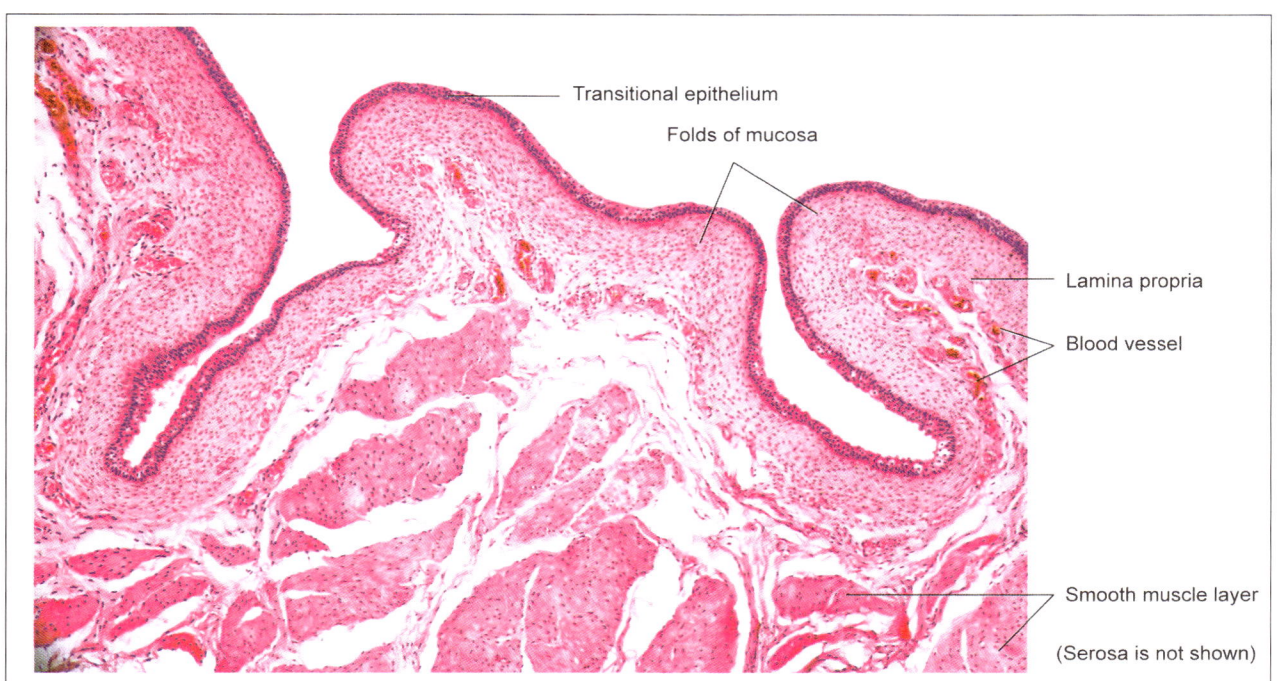

Fig. 20.14: Photomicrograph. Histology of transverse section of urinary bladder (low magnification, *H&E* stain).

- *Lamina Propria:* Transitional epithelium rests on thick coat of lamina propria (loose connective tissue).
- *Mucosal folds:* Empty bladder shows numerous mucosal folds that disappear on distention of bladder.
- Thickness of transitional epithelium in empty bladder may range up to six cell-layered and on distention, it may reduce to three cell-layered because of stretching of cells.

Muscle Coat/Detrusor Muscle

- Urinary bladder has **thick** muscle coat that forms a meshwork (fibers running in all directions).
- Usually, inner and outer layers are arranged longitudinally, and middle fibers run obliquely.
- At the junction of bladder with urethra, smooth muscle fibers are arranged circularly to form *sphincter vesicae.*

Serous Layer

- External surface of bladder is covered by connective tissue as follows:
  - Only superior surface and part of posterior surface is covered by peritoneum (serosa).
  - Rest of the surfaces are covered by adventitia.
- *Note:* In the region of *trigone* (smooth area), the mucosa is thin and firmly adherent to muscle coat.[Neet] Trigone is derived from absorption of mesonephric ducts, whereas remaining bladder form cloaca.[Neet]

Clinical Correlation

- **Ectopia vesicae** is a developmental deficiency of anterior abdominal wall and anterior wall of urinary bladder. In this condition, interior of bladder is exposed.
- **Cystitis:** It is inflammation of urinary bladder.
- **Bladder stones:** Urinary stones may develop in urinary bladder because of crystallization of urinary waste products.

URETHRA

- Urethra is *mucomuscular* tube that carries urine from urinary bladder to the exterior.
- Male urethra (20 cm) is longer than female urethra (4 cm).
- Urethra consists of three coats (Flowchart 20.8)
  - Inner *mucous membrane*
  - Middle *submucosa*
  - Outer *muscle layer*

Mucous Membrane

- Urethra is mostly lined by *pseudostratified columnar epithelium* except at the following sites (Figs 22.7 and 22.8):[Neet]
  - Adjacent to urinary bladder – lined by transitional epithelium
  - Near external opening – lined by stratified squamous epithelium

Submucosa

- It consists of loose connective tissue.

Muscle Coat

- It consists of inner longitudinal and outer circular coat of smooth muscle fibers.
- Terminal part of urethra is surrounded by striated muscle fibers that form *external urethral sphincter.*

Flowchart 20.8: Histology of urethra

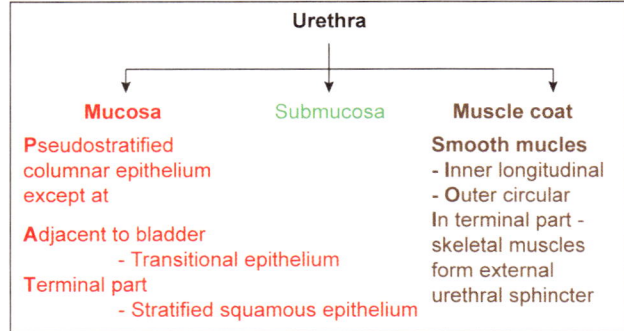

CHAPTER 21

Male Reproductive System I: Testis, Epididymis, Ductus Deferens

Chapter Outline
- Testis
- Spermatogenesis
- Epididymis
- Ductus deferens

Competency achievement: The student should be able to:
AN52.2 Describe and identify the microanatomical features of male reproductive system: Testis, epididymis, vas deferens

INTRODUCTION

- Male reproductive system consists of (Fig. 21.1)
  - Pair of testes
  - Genital ducts (epididymis, ductus deferens, and ejaculatory ductus)
  - Accessory sex glands: Seminal vesicles, prostate, and bulbourethral glands
  - Male urethra
  - Penis
- Main functions of male reproductive organs are
  - Production of sperms (spermatogenesis)
  - Production of sex steroid hormones (testosterone)
  - Helps in deposition of sperms in the female reproductive tract

TESTIS

- Testes are paired ovoid masses (organs) that lie in the sac of scrotum.
- Testis develops from intermediate mesoderm of genital ridge in the abdomen and migrated primordial germ cells of yolk sac. Later, testis descends to lie in the scrotum.

Some Interesting Facts

- Scrotum helps to maintain *2–3°C* less temperature than the body temperature. This is essential for spermatogenesis, but not for testosterone production.
- Presence of Y chromosome/*SRY gene* (sex-determining region of Y chromosome) is essential for differentiation of testis. The SRY gene codes *testis-determining factor*.
- Leydig cells produce testosterone, whereas Sertoli cells produce Mullerian inhibiting factor (that inhibits the development of female reproductive organs).*Neet*
- Cryptorchidism (undescended testis) can result in loss of sperm production. Cryptorchidism can be treated with orchidopexy by 2 years of age to prevent irreversible histological changes.*Neet*
- Testicular artery and surrounding pampiniform plexus of veins circulate, blood in opposite directions and maintains the required temperature for spermatogenesis.

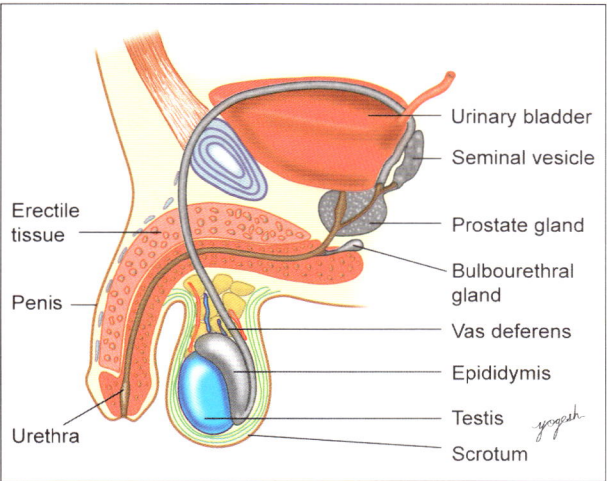

Fig. 21.1: Parts of male reproductive system.

Structure of Testis (Figs 21.2 to 21.4)

- *Tunica albuginea:* Testis is surrounded by thick connective tissue capsule called *tunica albuginea.*
- *Tunica vasculosa:* It is a vascular connective tissue coat that lies just deep to the tunica albuginea.

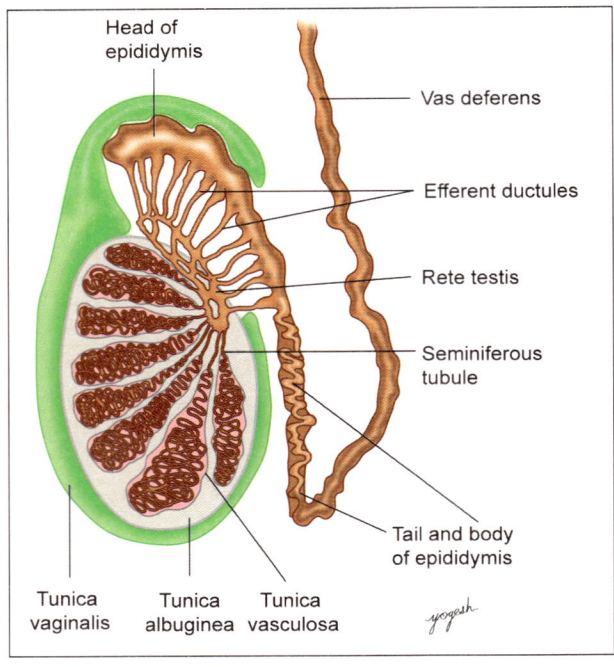

Fig. 21.2: Parts of male reproductive system

- *Connective tissue septa* and *lobules:* Connective tissue septa arising from the capsule, divide the testis into more than 250 incomplete lobules.
- *Mediastinum testis:* It is the thickened part of tunica albuginea that gives passage to vessels and ducts of testis.
- *Seminiferous tubules:* Each lobule of testis consists of 1–4 highly coiled seminiferous tubules.
- Each seminiferous tubule is surrounded by connective tissue stroma.
- *Leydig (interstitial) cells* lie in connective tissue stroma.
- *Straight tubules* (tubuli recti): It is the terminal straight part of the seminiferous tubules that lie near mediastinum testis.
- *Rete testis:* Straight tubules form a network in the mediastinum. This network is called *rete testis.*
- *Efferent ductules:* Rete testis give rise to 12–30 efferent ductules at its upper end. Efferent ductules enter the epididymis (highly coiled tubules) that later continue as ductus deferens.
- Passage of sperm in the male reproductive tract is listed in Flowchart 21.1.

Microscopic Structure of Testis

Seminiferous Epithelium (Fig. 21.5)

- Seminiferous tubules are lined by *complex stratified epithelium* called seminiferous epithelium.

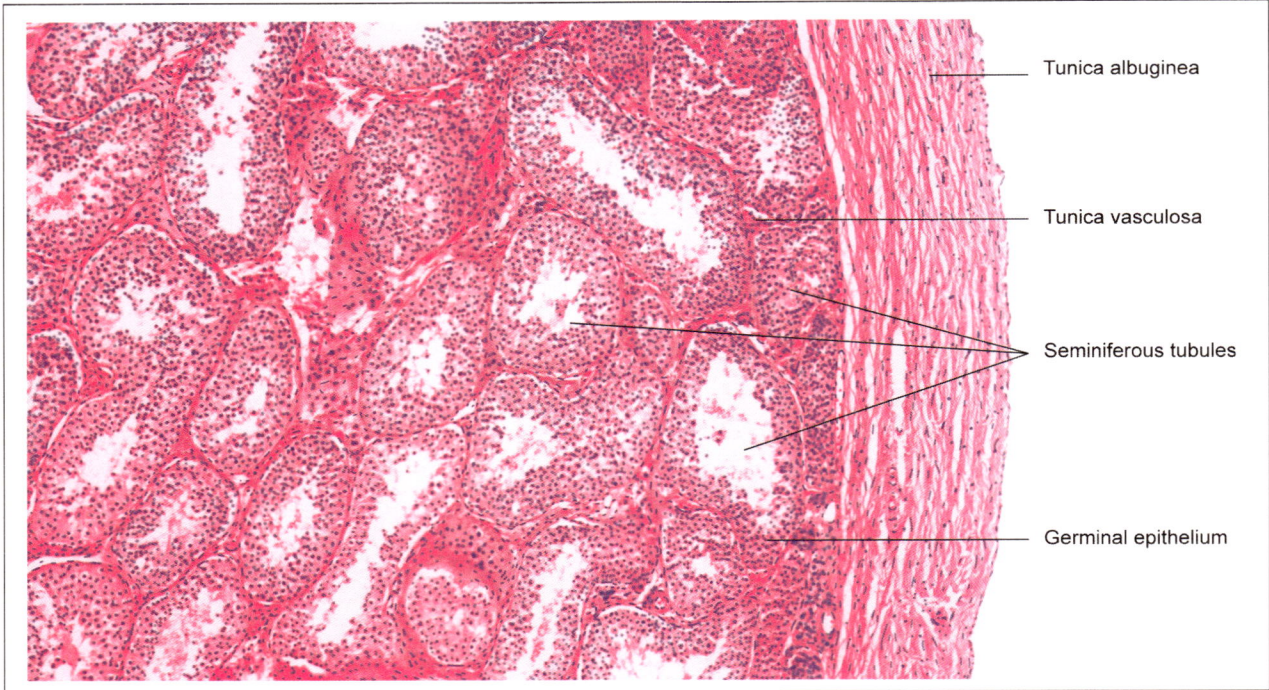

Fig. 21.3: Photomicrograph. Histology of testis (low magnification, *H&E* stain).

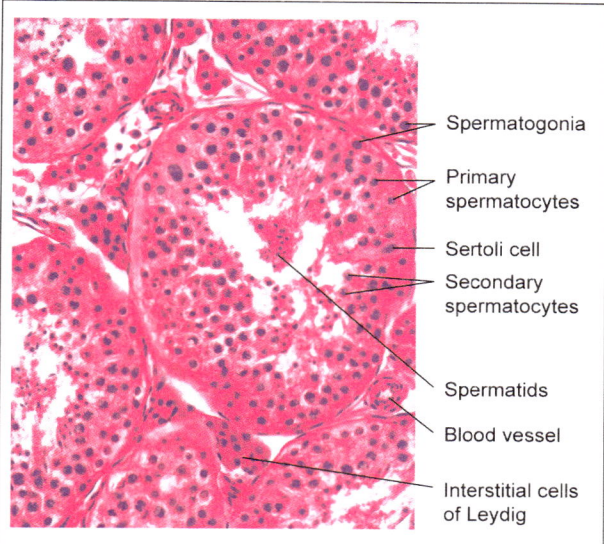

Fig. 21.4: Photomicrograph. Seminiferous tubule (high magnification, H&E stain).

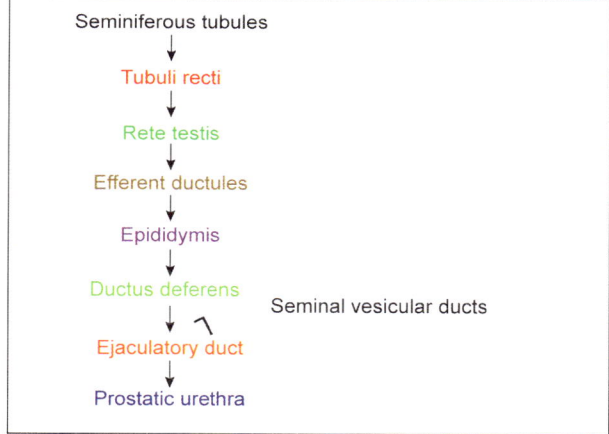

Flowchart 21.1: Passage of sperms

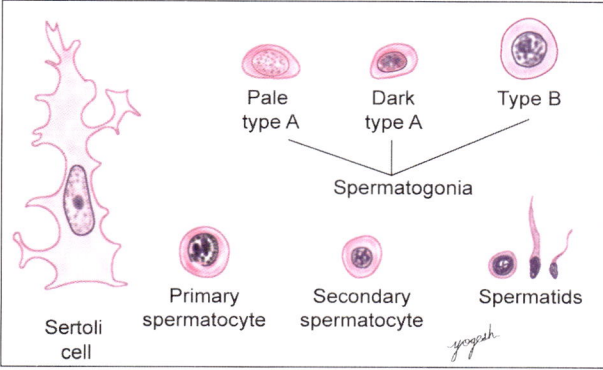

Fig. 21.5: Types of cells in seminiferous tubules (high magnification, practice figure).

- It consists of two types of cells
  1. Sertoli cells
  2. Spermatogenic cells
- Each seminiferous tubule is approximately 50 cm long and 150–200 µm in diameter.
- *Sertoli cells (sustentacular cells)*
  - These are supporting cells [Enrico Sertoli, 1842–1910, Italian physiologist and histologist].
  - They are columnar or pyramidal in shape with light staining euchromatic nucleus. *Note:* On H&E staining, these cells cannot be distinguished.
  - Sertoli cells represent the true epithelium of seminiferous tubules.*Viva*
  - *Charcot-Böttcher inclusion bodies:* These are inclusion bodies found in the basal cytoplasm of Sertoli cells. They consist of microfilaments. [Jakob Ernst Arthur Böttcher, 1831–1889, German pathologist and anatomist; Jean-Martin Charcot, 1825–1893, French anatomical pathologist].
  - *Sertoli cell-to-Sertoli cell* junctional complex form *blood-testis barrier* that isolates haploid germ cells from the immune system.*Neet*
  - Sertoli cells have follicle stimulating hormone/FSH receptors on their surface. FSH activates Sertoli cells that result in secretion of anti-Müllerian hormone.*Neet*
  - Functions
    - Secretion of *androgen-binding protein* (ABP): It helps to bind and increase concentration of testosterone in seminiferous tubules (essential for spermatogenesis).
    - Secretion of *inhibin* that inhibits FSH release by adenohypophysis (anterior pituitary).
    - Secretion of *plasminogen activator* and transferrin (iron-transporting protein).
    - Support and nourishes germ cells.
    - Phagocytosis of residual bodies after spermiogenesis.
- **Spermatogenic cells** (Germ cells) (Figs 21.5 and 21.6)
  - These are derived from primordial germ cells.
  - They replicate and form various stages of spermatogenesis.
  - They are arranged in stratified manner from basal lamina to luminal area as follows: Spermatogonia, spermatocytes, spermatids, and spermatozoa.
  - In any one cross-section of seminiferous tubules, all these cells may not be seen.
  - *Spermatogenic cycle:* It is a wave of germ cell maturation that reverses along the length of seminiferous tubule.*Viva*

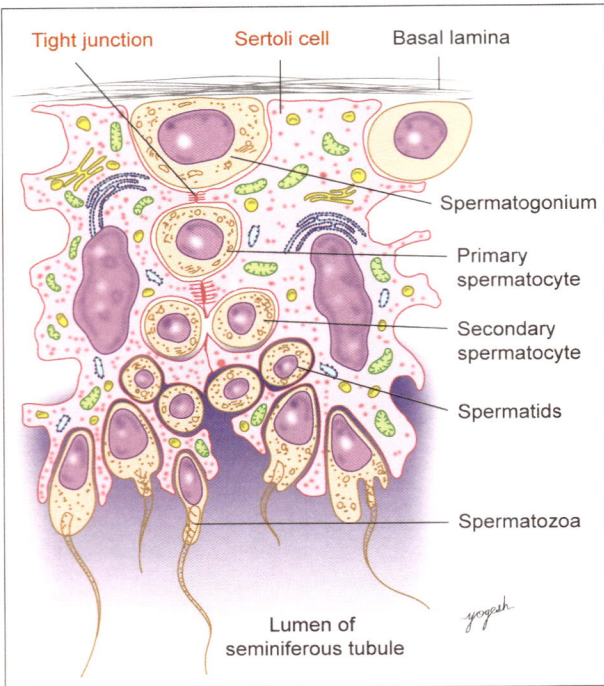

Fig. 21.6: Ultrastructure of Sertoli cell and its relation with various germ cells.

Lamina (Tunica) Propria

- It is a thin layer of vascular connective tissue that surrounds each seminiferous tubule.
- Lamina propria do not contain fibroblasts.^MCQ
- It consists of few layers of contractile *myoid* or *peritubular cells,* external to basal lamina of seminiferous tubules.
- Rhythmic contractions of myoid cells help in expulsion of sperms and seminiferous tubule secretions.
- **Leydig (interstitial) cells** [Franz von Leydig, 1821–1908, German anatomist]
  - Leydig cells lie in the connective tissue between adjacent seminiferous tubules.
  - These are large, polygonal *eosinophilic* cells with round nucleus.
  - Leydig cells have luteinizing hormone (LH) receptors. LH stimulates Leydig cell for production of testosterone.^Neet
  - Leydig cells secrete steroid. These cells have foamy eosinophilic cytoplasm, because Leydig cells have well developed smooth endoplasmic reticulum. Leydig cells also have lipofuscin pigments.
  - Function: *Testosterone synthesis.*
  - *Crystals of Reinke:* These are rod-shaped cytoplasmic crystals (unknown function) present in Leydig cells.^Neet [Friedrich Reinke 1862–1919, German anatomist]
  - Leydig cells are active in the following phases:
    1. Embryonic life: Leydig cells are active in embryonic life (by 5 months) till birth.
    2. After puberty: Leydig cells get reactivated by gonadotropic hormones at puberty and remain active throughout the life.

Spermatogenesis (Flowchart 21.2)

- Spermatogenesis is the formation of spermatozoa from spermatogonia.
- Spermatogenesis occurs in three phases: Spermatocytosis, meiosis, and spermiogenesis.

Spermatocytosis

- It is the conversion of spermatogonia into primary spermatocyte.
- Human spermatogonia are classified into three types based on the appearance of nuclei in *H&E* staining as follows (Figs 21.5 and 21.6):
  - *Type A dark spermatogonia:* It has an ovoid nucleus with dark basophilic chromatin.
  - *Type A pale spermatogonia:* It has a spherical nucleus with clumsy chromatin and central nucleolus.
  - Type A dark spermatogonia (behave similar to stem cell) divide mitotically to form type A pale spermatogonia and later divide to form type B spermatogonia
  - *Type B spermatogonia* on mitosis form primary spermatocyte (46,XY). These are largest cells with a spherical nucleus. These cells occupy the middle region of seminiferous tubules.

Flowchart 21.2: Spermatogenesis.

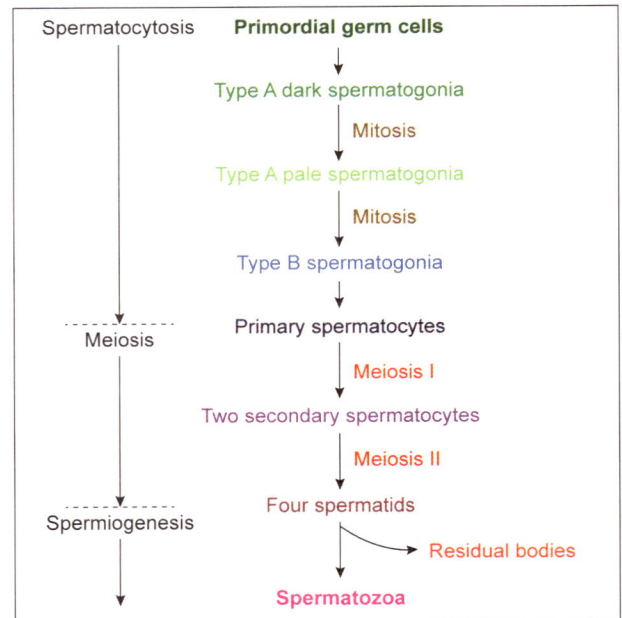

Meiosis (Spermatocyte) Phase

- It involves conversion of primary spermatocyte into spermatids (23,X and 23,Y).
- *Primary spermatocyte* on meiosis form two *secondary spermatocytes* that later undergo meiosis II to produce four spermatids (23,X; 23,X; 23,Y, and 23,Y).^{Neet}
- Each spermatid contains a single standard haploid DNA (1n).

Spermiogenesis (Spermatid Phase) (Fig. 21.7)

Q. Write a short note on spermiogenesis.

- Spermiogenesis is the process of metamorphosis of spermatids by which they get converted into a spermatozoon.
- Metamorphosis is the change in form of cell.
- Four phases of spermiogenesis are as follows:
  1. Golgi phase: Golgi complexes coalesce to form an acrosomal vesicle that determines the anterior pole of sperm. Centrioles migrate to posterior pole.
  2. Cap phase: Acrosomal vesicle covers anterior half of nucleus to form an acrosomal cap.
  3. Acrosome phase: Tail (flagellum) extends and nucleus condenses. Centriole modifies to form flagellum.
     Nine coarse fibrils develop from the centriole extend in tail. Mitochondria migrate in the middle piece.
     Part of tail covered by fibrous sheath forms principal piece, whereas distal to it forms the end piece of tail.
  4. Maturation phase: Most of the cytoplasm of spermatid is shed as *Raynaud residual body*. [Sertoli cell phagocytose residual bodies]. *Spermiation:* Finally, spermatozoa are released into lumen of seminiferous tubules. This is spermiation.

Structure of Mature Sperm

Q. Write a short note on structure of spermatozoa or sperm.

- Mature spermatozoa have head, neck, middle piece, and tail (Fig. 21.8).
- Length: 50–60 μm.
- Count: In a single ejaculum, 200–300 million sperms are emitted in a volume of 2.5 ml semen.

Head of Sperm

- It is pyriform (flattened and pointed).
- Acrosomal cap covers the anterior two-thirds of the nucleus. Acrosome contains digestive enzymes (hyaluronidase, acrosin) that help to break the outer wall of ovum.

Tail

- Tail of sperm is divided into neck, middle, and end piece (Pawlina W, Histology, 7th Ed.].
- *Neck* contains proximal centriole.
- *Middle piece* shows axial filament surrounded by spirally arranged mitochondrion.^{Neet}

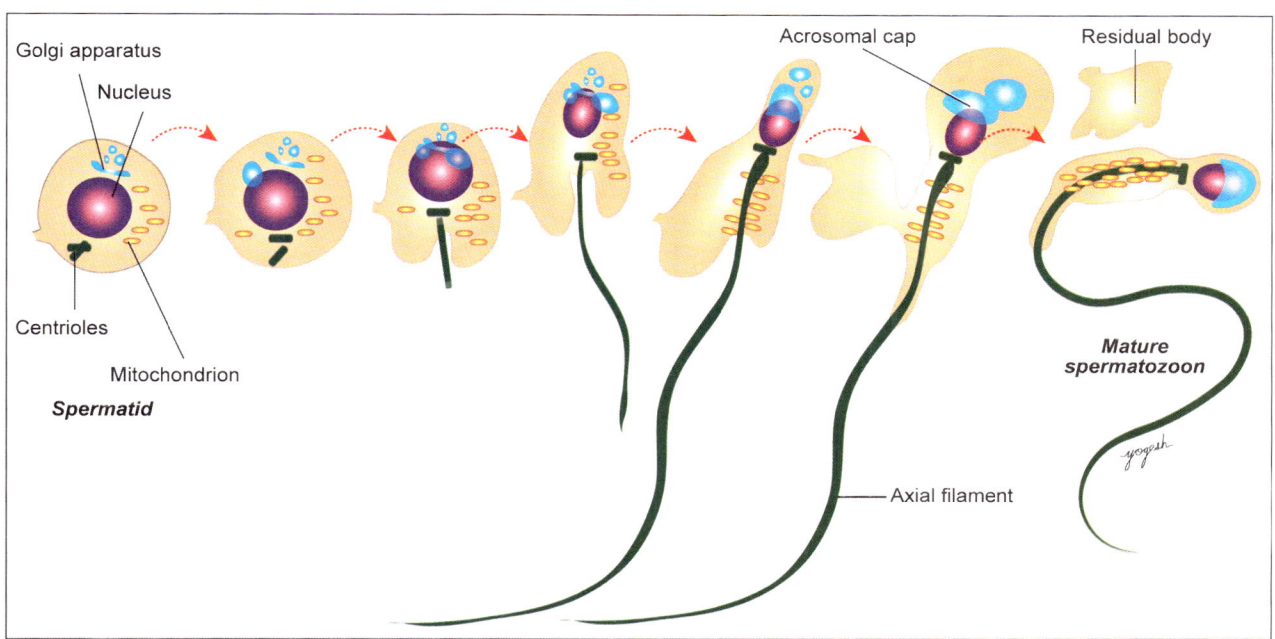

Fig. 21.7: Process of spermiogenesis (Source: Textbook of Human Embryology, Yogesh Sontakke, 1st Edn, CBS Publishers).

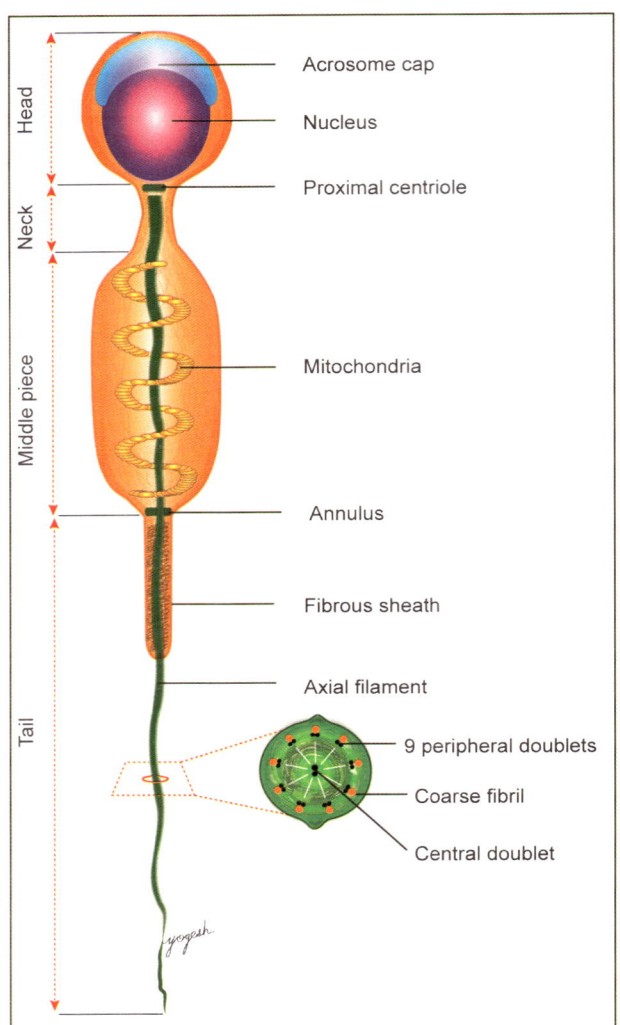

Fig. 21.8: Structure of sperm (Source: Textbook of Human Embryology, Yogesh Sontakke, 1st Edn, CBS Publishers).

- At the junction of middle piece with principal piece, distal centriole is present in the form of annulus (ring-like structure).
- *Principal piece* shows axial filament covered by a fibrous sheath. End piece has no fibrous covering over the axial filament.
- *Axial filament* (axonemal complex) consists of the central doublet of fibril surrounded by nine doublets of fine fibrils and nine coarse fibrils.

Maturation and Capacitation of Spermatozoa

- Sperms released from Sertoli cells are nonmotile. They get partial motility in epididymis.
- **Capacitation:** After ejaculation, sperms in the female reproductive tract undergo capacitation. It is the maturation of sperm. It involves removal of glycoprotein coat from sperm. It enhances sperm motility and makes the acrosome ready to release lysosomal enzymes.

Duct System of Testis

- Seminiferous tubules drain as follows:
  Seminiferous tubules → straight tubules → rete testis → efferent ductules → epididymis

Straight Tubule (Tubuli Recti)

- Short terminal part of seminiferous tubule forms straight tubules (tubuli recti).
- Their proximal part is lined by *simple columnar cells* and Sertoli cells, whereas distal part is lined by *simple cuboidal cells.*

Rete Testis

- It is a complex series of *anastomosing* tubules in mediastinum.
- They are lined by *low cuboidal* or *low columnar* cells with a *single flagellum.*[Neet]

Efferent Ductules

- Efferent ductules collect sperms from rete testis.
- It consists of 12–15 ducts.
- These are lined by *simple ciliated columnar epithelium* resting on thin lamina propria and circular smooth muscles.

Summary (Examination Guide)
(Flowchart 21.3, Figs 21.3, 21.4 and 21.9)

- Testis is covered by fibrous *tunica albuginea* and vascular *tunica vasculosa.*
- Septae divide the testis into approximately 250 *incomplete lobules.*
- Each lobule contains 1–3 highly coiled *seminiferous tubules* that are surrounded by lamina propria, blood vessels, lymphatics, and Leydig cells.
- *Seminiferous tubules* are lined by seminiferous epithelium with two types of cells: Spermatogenic cells (spermatogonia, spermatids, and sperms) and Sertoli cells.
- *Sertoli cells* are tall columnar cells that support development of spermatogenic cells.
- *Leydig (interstitial) cells* are polyhedral eosinophilic cells that lie in clusters and produce testosterone. These cells are epithelioid cells.[Neet] These cells contain Reinke's crystals and lipofuscin pigment.[Neet]
- Seminiferous tubules drain into straight tubules (lined by Sertoli cells) and then into rete testis (lined by simple cuboidal to columnar epithelium).

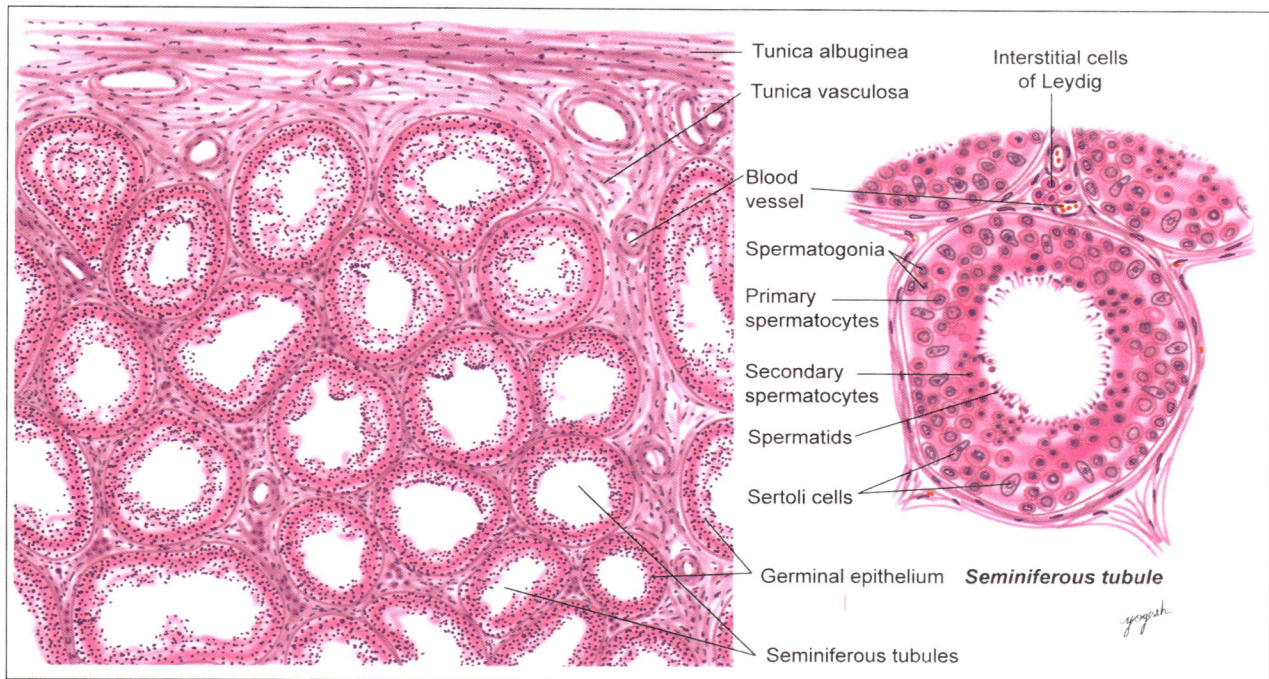

Fig. 21.9: Histology of testis (low magnification on left) and seminiferous tubule (high magnification on right, practice figure).

Flowchart 21.3: Histology of testis

```
                                    Testis
        ┌──────────────┬─────────────────┬─────────────────┬──────────────┐
    Coverings and   1-3 seminiferous    Interstitial/    Straight tubules
    lobules         tubules             Leydig cells     (lined by sertoli
                    in each lobule      - Polygonal      cells)
    Tunica                              cells with
    albuginea                           round nucleus
    Tunica         Spermatogonic   Sertoli cells  - Lie in clusters    Rete testis
    vasculosa      cells           - Large,         between            (lined by simple
                   - Spermatogonia   pyramidal      seminiferous       cuboidal to
    Incomplete       (type A dark,   cells          tubules            columnar cells)
    lobules          type A pale,  - Supporting
                     type B)         cells
                   - Spermatocytes - Removes
                     (Primary,       residual body
                     secondary)
                   - Spermatids,
                     spermatozoa
```

EPIDIDYMIS

- Epididymis is a crescent-shaped structure present along the posterior and superior surfaces of testis.
- Length: 7.5 cm.
- In epididymis, sperms acquire motility. *Viva, MCQ*
- Parts of epididymis: Head, body, and tail.
- Head is occupied by efferent ductules.
- Body and tail accommodate a single, highly coiled duct of epididymis
- *Duct of epididymis* (Flowchart 21.4, Figs 21.10 and 21.11)
  - Length: 4–6 cm.
  - Lining epithelium: *Pseudostratified columnar epithelium.* It has tall principal cells and short basal cells.
  - Principal cells have numerous, long modified microvilli called *stereocilia.*
  - *Halo cells:* These are few intraepithelial lymphocytes found in the epididymis. *Neet*

Flowchart 21.4: Histology of epididymis

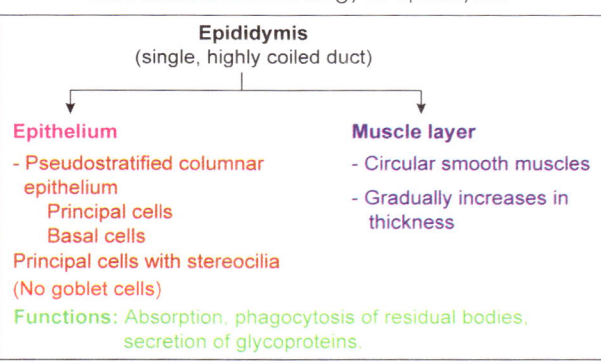

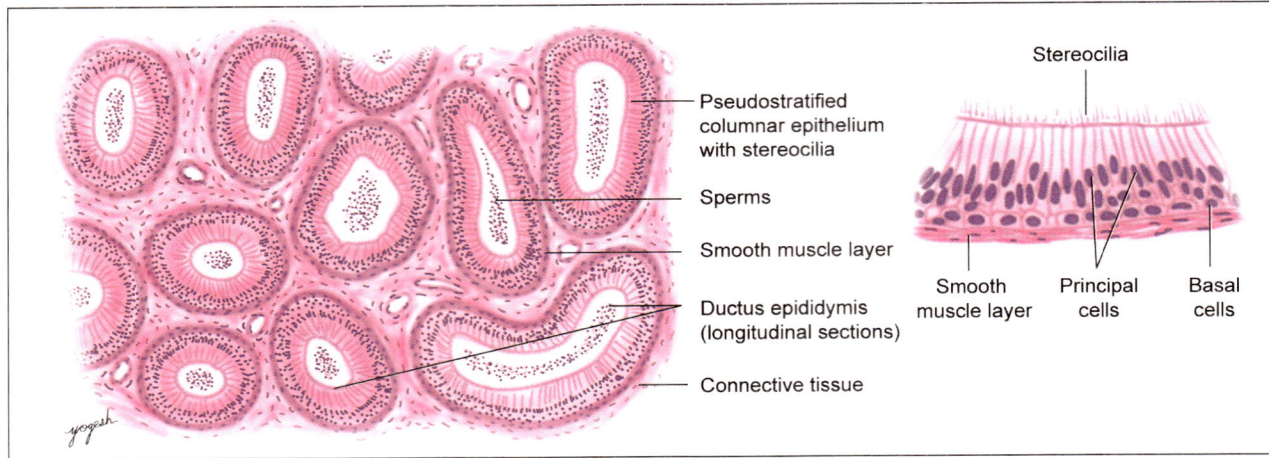

Fig. 21.10: Histology of epididymis (low magnification on left and high magnification on right, practice figure).

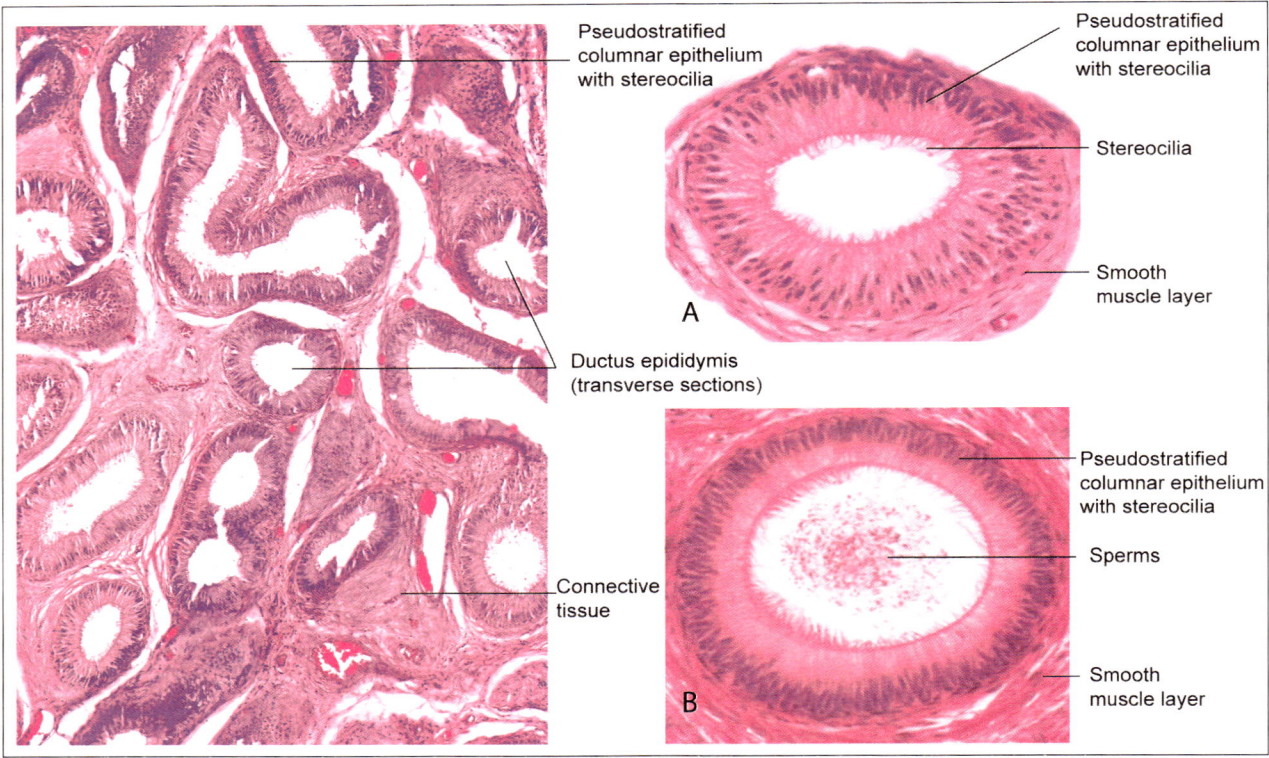

Fig. 21.11: Photomicrograph. Histology of epididymis (low magnification on left and A, section of epididymis without sperms; B, section of epididymis with sperms, high magnification on right, *H&E* stain).

- *Muscle coat:* It consists of thin layers of circular smooth muscle cells. They help in propulsion of sperms into the epididymis from efferent ductules and also help in ejaculation.

Functions
- Epididymis is a *reservoir of sperms.*
- Absorption of excess fluid secreted by testis.
- Phagocytosis of residual bodies and defective sperms.
- Secretion of surface-associated *decapacitation factor* (glycoprotein) that coats sperms. This factor is removed during capacitation of sperms.

> **Box 21.1:** Blood–testis barrier (Sertoli cell barrier)
>
> - Blood–testis barrier is a physical barrier between seminiferous tubules and blood vessels.
>
> **Structure**^{Neet}
> - Adjacent walls of Sertoli cells has junctional complexes that divide seminiferous epithelium into two compartments: Basal and luminal.^{Neet}
> - Basal compartment is present between basement membrane and junctional complexes. It contains spermatogonia and primary spermatocytes.
> - Adluminal (luminal) compartment: It lies toward the luminal side of junctional complexes. It contains secondary spermatocytes and spermatids.
> - Primary spermatocyte moves from basal to luminal compartment by breakage of luminal junctional complex and formation of new basal junctional complex.
>
> **Function**
> - Blood–testis barrier separate haploid germ cells from immune system and prevents formation of sperm-specific antibodies.

Clinical Correlation

- *Immotile cilia syndrome (Kartangener syndrome)* is an autosomal recessive disorder with impaired ciliary motility causing abnormal mucociliary clearance and immotile sperms (causing infertility). Cause: Genetic defect of dynein protein that is essential for the formation of cilia flagella.
- *Cryptorchidism and infertility:* For normal spermatogenesis, temperature should be ~2–3°C below the body temperature (that is, below 37°C). In undescended testis, germ cells cannot undergo cell division due to a higher temperature but testosterone production, on by Leydig cell continue normally. Hence, such cases become infertile (azoospermia) with normal secondary sexual characters because of testosterone.
- Factors affecting spermatogenesis
  1. Dietary factors
  2. Environmental factors
  3. Developmental disorders
  4. Infections
  5. Steroid hormones
  6. Toxic agents
  7. Ionizing radiations

DUCTUS DEFERENS/VAS DEFERENS

- Ductus deferens is the continuation of epididymis.
- It is a thick-walled *muscular tube* that extends from epididymis to ejaculatory duct.
- It ascends along the posterior pole of testis in the spermatic cord.
- In addition to vas deferens, the spermatic cord contains testicular artery, artery to vas deferens, cremaster muscle, pampiniform venous plexus, lymphatic vessels, and nerves.
- Terminal part of vas deferens is dilated and called ampulla.

Histology of Ductus Deferens

- Ductus deferens consists of three layers: Mucosa, muscle coat and adventitia (Figs 21.12 and 21.13).

Mucosa

- Lumen of vas deferens is star-shaped because of longitudinal folding of mucosa.
- Lining epithelium: Pseudostratified columnar epithelium with stereocilia.
- Epithelium shows two types of cells as follows:
  – Tall columnar cells with stereocilia: Extends from basal lamina to lumen of ductus deferens.

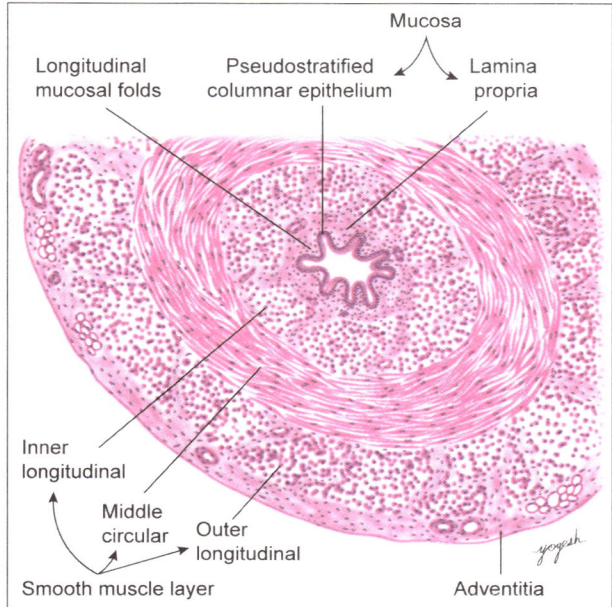

Fig. 21.12: Histology of transverse section of vas deferens (low magnification, practice figure).

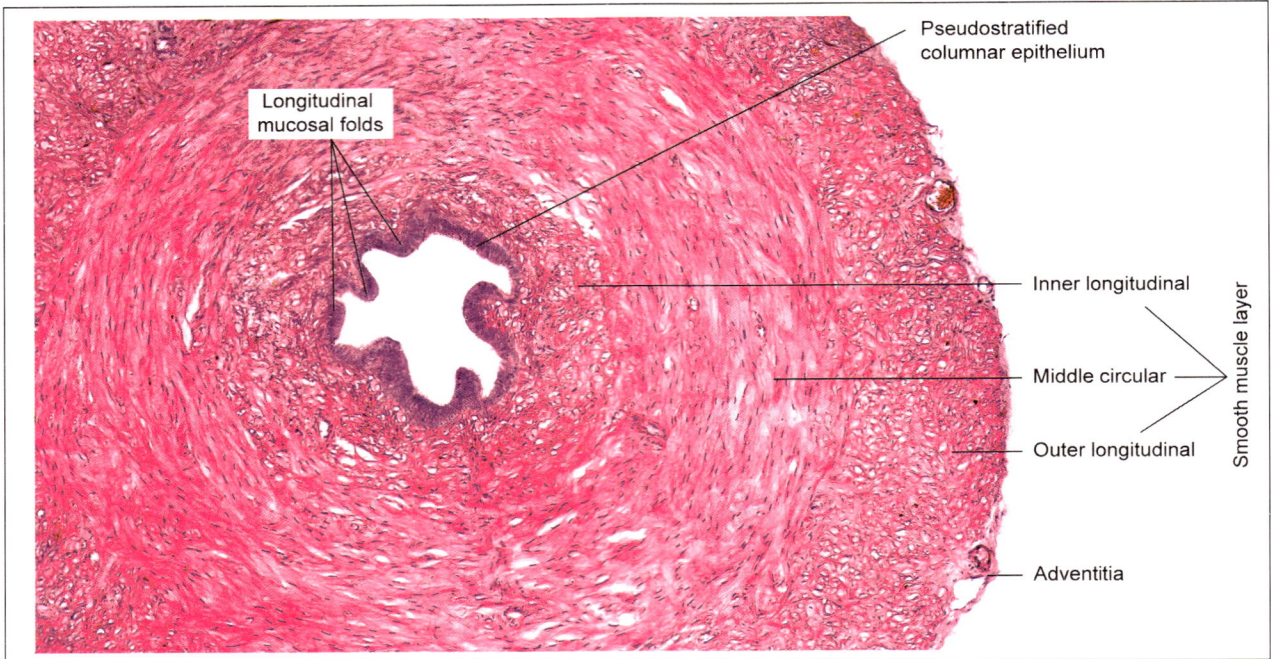

Fig. 20.13: Photomicrograph. Histology of transverse section of vas deferens (low magnification, H&E stain).

- Basal cells: Short, rest on basal lamina and acts like germinal cells.
- Lamina propria: Epithelium is surrounded by thin layer of connective tissue.

Muscle Coat

- It consists of three layers of smooth muscles as inner and outer longitudinal and thick middle circular layer.
- Muscle coat is much thicker than mucosa.
- Peristaltic contractions of muscle layer help in propulsion of sperms.

Adventitia

- It is made up of loose areolar tissue that contains blood vessels and nerves.

Functions

- Peristatic contractions of ductus deferens help in rapid propulsion of sperms during ejaculation.
- Note: It does not store the sperms.

Flowchart 21.5: Histology of vas deferens

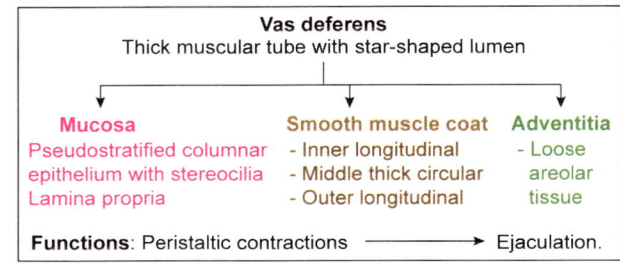

Summary (Examination Guide) (Flowchart 21.5)

Vas deferens is a thick-walled muscular tube (star-shaped lumen) having three layers:
- Mucosa: Lined by pseudostratified columnar epithelium with stereocilia
- Smooth muscle coat arranged as inner and outer longitudinal and middle thick circular layers
- Adventitia consists of loose areolar tissue.

Function: Ejaculation of sperms.

CHAPTER 22

Male Reproductive System II: Accessory Sex Glands and Penis

Chapter Outline
- Accessory sex glands
- Seminal vesicles
- Prostate gland
- Bulbourethral gland
- Penis

Competency achievement: The student should be able to:

AN52.2 Describe and identify the microanatomical features of prostate and penis

ACCESSORY SEX GLANDS

SEMINAL VESICLES

- Seminal vesicles are paired, elongated, and highly folded glands with irregular lumen.
- They are located at the base of urinary bladder.
- Each gland consists of a single folded duct (12–15 cm length, 3–4 mm diameter).
- Duct of seminal vesicle joins with ductus deferens to form ejaculatory duct.

Histology of Seminal Vesicle

- Wall of seminal vesicle consists of three layers: Mucosa, muscle layer, and adventitia (Fig. 22.1 and Flowchart 22.1).

Mucosa

- Mucosa of seminal vesicle is thrown into numerous folds that form many crypts and cavities (chambers). However, these crypts and cavities communicate with the lumen.
- *Lining epithelium:* Pseudostratified columnar (nonciliated) epithelium rests on lamina propria. It is composed of low columnar or cuboidal larger *principal cells* and few interspersed, small, and round *basal cells.*
- *Lamina propria:* It consists of loose connective tissue, elastic fibers, and few smooth muscle cells.

Muscle Layer

- It consists of a thin layer of smooth muscles.
- It is arranged in *inner circular* and *outer longitudinal* layers (IC-OL).
- Contraction of these muscles helps in expulsion of glandular secretions (seminal fluid) into ejaculatory duct.

Adventitia

- It consists of a thin layer of loose connective tissue.

Functions

- Seminal vesicles produce *seminal fluid.*
- Seminal fluid is rich in fructose (main energy source for sperms) and prostaglandins.
- Seminal fluid is alkaline in nature that helps to neutralize vaginal secretions.
- Seminal fluid contains *lipochrome pigments* that impart yellowish color to semen.

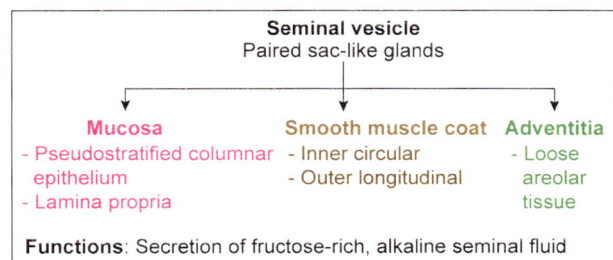

Flowchart 22.1: Histology of seminal vesicles

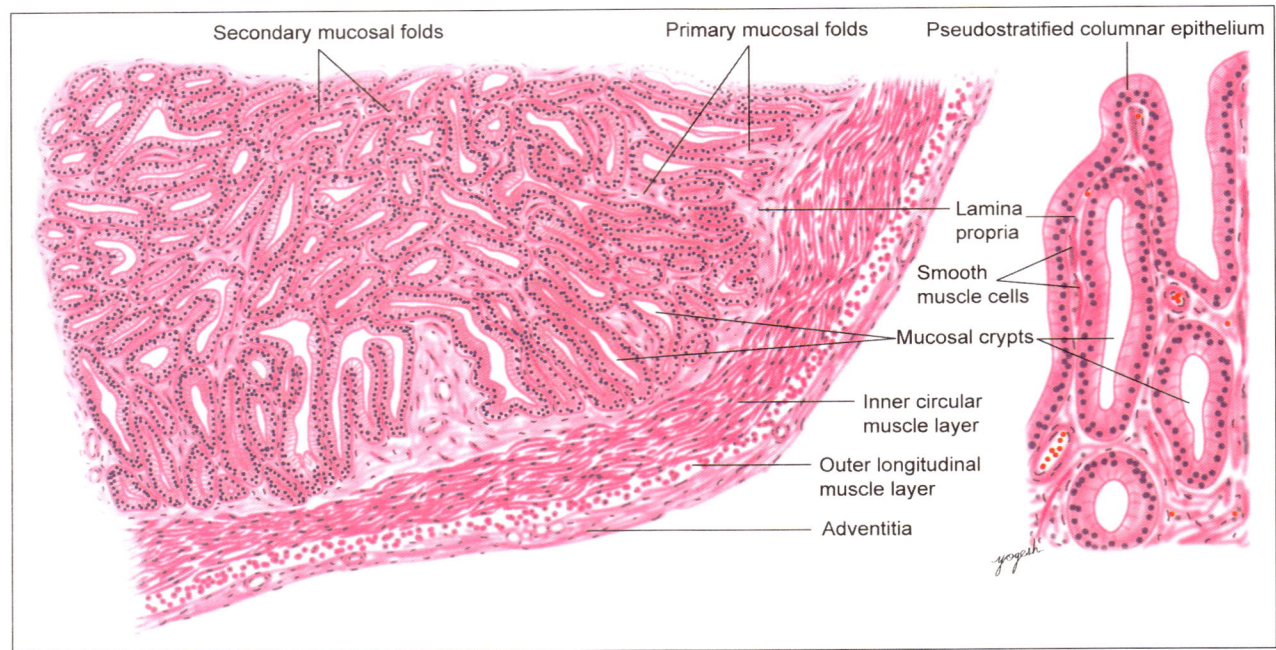

Fig. 22.1: Histology of transverse section of seminal vesicle (low magnification on left, high magnification on right, *H&E* stain).

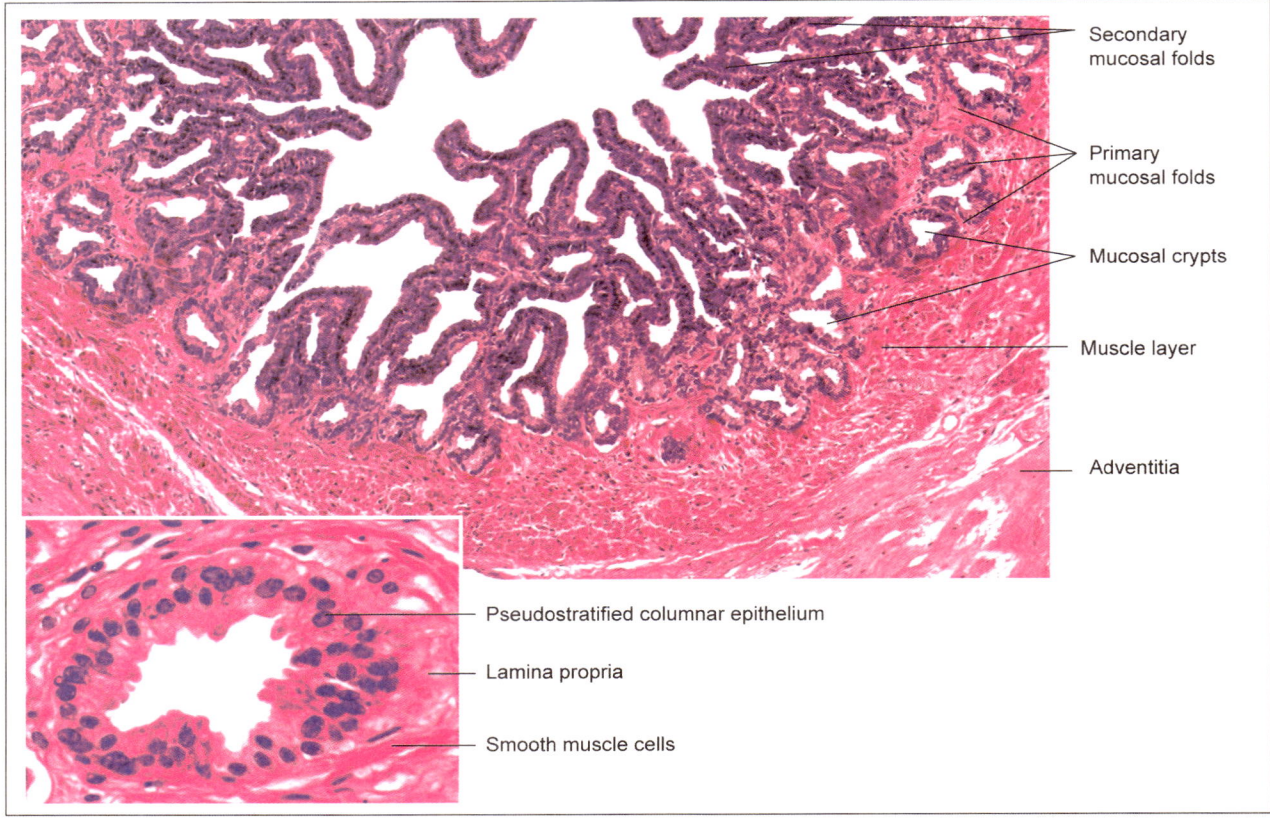

Fig. 22.2: Photomicrograph. Histology of seminal vesicle (low magnification on top, epithelial lining at high magnification in bottom, *H&E* stain).

Summary (Examination Guide)
- Seminal vesicle is a sac-like glandular structure that has following three layers:
- *Mucosa:* Lined by pseudostratified columnar epithelium resting on lamina propria. Mucosa is highly folded and occupies most of the lumen.
- *Smooth muscle coat:* Arranged as inner circular and outer longitudinal layers.
- *Adventitia:* Loose connective tissue.
- *Functions:* Secretions of fructose-rich, alkaline seminal fluid.

PROSTATE GLAND

- Prostate is the largest accessory sex gland of male reproductive system.
- Its size is about that of a walnut.
- It surrounds the beginning of urethra (prostatic urethra).
- It consists of 30–50 tubuloalveolar glands.

Histology of Prostate Gland

Parenchyma (Figs 22.3, 22.4, and 22.5)
- Prostate is surrounded by a thick *capsule*.
- Prostate consists of 30–50 *tubuloalveolar glands* embedded in fibromuscular stroma.

- Parts of prostatic gland can be grouped as follows (Fig. 22.3):
  1. *Mucosal glands:* Small tubular glands located in the mucosa. These glands open directly into the prostatic urethra.
  2. *Submucosal glands:* These are tubuloalveolar glands and situated deep into the mucosa. These open through ducts into prostatic urethra.
  3. *Main prostatic glands:* These are located in the outer zone of prostate and opens through ducts into the prostatic urethra.

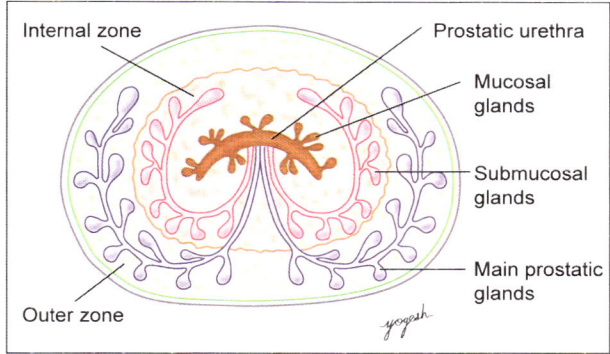

Fig. 22.3: Group of prostatic glands.

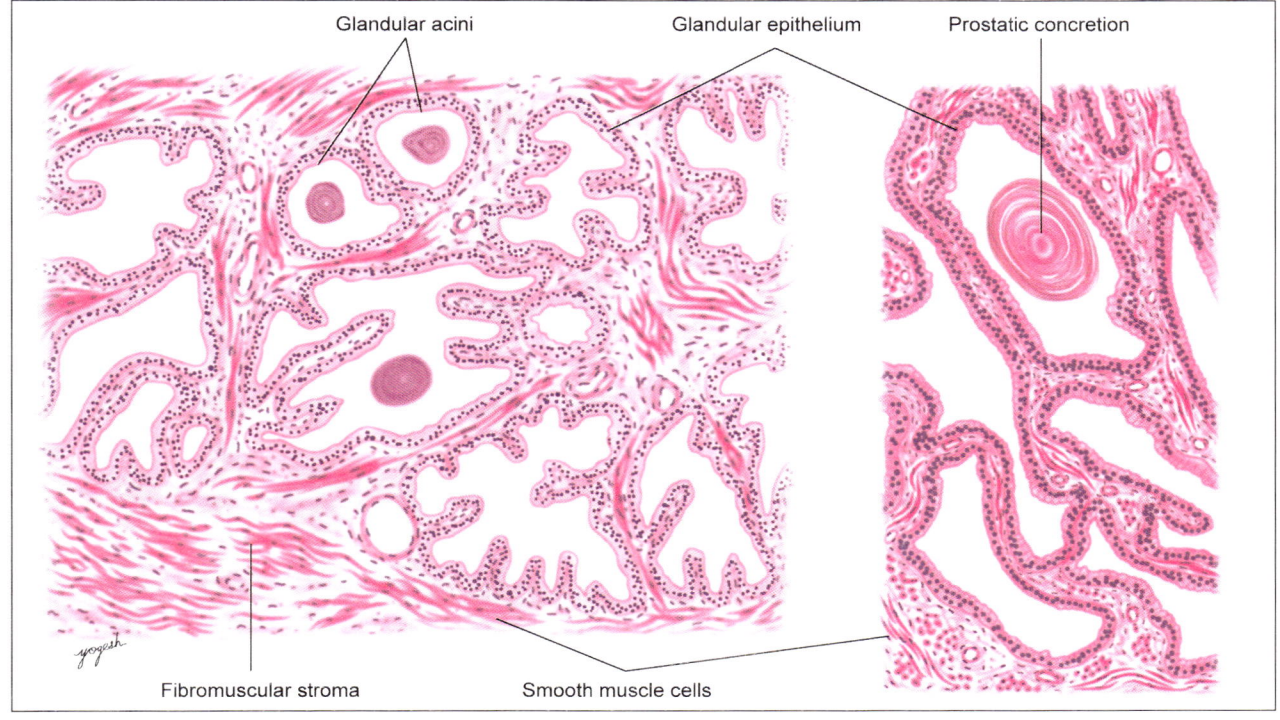

Fig. 22.4: Histology of prostate gland (low magnification on left, high magnification on right).

- *Epithelial lining of alveoli:* Alveoli of glands are lined by *pseudostratified columnar epithelium.*^{Neet}
- Epithelial lining of ducts: Ducts of prostate gland (12–20 in number) are lined by stratified columnar epithelium having superficial columnar cell layer and deep cuboidal cell layer.

Stroma

- Alveoli of prostate gland are surrounded by fibromuscular stroma.^{Viva}
- Stroma consists of smooth muscles, collagen, and elastic fibers running in different directions.^{Viva, Identification feature}
- Stroma also contains blood vessels, nerve fibers and lymphatics.

Corpora Amylacea (Prostatic Concretions)^{Neet}

- In *older men,* some of the prostatic alveoli show *concentric lamellated bodies* called *corpora amylacea.*
- This is a *glycoprotein* precipitate and after precipitation gets calcified. It stains pink (eosinophilic).^{Neet}
- It shows concentric lamellar arrangement.
- Number of corpora amylacea increases with advancing age.

Prostatic Urethra

- Prostatic urethra is lined by *transitional epithelium* in its upper part, whereas *stratified columnar epithelium* in its lower part.

Functions

- ***Prostatic fluid*** forms major part of semen (10–30%).
- Prostatic alveoli secrete prostatic fluid that contains prostatic acid phosphatase (PAP), *fibrinolysin,* citric acid and *prostate-specific antigen* (PSA).
- Prostatic secretions are pumped by contractions of smooth muscles that lie in fibromuscular stroma.
- Prostatic fibrinolysin helps in liquefaction of semen.

Summary (Examination Guide) (Flowchart 22.2)

- Prostate is the largest accessory sex glands in male.
- It consists of 30–50 tubuloalveolar glands embedded in fibromuscular stroma.
- Glandular epithelium: Simple columnar to pseudostratified columnar epithelium.
- Ducts are lined by simple columnar or stratified columnar epithelium (opens into prostatic urethra).
- Fibromuscular stroma: Contains smooth muscles, collagen fibers, elastic fibers, blood vessels, and lymphatics.
- Corpora amylasea are concentric lamellated eosinophilic structures that lie in prostatic alveoli in old age.

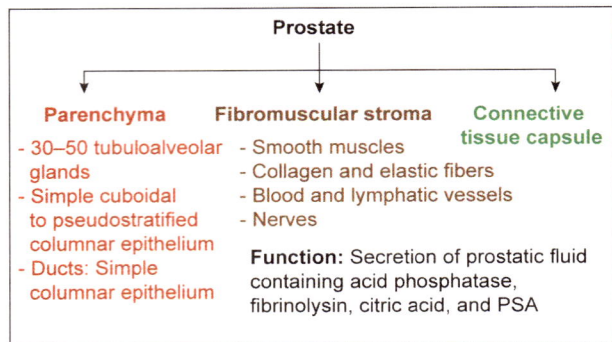

Flowchart 22.2: Histology of prostate

Clinical Correlation

- Prostatitis is inflammation of prostate gland.
- Benign prostatic hyperplasia (BHP) (Flowchart 22.3)
  - BHP is a noncancerous enlargement of prostate gland.
  - Cause: BHP is caused because of dihydrotestosterone (DHT).
  - BHP occurs usually over 50 years of age.
  - If symptoms are mild, BHP can be treated with medicines (selective α-1 blockers, 5α-reductase inhibitors) and in severe cases, surgical removal of prostate is required (transurethral resection of prostate/TURP).
- Prostatic cancer is the second most common cancer in males.^{Neet}
- Adenocarcinoma of prostate is a cancer that develops from parenchyma of prostate.
- Prostate-specific antigen (PSA)/kallikrein-3 is a glycoprotein enzyme secreted by prostatic epithelium.
- In prostatic cancers, PSA level increases significantly.

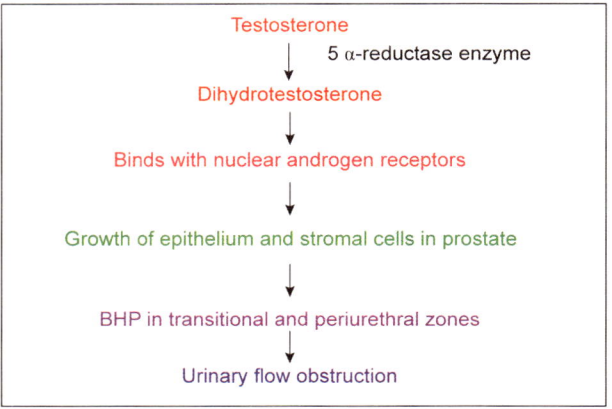

Flowchart 22.3: Pathogenesis of BHP

Box 22.1: Benign prostatic hypertrophy

- Robbins pathology (Tenth Edn): Adult prostate gland has central zone (CZ), peripheral zone (PZ), transitional zone (TZ), and periurethral zone. Peripheral zone is palpable on per-rectal examination. Carcinomas are common in peripheral zone.[Neet]
- Benign hypertrophy of prostate is common in transitional and periurethral zones, and produces urethral obstruction.[Neet]

Box 22.2: Cowper's/bulbourethral gland

- Cowper's glands are paired pea-sized glands. [William Cowper, British Anatomist, 1666–1709].
- They lie in the urogenital diaphragm.
- These are tubuloalveolar glands.
- Lining epithelium: Simple columnar epithelium.
- Gland has connective tissue capsule.
- Function: Mucus-like secretion containing galactose, galactosamin, galacturonic acid, sialic acid, and methyl-pentose. This constitutes preseminal fluid that lubricate penile urethra.

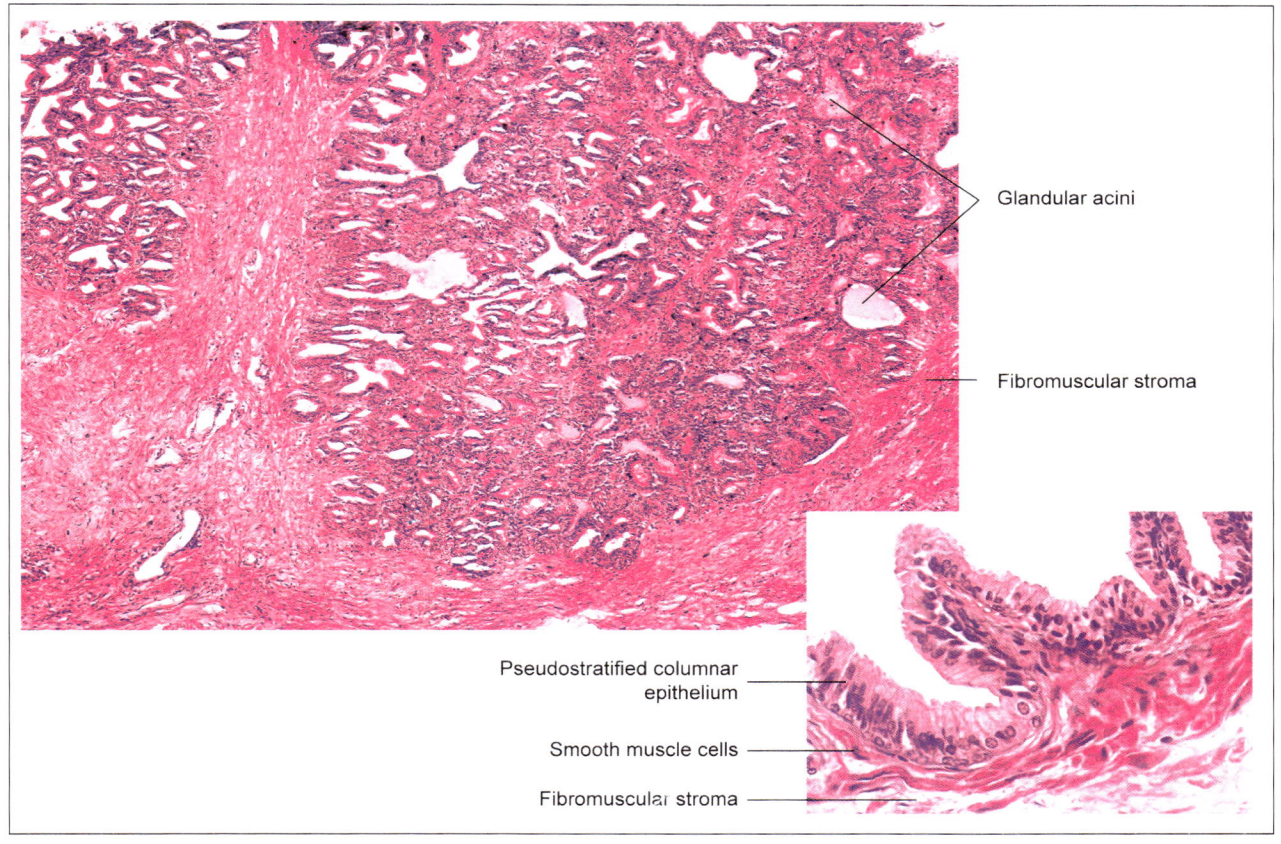

Fig. 22.5: Photomicrograph. Histology of prostate gland (low magnification on left, high magnification on right, *H&E* stain).

PENIS

Q. Write a short note on histology of penis.

- Penis is the erectile organ of copulation in males.
- It consists of *root* (fixed to perineum) and body (free part).
- Penis consists of *three masses of erectile tissues* (Figs 22.6, 22.7, and 22.8):
  - Two dorsal masses called *corpora cavernosa*
  - A single ventral mass called *corpus spongiosum*

Structure of Erectile Tissue

- Corpora cavernosa contain numerous vascular spaces lined with vascular endothelium and covered by thin smooth muscle layer.
- Corpus spongiosum is sponge-like tissue that surrounds the penile urethra.
- Tunica albuginea: It is a thick connective tissue sheath that binds three erective masses together and also partially separates two corpora cavernosa.
- Skin and connective tissue: Tunica albuginea is covered by a thin layer of connective and skin that is devoid of hairs. Connective tissue of the penis is called Buck's fascia and it is devoid of fat.[MCQ] [Gurdon Buck, 1807–1877, American plastic surgeon].
- Penile urethra is lined by pseudostratified columnar epithelium except at terminal part that is lined by stratified squamous epithelium.
- Near the terminal part, penile urethra is surrounded by glands of Littre (mucus secreting glands).[MCQ] [Alexis Littre, French Anatomist, 1654–1726].

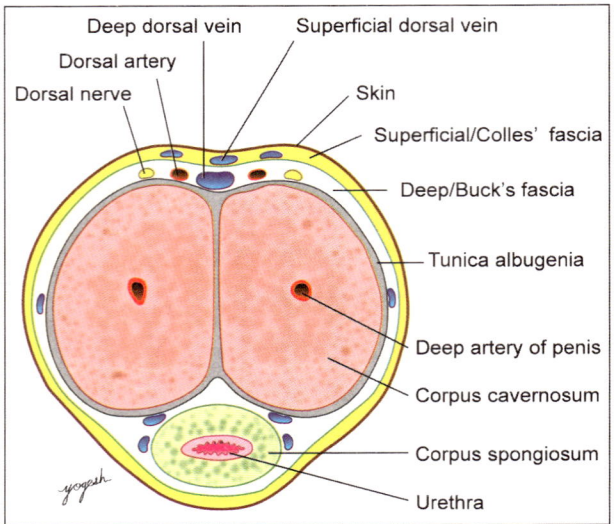

Fig. 22.6: Transverse section of penis.

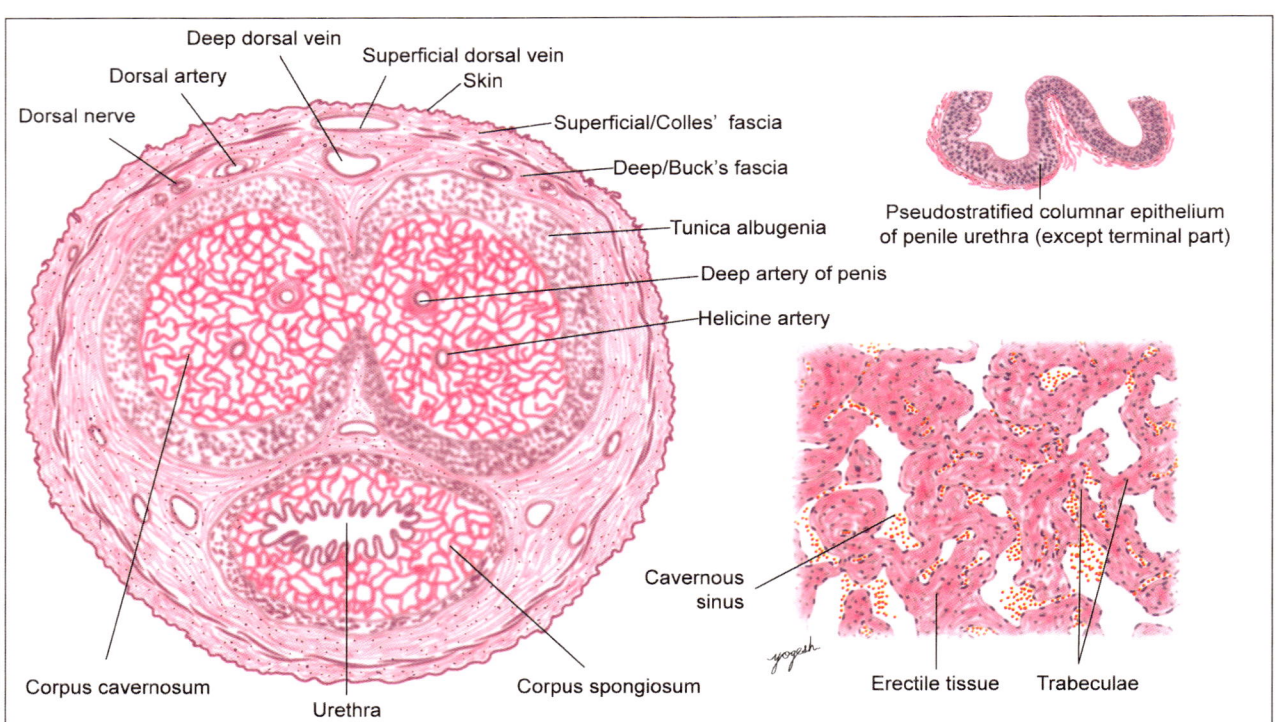

Fig. 22.7: Histology of penis (transverse section, panoramic view on left), lining epithelium of penile urethra (on upper right), and erectile tissue (high magnification, on right lower corner, practice figure).

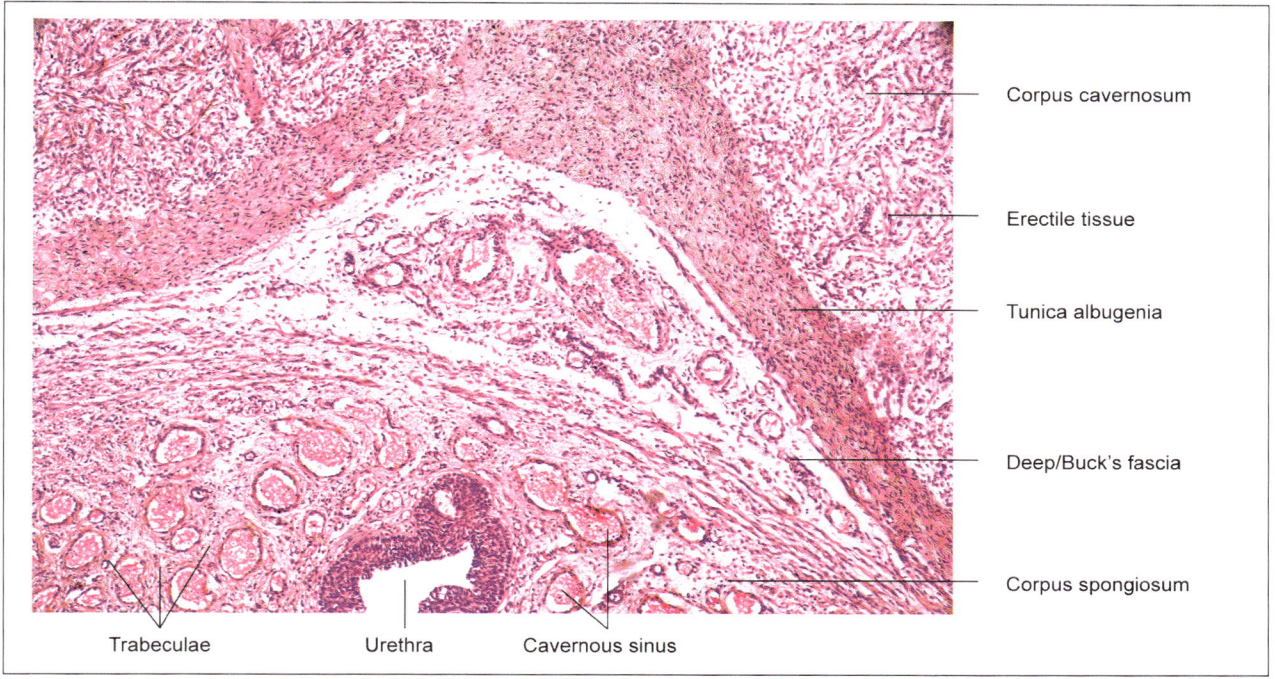

Fig. 22.8: Photomicrograph. Histology of penis (low magnification, *H&E* stain).

Mechanism of Erection
- Cavernous spaces of erectile penile tissue are supplied by helicine arteries (branches of central deep arteries).
- Vein draining cavernous spaces lie deep to tunica albuginea and obliquely traverses tunica albuginea.
- Neuropsychological stimulation causes arterial dilation, increased blood supply to cavernous spaces, and expansion of cavernous spaces because of blood. It causes compression of veins against tunica albuginea, reduces venous return and accumulation of blood in cavernous spaces, and finally erection of penis.

CHAPTER 23

Female Reproductive System I: Ovary, Uterus and Vagina

Chapter Outline
- Ovary
- Fallopian tube
- Uterus
- Cervix of uterus
- Vagina

Competency achievement: The student should be able to:

AN52.2 Describe and identify the microanatomical features of female reproductive system: Ovary, uterus, uterine tube, cervix

AN52.3 Describe and identify the microanatomical features of corpus luteum

INTRODUCTION

- Female reproductive system consists of the following parts:
  - Internal genital organs are located in the pelvis. They are ovaries, uterine tubes, uterus, and vagina (Fig. 23.1 and Flowchart 23.1)
  - External genital organs are located in perineum. They are mons pubis, labia majora, labia minora, clitoris, vestibule, and vaginal opening.
  - Accessory sex glands: Mammary gland, skene's (lesser vestibular) glands, Bartholin's (greater vestibular) glands, and pregnancy-related structures, such as placenta, umbilical cord.

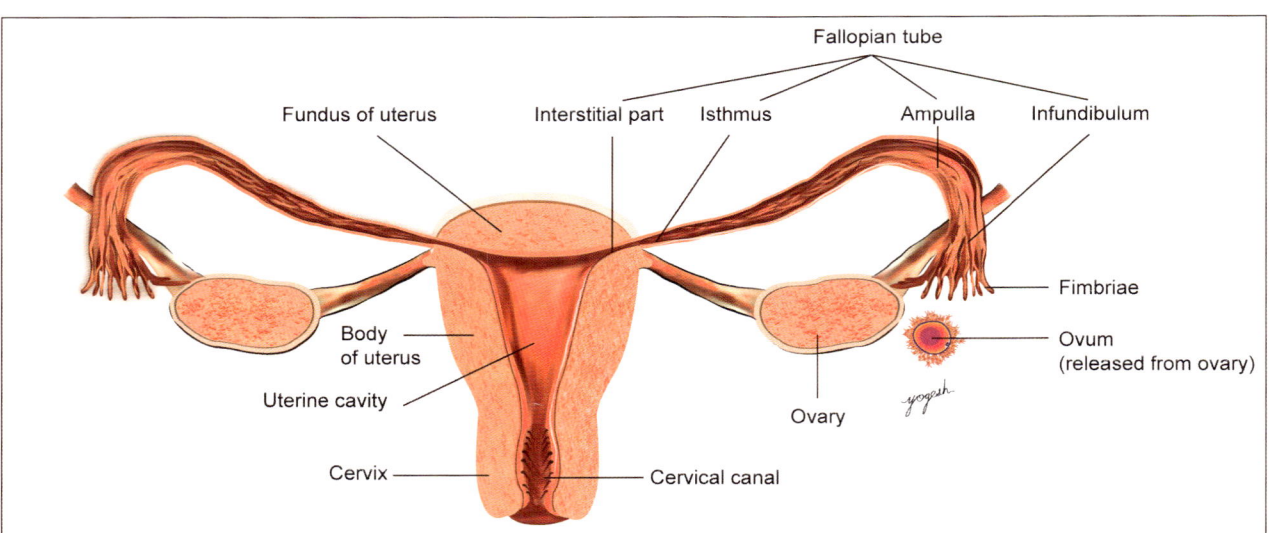

Fig. 23.1: Schematic representation of female reproductive system showing uterus, fallopian tube, and ovary (Source: Textbook of Human Embryology, Yogesh Sontakke, 1st edn, CBS Publishers).

Flowchart 23.1: Parts of female reproductive system

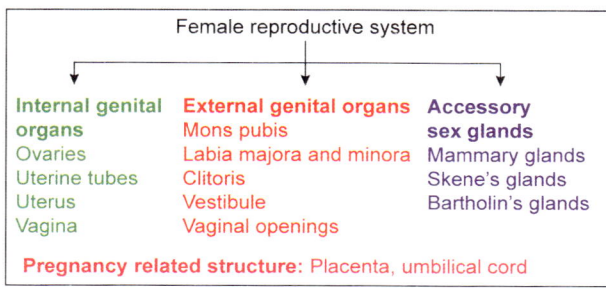

- Menstrual cycle: Ovary and uterus show cyclic changes under control of hormones. These changes are called menstrual cycle.
- Menarche: It is the initiation of menstrual cycle. It occurs at 9–14 years of age.
- Menopause (*Climacterium*): It is the termination of menstrual cycles. It occurs by the age of 45–55 years.
- Average length of each menstrual cycle is 28–30 days. It varies from female to female.

OVARY

Q. Write a short note on histology of ovary.

- Ovaries perform two major functions:
  1. Gametogenesis: Production of ova (female gametes).
  2. Steroid hormone secretion:
     Estrogens: It promotes growth of reproductive organs and mammary glands.
  3. Progesterone: It prepares the internal genital organs for reproduction in each menstrual cycle.
- Ovaries are almond-shaped, pinkish-white paired organs.
- Each ovary lies in broad ligament.
- Dimensions: 3 cm in length, 1.5 cm in width, and 1 cm in thickness.

General Structure of Ovary

- Each ovary consists of the following components (Figs 23.2, 23.3 and Flowchart 23.2):

Flowchart 23.2: General structure of ovary

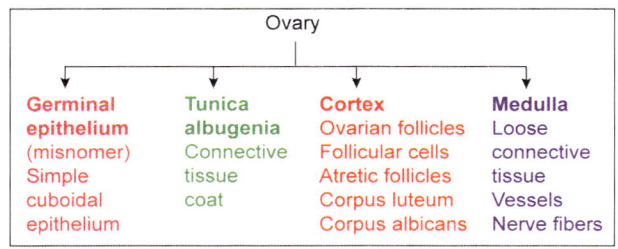

Germinal Epithelium

- Surface of ovary is covered by a single layer of cuboidal epithelium (germinal epithelium).*Viva*
- Note: This epithelium does not give rise to female gametes. It is a misnomer.*Viva*
- Primordial germ cells migrating from yolk sac give rise to female gametes.
- Germinal epithelium is continuous with mesothelium of peritoneum

Tunica Albuginea

- Germinal epithelium rests on a connective tissue layer called tunica albuginea. Note: Tunica albuginea of testis is much thicker and denser than that of ovary.*Viva*

Cortex

- It is the peripheral portion of ovary that lies just beneath the tunica albuginea.
- It consists of various stages of ovarian follicles with oocytes (germ cells) in cellular connective tissue stroma.
- Stromal cells of cortex surround the ovarian follicles and form follicular cells, corona radiata, cumulus oophorous, granulosa cells, theca interna, and theca externa cells.
- Cortex also contains corpus luteum, corpus albicans and atretic follicles.

Medulla

- It is located in central portion of ovary and mainly consists of loose connective tissue, blood vessels, lymphatic vessels, and nerve fibers.
- Hilum of ovary: It is a part of ovary through which blood vessels enter ovarian medulla. Histologically, there is no clear demarcation between cortex and medulla.

Ovarian Follicles (Oogenesis) (Figs 23.4 to 23.7 and Flowchart 23.3)

- Ovarian cortex shows various stages of developing follicles as follows: Primordial follicle, secondary follicle, Graafian follicle, corpus luteum, corpus albicans, and atretic follicles.

Oogonia

- Primordial germ cells give rise to oogonia before the birth of female (in fetal life).
- Oogonia multiply mitotically, enlarge and form primary oocytes.
- Primary oocytes complete prophase of first meiotic division and get arrested at dictyotene (diplotene)

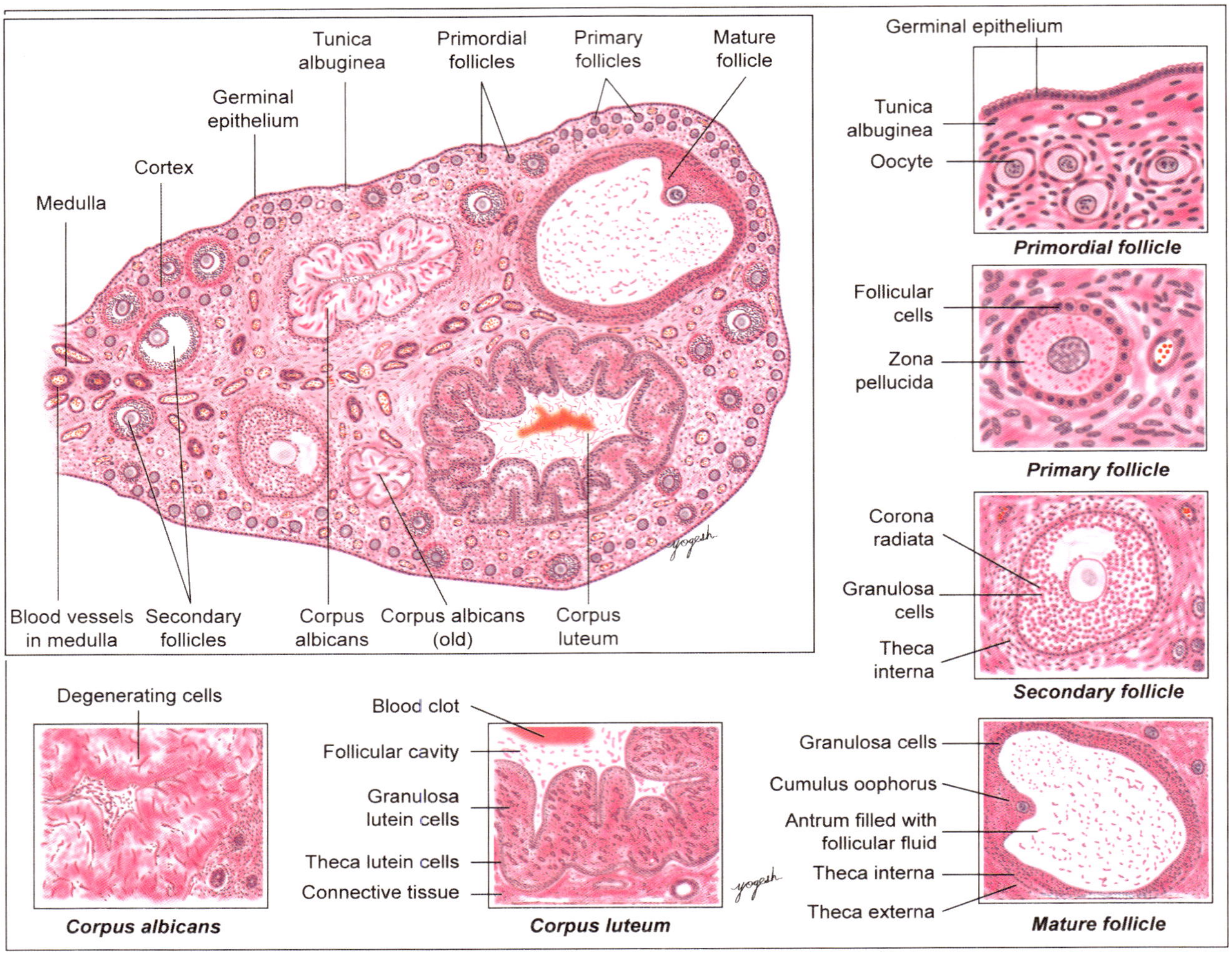

Fig. 23.2: Histology of ovary and various components of ovary at high magnification in insets (practice figure).

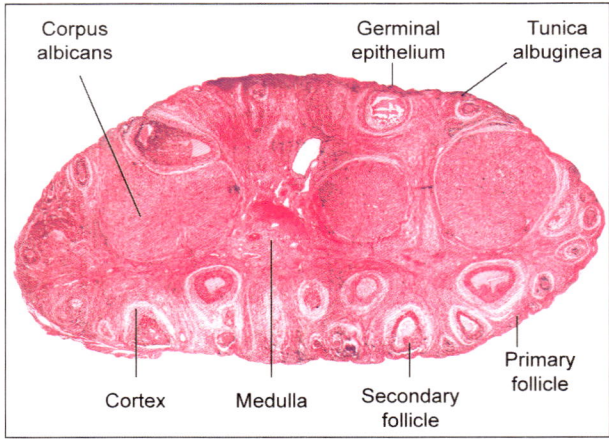

Fig. 23.3: Photomicrograph. Histology of ovary, panoramic view (X40, H&E stain).

stage at birth by oocyte maturation inhibitor (OMI) factor till puberty.^{Next}
- Out of 2 million primary oocytes, four lakhs persist up to puberty and only 500 ovulate.^{Next}
- From birth to puberty, follicles remain in dormant phase.

Primordial Follicle

- These are located just beneath tunica albuginea in the cortex of ovary (Fig. 23.8).
- It consists of
  - Oocyte (30 μm size): It has eccentric nucleus, cytoplasm, and **Balbiani body.**^{MCQ} The Balbiani body is a membraneless ball of mitochondria, other organelles, and proteins. [Édouard-Gérard Balbiani, French embryologist, 1823–1899].
  - Follicular cells: Oocyte is surrounded by single layer of squamous (flat) follicular cells.

Primary Follicle

- Primordial follicle enlarges and surrounding follicular cells proliferate and become cuboidal to form primary follicle (Fig. 23.8).
- Oocyte starts secreting homogeneous, deeply staining acidophilic (pink) layer between oocyte

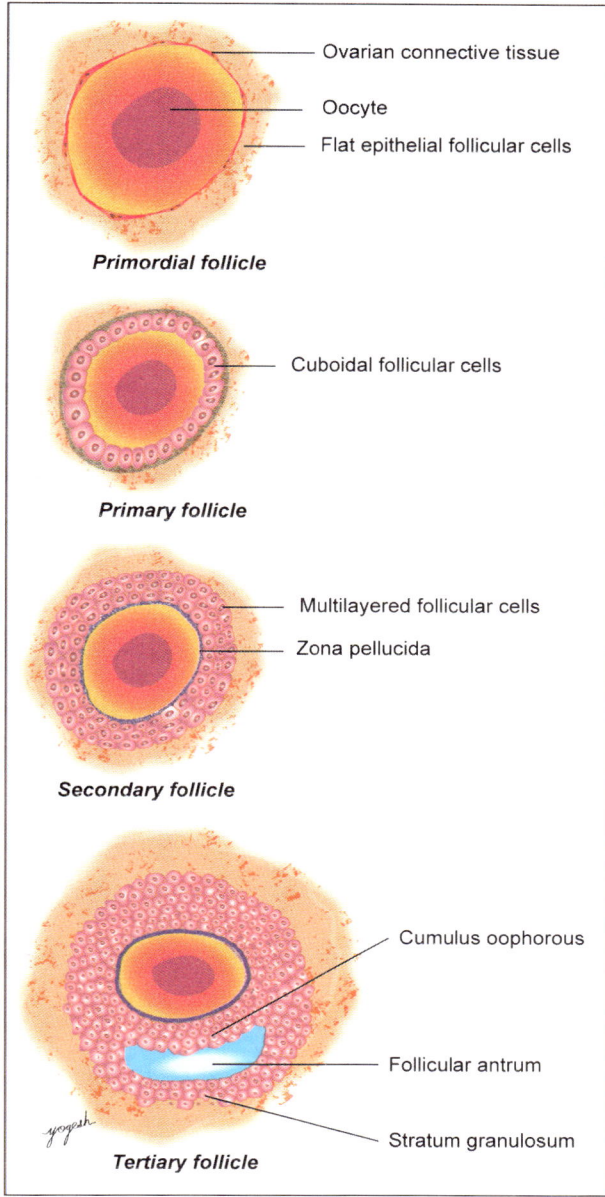

Fig. 23.4: Developing ovarian follicles.

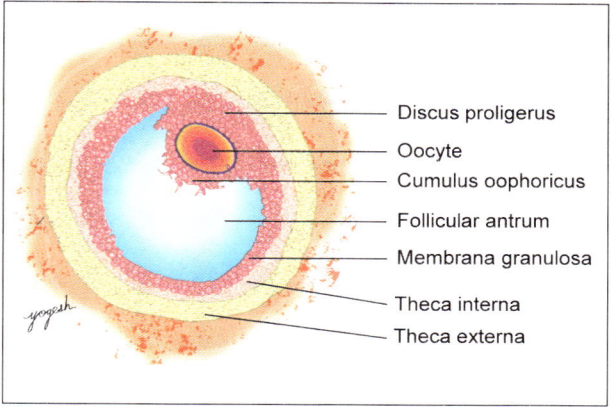

Fig. 23.5: Mature ovarian follicle (Source: Textbook of Human Embryology, Yogesh Sontakke, 1st edn, CBS Publishers).

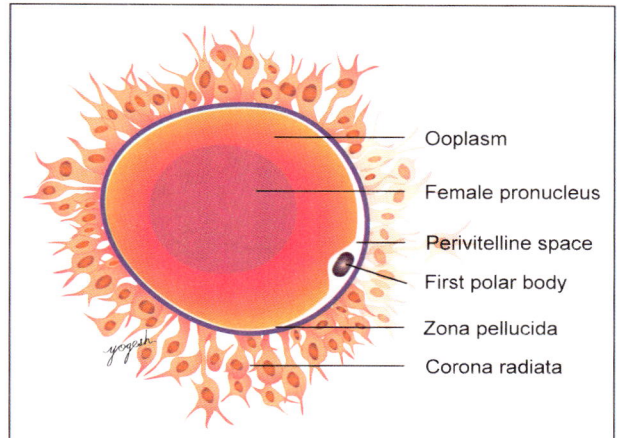

Fig. 23.6: Structure of ovum at the time of ovulation (Source: Textbook of Human Embryology, Yogesh Sontakke, 1st edn, CBS Publishers).

and follicular cells. This layer is called *zona pellucida.*
- Zona pellucida is rich in glycosaminoglycans and glycoproteins. Hence, stains with periodic acid–Schiff (PAS) reagent (deep magenta color).

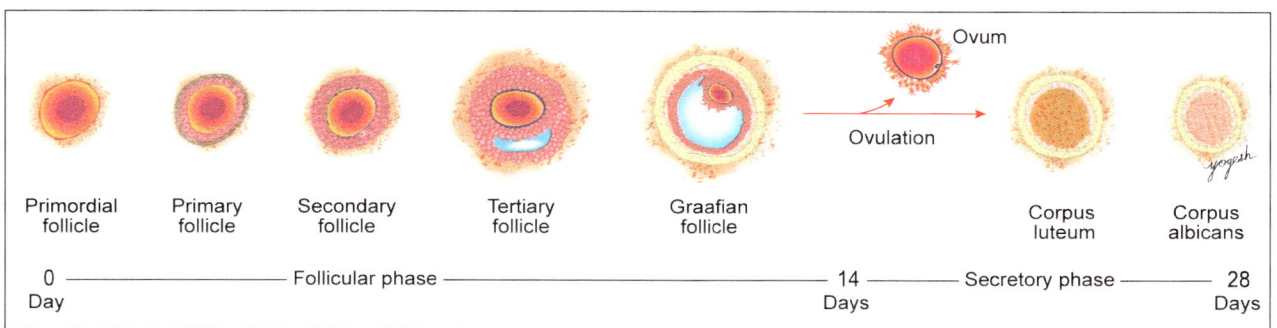

Fig. 23.7: Various ovarian follicles (Source: Textbook of Human Embryology, Yogesh Sontakke, 1st edn, CBS Publishers).

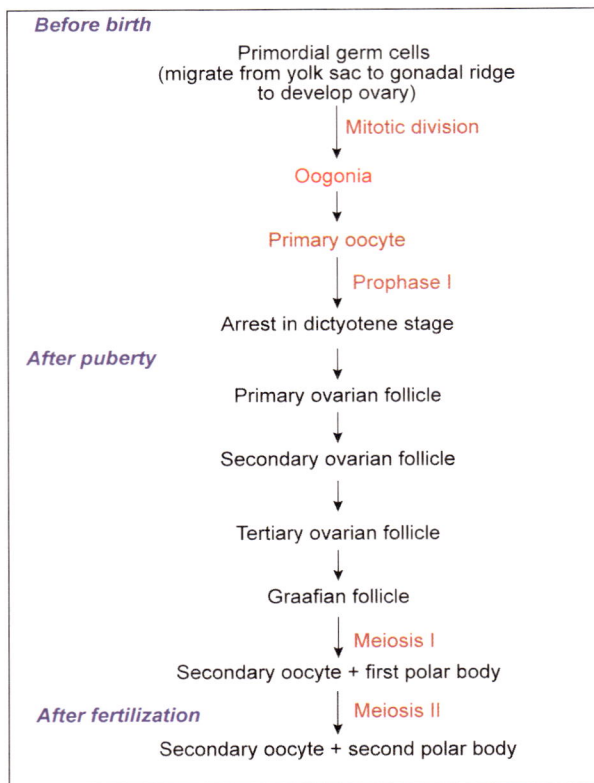

Flowchart 23.3: Oogenesis.

Secondary Follicle (Fig. 23.9)

- With the growth of follicle, granulosa cells proliferate, and fluid-filled cavities start appearing among these cells.
- These small cavities fuse to form a large fluid-filled cavity called *antrum* and fluid is called *liquor folliculi*. The follicle with antrum (cavity) is called *secondary follicle*.
- Oocyte enlarges up to 125 µm diameter and its further growth gets arrested by *oocyte maturation inhibitor* (OMI) factor secreted by granulosa cells.
- On appearance of follicular antrum, some granulosa cells form *cumulus oophorous* layer. It surrounds the oocyte (future corona radiata cells).
- *Call–Exner bodies:* These are extracellular bodies (PAS positive) consisting of hyaluronic acid and proteoglycans secreted by granulosa cells. [Emma Call, American physician, 1847–1937; Sigmund Exner, Austrian physiologist, 1846–1926].

Graafian Follicle (Figs 23.5 and 23.9)

- Its diameter is about 10 mm or even more.
- Primary oocyte completes first meiotic division to form secondary oocyte and the first polar body.
- Follicular antrum increases in size and granulosa cells of cumulus oophorous surrounding the oocyte form a layer called *corona radiata.*
- Graafian follicle bulges on the surface of ovary.
- Theca interna cells secrete androgens, whereas granulosa cells convert these androgens into estrogens.
- Granulosa cells proliferate under the influence of estrogen and increase follicle size.

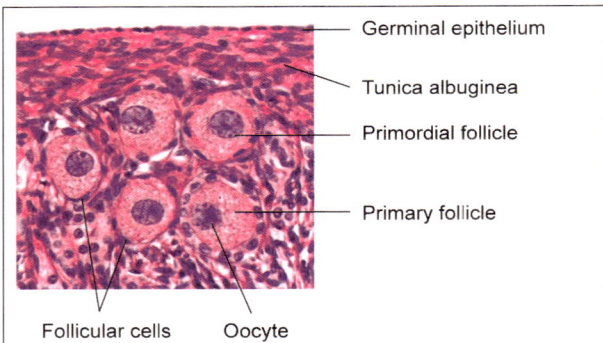

Fig. 23.8: Photomicrograph. Primordial and primary follicles (high magnification, *H&E* stain).

- Follicular cells multiply to form membrane granulosa cells (stratum granulosum). These are cuboidal cells. Outermost layer rests on basal lamina.
- Surrounding stromal cells differentiate into
  - *Theca interna:* This is inner, highly vascular layer of cuboidal cells.
  - *Theca externa:* This is outer, connective tissue layer that consists of smooth muscle cells and bundles of collagen fibers.

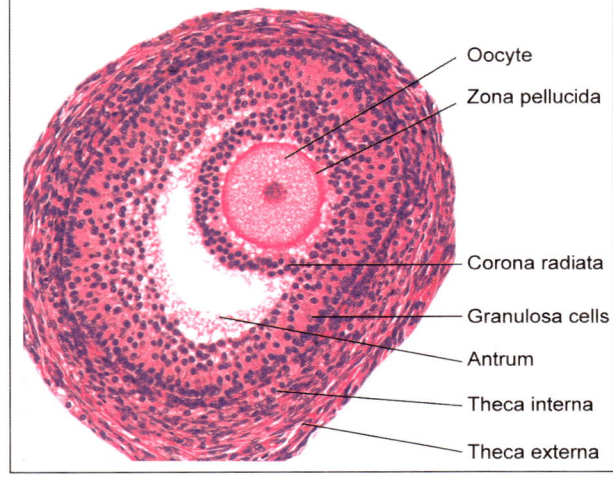

Fig. 23.9: Photomicrograph. Maturing follicle (stage between secondary and Graafian follicles, High magnification, *H&E* stain).

Ovulation

- Ovulation is the release of secondary oocyte from Graafian follicle.
- Factors responsible for ovulation
  1. Increased volume of follicular fluid
  2. Plasminogen causing proteolysis of follicular cells
  3. Prostaglandin-induced smooth muscle contractions of theca externa layer
- *Macula pellucida or stigma:* At the surface of ovary covering the bulging follicle, blood supply of germinal epithelium ceases, and it leads to formation of small necrotic zone called macula pellucida or stigma. The oocyte comes out through macula pellucida.
- After ovulation, secondary oocyte is viable for 24–48 hours. If fertilization does not occur, secondary oocyte degenerates.[Neet]
- Secondary oocyte begins second meiotic division but gets arrested at metaphase. It completes second meiotic division only if it gets fertilized (Fig. 23.6).[Neet]

Corpus Luteum/Luteal Gland

- On ovulation, the follicle collapses, and its wall becomes enfolded to form corpus luteum (yellow body) (Fig. 23.10).
- Cells of stratum granulosa and theca interna layers enlarge in the size and get filled with lipid pigment called lipochrome (yellow-colored).
- Cells of corpus luteum:
  - Granulosa luteum cells: Large, centrally located cells
  - Theca lutein cells: Small, peripherally located cells
- Granulosa lutein cells secrete progesterone, whereas theca lutein cells secrete estradiol.

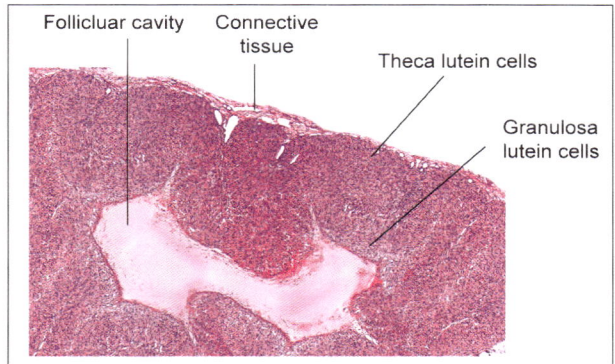

Fig. 23.10: Photomicrograph. Corpus luteum (low magnification, H&E stain).

- If fertilization does not occur, the corpus lutetium undergoes degeneration to form *corpus albicans.*
- Cells of corpus luteum become swollen, thin, pyknotic and get replaced with a scar of connective tissue after complete autolysis. This white scar is called *corpus albicans.*
- Scar slowly sinks deeper into the ovarian cortex and disappears in several months.

Follicular Atresia

- Most of the ovarian follicles degenerate and undergo follicular atresia.
- Events in follicular atresia:
  1. Initiation of apoptosis by granulosa cells
  2. Autolysis of granulosa cells by proteolytic enzymes
  3. Hypertrophy of theca interna cells
  4. Replacement of follicular cells by connective tissue
- Macrophages remove degenerating follicular cells, oocyte, and zona pellucida by phagocytosis.
- Basement membrane separating theca interna and granulosa cells become thick to form wavy hyaline glassy membrane. It is a characteristic of degenerating follicle.[Neet]

Some Interesting Facts

- Ovary is supplied by the ovarian artery (branch of abdominal aorta) and ovarian branches of uterine artery. Helicine artery is the largest ovarian branch of uterine artery.
- All arteries supplying ovary are covered by pampiniform plexus that joins to form ovarian vein.

Interstitial glands of ovary

- Some luteal cells of atretic follicle do not degenerate and persist as cords of cells that form interstitial glands of ovary.
- These glands produce steroid hormones (estrogen).

Ovarian hilar cells

- These cells are found in the hilum of ovary.
- These are similar to the interstitial Leydig cells of testis.[Neet, Viva]
- Hilar cells of ovary contain Reinke crystalloids (rod-like inclusions, also found in Leydig cells of testis) [FB Reinke, German anatomist, 1862–1919].
- Function: Secretion of androgens

> **Summary (Examination Guide)** (Fig. 23.2 and Flowchart 23.4)
> - Ovary has an outer cortex that shows follicles of various sizes and an inner medulla that consists of connective tissue, blood vessels, and nerves.
> - Ovary is covered with cuboidal germinal epithelium.
> - A layer of connective tissue that lies deep to germinal epithelium is called *tunica albuginea*.
>
> **Ovarian follicles:**
> - *Primordial follicle:* Primary oocyte covered by a flattened layer of follicular cells.
> - *Primary follicle:* Primary oocyte covered by zona pellucida and single cell thick cuboidal follicular cells.
> - *Secondary follicle:* In secondary follicle, the primary oocyte is covered by zona pellucida, granulosa cells with follicular antrum, theca interna (vascular), and theca externa (fibrous) layers.
> - *Graafian follicle:* It is about 10 mm or more in size and shows secondary oocyte with first polar body.
> - *Corpus hemorrhagicus:* It is a follicle just after ovulation. It is filled with blood.
> - *Corpus luteum:* Follicle after ovulation, consists of luteal cells (yellow pigments in cytoplasm), secretes progesterone.
> - *Corpus albicans:* If ovum does not get fertilize, the corpus luteum degenerates and forms fibrous corpus albicans (white body).

Flowchart 23.4: Histology of ovary

Ovary	Ovarian follicles					
	Primordial	Primary	Secondary	Graafian	Corpus luteum	Corpus albicans
Germinal epithelium - Simple cuboidal						
Tunica albuginea	Primary oocyte Flat follicular cells	Primary oocyte Zona pellucida Cuboidal follicular cells	Primary oocyte Granulosa cells Theca interna and externa	Secondary oocyte First polar body Corona radiata Cumulus oophorus	Luteal cells with lipid pigments	Small fibrous mass
Outer cortex - Ovarian follicles						
Inner medulla - Connective tissue - Vessels and nerves	Graafian follicle →(Ovulation)→ Ovum			Corpus hemorrhagicus (follicle filled with blood) → Corpus luteum		

FALLOPIAN TUBE (UTERINE TUBES)

Q. Write a short note on histology of fallopian tube.

- These are a pair of *mucomuscular tubes* that convey ova from ovaries to uterine cavity and serves as the site for fertilization.
- Length: 10–12 cm
- It has 4 parts:
  1. *Infundibulum:* It is funnel-shaped part that lies adjacent to ovary. It has finger-like projections called *fimbriae*.
  2. *Ampulla:* It is longest, thin-walled, dilated part. It serves as the site of fertilization.
  3. *Isthmus:* It is the narrowest part.
  4. *Uterine or interstitial part:* It lies within the wall of uterus and communicates with uterine cavity.

Histology of Fallopian Tube (Figs 23.11, 23.12 and Flowchart 23.5)

- Wall of fallopian tube shows three layers from inside outwards: Mucosa, muscle layer, and serosa.

Mucosa

- It consists of thin projecting longitudinal folds that fill the lumen. These folds are more numerous in ampulla.
- Epithelial lining
  – It is lined by *simple ciliated columnar epithelium* and consists of two types of cells[Neet]

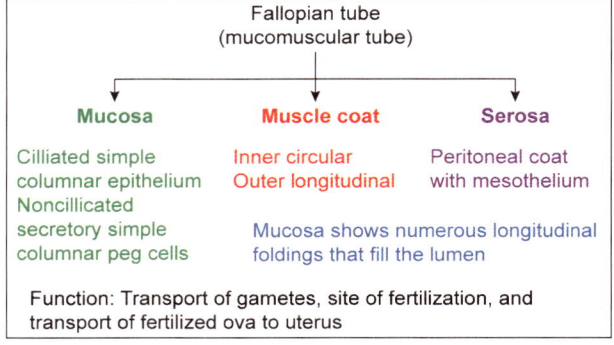

Flowchart 23.5: Histology of fallopian/uterine tube.

Female Reproductiave System I: Ovary, Uterus and Vagina

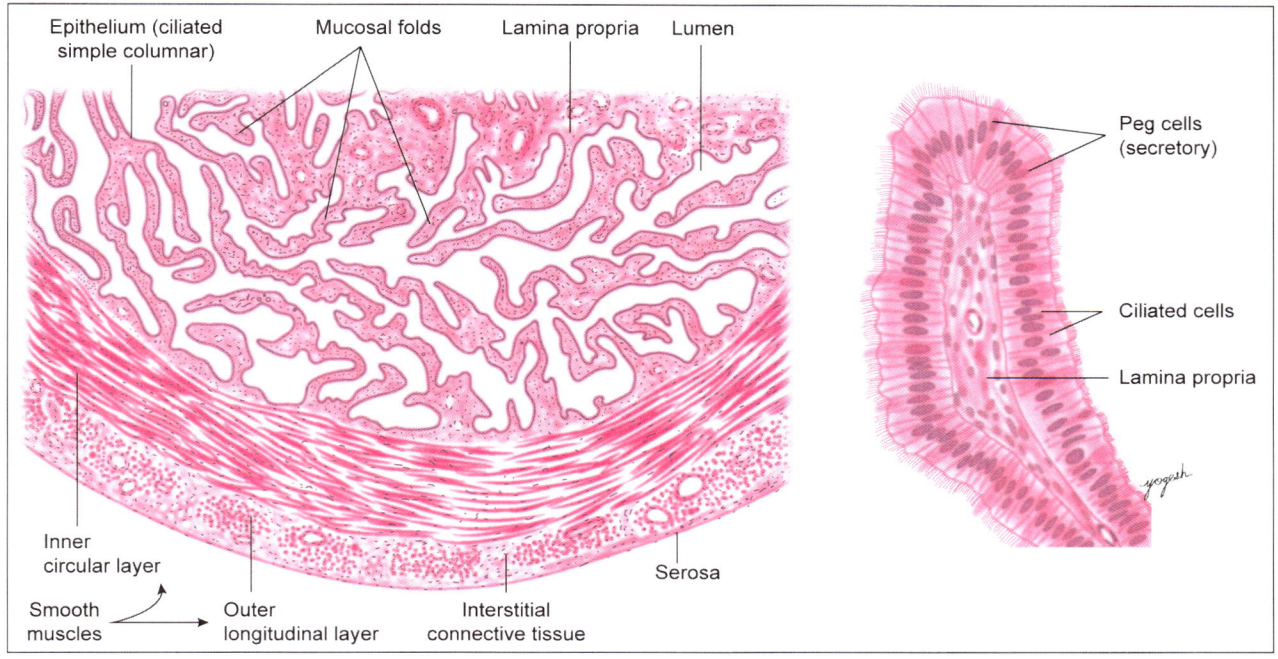

Fig. 23.11: Histology of uterine tube (low magnification on left, high magnification showing mucosa on right).

Ciliated columnar cells: These cells show cilia that beat toward uterus.

Nonciliated columnar peg cells: They secrete fluid that nourishes spermatogonia and fertilized egg. They provide environment for capacitation of sperms (maturation).^{Neet}
- Lining epithelium shows cyclic changes in menstrual cycle.
- Core of mucosal fold consists of highly cellular and vascular connective tissue.

Muscle Layer

- Muscle coat consists of two layers of smooth muscle: Inner thick circular and outer thin longitudinal layers.
- Circular muscle layer is thickest in isthmus. It controls passage of fertilized ovum from fallopian tube to uterus.

Serosa/Peritoneal Coat

- Fallopian tube is covered by a thin layer of connective tissue and mesothelium.

Function

- Bidirectional transport: Sperms toward ampulla, and ovum and fertilized egg toward uterus.
- *Note:* There is no mucularis mucosae and submucosa in the fallopian tubes.

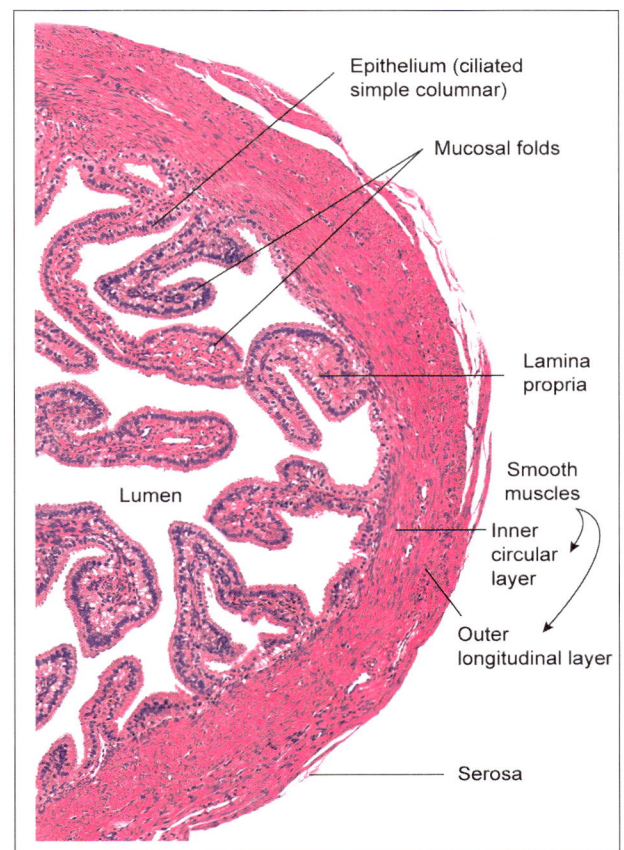

Fig. 23.12: Photomicrograph. Histology of uterine tube (low magnification, *H&E* stain).

> **Clinical Correlation**
> - Fallopian tube is the commonest site of *ectopic pregnancy*. Usual site of implantation is endometrium of upper uterine segment (mostly on posterior wall).[Neet]
> - Other sites of ectopic pregnancy are lower uterine segment (placenta previa), ovary, abdominal cavity, or musculature of uterus (interstitial implantation).

UTERUS

- Uterus is a muscular organ located in pelvic cavity.
- It is a pear-shaped organ that has the following parts:
  1. *Body:* It is flat part of uterus that extends between cervix and openings of the fallopian tubes.
  2. *Fundus:* It is the uppermost dome-shaped part of the uterus that lies above the openings of fallopian tubes.
  3. *Cervix:* It is the lowest part of uterus. It is barrel-shaped and separated from body of uterus by a constriction called *isthmus*.
- The canal of cervix opens into the uterine cavity through *internal os*, whereas into the vagina through *external os*.

Histology of Uterus

- Uterine wall consists of three layers (from within outside):
  1. Endometrium
  2. Myometrium
  3. Perimetrium

Endometrium

- Mucosal lining of uterus is called *endometrium*.[MCQ]
- Endometrium consists of
  - Lining epithelium: Simple columnar epithelium
  - *Uterine glands:* Simple tubular glands lined by simple columnar epithelium
  - *Endometrial stroma:* Highly vascular and contains endometrial/uterine glands

Myometrium

- Myometrium consists of *smooth muscle* cells.
- It is the thickest layer of uterine wall.
- Its muscles are arranged into three layers:
  - Inner longitudinal layer
  - Middle irregular cell layer: Muscle fibers are oriented in circular or spiral pattern. As this middle layer contains numerous vessels, it is also called *stratum vascularae*.
  - Outer longitudinal layer
- During pregnancy, smooth muscle cells of myometrium can undergo hypertrophy (enlargement of cell size) and hyperplasia (increase in number of cells). Myometrium can contract on release of oxytocin from posterior pituitary and helps in expulsion of fetus from uterus.

Perimetrium

- Uterus is covered by perimetrium.
- Perimetrium has two layers
  - Outer layer of mesothelium (simple squamous epithelium)
  - Inner layer of vascular connective tissue

> **Box 23.1:** Endometrium in menstrual cycle
> - Endometrium shows cyclic changes in each menstrual cycle under the influence of ovarian hormones.
> - Uterine cyclic changes are divided into three phases (for 28 day cycle) as follows:
>   1. Follicular phase/proliferative phase/preovulatory phase: Endometrium shows changes under influence of estrogen from 4th to 14th day of menstrual cycle (follicular phase).
>   2. Secretory phase: Endometrium shows changes under influence of progesterone from 15th to 28th days of menstrual cycle.
>   3. Menstrual (bleeding) phase: Endometrium shed off in absence of estrogen and progesterone for first 3–4 days of menstrual cycle.

Strata of Endometrium

- Endometrium shows three strata (from within outside) as:
  1. Stratum compactum: It is the superficial layer containing necks of uterine glands.
  2. Stratum spongiosum: It is the middle layer consisting of loose areolar tissue.
  3. Stratum basale: It is the deep layer that lies adjacent to myometrium.

Histological Changes in Endometrium (Figs 23.13 to 23.15)

Proliferative Phase (Fig. 23.14)

- This phase involves repair of damaged endometrium by proliferation of cells of stratum basale.
- Glandular epithelium proliferates to cover entire endometrium. The glands become straight and have narrow lumen.
- Endometrial stroma proliferates to make endometrium 3–4 mm thick
- Spiral arteries elongate and reach the middle of endometrium.

Female Reproductiave System I: Ovary, Uterus and Vagina

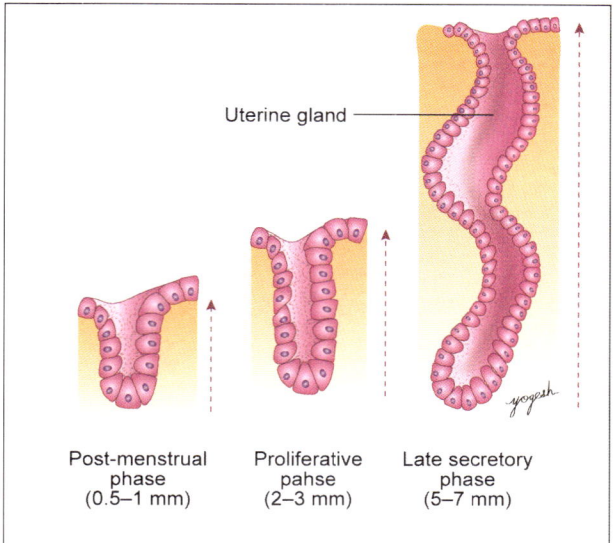

Fig. 23.13: Changes in uterine endometrium during menstrual cycle (Source: Textbook of Human Embryology, Yogesh Sontakke, 1st edn., CBS Publishers).

Secretory Phase (Fig. 23.14)

- This phase is under control of progesterone and endometrium shows the following changes.

- Changes in glands
  - Uterine glands become more coiled and tortuous (produces sawtooth appearance).*Identification feature*
  - Glandular epithelium starts accumulating glycogen. Glands secrete carbohydrate-rich fluid.
- Changes in stroma
  - Spiral arteries become more tortuous.
  - Vascularity of endometrium enhances.
  - Uterine fluid starts accumulating in stroma and makes it edematous and thick.
  - Stromal cells accumulate glycogen and lipid droplets in their cytoplasm. This is called *decidual reaction.**Viva, MCQ*

Menstrual Phase

- In later part of the secretory phase, because of low levels of estrogen and progesterone, spiral arteries undergo constriction. This results in decreased blood supply (ischemia) of endometrium.
- Ischemia, released prostaglandins, and proteolytic enzymes cause menstrual bleeding.
- Epithelium of stratum compactum, and stratum basale remains intact because these layers are supplied by straight arteries rather than spiral arteries.

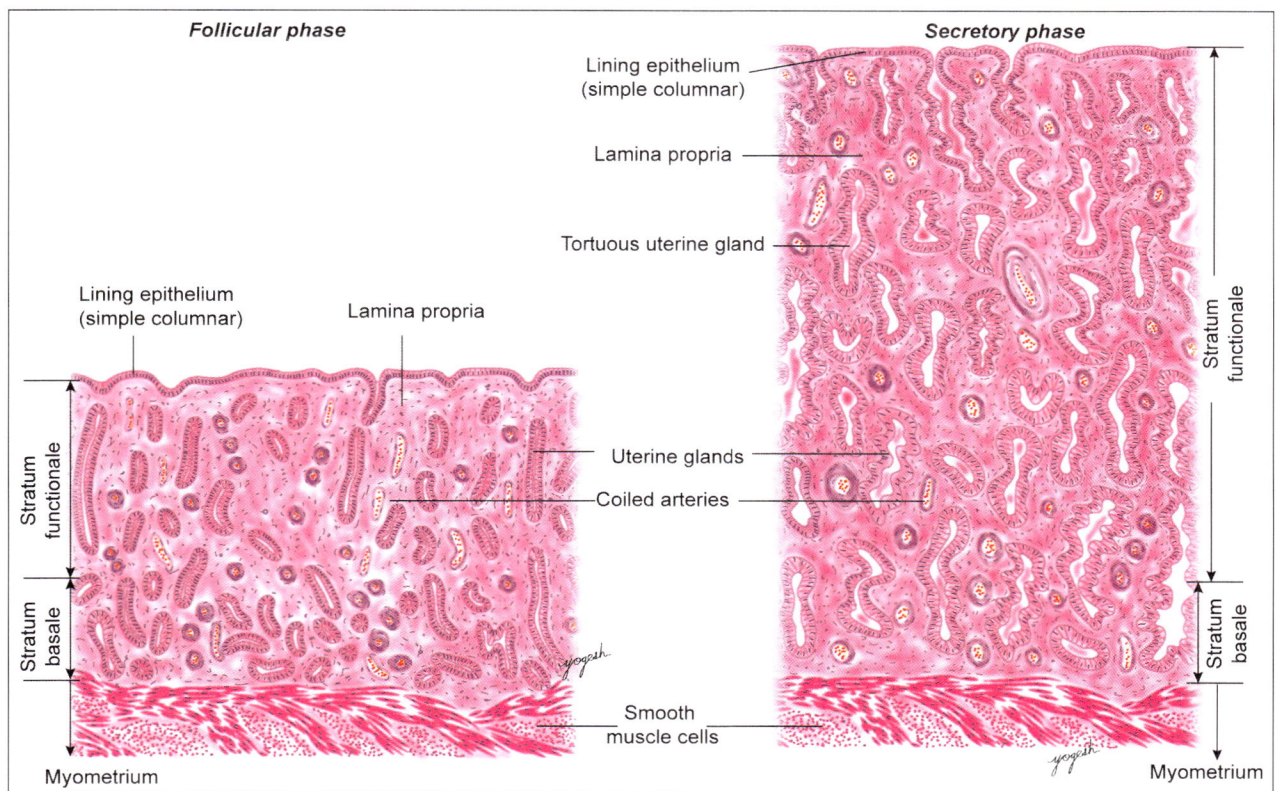

Fig. 23.14: Histology of uterus (follicular phase on left and secretory phase on right).

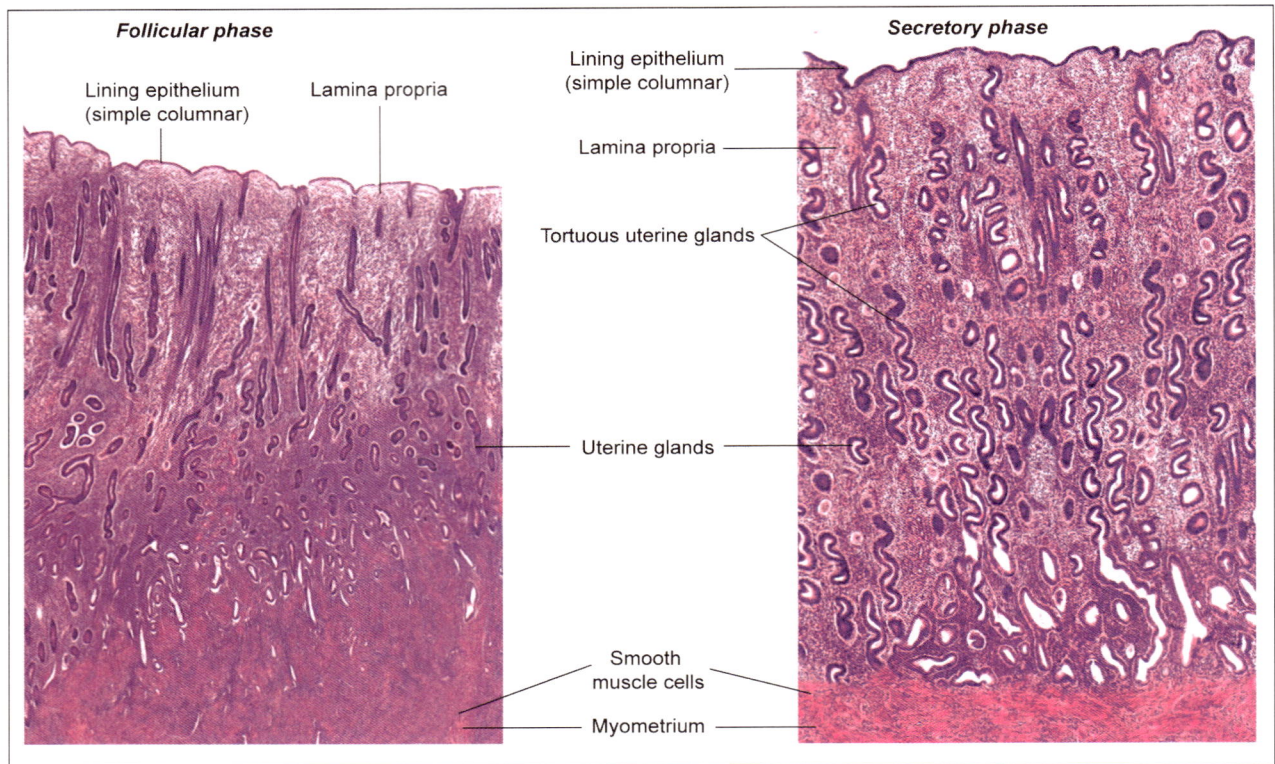

Fig. 23.15: Photomicrograph. Histology of uterus (follicular phase on left and secretory phase on right).

Differences between endometrium of proliferative and secretory phase are listed in Table 23.1.

Q. List the differences between endometrium of proliferative and secretory phases.

Table 23.1: Differences between endometrium of proliferative and secretory phases

Features	Proliferative/follicular/ preovulatory phase	Secretory/luteal/ postovulatory/ presentational phase
Predominant hormone	Estrogen	Progesterone
Endometrial thickness	3–4 mm	6–7 mm
StraTA	At the beginning, only stratum basale is present	All strata of endometrium are present
Uterine glands	Straight, long, widely separated from each other with narrow lumen	Coiled (cork-screw-shaped), closely placed to each other, with wide lumen
Secretion in glands	Scanty secretions	Lumen of glands may be filled with secretions
Decidual reaction	Absent	Present
Accumulation of intra-cellular glycogen	Absent (minimal)	Present
Spiral arteries	Less coiled	More coiled

Summary (Examination Guide)
(Figs 23.13, 23.14, Flowcharts 23.6 and 7)

- Uterus is pear-shaped muscular organ having three parts: Fundus, body, and cervix.
- Uterus has three layers: Endometrium, myometrium, and perimetrium.
- Endometrium consists of simple columnar epithelial lining, simple tubular glands, and connective tissue stroma.
- Myometrium consists of smooth muscle cells showing inner and outer longitudinal fibers and middle spirally arranged fibers.
- Perimetrium consists of connective tissue layer covered by mesothelium.
- Endometrium shows cyclic changes as follows:
  - In proliferative phase, glands are long with narrow lumen; thick stroma with less coiled spiral arteries.
  - In secretory phase, glands are highly coiled with wide lumen and secretions, stroma with coiled spiral arteries.

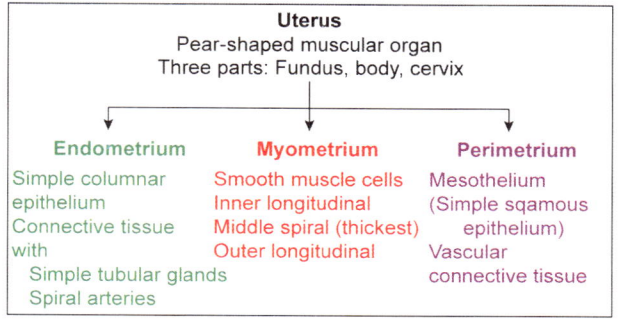

Flowchart 23.6: Histology of uterus

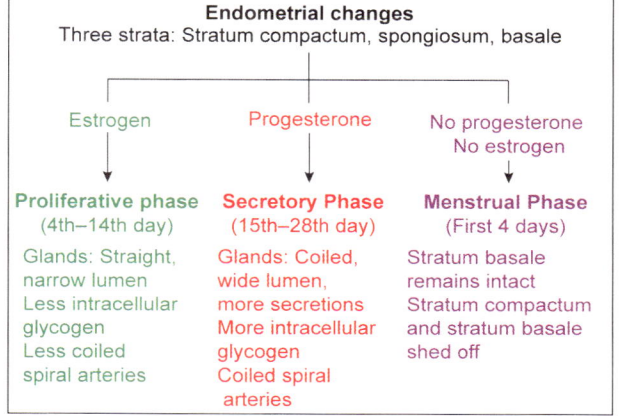

Flowchart 23.7: Endometrial changes

CERVIX OF UTERUS

- Cervix is a lower part of the uterus.
- Cervix has a narrow cavity called *cervical canal*.
- Cervical canal lumen communicates with cavity of uterine body through *internal os*, whereas with the vagina through *external os*.
- Lower projecting part of cervix in the vagina is called *portio vaginalis*.^{MCQ}

Histology of Cervix

- Cervix shows endocervix (mucous membrane) and muscle layer.

Endocervix

- Cervical canal is lined by *tall columnar* mucus secreting epithelium.
- Epithelium rests on *lamina propria* (loose areolar tissue).
- *Cervical glands:* These are small, branched tubular glands that lie in lamina propria. These glands secrete cervical mucus that is rich in lysozyme.

Muscle Coat

- Mucosa rests on thick layer of fibroelastic tissue and smooth muscles (6%–25%). The elastic component of cervix is essential for stretching of the cervix during childbirth.^{Neet}

Ectocervix/Portio Vaginalis

- Portion of cervix that projects into the vagina is called ectocervix.
- Ectocervix shows transformation zone where simple columnar epithelium of cervical canal become stratified squamous epithelium that continues with vaginal epithelium.

Clinical Correlation

- *Cervical mucous*
  Cervical glands secrete mucus that changes its quality according to the phase of menstrual cycle as follows:
  – In mid-cycle: Mucus is less viscous and favorable for sperm transport.
  – In other days of cycle: Mucus is thick, less viscous, and unfavorable for sperm transport.
- *Nabothian cyst:* Blockade of openings of cervical mucous glands result in retention of secretions and formation of cyst, called *Nabothian cyst*.^{Neet}
- *Pap (Papanicolaou) smear*
  – Cervical epithelial cells are constantly shed off *(exfoliated)* into the vagina.
  – These cells can be collected, stained, and observed for routine screening and diagnosis of cancerous conditions of cervix. These smear of cells on glass side is called pap smear. [Georgios Papanikolaou, Greek cytopathologist, 1883–1962].

VAGINA

Q. Write a short note on histology of vagina.

- Vagina is a fibromuscular elastic tube.
- It is about 8 cm long and extends from external cervical os to the external genitalia.

Histology of Vagina (Fig. 23.16 and Flowchart 23.8)

- Vagina has three layers: Mucosa, muscle layer, and adventitia.

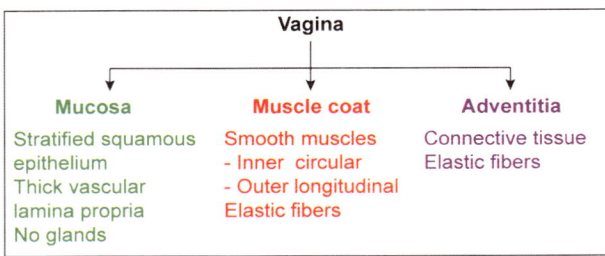

Flowchart 23.8: Histology of vagina

Mucosa

- Mucosa shows numerous longitudinal folds.
- Lining epithelium: *Nonkeratinized stratified squamous epithelium* (may show keratinization).[Neet]
- In follicular phase, epithelium accumulates intracellular glycogen. In secretory, glycogen content diminishes.
- *Lamina propria* is broad and highly vascular.

Muscular Layer

- Muscle layer consists of *smooth* muscle fibers arranged as inner circular and outer longitudinal layers.
- Muscle layer also contains many elastic fibers.
- Terminal part of vagina is guarded by fibers of bulbospongiosus muscle (striated muscle).

Adventitia

- Vagina is surrounded by adventitia that is made up of connective tissue and blood vessels

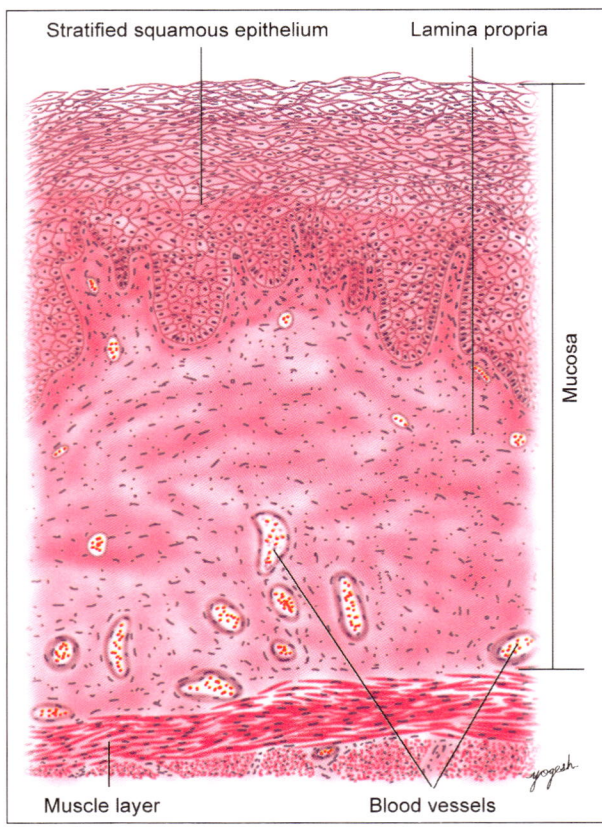

Fig. 23.16: Histology of vagina (practice figure).

Some Interesting Facts

- Wall of vagina does not have glands. Vagina remains moist due to secretions of cervical glands.[MCQ]
- In virgin, external opening of vagina may be surrounded by a fold of mucous membrane called *hymen*.
- Acidic pH of vagina: Bacteria act on the glycogen to produce lactic acid in vagina. It helps to maintain acidic pH of vagina.
- Vaginitis: Inflammation of vagina is called vaginitis. Candida (fungus) infection is the commonest cause of vaginitis.[MCQ]
- Bartholin (greater vestibular) glands are homologous to bulbourethral gland of Cowper in males. Its duct opens external to hymen on inner side of labia minora. The epithelium of duct is cuboidal near acini, transitional in mid portion, and becomes squamous near the mouth of duct.[Neet] Bartholin gland secretes mucus that provide vaginal lubrication [Caspar Bartholin the Younger, 1655–1738, Danish anatomist; William Cowper, 1666–1709, English surgeon and anatomist].
- No gland opens in vagina. Vaginal secretions are derived from mucous discharge of cervix and transduction through vaginal epithelium.[Neet]

CHAPTER 24

Female Reproductive System II: Mammary Gland, Placenta and Umbilical Cord

Chapter Outline
- Mammary gland
- Placenta
- Umbilical cord

Competency achievement: The student should be able to:

AN52.2 Describe and identify the microanatomical features of placenta and umbilical cord

MAMMARY GLAND

Q. Write a short note on histology of mammary gland.

- Mammary gland is the classical feature of mammals.
- Mammary glands develop from epidermal thickenings (mammary ridges/milk lines).^{MCQ}
- In males, mammary glands remain rudimentary throughout life.
- In female, postpuberty mammary glands enlarge and develop under the influence of ovarian hormones.
- Mammary glands produce milk on prolactin stimulation (hormone of anterior pituitary), whereas ejection of milk is under the control of oxytocin (posterior pituitary hormone).
- Mammary glands are *modified sweat glands* that lie in the superficial fascia.^{Neet}
- Skin covering the mammary gland shows (Fig. 24.1)
  - *Areola:* Dark pigmented circular area.
  - *Nipple:* Projection at the center of areola.
  - *Tubercles of Montgomery:* At periphery of areola, these are elevations produced because of enlarged *sebaceous* glands.^{MCQ} [William Montgomery, 1797-1859, Irish obstetrician].
- Fascia underlying the gland is connected with skin by suspensory *ligaments of Cooper* (Fig. 24.1). [Sir Astley Cooper, 1768–1841, British surgeon and anatomist].
- Glandular tissue of mammary gland consists of 15–20 lobes. Each lobe has number of lobules that are separated by dense connective tissue.
- Each lobe is drained by *lactiferous duct* that opens at the nipple as milk pores.
- Lactiferous duct shows dilatation (near its opening) called *lactiferous sinus*.
- Lactiferous duct divides into interlobular ducts, intralobular ducts and finally into alveolar ductule.
- Each alveolar ductule drains number of alveoli that lies in the form of clusters. These clusters of alveoli form small lobules of mammary gland.

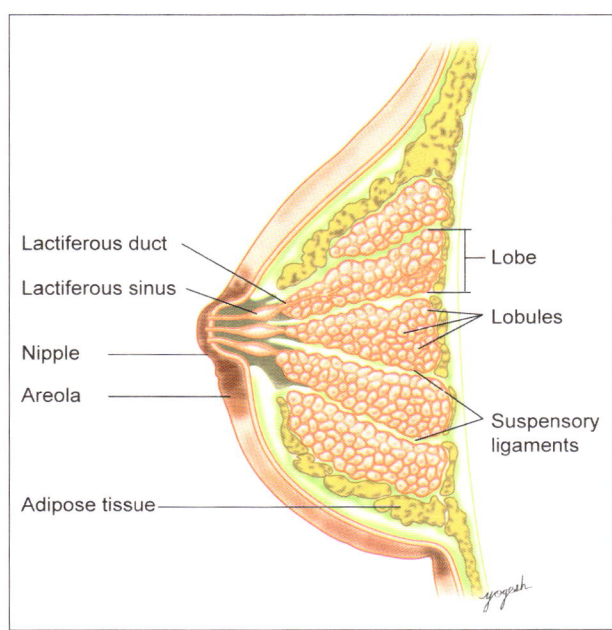

Fig. 24.1: Section of mammary gland.

- Mammary gland shows change in its structure according to its activeness (lactation).

Histology of Non-lactating (Inactive) Gland

- Inactive mammary gland mainly consists of ducts and their branches that lies in connective tissue stroma (Figs 24.2, 24.3 and Flowchart 24.1).
- Each lobule of inactive mammary gland shows:
  – *Intralobular duct* that is lined by cuboidal epithelium and few myoepithelial cells.
  – *Inactive alveoli* (even may be absent) that are made up of spherical masses or cords of epithelial cells.
  – Intralobular connective tissue: Ducts are surrounded by loose connective tissue (more cells, few fibers).
  – Interlobular connective tissue: Adjacent lobules are separated from each other by interlobular *dense connective tissue*.

Histology of Lactating (Active) Gland

- Active mammary gland develops under influence of ovarian hormones – estrogen and progesterone during pregnancy (Figs 24.2, 24.3 and Flowchart 24.1).
- Under influence of these hormones,
  – Ducts of mammary gland and acini develop
  – Fat deposits in interlobular connective tissue
  – Acini enlarge in size
  – Many new acini appear and occupy intralobular spaces
- Alveoli are lined by *low columnar (cuboidal) epithelium* and myoepithelial cells resting on basal lamina with

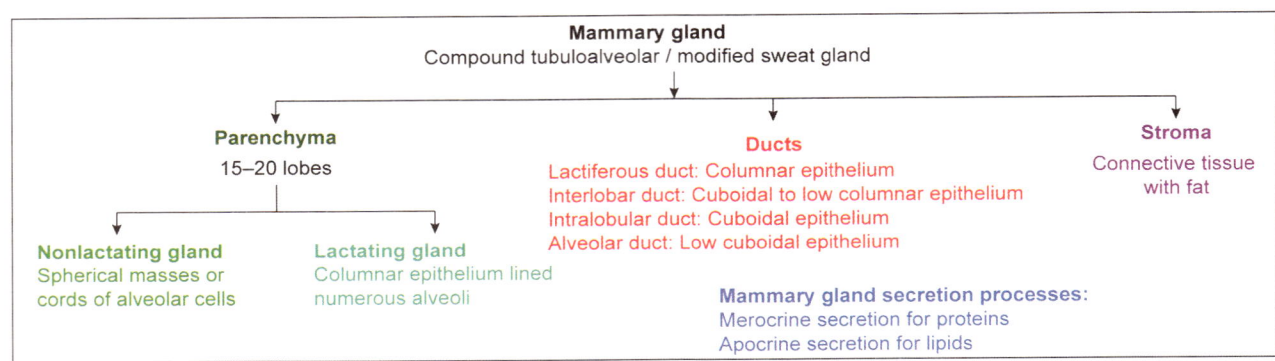

Flowchart 24.1: Histology of mammary gland.

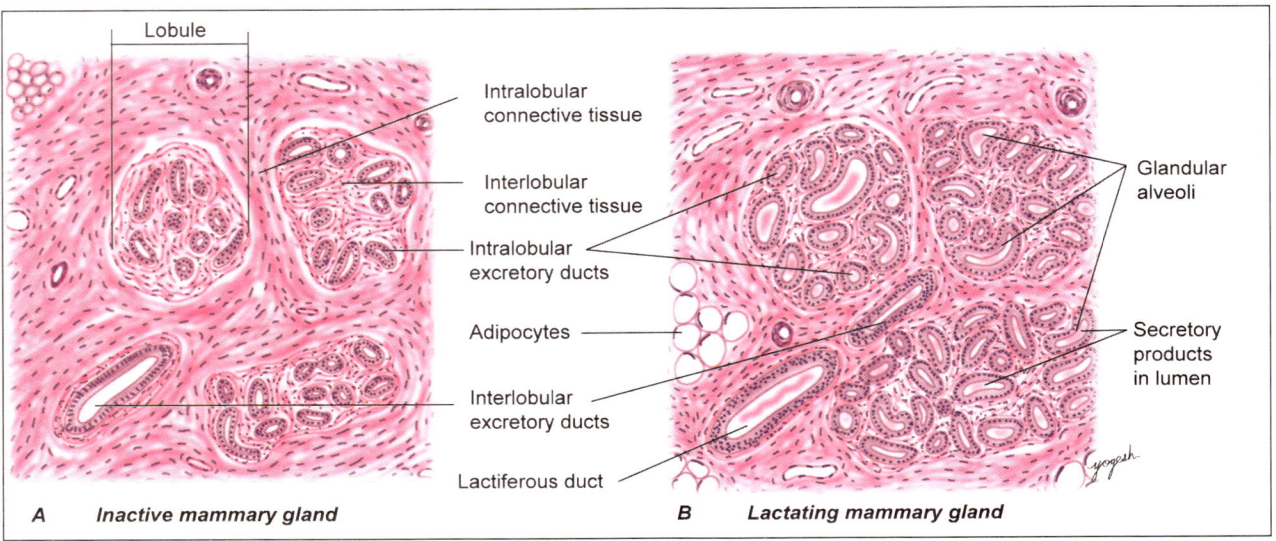

Fig. 24.2: Histology of mammary gland. A. Inactive mammary gland. B. Lactating mammary gland (practice figure).

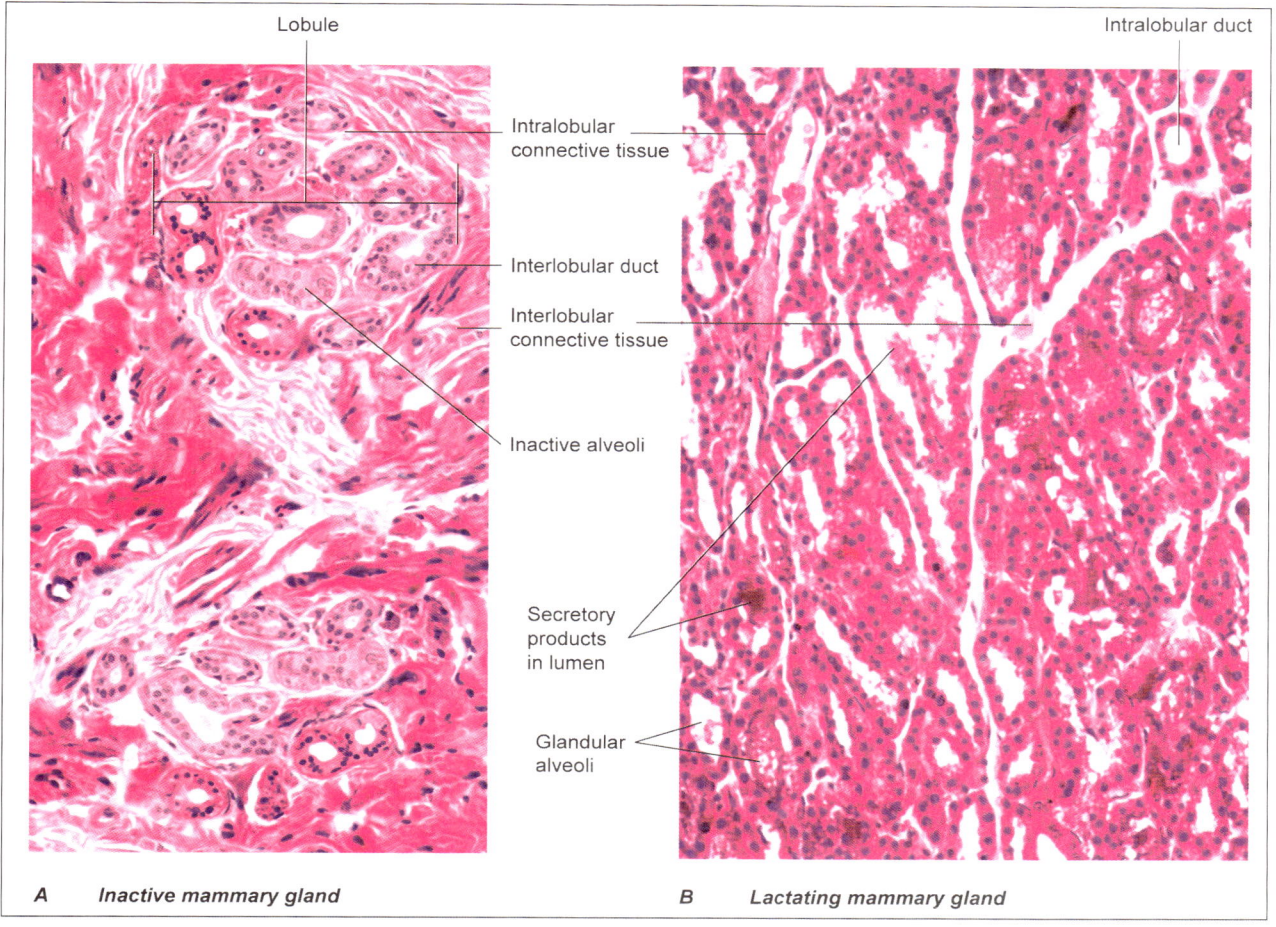

Fig. 24.3: Photomicrograph. Histology of mammary gland. (A) Inactive mammary gland. (B) Lactating mammary gland (high magnification, *H&E* stain).

narrow lumen. Lumen of alveoli is mostly filled with precipitated secretory products.
- Cells of acini show basal basophilia and apical eosinophilia with spherical nucleus.
- Basal lamina of acini is surrounded by *myoepithelial cells*.^{MCQ} Note: Myoepithelial cells are difficult to identify even at higher magnification with *H&E* staining.
- Electron microscopy: Alveolar secretory cells show lipid droplets, secretory vesicles, rough endoplasmic reticulum (basal basophilia on *H&E*), and well-developed Golgi complex (apical eosinophilia on *H&E* staining)

Duct System of Mammary Gland

- Alveolar ducts are lined by low cuboidal epithelium.
- Intralobular ducts are lined by cuboidal to low columnar epithelium.
- Lactiferous ducts are lined by columnar epithelium. Their terminal part shows transformation from simple columnar to pseudostratified columnar to stratified squamous epithelium.
- Ducts are surrounded by myoepithelial cells and basal lamina.

Mode of Milk Secretion

- Mammary gland uses the following two modes of secretion in production of milk:
  - **Merocrine secretion:** *Proteins* packed in secretory vesicles get released by fusion of vesicles with plasma membrane.^{Next}
  - **Apocrine secretion:** *Lipid* droplets fuse to form a large droplet. These large droplets along with a small quantity of cytoplasm get expelled out with a part of plasma membrane.^{Next}

Clinical Correlation

- *Colostrum/premilk* is alkaline, yellowish secretions of mammary gland released for first few days after birth of child (delivery). It is rich in *antibodies* (provide passive immunity to newborn), proteins, and vitamins.^MCQ
- *Brest cancer:* Cancerous proliferation of lining epithelium of ducts and alveoli produces breast cancer. These are the *commonest cancer of human* in the world and its early detection is possible on self-examination of breast.^MCQ
- *Fibroadenoma* is a benign tumor of mammary glands.
- Estrogen promotes duct proliferation, whereas progesterone promotes alveolar growth.

Box 24.1: Milk ejection reflex

- It is a neurohormonal reflex that initiates ejection of milk from mammary gland (Flowchart 24.2).
- Suckling of nipple sends impulses to hypothalamus that releases oxytocin via posterior pituitary and stops release of prolactin-inhibitory factor.
- Anterior pituitary secretes prolactin in absence of prolactin inhibitory factor.
- Prolactin induces milk secretion by alveolar cells, whereas oxytocin causes contraction of myoepithelial cells and induces milk ejection from the gland.

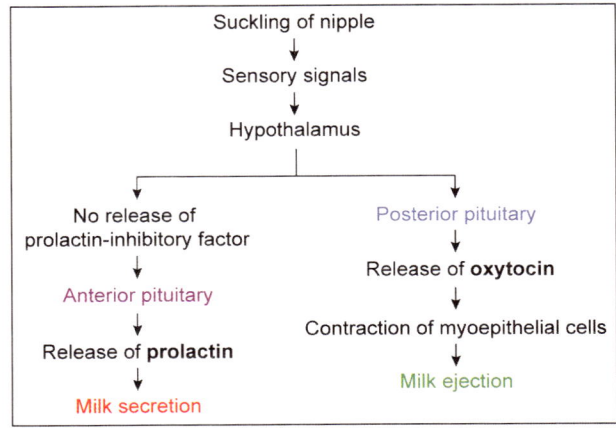

Flowchart 24.2: Milk ejection reflex

Summary (Examination Guide)

- Mammary gland is a *modified apocrine sweat gland.*
- It is composed of ducts, parenchyma, and stoma.
- Ducts: Mammary gland has the following order of ducts:
  - Lactiferous duct: Lined by columnar epithelium (terminal part shows transformation from columnar to stratified squamous epithelium).
  - Interlobular ducts: Lined by cuboidal to low columnar epithelium.
  - Intralobular ducts: Lined by cuboidal epithelium.
  - Alveolar ducts: Lined by low cuboidal epithelium.
- Parenchyma
  - Each gland shows 15–20 lobes of *compound tubuloalveolar gland.*
  - Non-lactating inactive glands: Shows spherical masses or cords of alveolar cells.
  - Lactating active glands: Shows numerous branched ducts with clusters of alveoli that are lined by simple columnar epithelium.
- Stroma: Consists of interlobular, intralobar, and interlobar connective tissue.

PLACENTA

- Placenta is a fetomaternal organ that is meant for nourishment of fetus.
- It grows during pregnancy in the uterus.
- Shape: Disk-like
- Weight: ~500 g
- Surfaces: It has two surfaces (Fig. 24.4)
  - Fetal surface: Smooth, shining, and covered by the amnion
  - Maternal surface: Rough, lobulated, shows 15–20 cotyledons. [for details refer Chapter 9: Placenta from Textbook of Human Embryology by Yogesh Sontakke before reading histology of placenta.]

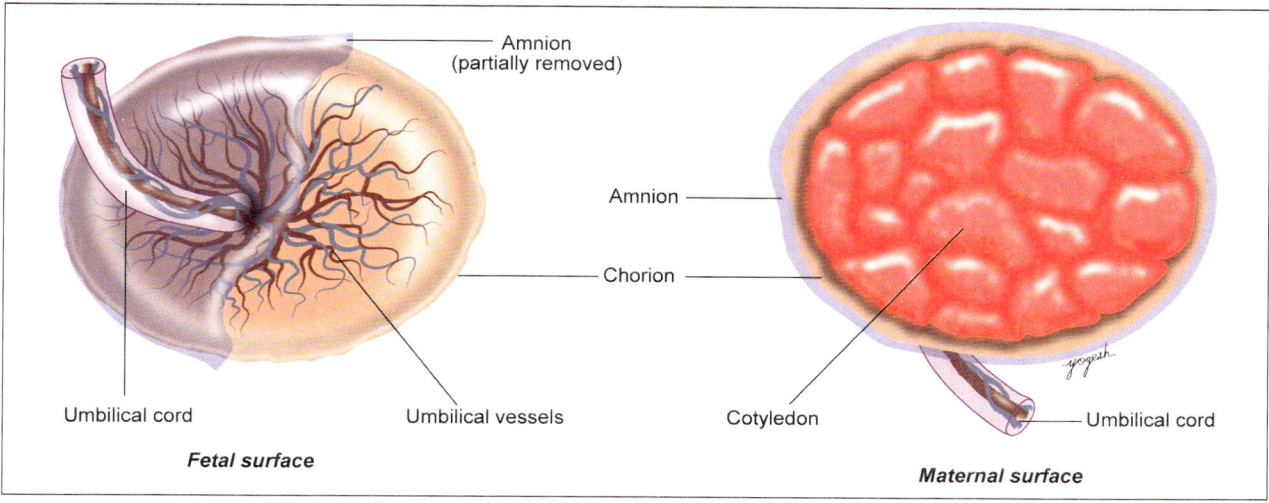

Fig. 24.4: Surfaces of placenta. Placenta has two surfaces – fetal and placental. Fetal surface is smooth, covered by translucent layer of amnion and shows attachment of umbilical cord. Maternal surface shows 15–30 polygonal cotyledons (Source: Textbook of Human Embryology, Yogesh Sontakke, 1st edn., CBS Publishers).

Components of Placenta (Flowchart 24.3)

- As placenta is a fetomaternal organ, it has fetal component – chorion and maternal component – decidua.

Decidua

- Uterine endometrium is known as *decidua* on implantation of blastocyst (fertilized ovum).

Flowchart 24.3: Structure of placenta (Source: Textbook of Human Embryology, Yogesh Sontakke, 1st edn., CBS Publishers)

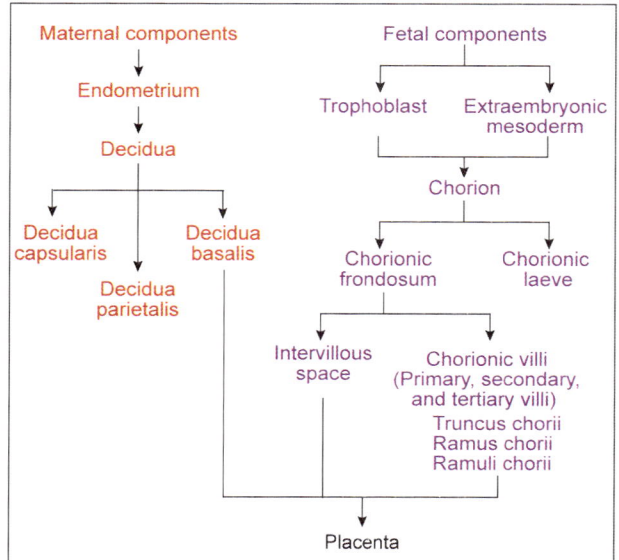

- Decidua has three components (Fig. 24.5):
  - *Decidua basalis:* It underlies blastocyst and takes part in the formation of placenta
  - *Decidua capsularis:* It surrounds blastocyst

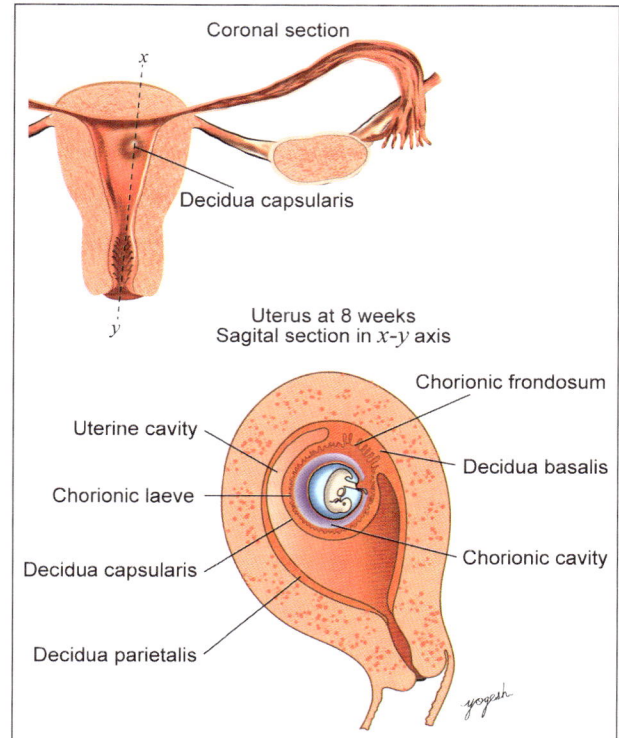

Fig. 24.5: Fusion of decidua capsularis and parietalis. By the end of eighth week, decidua shows three zones called decidua basalis, capsularis, and parietalis (Source: Textbook of Human Embryology, Yogesh Sontakke, 1st edn., CBS Publishers).

- *Decidua parietalis*: It covers rest of the uterine wall
- *Decidualization* involves enlargement of endometrial cells. These cells become round-shaped.
- *Placental septa*: These are wedge-shaped extensions of decidua into the placenta.

Chorion and Trophoblast

- Blastocyst is consisting of outer trophoblast (trophoectoderm) and inner embryoblast (inner cell mass).
- Embryoblast gives rise to embryo. In initial stages, embryoblast forms epiblast, hypoblast, amnion, Heuser's membrane, amniotic cavity, primary yolk sac, and extraembryonic mesoderm.
- Trophoblast forms outer syncytiotrophoblast and inner cytotrophoblast layer.
- Extraembryonic mesoderm and trophoblastic layer form chorion surrounding the embryo.
- Chorion has two parts
  - *Chorionic frondosum*: It is a part of chorion toward placenta or decidua basalis.
  - *Chorionic laeve*: It is a part of chorion toward decidua capsularis.

Placental Villi

- Chorionic frondosum gives rise to 40–60 stem villi (*truncus chorii*) that branches to form *ramus chorii*.
- Spaces surrounding the villi are called *intervillous spaces* that contain maternal blood (Figs 24.6 and 24.7).
- Developmentally villi are of three types[Viva, MCQ]
  - *Primary villi* have outer syncytiotrophoblast and inner cytotrophoblast.

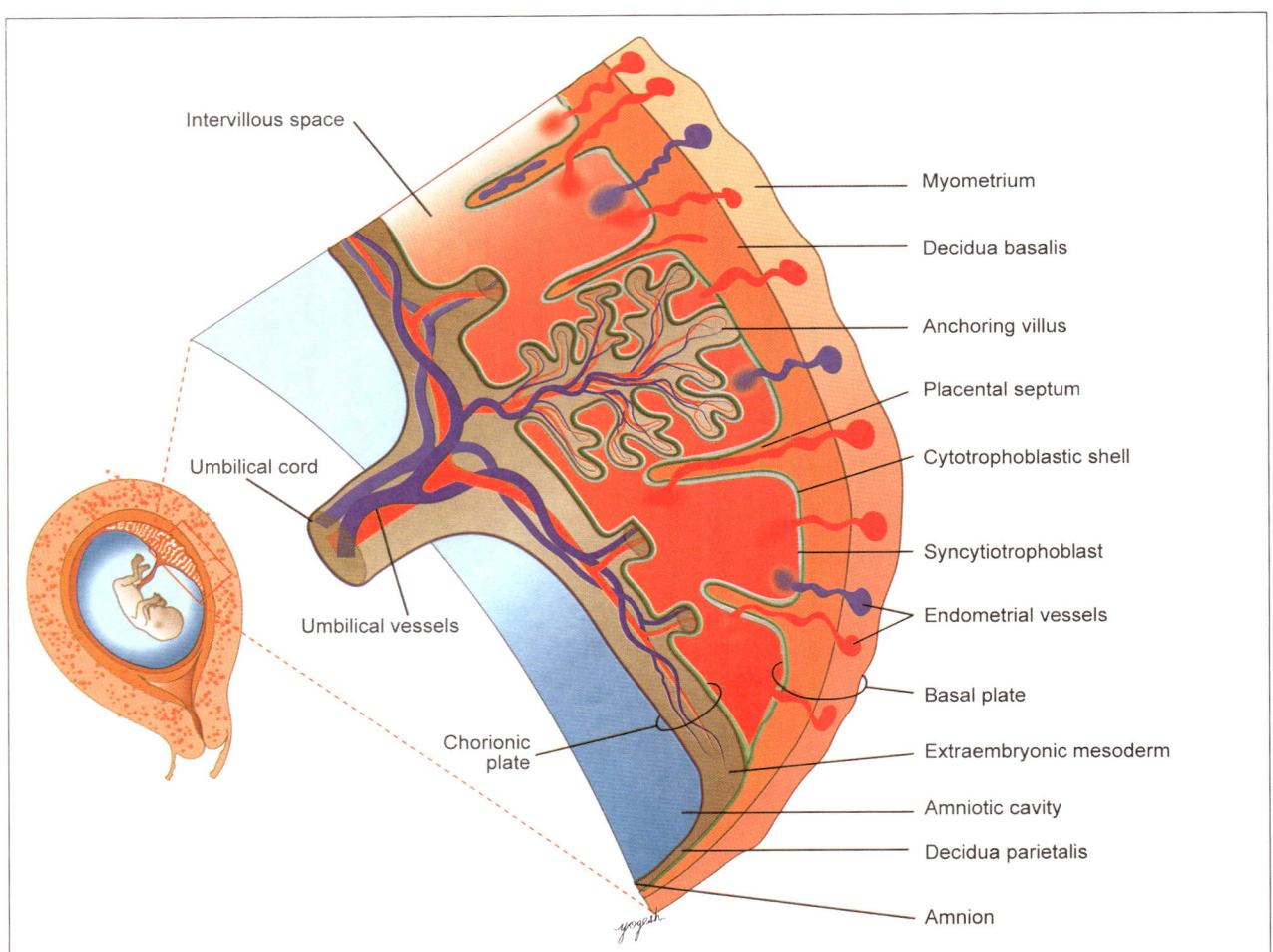

Fig. 24.6: Structure of placenta. Intervillous spaces are filled with maternal blood. Cotyledons are partially separated by decidual septa. Anchoring villi extend between basal plate and chorionic plate. Branches of anchoring villus contain fetal blood vessels. Endometrial arteries bring oxygenated blood to intervillous space and drained by endometrial veins (Source: Textbook of Human Embryology, Yogesh Sontakke, 1st edn., CBS Publishers).

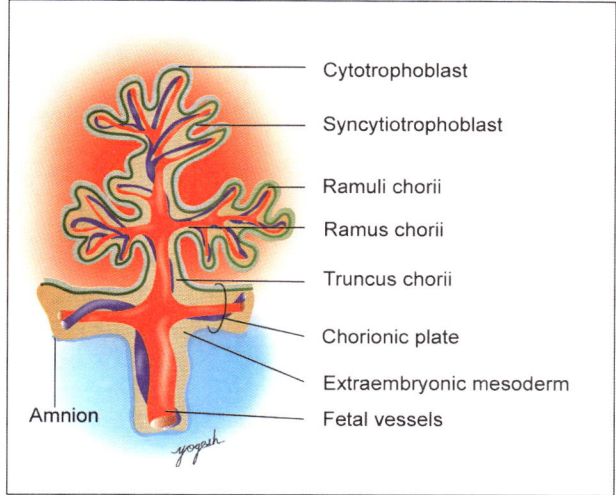

Fig. 24.7: Branching pattern of villi. Villi are truncus chorii, ramus chorii, and ramuli chorii (Source: Textbook of Human Embryology, Yogesh Sontakke, 1st edn., CBS Publishers).

- *Secondary villi* have central core of extraembryonic mesoderm surrounded by cytotrophoblast and syncytiotrophoblast.
- *Tertiary villi* have fetal blood vessels in the mesodermal core of secondary villi.

Placental Barrier^{Viva, MCQ}

- Placental barrier separates maternal blood from fetal blood but allows the exchange of nutrients.
- It consists of (Fig. 24.8)
  - Syncytiotrophoblast
  - Cytotrophoblast and its basal lamina
  - Extraembryonic mesoderm (connective tissue)
  - Basal lamina of fetal blood vessels
  - Endothelium of fetal capillaries (non-fenestrated)

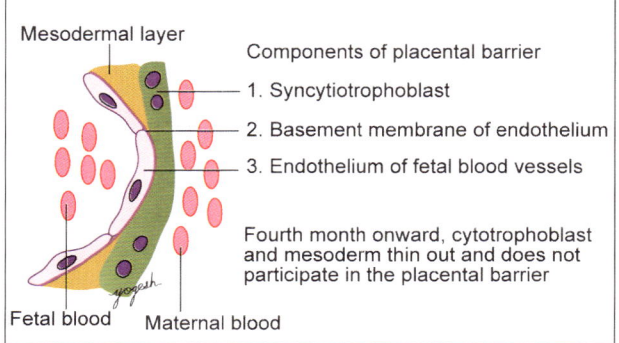

Fig. 24.8: Placental barrier (Source: Textbook of Human Embryology, Yogesh Sontakke, 1st edn., CBS Publishers) (practice figure).

Some Interesting Facts

- *Hofbauer cells:* These are macrophages found in mesodermal connective tissue of villi [J Isfred Isidore Hofbauer, 1878–1961, an American gynecologist].^{Neet}
- HIV virus is primarily localized in Hofbauer cells and syncytiotrophoblast.^{Neet}
- *Trophoblastic shell:* Cytotrophoblast covers and separates syncytiotrophoblasts from maternal decidua. This layer of cytotrophoblasts is called trophoblastic shell.^{MCQ} It prevents further growth of placenta and restricts placenta in endometrium.^{Viva}
- Delivery of placenta: Placenta gets delivered approximately 30 minutes after birth.^{MCQ} Placenta, fetal membranes, and placental septa (part of decidua) get expelled together.
- *Lochia rubra:* In first week of delivery, remnants of decidua are shed and called lochia rubra.^{MCQ}

Histology of Placenta (Fig. 24.9, 24.10 and Flowchart 24.4)

- Placenta extends from smooth amnion-covered *fetal surface* to rough decidual *maternal surface*.
- Amnion consists of a layer of *simple cuboidal epithelium* and underlying connective tissue.
- Underneath the amniotic connective tissue, extraembryonic mesodermal connective tissue is present. Amnion, amniotic connective tissue, and extraembryonic connective tissue together form *chorionic plate*.
- Chorionic plate shows fetal blood vessels. These vessels do not show distinctive features of artery and veins.
- Remaining part of placenta consists of *chorionic villi* of different sizes.^{Identification feature} Usually placental section shows floating/free villi surrounded by intervillous space.
- On maternal side of placenta, *basal plate* (decidua basalis) is present.
- Basal plate consists of connective tissue and some decidual cells.
- *Decidual cells* are present in clusters and have an epithelial appearance.^{Identification feature}
- *Placental septa* (connective tissue) arise from basal plate and enters into the substance of placenta. These septa do not contain fetal vessels. Stem villi have fetal vessels.

Microscopy of Villi

- Placenta shows villi of different sizes that are surrounded by intervillous spaces.

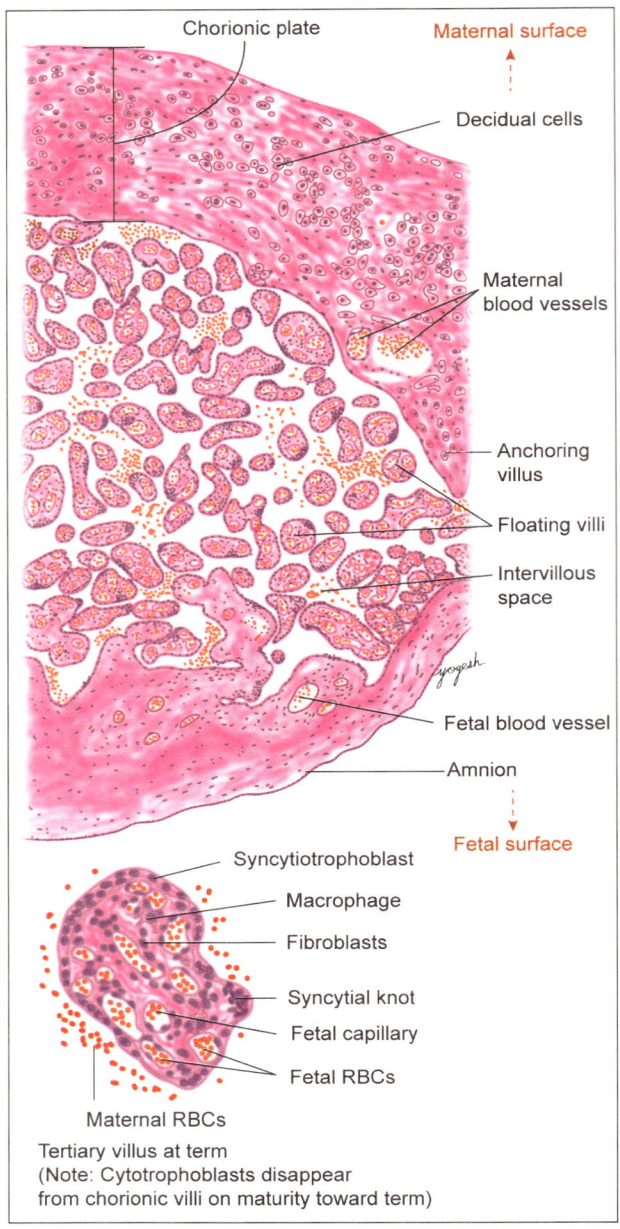

Fig. 24.9: Histology of placenta (practice figure).

- Villi are covered by a layer of syncytiotrophoblasts that looks similar to cuboidal epithelium on *H&E* staining. There are no intercellular margins as syncytiotrophoblast are a protoplasmic multinucleated mass.
- *Syncytial knots:* In some regions of placenta, nuclei of syncytiotrophoblast gather to form clusters called *syncytial knots*. Even in some areas, syncytiotrophoblast thin out and may be free of nuclei.
- Syncytiotrophoblast may has striated border as it has projecting microvilli into intervillous space.
- *Cytotrophoblasts*
  - Early placenta: Cytotrophoblast is located by the side of syncytiotrophoblasts.
  - Mature placenta: Cytotrophoblastic cells are present on inner side of syncytiotrophoblast.
- Mesodermal core and fetal blood vessels
  - Core of each villus shows connective tissue, intercellular matrix, occasional Hofbauer cells (phagocytic cells), and fetal vessels.
  - Small villi may show only thin syncytiotrophoblasts layer and fetal vessels.
  - Fetal vessels and intervillous spaces show RBCs and other blood cells.

Summary (Examination Guide)

- Placenta is a fetomaternal organ.
- It has *chorionic* plate that consists of amnion (cuboidal epithelium), connective tissue layer, and fetal blood vessels.
- It also has *basal plate* that shows connective tissue, decidual cells, and placental septa.
- Core of placenta consists of chorionic villi and intervillous spaces.
- Chorionic villi show outer syncytiotrophoblasts (multinucleated protoplasm), occasional cytotrophoblast, connective tissue, fetal vessels, and occasional Hofbauer (phagocytic) cells.
- Intervillous spaces are filled with maternal blood.

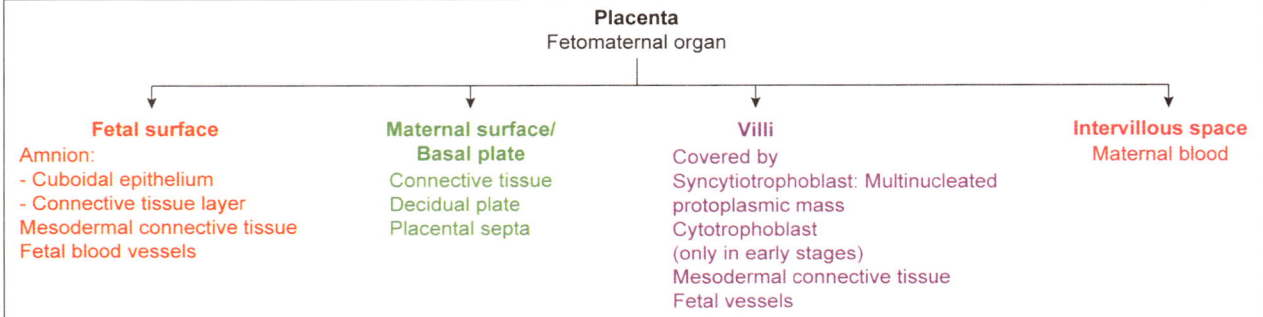

Flowchart 24.4: Histology of placenta

Female Reproductive System II: Mammary Gland, Placenta and Umbilical Cord

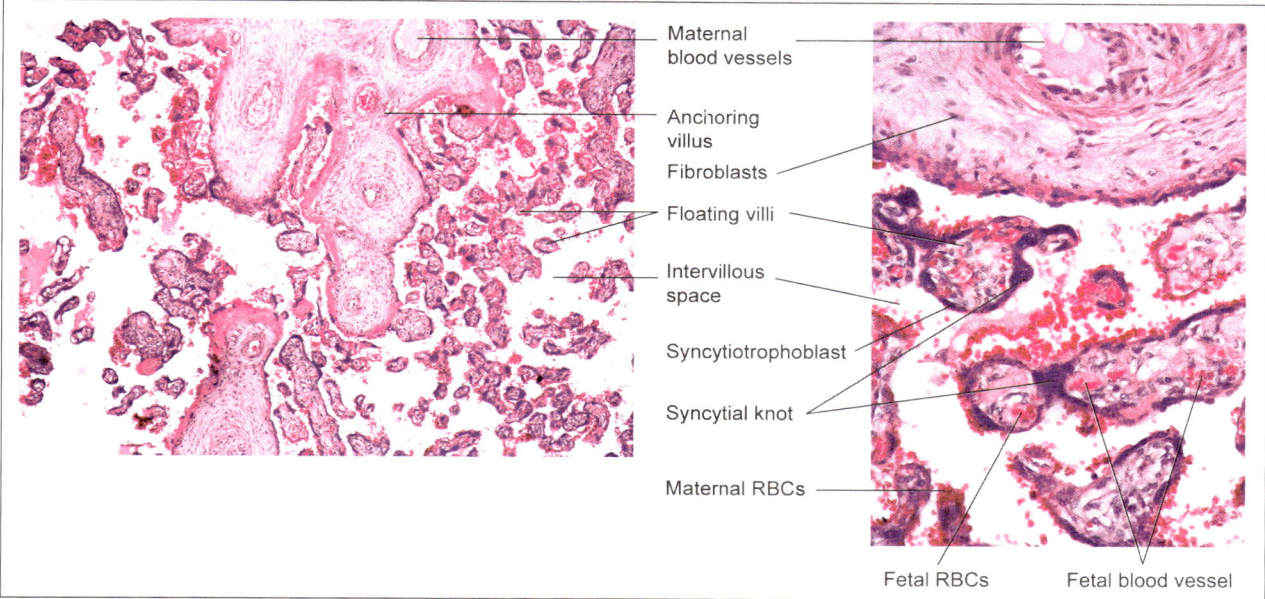

Fig. 24.10: Photomicrograph. Histology of placenta (low magnification on right, High magnification on left).

Functions of Placenta

1. Gaseous exchange: O_2 and CO_2 exchange takes place across placenta through simple diffusion. Fetal hemoglobin has high affinity for oxygen and high hemoglobin concentration in fetus facilitates transfer of oxygen from mother to the fetus.
2. Transport of nutrients such as glucose, fatty acids, amino acids, and electrolytes such as sodium, potassium, and chloride.
3. Excretion of urea, uric acid and creatinine from fetal blood into maternal blood.
4. Passive immunity: Maternal antibodies (immunoglobulins) pass placental barrier by pinocytosis of syncytiotrophoblast. These antibodies provide passive immunity to fetus against diphtheria, measles, smallpox, and so on. Maternal antibodies do not protect newborn from chickenpox and whooping cough.*MCQ*
5. Placental barrier: It prevents entry of many drugs and bacteria. However, almost all viruses can cross placental barrier. Some of fetal blood cells may cross placental barrier and circulate in maternal blood.
6. Storage: Placenta stores glycogen, calcium, and iron.
7. Endocrine function:
   Placenta secretes following hormones:
   – Human chorionic gonadotropin
   – Placental estrogen
   – Placental progesterone
   – Placental lactogen

Source: Textbook of Human Embryology, Yogesh Sontakke, 1st edn, CBS Publishers.

UMBILICAL CORD

Q. Write a short note on histology of umbilical cord.

- Umbilical cord is a communicating stalk between fetus and placenta.
- It carries oxygenated blood from placenta to fetus through *single umbilical artery* and deoxygenated blood from fetus to placenta through *two umbilical veins* (Fig. 24.11).*Neet*
- Vessels of umbilical cord are embedded in loose connective tissue called *Wharton's' jelly.*
- Length: 50–60 cm, Thickness: 12 mm

Histology of Umbilical Cord

- Umbilical cord is covered by a simple squamous epithelium and it floats in amniotic fluid (Figs 24.12, 24.13 and Flowchart 24.5).

Umbilical Artery

- Umbilical artery consists of tunica intima and media.
- Tunica intima has
  – Endothelial lining: *Simple squamous epithelium*

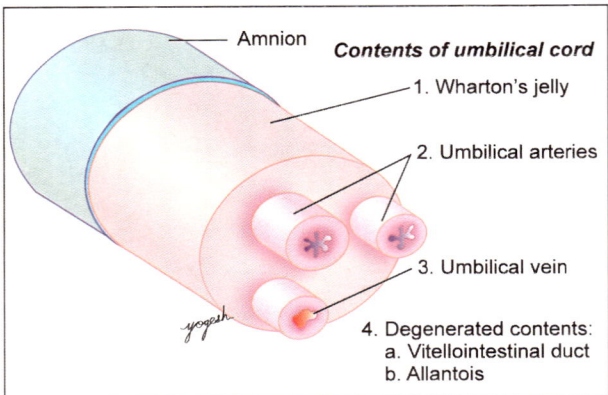

Fig. 24.11: Structure of umbilical cord (Schematic representation) (Source: Textbook of Human Embryology, Yogesh Sontakke, 1st edn, CBS Publishers).

Flowchart 24.5: Histology of umbilical cord

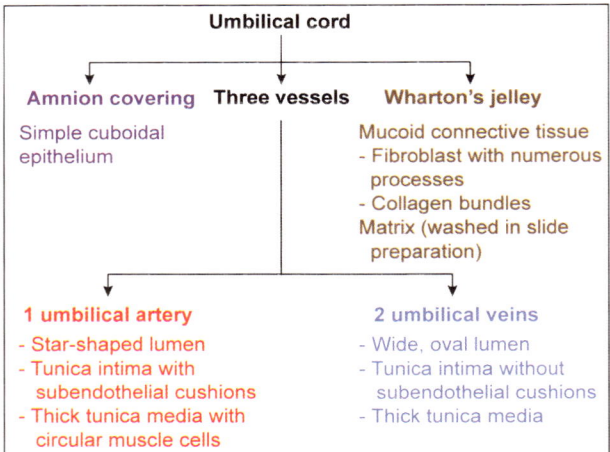

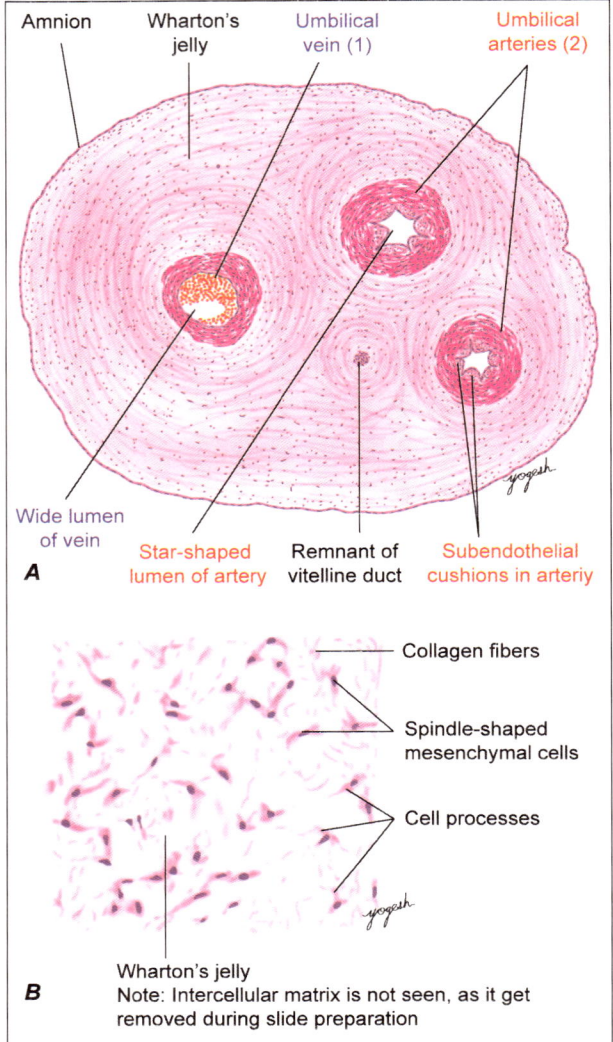

Fig. 24.12: Histology of umbilical cord. (A) Transverse section of umbilical cord. (B) Wharton's jelly at high magnification (practice figure).

- *Subendothelial cushions:* They consist of connective tissue thickenings that produce folding of tunica intima; hence, star-shaped lumen of the umbilical arteries.
- Tunica intima: It contains number of elastic lamellae.
- Tunica media: It consists of smooth muscle cells and interspaced elastic fibers.

Umbilical Veins

- They consist of tunica intima and tunica media.
- Tunica intima: It shows simple squamous endothelium and small amount of subendothelial connective tissue layer. Umbilical veins show well-defined internal elastic lamina and regular (oval) lumen (Fig. 24.14).
- Tunica media: It consists of circularly arranged smooth muscle cells.

Wharton's Jelly/Mucoid Connective Tissue

- Umbilical vessels are surrounded by a mucoid connective tissue.
- It consists of highly branched fibroblasts, collagen fibers, and ground substance.
- During *H&E* preparation, the ground substance gets removed; hence, Wharton's jelly shows only collagen fibers and fibroblasts.

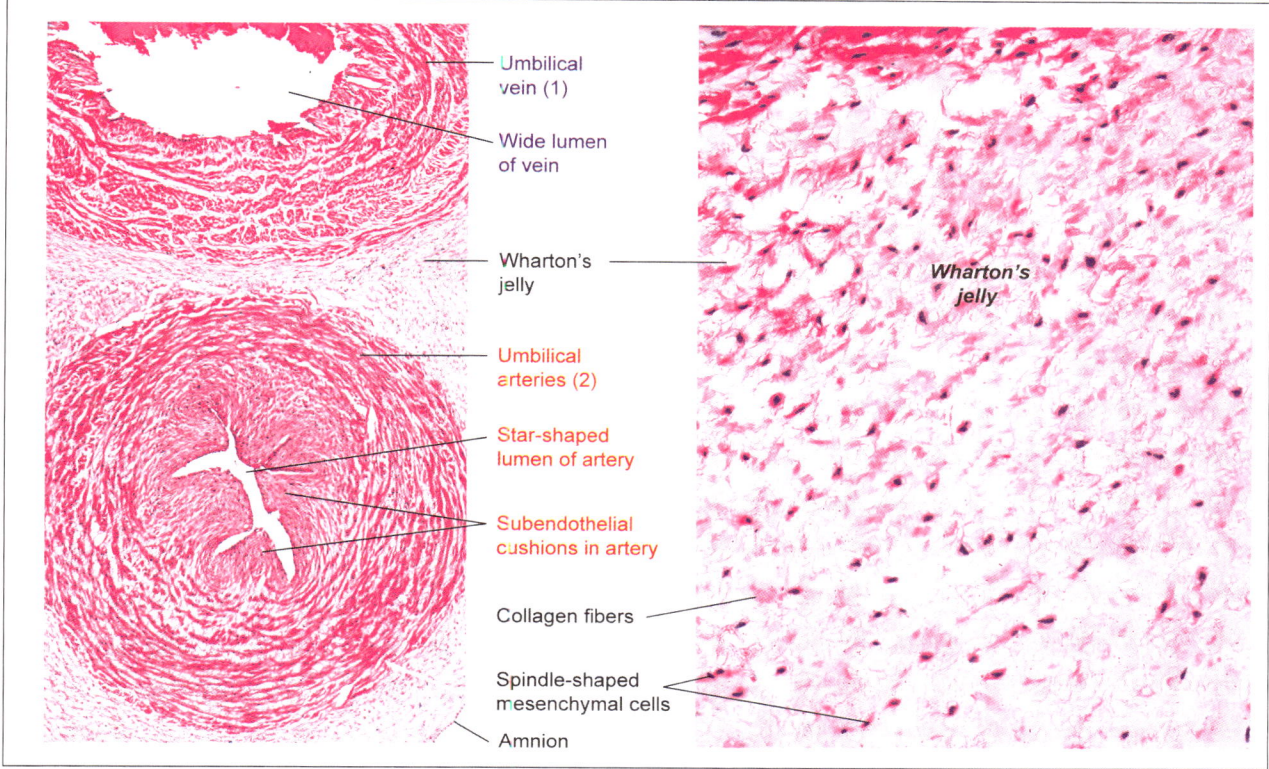

Fig. 24.13: Photomicrograph. Histology of umbilical cord. (low magnification on left showing umbilical vein and artery, high magnification on right showing Wharton's jelly, H&E stain).

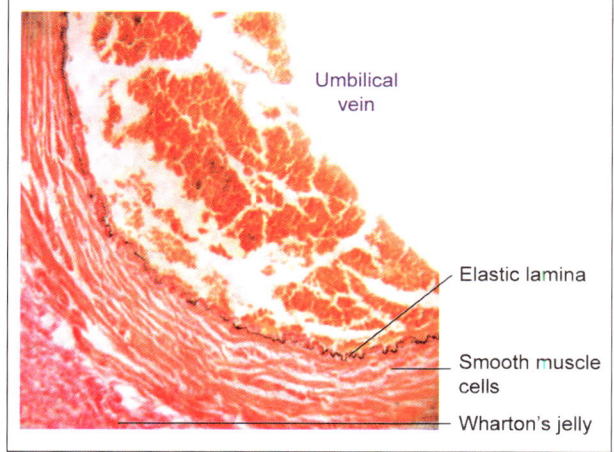

Fig. 24.14: Photomicrograph. Umbilical vein. (high magnification, orcein stain, Cells – yellow, Collagen – pink, Elastic fibers – black).

Some Interesting Facts

- Lumen of umbilical artery is star-shaped because of presence of subendothelial cushion. Lumen of umbilical veins is wide (oval or regular). *Identification feature*
- Umbilical veins are thin walled than umbilical arteries. *Identification feature*
- Post birth, umbilical arteries constrict and causes obstruction of the lumen by approximation of subendothelial cushions.
- Umbilical cord does not possess any nerve or lymphatics. *Neet*
- Helical course of umbilical arteries decreases the possibilities of kinking of vessels around vein.
- Unlike other blood vessels, the umbilical vessels do not have tunica adventitia.

Summary (Examination Guide)

- Umbilical cord is a communication between the fetus and placenta.
- It consists of two umbilical veins and one umbilical artery embedded in Wharton's jelly.
- Umbilical artery has tunica intima (endothelium and subendothelial cushions) and tunica media (circular smooth muscles) with number of elastic laminae.
- Umbilical vein also has tunica intima and media without subendothelial cushions.
- Lumen of umbilical artery is star-shaped, whereas lumen of umbilical vein is wide (oval).
- Wharton's jelly is a mucoid connective tissue that has fibroblasts, collagen fibers, and extracellular matrix.

CHAPTER 25

Endocrine System

Chapter Outline
- Pituitary gland
- Thyroid gland
- Parathyroid gland
- Adrenal gland
- Pineal gland

Competency achievement: The student should be able to:

AN43.2 Identify, describe and draw the microanatomy of: Pituitary gland, thyroid, parathyroid gland
AN52.1 Describe and identify the microanatomical features of gastrointestinal system: Suprarenal gland

INTRODUCTION

- Endocrine system involves production of *hormones* secreted *directly into the bloodstream*. These hormones regulate activities of various cells, tissues, and organs. (*Hormaein* = to excite, in Greek).
- Endocrine system (hormones) produces slower and prolonged response than the nervous system.
- Endocrine tissues are *highly vascular.*

Distribution of Endocrine Cells

Endocrine cells are present in the form of endocrine glands or a cluster of cells in organs or may occur singly (Flowchart 25.1).

Hormone

- *Definition:* Hormone is a *biological substance* secreted by an endocrine tissue that acts on specific target cells through *cell receptors.*
- Blood and interstitial fluid act as a *medium* for transport of hormones.
- Hormones can be classified according to their chemical nature (Flowchart 25.2).
- Hormone exerts its effect on interaction with hormone-specific receptors that are located on target cells.
- There are two types of *hormone receptors*
  A: Cell surface receptors
  B: Intracellular receptors

Mechanism of Hormone Action

A. Protein hormones bind with *cell surface receptors* that activate production of second messengers such as cyclic adenosine monophosphate (cAMP), 1,2-diacylglycerol (DAG) or calcium ions. Second messenger amplifies and produces physiological effects.
B. *Intracellular receptors:* Steroid and thyroid hormones can

Flowchart 25.1: Distribution of endocrine cells

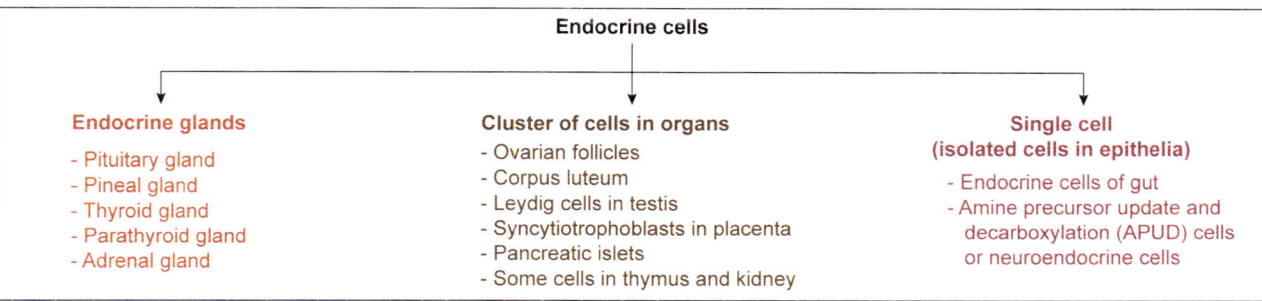

Flowchart 25.2: Classification of hormones

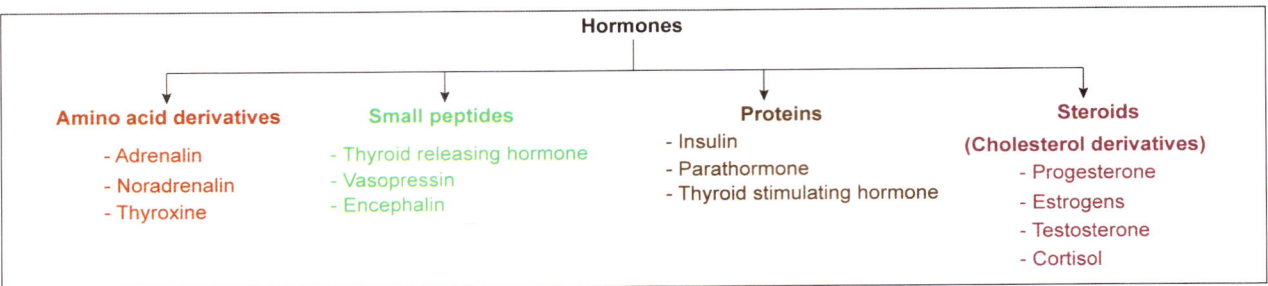

penetrate cell membrane and nuclear membrane to reach intracellular receptors. When these hormones bind to these receptors, mRNA is produced, and new protein is formed. The newly formed proteins cause physiological effects.

PITUITARY GLAND (HYPOPHYSIS CEREBRI)

Q. Draw a well-labeled diagram of histology of pituitary gland.

- The hypophysis cerebri is a small endocrine gland that lies in the hypophyseal fossa or *sella turcica of sphenoid bone.*^MCQ
- The gland is about the size of a pea.
- It is suspended from floor of the third ventricle of the brain by infundibulum (a connecting stalk).
- Hypophysis cerebri is also called *"master of endocrine glands"* as its secretions the influence activity of most of the endocrine glands.

Parts/Subdivisions of Pituitary Gland

- Hypophysis cerebi is divided into two functional components (Figs 25.1, 25.2 and Flowchart 25.3):
  A. *Adenohypophysis* (anterior lobe) that consists of glandular epithelium
  B. *Neurohypophysis* (posterior lobe) that consists of neurosecretory tissue
- Adenohypophysis has three parts:
  1. Pars distalis
  2. Pars intermedia
  3. Pars tuberalis (collar or sheath around infundibulum)
- Neurohypophysis has two parts:
  1. Pars nervosa
  2. Infundibulum or hypothalamo-hypophyseal tracts

Development of Pituitary Gland

- Anterior lobe is derived from an evagination of ectoderm of oropharynx (*Rathke's pouch*), whereas posterior lobe is derived from the downward growth of neuroectoderm from the floor of the third ventricle (diencephalon).

Flowchart 25.3: Parts of pituitary gland

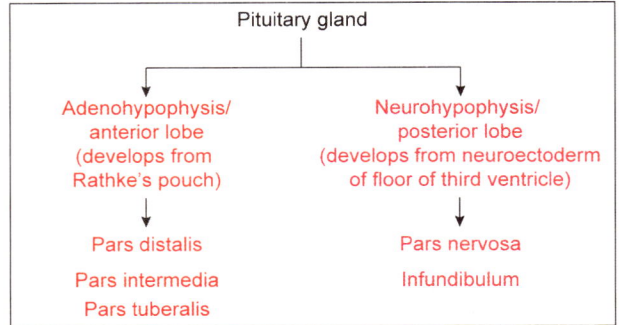

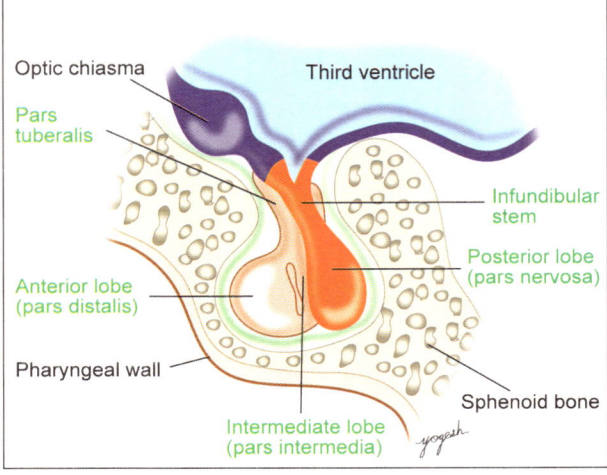

Fig. 25.1: Subdivisions of pituitary gland (as seen at birth).

Endocrine System

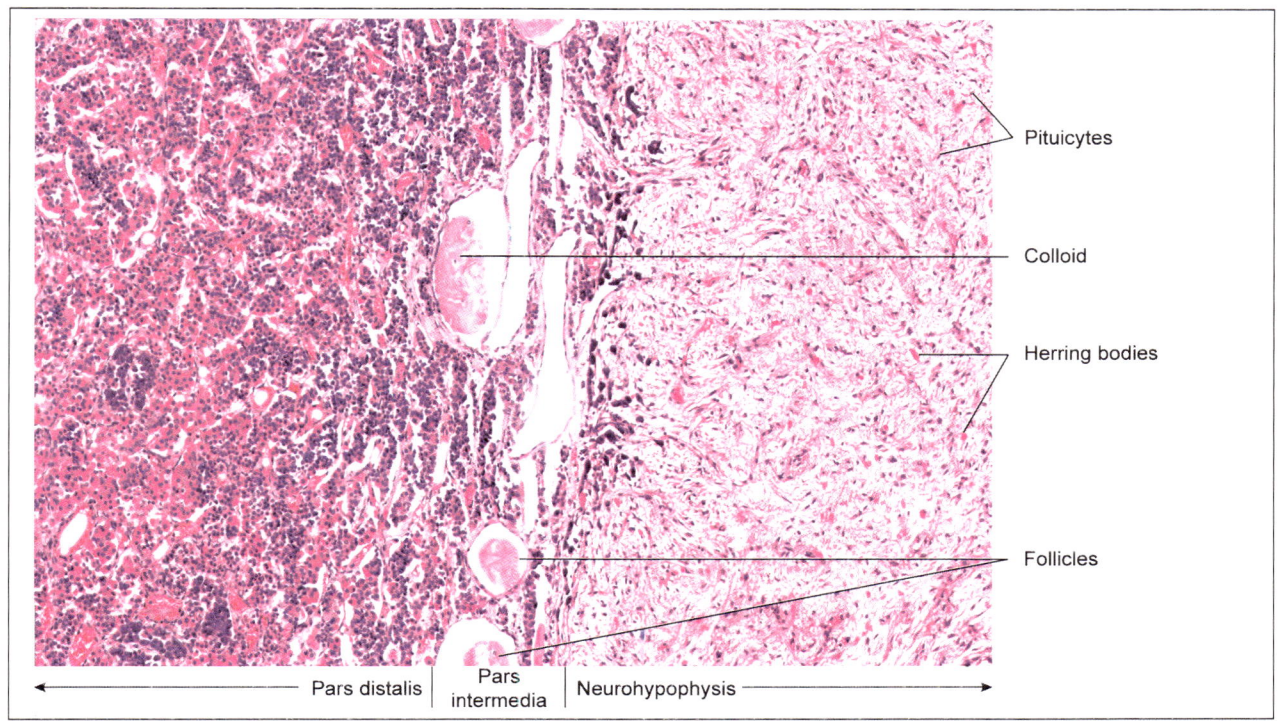

Fig. 25.2: Photomicrograph. Histology of pituitary gland (low magnification *H&E* stain).

> **Box 25.1:** Hypothalamo-hypophyseal portal system
>
> - Pituitary gland receives blood supply from internal carotid artery through (Fig. 25.3)
> - – Superior hypophyseal artery for pars tuberalis and infundibular stem
> - – Inferior hypophyseal artery for neurohypophysis
> - Arteries that supply pars tuberalis, median eminence, and infundibular stem form *fenestrated capillary plexus.* These capillaries join to form *hypophyseal portal veins* (Flowchart 25.4).
> - Hypophyseal portal veins form *secondary capillary plexus* in pars distalis.
> - Thus, hypothalamic hormones are carried toward pars distalis via hypophyseal portal veins.
> - Finally, pituitary drains into the cavernous sinus through *hypophyseal veins.*

Histology of Pituitary Gland

Adenohypophysis (Figs 25.4, 25.2 and 25.5)

- It consists of clumps or cords of cells separated by fenestrated sinusoidal capillaries (Flowchart 25.5).

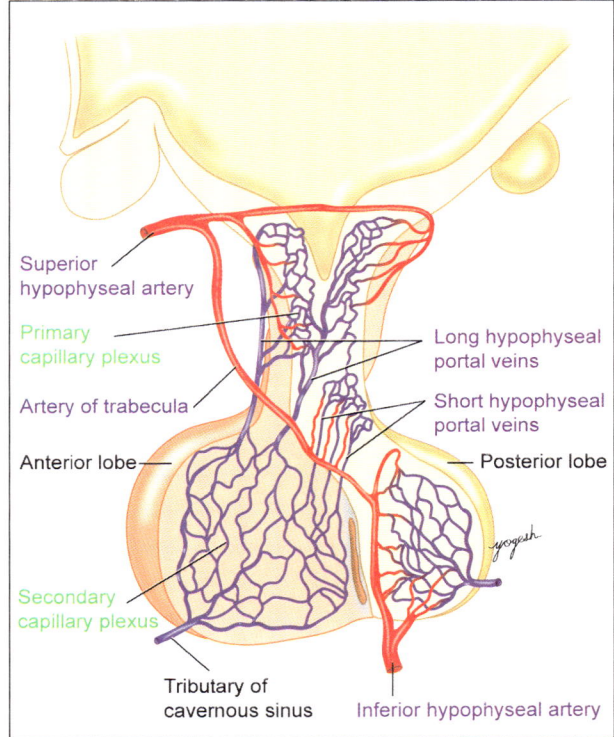

Fig. 25.3: Hypothalomo-hypophyseal portal circulation.

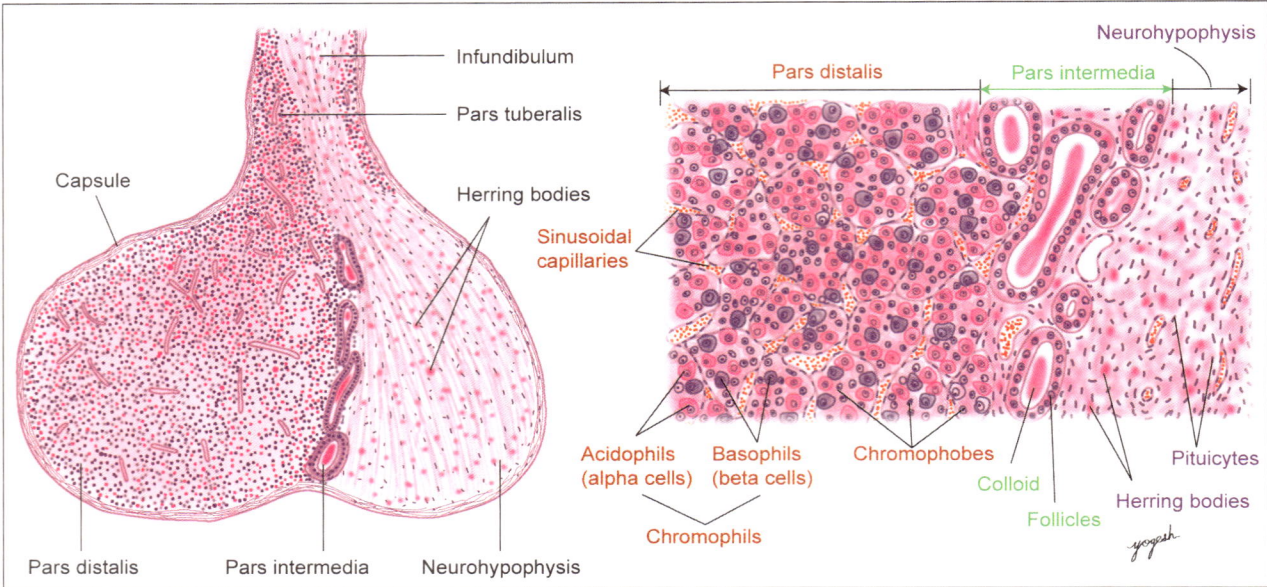

Fig. 25.4: Histology of pituitary gland (low magnification on left, high magnification on right, practice figure).

Flowchart 25.4: Hypothalamo-hypophyseal portal system

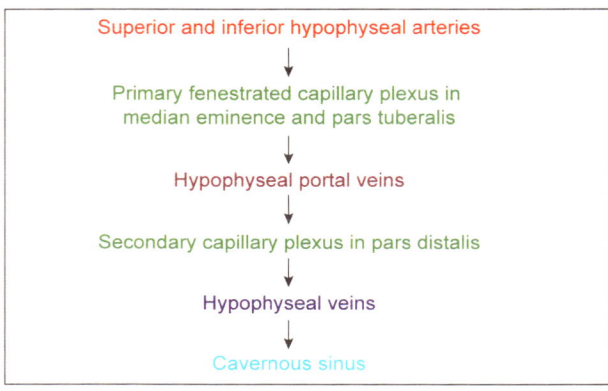

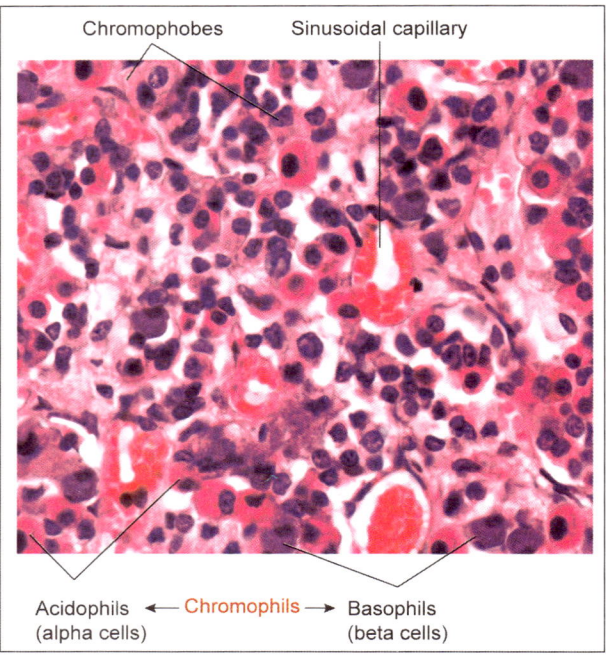

Fig. 25.5: Photomicrograph. Histology of anterior pituitary gland (high magnification *H&E* stain).

- *H&E staining:* On routine staining, cells of anterior pituitary are grouped as *Identification feature*

  Chromophils have brightly stained granules
  - *Basophils* (10%): Their granules stain with basic dye (Hematoxylin), hence blue colored and also with periodic acid–Schiff (PAS) stain.
  - *Acidophils* (40%): Their granules stain with acidic dyes such as eosin, hence bright pink colored.

  Chromophobes (50%) have no granules.

- Histochemical and immunohistochemical staining: Depending on secretory proteins and peptides, acidophils and basophils are further classified as follows:

  Acidophils:
  - *Somatotrophs* (GH cells): These constitute 50% of anterior pituitary and produce growth hormone or somatotropin. Growth hormone regulates body growth before puberty and its excess secretion causes gigantism in children and acromegaly in adults.[MCQ]
  - *Lactotrophs* (mamotropes): These constitute about 15–20% of anterior pituitary and produce prolactin (PRL). During pregnancy and lactation,

Flowchart 25.5: Cells and hormones of pituitary gland^(Viva, Neet)

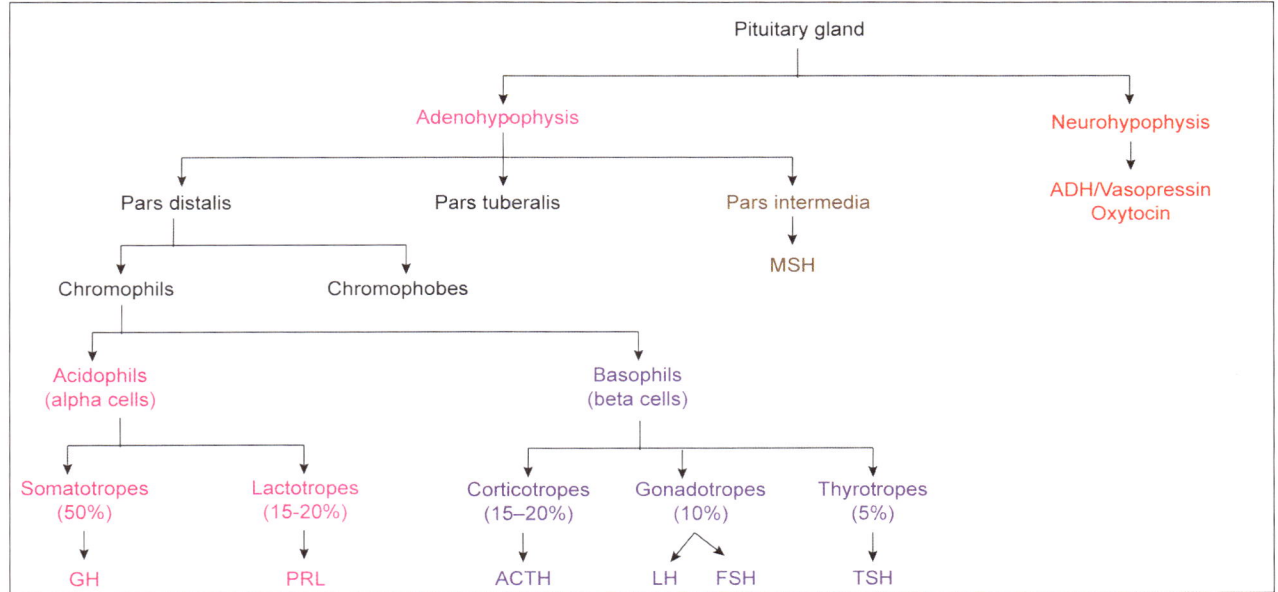

GH: growth hormone, ACTH: adrenocorticotropic hormone, LH: luteinizing hormone, FSH: follicle stimulating hormone, TSH: thyroid stimulating hormone, MSH: melanocyte stimulating hormone, ADH: antidiuretic hormone.

lactotropes undergo hypertrophy and result in increased size of pituitary gland, especially in multiparous females.^(MCQ)

Basophils:
- *Corticotropes:* These constitute about 15–20% of anterior pituitary and secrete adrenocorticotropic hormone (ACTH) or pro-opiomelanocortin (POMC) (ACTH precursor). POMC is converted into ACTH, β-lipotropic hormone, melanocyte stimulating hormone, β-endorphin, and enkephalin. Corticotropes are strongly *PAS positive* because of carbohydrate content of POMC.
- *Gonadotropes* (delta basophils): These constitute about 10% of anterior pituitary and secrete luteinizing hormone (LH) and follicle stimulating hormone (FSH).
- *Thyrotropes:* These constitute about 5% of anterior pituitary and secrete thyroid stimulating hormone (TSH).

Pars intermedia
- It is located between pars distalis and pars nervosa.
- It is not well developed in humans.
- It consists of a series of *colloid filled vesicles.*^(Viva, Identification feature)
- Cavity of these vesicles represents residual lumen of *Rathke's pouch.*^(MCQ)
- Cells of follicle/vesicles are basophils and chromophobes.
- These cells secrete *melanocyte stimulating hormone* (MSH) that stimulates production of skin pigments by melanocytes.

Pars tuberalis
- It is an extension of anterior pituitary that wraps around infundibular stalk.
- It is highly vascular region and has primary capillary plexus of hypothalamo-hypophyseal portal system.^(MCQ)
- Pars tuberalis consists of small clusters or cords of cells (both acidophils and basophils).

Neurohypophysis/Posterior Lobe of Pituitary Gland
- It consists of pars nervosa and infundibulum.
- It consists of about 1 lakh *nonmyelinated axons* of neurosecretory neurons.^(Viva)
- Bodies (soma) of these neurons are located in *supraoptic* and *paraventricular nuclei* of hypothalamus.^(Neet)
- These axons do not synapse with other neurons.
- These axon terminals secrete neurosecretory vesicles into adjacent fenestrated capillaries.
- *Note:* Posterior lobe of pituitary gland is a storage site of neurosecretions of supraoptic and paraventricular nuclei (not similar to other endocrine glands)
- *Pituicytes*
  - These are specialized *glial cells* of neurohypophysis associated with nerve endings and fenestrated capillaries.

- Pituicytes constitute 25% volume of neurohypophysis and they have many elongated processes similar to that of astrocytes.
- On *H&E* staining, cytoplasm of pituicytes cannot be distinguished from nonmyelinated nerve fibers. *Identification feature*

- *Electron microscopy:* Axon terminal contains secretory vesicles.
- *Herring bodies*
  - These are collection of secretory vesicles in dilated terminal portion of axons in the neurohypophysis. *Neet, Viva*
  - On *H&E* staining, Herring bodies take eosin (*pink*) staining.
  - On aniline blue staining, the Herring bodies look similar to dark black islands (granular appearance because of accumulated secretory vesicles).

Functions

Neurohypophysis produces two polypeptide hormones:

1. *Oxytocin:* It promotes contraction of smooth muscles of uterus during orgasm, menstruation, and parturition. It also promotes contraction of myoepithelial cells of mammary gland and helps in ejection of the milk.
2. *Vasopressin or antidiuretic hormone* (ADH): It decreases the urine volume by increasing renal water reabsorption by collecting ducts and thus increases blood pressure by increasing the blood volume.

Box 25.2: Hypothalamic control over anterior pituitary

- Hypothalamus produces several polypeptide hormones that regulate secretion of various hormones by adenohypophysis (Figs 25.4, 25.6 and Flowchart 25.6).
- Even hypothalamus works under feedback control by the levels of hormones of adenohypophysis.

Summary (Examination Guide)

- Pituitary gland consists of (Fig. 25.4)
  - Adenohypophysis that have pars distalis, pars intermedia, and pars tuberalis
  - Neurohypophysis
- *Adenohypophysis* shows clumps or cords of cells separated by fenestrated capillaries. These cells consist of Acidophils: Having pink granules
  - Somatotrophs (50%) secrete growth hormone
  - Lactotropes (15–20%) secrete prolactin
  Basophils: Having dark blue granules
  - Corticotropes (15–20%) secrete ACTH
  - Gonadotropes (10%) secrete LH and FSH
  - Thyrotropes (5%) secrete TSH
- *Pars intermedia* consists of a series of colloid-filled cysts/vesicles that secrete MSH.
- *Neurohypophysis* consists of nonmyelinated axons and pituicytes. Bodies of these neurons lie in supraoptic and paraventricular nuclei of hypothalamus. Neurohypophysis secretes vasopressin/ADH and oxytocin.

Clinical Correlation

- *Gigantism:* It occurs because of over secretion of growth hormone (GH) prior to epiphyseal closure (in prepubertal boys and girls). Clinical features are excessive and proportionate growth of the child, enlargement, and thickening of the bones, increase in height, and enlarged thoracic cage.
- *Acromegaly:* It occurs owing to the over secretion of GH in adults (after epiphyseal closure). Clinical features include growth of extremities (enlargement of hands and feet), coarseness of facial features, prominent supraorbital ridges and lower jaw, and protrusion of the lower teeth in front of upper teeth (prognathism).
- *Diabetes insipidus:* It occurs owing to the reduced secretion of ADH. Clinical features include excretion of high volume of dilute urine (polyuria) and polydipsia.

Flowchart 25.6: Hypothalamic regulating hormones

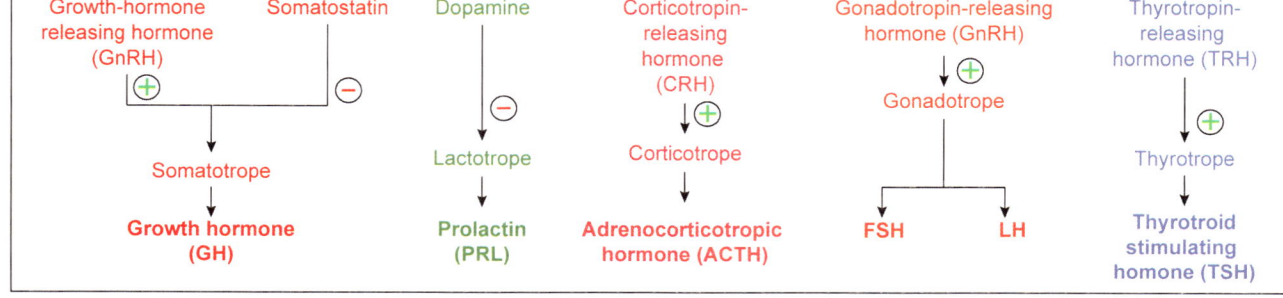

Endocrine System

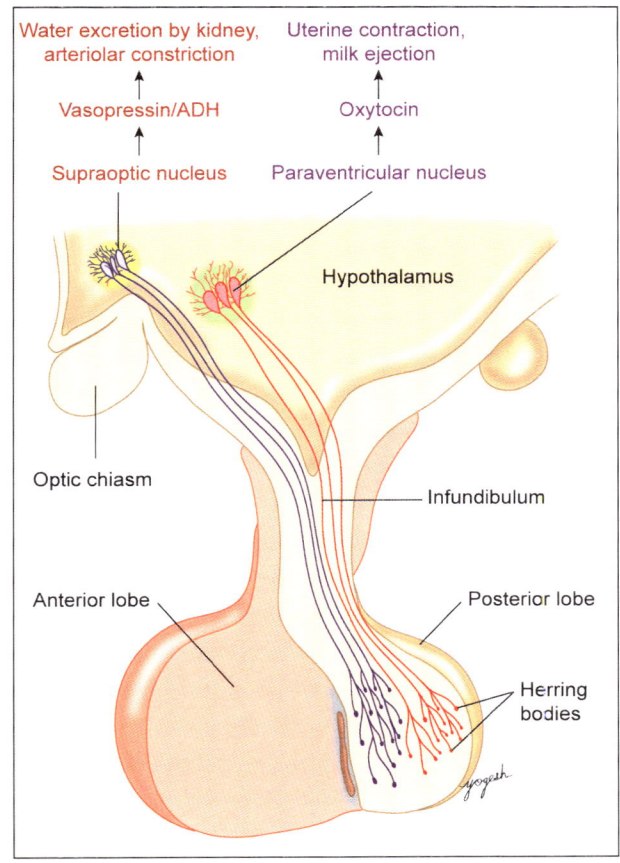

Fig. 25.6: Role of hypothalamus in secretions of posterior pituitary.

THYROID GLAND

Q. Draw a well-labeled diagram of histology of thyroid gland.

Q. List the identification features of histology of thyroid gland.

- Thyroid gland lies in the lower part of front and sides of neck. It consists of right and left lobes that are joined to each other by isthmus (Fig. 25.7).
- The gland weighs about 20–30 g. It is larger in females than males and increases further during menstruation and pregnancy.
- *Follicles of thyroid gland* develop from the *thyroglossal duct* (arising from endoderm of pharynx), whereas *parafollicular cells* develop from *ultimobranchial bodies*.^MCQ

Histology of Thyroid Gland (Figs 25.8 and 25.9)

- *Capsule:* Thyroid gland is covered by a thin connective tissue (fibrous) capsule.

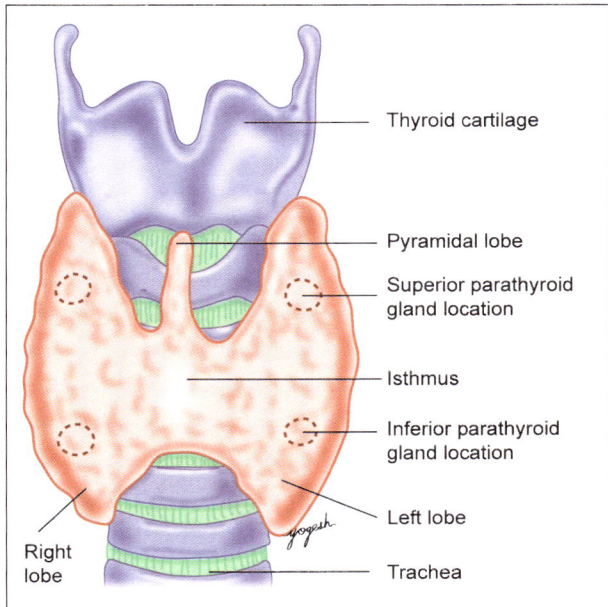

Fig. 25.7: Gross parts of thyroid gland.

- *Septa and lobules:* Connective tissue septa extend from the capsule and divide the gland (parenchyma) into number of lobules.
- *Follicles:* Parenchyma of each lobule consists of spherical masses called thyroid follicles (size 0.2–1.0 mm).
- *Follicular cells:* Each follicle is lined by *simple cuboidal or low columnar* follicular cells resting on a basement membrane (Fig. 25.10).^Identification feature
- *Colloid:* Center of each follicle contains gel-like acidophilic (*pink*) homogeneous material called colloid.^Identification feature
- *H&E staining:* Follicular cells shows slightly basal basophilic cytoplasm and single spherical nucleus with 1–2 nucleoli.^Identification feature
- *Interfollicular space:* It contains numerous blood vessels, lymphatics, and connective tissue fibers.
- *Parafollicular cells:*
  – Parafollicular cells or *C-cells* may be embedded within a follicle or between follicles.
  – Parafollicular cells are polyhedral cells with oval eccentric nuclei. These cells are not exposed to the follicular lumen.
  – C-cells lie single or in small clusters. These cells are *difficult to identify under light microscopy.*
  – Electron microscopy: Parafollicular cells show numerous secretory vesicles.
- Function: Follicular cells secrete thyroxine (T4) and triiodothyronine (T3). Note: Parafollicular/C-cells secrete calcitonin.

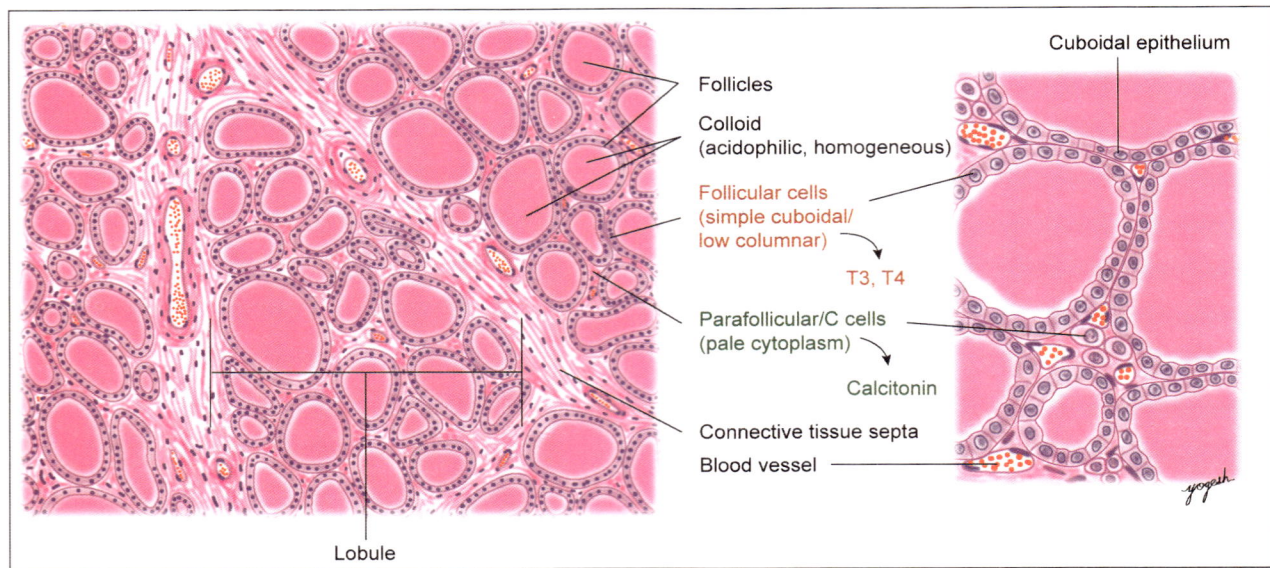

Fig. 25.8: Histology of thyroid gland (low magnification on left, high magnification on right, practice figure).

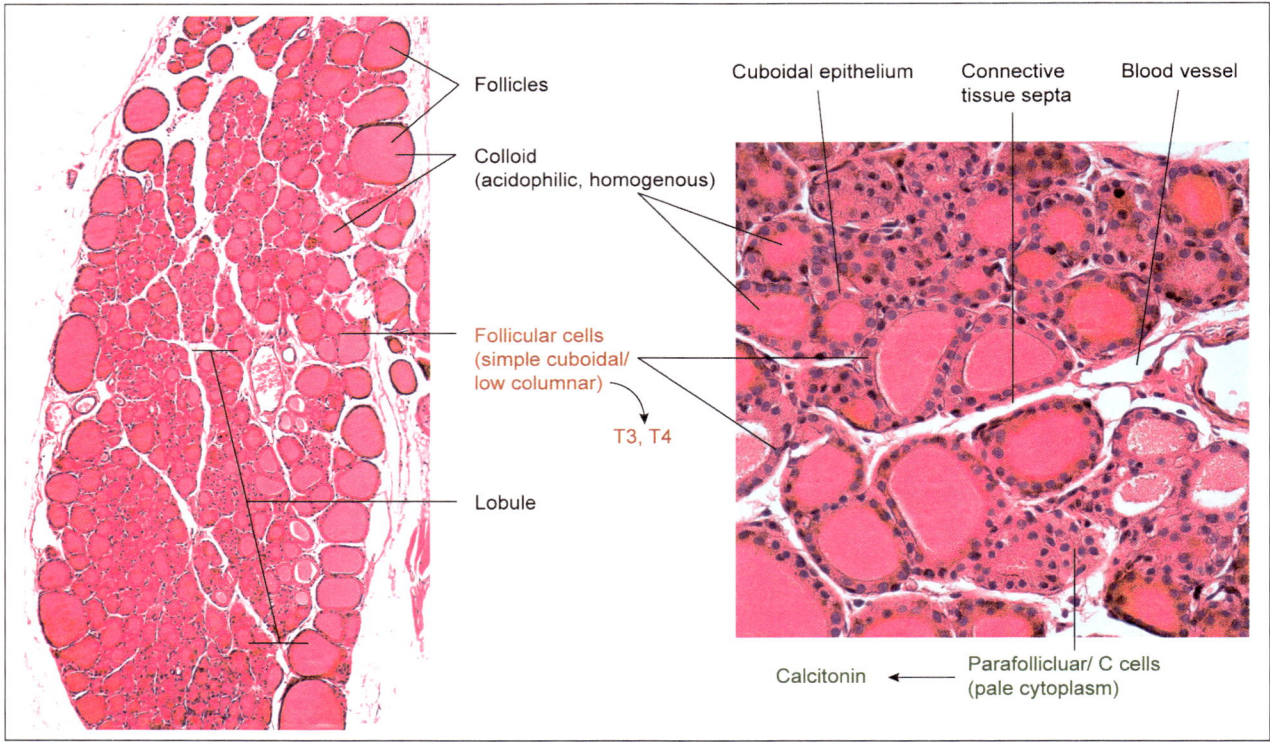

Fig. 25.9: Photomicrograph. Histology of thyroid gland (low magnification on left, high magnification on right, *H&E* stain).

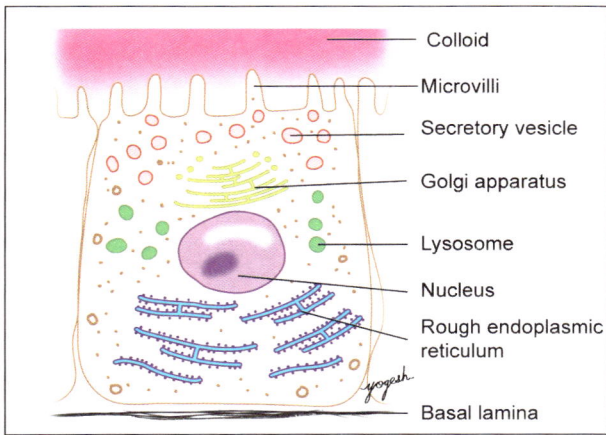

Fig. 25.10: Ultrastructure of follicular cells of thyroid gland.

Box 25.3: Follicular cells and activity of thyroid gland^{MCQ, Viva}

- Follicular cells secrete thyroid hormones (T3 and T4) (Fig. 25.11).
- The shape of follicular cells depends on activity of the cells.
- *Resting/inactive cells:* These are *squamous.* Inactive follicles contain *large quantity of colloid.*
- *Secretory/active cells:* Under the influence of thyroid stimulating hormone, follicular cells become *cuboidal* or *low columnar* with large vesicular nucleus (even tall columnar epithelium is also seen). Active follicles contain less colloid.^{Neet}
- *Scalloping of colloid:* Moth-eaten edges or scalloped colloid is an indicator of active thyroid gland. It is mostly seen in Graves' disease (hyperthyroidism).^{MCQ}

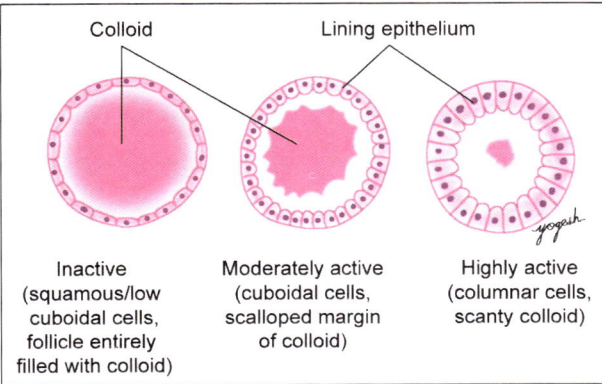

Fig. 25.11: Thyroid follicle appearance in various stages of activity.

Some Interesting Facts

- The main component of colloid is *thyroglobulin.*
- Thyroglobulin is an iodinated glycoprotein. It is an inactive storage form of thyroid hormone.
- Staining property of colloid: *H&E* stain – pink, PAS positive – magenta color.
- Thyroid gland is the only endocrine gland that stores its secretions extracellularly.
- Steps of synthesis of thyroid hormone are listed in Flowchart 25.7.
- T3 is five times more active than T4.^{Viva}
- Synthesis of T3 and T4 is controlled by negative feedback mechanism on *thyrotropin releasing hormone* (TRH) and *thyroid stimulating hormone* (TSH).
- Fetal thyroid begins to function during the fourteenth week of gestation.^{Neet}

Functions of Thyroid Gland

- Thyroid gland secretes T3, T4, and calcitonin hormones (Table 25.1).
- T3/T4 hormones control metabolic rate of the body.
- In fetal life and early childhood, thyroid hormones promote CNS development and growth.
- Calcitonin lowers the blood calcium levels by increasing calcium deposition in bones and inhibiting bone resorption by osteoclasts.

Clinical Correlation

- Irrespective of the cause, enlargement of thyroid gland is called *goiter.*
- *Hyperthyroidism/thyrotoxicosis:* It is excess production of thyroid hormones causing increased metabolism.
  Causes of hyperthyroidism: Graves' disease (most common cause), multinodular goiter, toxic thyroid adenoma (tumor), long-acting thyroid stimulator antibodies.
- *Hypothyroidism:* It is the inadequate production of thyroid hormone or tissue resistance for activity of thyroid hormone.
  Hypothyroidism during the infancy or childhood causes *cretinism,* whereas in adulthood causes *myxedema* (mental and physical sluggishness, edema of connective tissue).
  Causes of hypothyroidism: Iodine deficiency (most common cause) and Hashimoto's thyroiditis (autoimmune disorder).

Flowchart 25.7: Synthesis of thyroid hormone

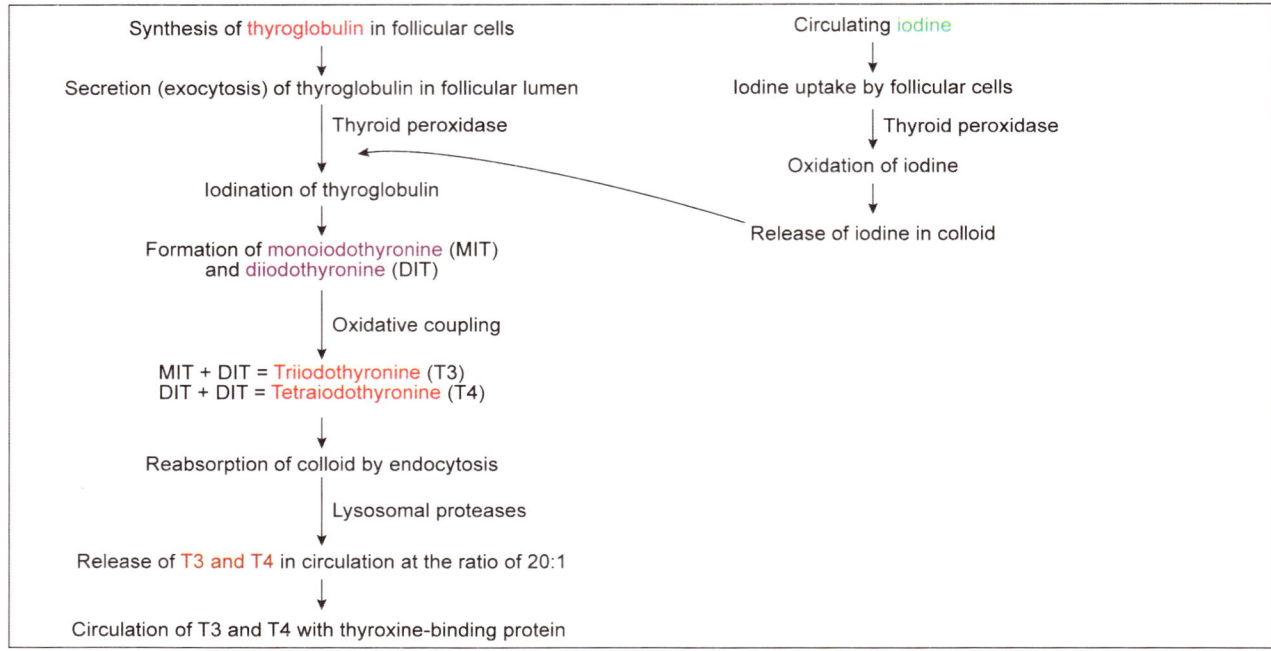

Summary (Examination Guide) (Fig. 25.8)

- Thyroid gland is covered by thin connective tissue *capsule*. *Septa* arising from capsule divide the gland into number of *lobules*.
- Thyroid gland is made up of *follicles* lined by *simple cuboidal epithelium* (ranges from squamous to low columnar) with rounded nuclei.
- Lumen of follicle contains pink homogeneous *colloid* material that consists of thyroglobulin.
- Few *parafollicular/C-cells* are present in relation to follicles. C-cells secrete *calcitonin* that reduces blood calcium levels.
- In between follicles, rich vascular connective tissue is present.

PARATHYROID GLANDS

Q. Draw a well-labeled diagram of histology of the parathyroid gland.

- Parathyroid glands consist of two pairs (superior and inferior) of small masses.
- They lie along the posterior border of thyroid gland within the false capsule.
- Superior parathyroid (parathyroid IV) develops from *fourth* pharyngeal pouch (endoderm), whereas *inferior parathyroid* (parathyroid III) develops from *third pouch*.^{MCQ}
- Each parathyroid gland is oval or lentiform in shape (about the size of split pea) and weighs about 50 mg.

Histology of Parathyroid Gland (Figs 25.12 and 25.13)

- Each gland is surrounded by a thin layer of connective tissue *capsule*.
- *Septa* extend from capsule and divide the gland into poorly defined *lobules*.
- *Glandular parenchyma* is richly supplied with numerous sinusoids.
- Cells of parathyroid gland include chief cells and oxyphil cells.
- *Chief cells (principal cells)*
  – These cells secrete parathyroid hormone.
  – These are more in number than oxyphilic cells.
  – *Light microscopy:* Chief cells are *small polygonal cells* (7–10 μm) with centrally located nucleus.
  – They have *dark staining* cytoplasm (based on parathyroid hormone content).
  – Depending on quantity of accumulated glycogen and lipofuscin, chief cells have three types: (1) Light, (2) Dark and (3) Clear cells.
  – *Electron microscopy:* Chief cells show abundant rough endoplasmic reticulum, Golgi apparatus, and secretory vesicles.
- Oxyphil (eosinophil) cells
  – These cells are *less in number* but much *larger in size* than chief cells.
  – These cells appear singly or in group.
  – *Light microscopy:* Oxyphil cells have *abundant, deeply eosinophilic (acidophilic) cytoplasm* because of large number of mitochondria.

Endocrine System

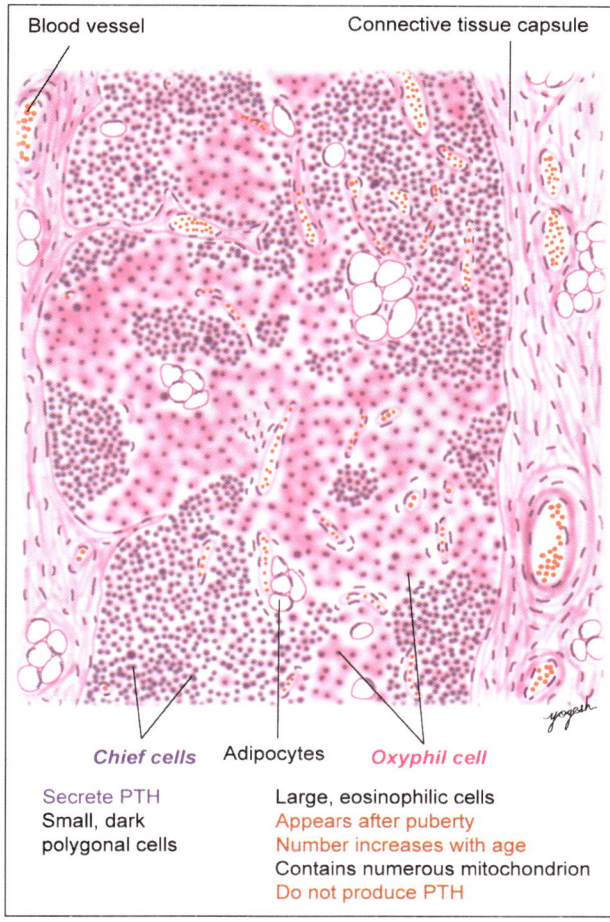

Fig. 25.12: Histology of parathyroid gland (practice figure).

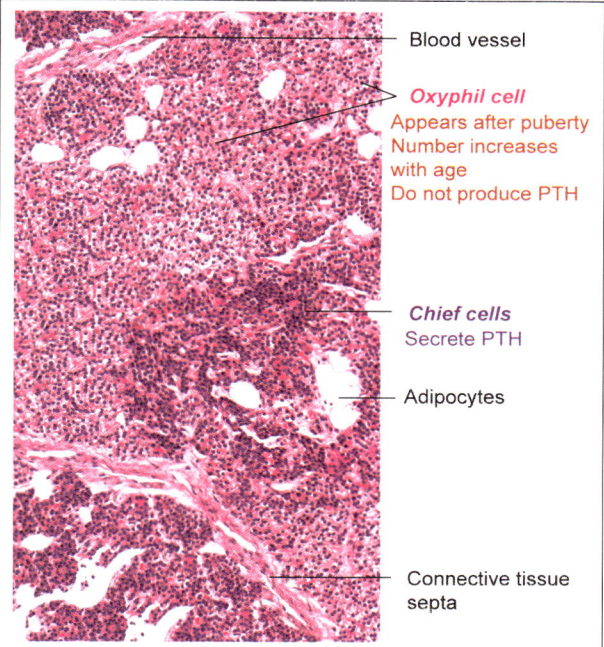

Fig. 25.13: Photomicrograph. Histology of parathyroid gland (low magnification, *H&E* stain).

– These cells do not show secretory vesicles and have very less rough endoplasmic reticulum. These cells do not have secretory function.

Functions

- *Chief cells* secrete *parathyroid hormone* (PTH) that *increases blood calcium* level (Table 25.1).
- PTH acts at the following sites: *MCQ*
  – Bone resorption: PTH activates osteoclasts and enhances bone resorption
  – Increases calcium reabsorption by kidney
  – Increases conversion of 25-OH vitamin D_3 to active 1,25-$(OH)_2$ vitamin D_3
  – Increases calcium absorption in intestine
  – Increases phosphate excretion by kidney
- *Note:* PTH and calcitonin have opposite roles in the regulation of blood calcium levels.

Summary (Examination Guide) (Fig. 25.12)

- Parathyroid gland shows cords or sheets of cells separated by numerous capillaries.
- It shows two types of cells: (1) chief and (2) oxyphil cells.
- Chief cells are more in number, small in size, and consist of a spherical nucleus with small amount of cytoplasm.
- They secrete PTH hormone.
- Oxyphil (eosinophilic) cells are less in number, larger in size, and small intense-staining nucleus with eosinophilic cytoplasm. They do not secrete any hormone. Oxyphilic cells appear just before puberty.

Clinical Correlation

- *Hyperparathyroidism:* Hyperparathyroidism is the *excessive* production of parathyroid hormone. It results in *high blood calcium levels.*
- *Hypoparathyroidism:* It is *decreased* secretion of parathyroid hormone. It results in *low blood calcium levels* that causes tetany, paresthesia, Chvostek's sign (tetany on tapping facial nerve), and Trousseau sign of latent tetany (occlusion of brachial artery with blood pressure cuff elicit tetany). *Neet, MCQ*

Table 25.1: Hormones of thyroid and parathyroid gland

Gland	Hormone	Source	Function
Thyroid	Thyroxine (T4), Triiodothyronine (T3)	Follicular cells	Regulates metabolism and growth of body. Also facilitates development of nervous system in fetus and young child
	Calcitonin	Parafollicular cells (C-cells)	Decreases blood–calcium level
Parathyroid gland	Parathyroid hormone	Chief (principal) cells	Increases blood–calcium level

Note: Removal of parathyroid glands results in rapid fall of blood calcium level.

ADRENAL/SUPRARENAL GLAND

Q. Draw a well-labeled diagram of histology of the adrenal gland.

- Adrenal glands (right and left) lie on superior pole of kidneys in the perirenal fat.
- Each adrenal gland is very small (5–7 g).

Histology of Adrenal Glands

- Gland is surrounded by a thin connective tissue *capsule* that sends *septa* inside the gland.
- *Parenchyma* of adrenal gland is organized into two zones: (1) superficial *cortex* (90%) and (2) deeper *medulla* (10%)
- Cortical mass is about 10 times that of the medulla.

Adrenal Cortex (Figs 25.11, 25.16 and 25.17)

- Adrenal cortex is divided into three zones: 1. zona glomerulosa (outermost, 15%), 2. zona fasciculata (middle, 80%) and 3. zona reticularis (inner, 5%).

Some Interesting Facts

- Cortical cells of adrenal gland originate from mesoderm (intermediate mesoderm), whereas medulla develops from neural crest cells.^{Neet}
- Each adrenal gland is supplied by suprarenal arteries (superior, middle, and inferior) that give rise to three sets of vessels (Fig. 25.14):
  – Capsular capillaries (supply capsule)
  – Fenestrated cortical sinusoidal capillaries (supply cortex)
  – Medullary arterioles (supply medullary sinusoids)
- *Cortical sinusoids* drain into *medullary sinusoids.*
- Blood from medullary sinusoids drains into single central *adrenomedullary vein.*
- Adrenomedullary vein has *longitudinally oriented smooth muscles* cells that help in squeezing the gland and ejecting hormone into the circulation.^{MCQ}

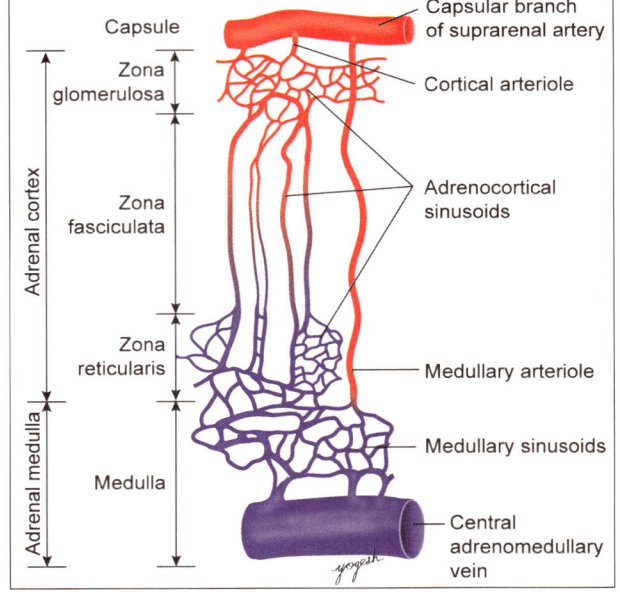

Fig. 25.14: Microvasculature of adrenal gland.

Zona Glomerulosa

- It is thin outermost zone situated just beneath the capsule.
- *Cellular arrangements:* In zona glomerulosa, cells are arranged in *ovoid clusters* such as glomeruli of kidney and in curved columns (inverted U-shaped).
- *Cells of zona glomerulosa:* They are small, *columnar or pyramidal* in shape with spherical nuclei.
- *Staining:* Acidophilic cytoplasm consisting of only few lipid droplets and dark-staining spherical nucleus.
- *Functions:* Cells of zona glomerulosa secrete *mineralocorticoids (aldosterone)* that regulate blood pressure through sodium-potassium homeostasis and water balance. Secretion of aldosterone is controlled by feedback mechanism of renin-angiotensin-aldosterone system (Flowchart 25.8).

Zona Fasciculata

- It is the middle zone of adrenal cortex constituting about 80% (middle three-fifth) of the cortex.

Endocrine System

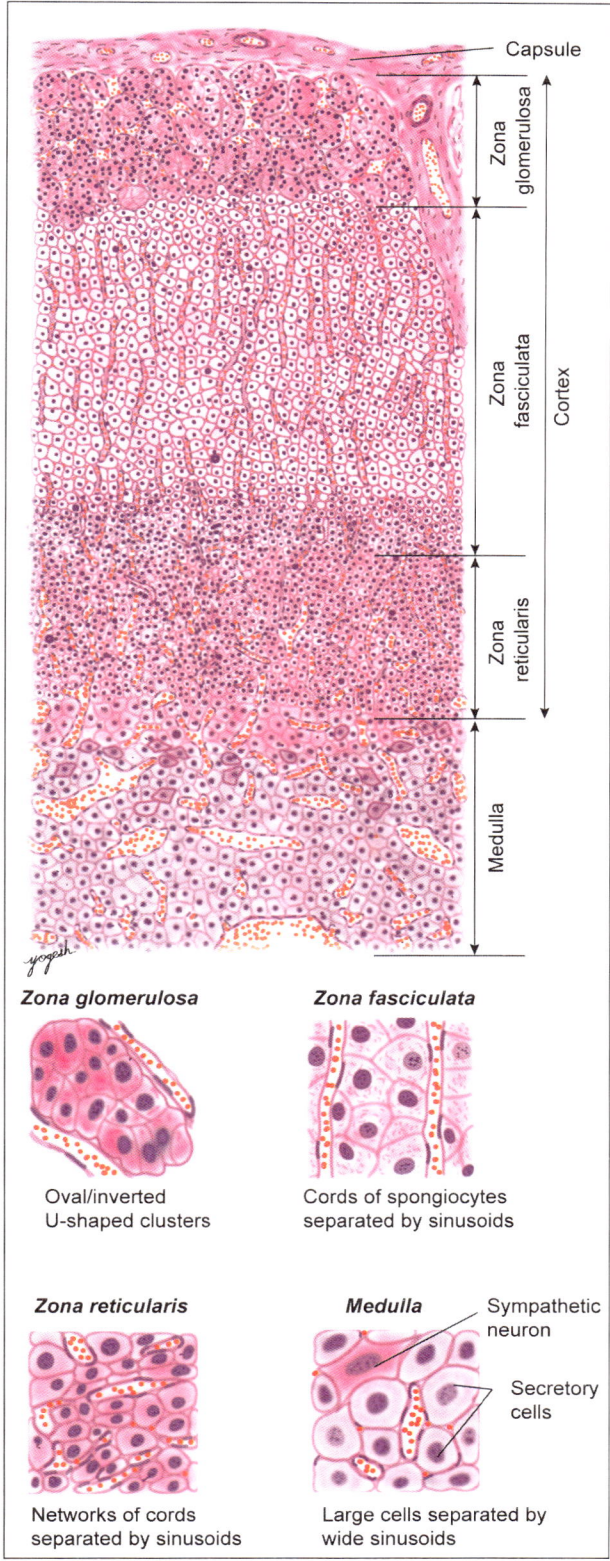

Fig. 25.15: Histology of suprarenal gland (practice figure).

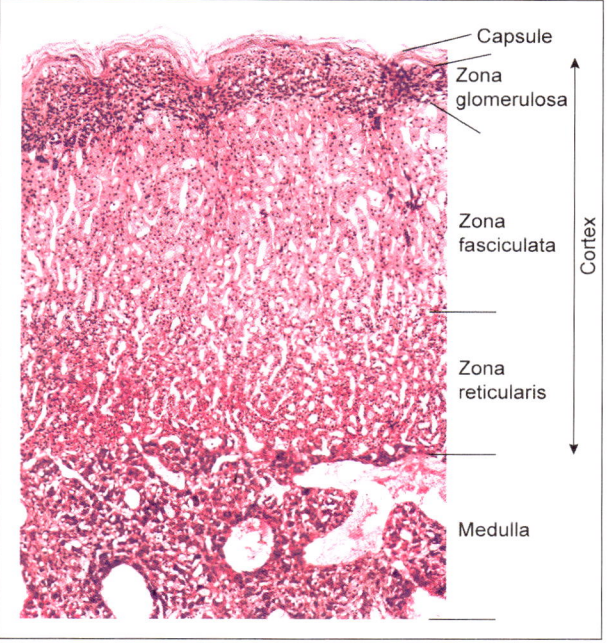

Fig. 25.16: Photomicrograph. Histology of suprarenal gland (low magnification, *H&E* stain).

Flowchart 25.8: Renin–angiotensin–aldosterone system

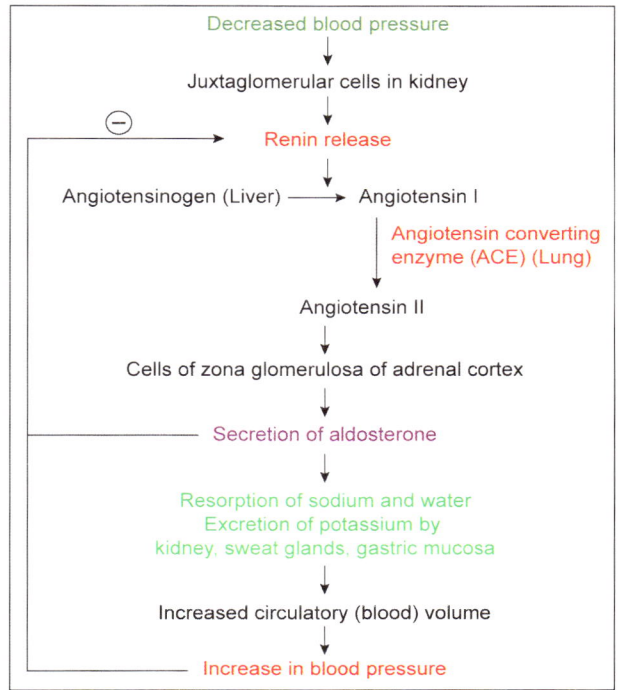

- *Cellular arrangement:* In zona fasciculata cells are arranged as two-cell thick and long straight *columns*. Adjacent columns are separated from each other by *sinusoidal capillaries*.

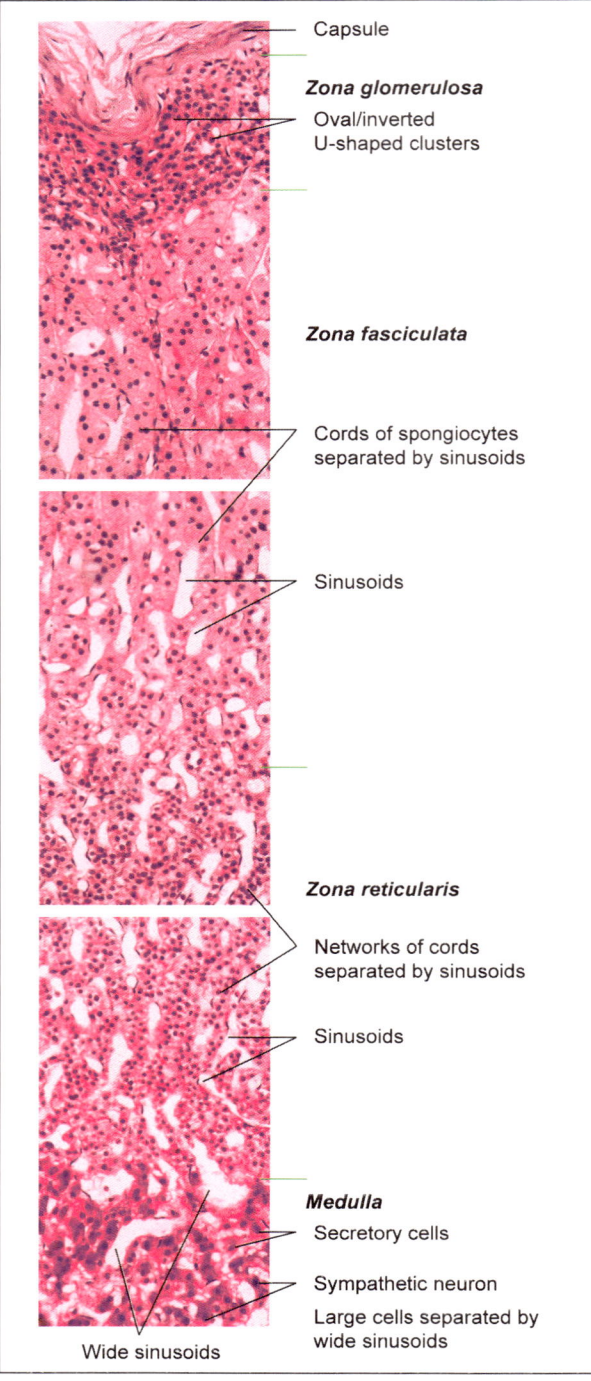

Fig. 25.17: Photomicrograph. Histology of suprarenal gland (high magnification, *H&E* stain).

- *Cells of zona fasciculata:* They are larger than cells of zona glomerulosa and *polyhedral* in shape.
- *Staining:* Cells have *light pink* (eosinophilic/acidophilic) *vacuolated cytoplasm* and light staining vesicular nucleus. Cells show vacuolated appearance of cytoplasm as they contain lipid droplets (hence, cells are also called as *spongiocytes*).^Viva
- Note: Lipid droplets are washed out during slide preparation; hence, on *H&E* staining, cells show empty or vacuolated cytoplasm.
- *Electron microscopy:* Cells of zona fasciculata show features of steroid-secreting cells such as well-developed smooth endoplasmic reticulum, Golgi apparatus, numerous lipid droplets, and mitochondria.
- *Functions:* Cells of zona fasciculata secrete *glucocorticoids* under the control of adrenocorticotropic hormone (ACTH) from anterior pituitary (Flowchart 25.9).

Zona Reticularis

- It is the inner most zone of adrenal cortex and constitutes about 5% of the cortex.
- *Cellular arrangements:* In zona reticularis, cells are arranged in *anastomosing cords* (forming reticulum – network). These cords are separated by *fenestrated capillaries*.
- *Cells of zona reticularis:* These are *smaller* than the cells of zona fasciculata because of less cytoplasm. These cells have *darkly stained nuclei*, well developed smooth endoplasmic reticulum, and few rough endoplasmic reticula.
- Cells contain abundant and large yellow-brown *lipofuscin pigment* granules.
- *Functions:* Cells of zona reticularis secrete *weak androgens* (dehydroepiandrosterone – DHEA) and small quantity of glucocorticoids (cortisol).

Suprarenal Medulla (Figs 25.15, 25.16 and 25.17)

- Central portion of adrenal gland is medulla.

Flowchart 25.9: Role of glucocorticoids

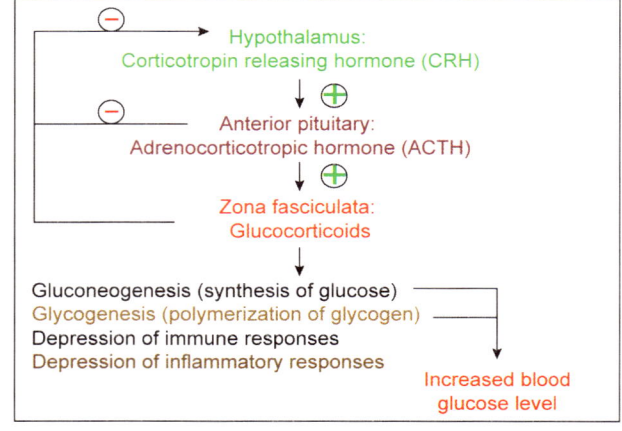

- *Cellular arrangements:* Cells are arranged in *ovoid and short interconnecting cords* separated by numerous sinusoidal capillaries.
- *Cells of adrenal medulla:* These are *pale-staining* epitheloid cells.
- These cells take potassium dichromate stain (salt of chromium); hence, also called *chromaffin cells* (*pheochromocytes*).^MCQ, Viva
- Note: Cells of adrenal cortex are not chromaffin cells.
- *Electron microscopy:* Cells of adrenal medulla show abundant rough endoplasmic reticulum and membrane-bound secretory granules/vesicles.
- Adrenal medulla may show *ganglion cells* that supply and control glucocorticoid secretion from adrenal cortex
- *Functions:* Adrenal medulla secretes *catecholamines* (20% norepinephrine and 80% epinephrine). They produce effects of sympathetic nervous system to prepare body for fight or flight mechanism. It includes increase in blood pressure (BP), heart rate, blood sugar levels, dilatation of coronary blood vessels, and so on → increase blood supply to heart and skeletal muscles → Preparation for *fight or flight* response (Flowchart 25.10).

Flowchart 25.10: Secretion of epinephrine and norepinephrine

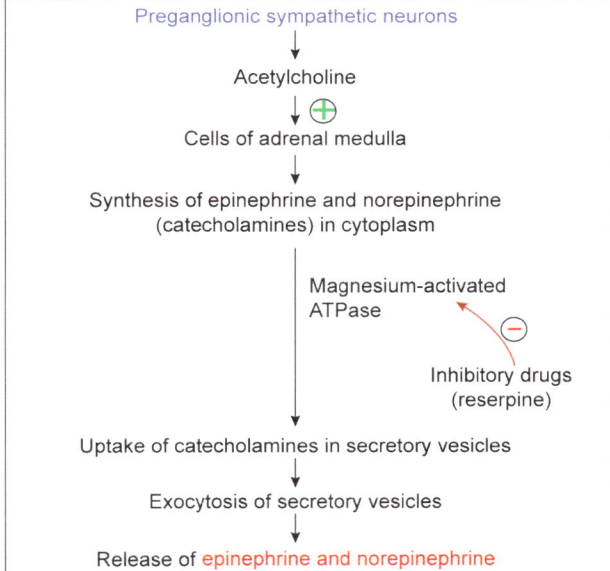

Note: Glucocorticoids secreted by adrenal cortex induce conversion of norepinephrine to epinephrine inducing conversion of norepinephrine to epinephrine by its methylation in chromaffin cells.

Some Interesting Facts
- Adrenal cortex develops from intermediate mesoderm, whereas adrenal medulla develops from neural crest cells.
- Chromaffin cells are modified neurons.
- Adrenal medulla is supplied by myelinated preganglionic sympathetic nerve fibers that stimulate release of catecholamines from pheochromocytes.
- Adrenal medullary pheochromocytes are a part of the amine precursor uptake and decarboxylation (APUD) system.
- Cells of adrenal medulla are equivalent to post-ganglionic sympathetic neurons; however, they do not have axons.^Viva
- Axonal growth of cells of adrenal medulla is inhibited by glucocorticoids of adrenal cortex.^Viva

Box 25.4: Chromaffin reaction^Viva
- Cells of adrenal medulla contain secretory vesicles of epinephrine and norepinephrine.
- Treatment of these cells with salts of chromium (potassium dichromate) causes oxidation of catecholamines and produce brown pigment. This is called *chromaffin reaction* (affinity for chromium).
- The cells that show chromaffin reaction are called *chromaffin cells* or *pheochromocytes.*
- Note: Enterochromaffin cells (Kulchitsky cells) become yellow on treatment with chromium salts. They are present in gastrointestinal tract epithelium. They are neuroendocrine in function and are not derivatives of neural cells.^Neet [Nikolai K Kulchitsky, 1856–1925, Russian anatomist and histologist].

Clinical Correlation
- *Pheochromocytoma*
  - It is the neuroendocrine tumor of medulla of adrenal gland.
  - It is catecholamine-producing tumor (increased adrenal blood levels).
  - It is usually benign (non-spreading) tumor.
  - It leads to high blood pressure, increased heart rate, palpitations, headache (most common symptom), and so on.
  - Surgical resection of the tumor is the treatment of choice.

- **Cushing's syndrome (Hyperadrenalism)**
  - It is produced by *excess* secretion of adrenal *cortical* hormones, mostly cortisol.
  - It may occur because of excess ACTH secretion of pituitary (Cushing's disease), tumors of adrenal cortex or ectopic ACTH secreting tumors.
  - Features of Cushing's syndrome include weight gain, buffalo hump (deposition of fat on the back of neck), moon face (deposition of fat on the face), excess sweating, facial plethora, decreased libido, thin skin, menstrual irregularities, abdominal red-purple stria, osteoporosis, and so on.
- Hypoadrenalism causes *Addison's disease* because of insufficient production of adrenocortical hormone. Features of Addison's disease include fatigue, weakness, anorexia, postural hypotension, hyperpigmentation, vitiligo, gastrointestinal disturbances, and so on.

Summary (Examination Guide) (Fig. 25.15)

- Adrenal gland is surrounded by thick connective tissue capsule, outer cortex, and inner medulla.
- *Adrenal cortex* shows
  - Outer *zona glomerulosa* (15%): Ovoid clusters or curved columns of small acidophilic cells.
  - Middle *zona fasciculata* (80%): Long straight columns of large polyhedral light-pink cells separated by sinusoidal capillaries.
  - Inner *zona reticularis* (5%): Anastomosing cords of small cells separated by fenestrated capillaries.
- *Adrenal medulla* consists of ovoid groups of pale-staining epithelioid cells (positive for chromaffin reaction; hence, called pheochromocytes).
- Secretions:
  - Zona glomerulosa – mineralocorticoids
  - Zona fasciculata – glucocorticoids
  - Zona reticularis – weak androgens
  - Adrenal medulla – catecholamines

PINEAL GLAND (EPIPHYSIS CEREBRI)

- Pineal gland is a small conical projection between two superior colliculi of midbrain. It arises from roof of the developing third ventricle.
- Pineal gland weighs about 0.1–0.2 g.
- It forms a part of epithalamus.
- It is a flat, pine cone-shaped structure (hence, named as pineal gland).

Histology of Pineal Gland (Fig. 25.18)

- Pineal gland is covered by *pia mater* that forms its capsule.

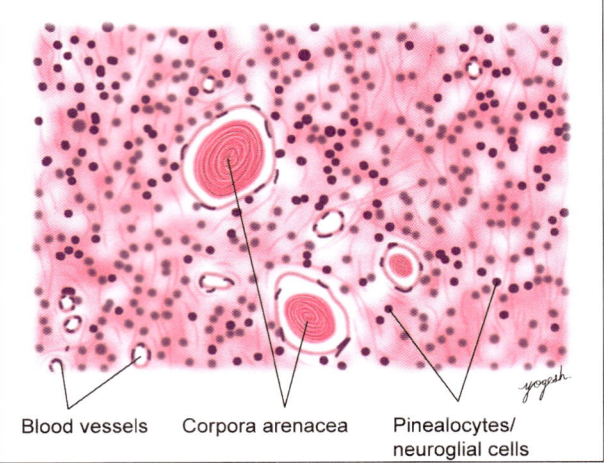

Fig. 25.18: Histology of pineal gland.

- Thin *septa* extend from capsule and divide the glandular parenchyma into small irregular cords or *lobules* of cells.
- Cells of pineal gland
  - Pinealocytes
  - Interstitial cells

Pinealocytes (95%)

- These are chief cells of the pineal gland.
- These are arranged in clumps or cords within the lobules.
- These are *pale-staining* epitheloid cells with large spherical nucleus (lighter than that of interstitial glial cells).
- Electron microscopy: Pinealocyte shows elongated cytoplasmic processes and secretory vesicles.
- Function: Secretion of *melatonin* hormone.

Interstitial (Glial Cells) (5%)

- These cells constitute about 5% of cells in gland.
- Their nuclei are smaller and more elongated than those of the pinealocytes.*identifying feature*

Corpora Arenacea/Brain Sand *Neet, Identifying feature*

- This is characteristic feature of pineal gland.
- It is *calcified concretions* (deposits).
- Corpora arenacea is present even in childhood and increases in number with age.
- Staining: On *H&E* staining, it takes *dark blue/hematoxylin* stain and shows *lamellated appearance*.
- Corpora arenacea is considered as identifying feature of the pineal gland histologically as well as radiologically.

Function

- Pineal gland secretes *melatonin* in relation to light intensity (Flowchart 25.11).

Flowchart 25.11: Role of melatonin and circadian rhythm

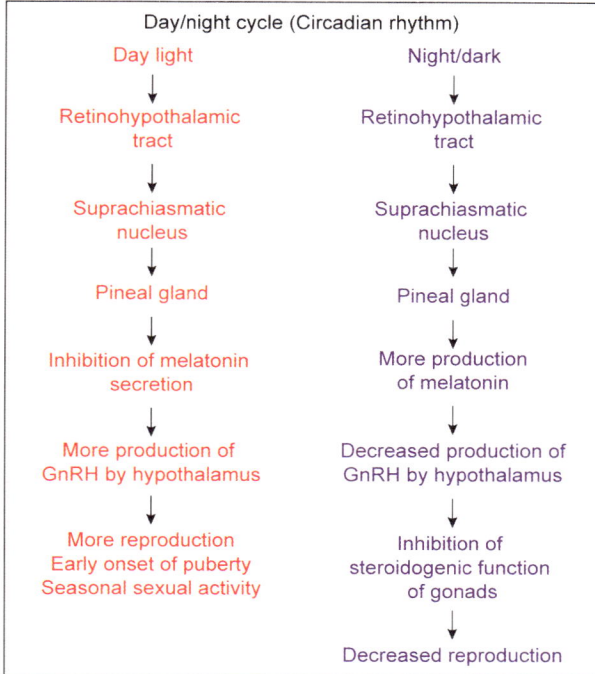

Summary (Examination Guide)
- Pineal gland is a cone-shaped gland that secretes melatonin.
- It shows:
  - *Pinealocytes* (95%) or chief cells that are arranged in clumps or cords (secretes melatonin).
  - *Glial cells* (interstitial cells) (5%) that have elongated, more darkly stained nucleus than pinealocytes.
  - *Corpora arenacea* or brain sand is the identifying feature of the gland. These are *calcified deposits* that increase with age.

Some Interesting Facts
- Pinealocytes give few long processes that show expanded terminal buds in relation to capillary walls.
- *Canaliculated lamellar bodies:* It is an unusual organ that is present in the pinealocytes. It consists of microfibrils and perforated lamellae.
- Supraoptic nucleus is the communication between retina (light) and pineal gland.

CHAPTER 26

Nervous System

Chapter Outline
- Spinal cord
- Cerebellum
- Cerebrum

Competency achievement: The student should be able to:
AN64.1 Describe and identify the microanatomical features of spinal cord, cerebellum and cerebrum

INTRODUCTION

- Nervous system consists of two parts:
  1. Central nervous system: Brain, spinal cord
  2. Peripheral nervous system: Peripheral nerves, sympathetic, and parasympathetic ganglia
- Peripheral nervous system is covered in Chapter 12.
- Central nervous system shows outer gray matter and inner white matter.
- *Gray matter:* It is a collection of neurons (body) and neuroglial cells.
- *White matter:* It is a collection of bundles of nerve fibers, mainly axons.
- *Nuclei:* These are the scattered masses of gray matter in the substance of white matter.
- The central nervous system is covered by three protective coatings: Dura, arachnoid, and pia maters.

SPINAL CORD

Q. Draw a well-labelled diagram of histology of spinal cord.
- Spinal cord is the long cylindrical mass that give rise to 31 pairs of spinal nerves.
- Length: 45 cm/18 inches.
- *Extent:* From upper border of atlas vertebra to lower border of first lumbar vertebra or upper border of second lumbar vertebra (in adults).
- Spinal cord is covered by three meninges: Outer dura mater, middle arachnoid mater, and inner pia mater.
- Spinal cord shows cervical enlargement (C4 to T1 segments) and lumbar enlargement (L2 to S3 segments).
- Spinal cord has (Fig. 26.1)
  - Deep anterior median fissure
  - Dorsal median sulcus
  - Venterolateral and dorsolateral sulci
  - Ventral motor roots of spinal nerves
  - Dorsal sensory roots of spinal nerves

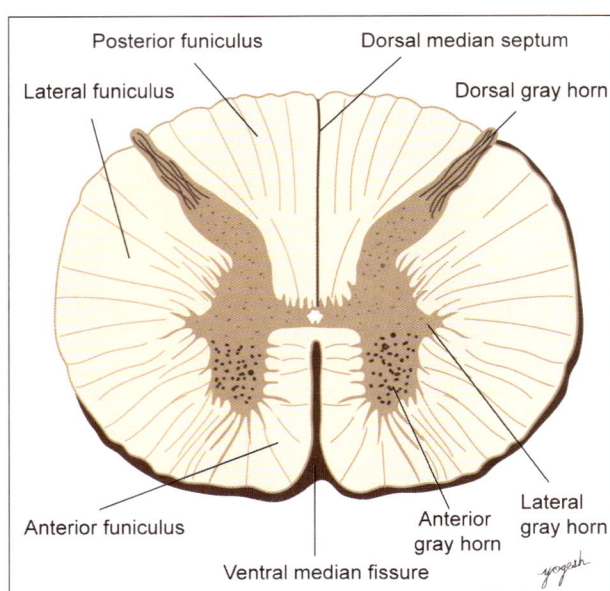

Fig. 26.1: Section of spinal cord showing main features.

Nervous System

- Lowest part of spinal cord is conical and is called *conus medullaris.*
- *Filum terminale* (modification of pia mater): It is a fibrous band. It is a continuation of conus medullaris.

Histology of Spinal Cord

- Section of spinal cord shows *central canal* lined by ependyma (Figs 26.1 to 26.3 and Flowchart 26.1).
- *Ependyma* consists of ciliated simple columnar epithelium.
- Central canal has surrounding gray matter and further outside white matter. *Identification feature*

Gray Matter

- Gray matter of spinal cord appears in the form of alphabet 'H' (Figs 26.1 and 26.2). *Identification feature*
- It has anterior and posterior gray horns.
- *Anterior gray horn* consists of large multipolar motor neurons. *Identification feature* These are called as anterior horn cells.
- *Anterior horn cells* have large, vesicular nuclei with prominent nucleolus, and numerous cytoplasmic Nissl granules.
- Axons of anterior horn cells exit spinal cord in the form of ventral root of spinal cord.
- Neurons of *posterior gray horn* are smaller in size.
- gray matter also contains many microglia and blood vessels.

White Matter

- White matter mainly consists of myelinated nerve fibers and neuroglial cells. *Identification feature*

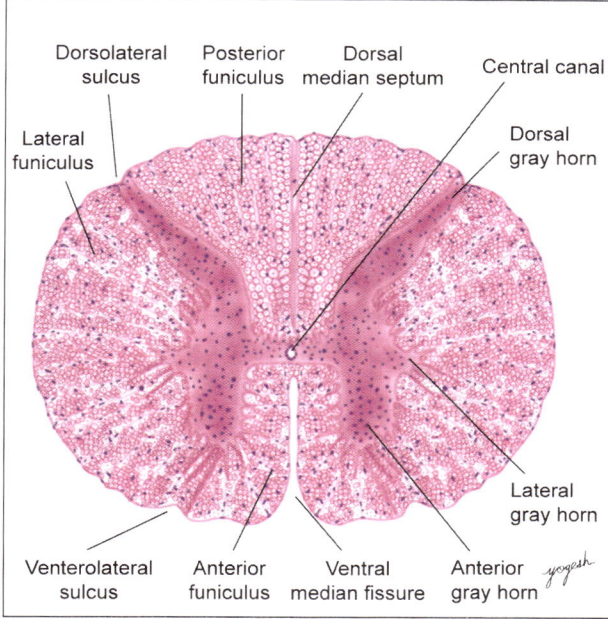

Fig. 26.2: Section of spinal cord (practice figure).

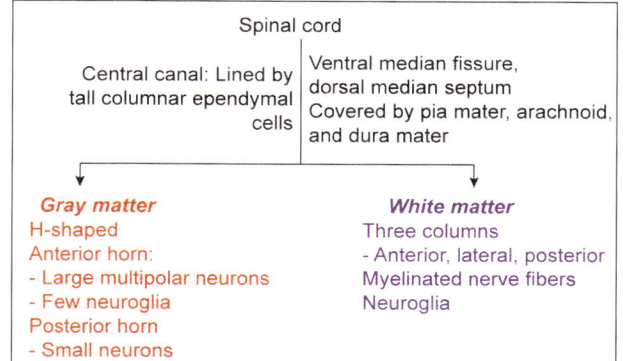

Flowchart 26.1: Histology of spinal cord

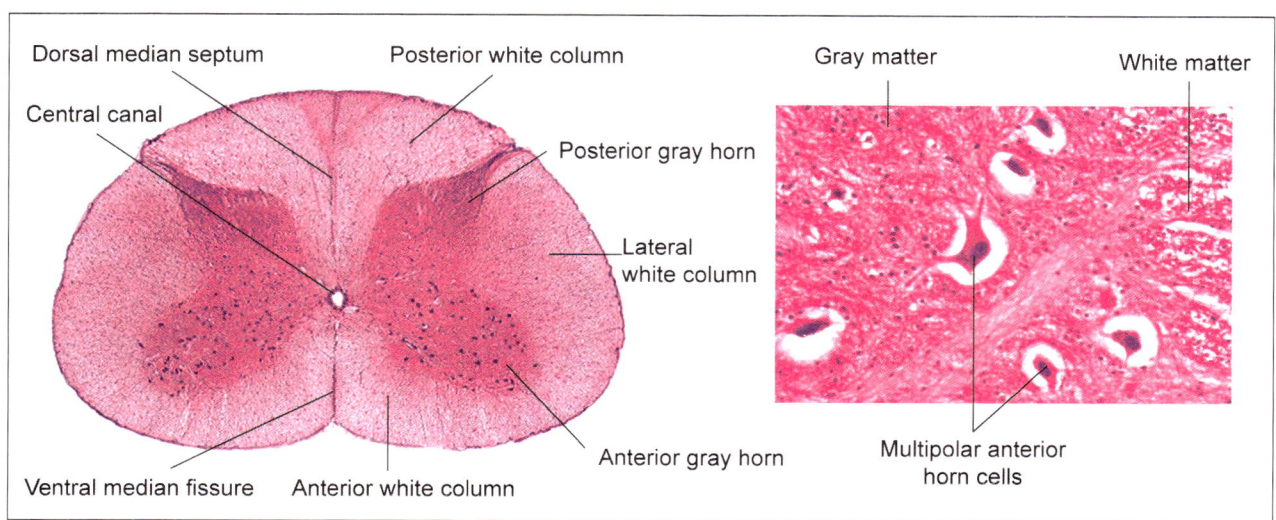

Fig. 26.3: Photomicrograph. Histology of spinal cord (low magnification on left, *H&E* stain), anterior horn cells (high magnification on right).

- The nerve fibers are covered by myelin sheath and a layer of fine connective tissue covering called epineurium.
- On *H&E* staining, myelin is removed during tissue processing; hence, axons are surrounded by a clear space. *Identification feature, Viva*
- White matter is divided into posterior, lateral, and anterior funiculus.
- Pia mater: Spinal cord is surrounded by a pale staining fibrous material called pia mater.

For segment identification, refer neuroanatomy textbook.

Clinical Correlation

Multiple sclerosis
- In multiple sclerosis, myelinated nerve fibers of brain and spinal cord are progressively damaged.
- It occurs because of damage to myelin.
- It may result in blindness, muscle weakness, loss of sensation, and so on.
- Its cause is unknown. It may be an autoimmune disorder.

Guillain Barré syndrome
- It is a rapid onset of muscle weakness [Georges Guillain, 1880–1961, French neurologist; Jean Barre, 1880–1967, French neurologist].
- It is an autoimmune disorder causing demyelination of peripheral nerves.
- It is characterized by rapid onset of numbness, muscular weakness, paralysis, and even death because of paralysis of respiratory muscles.

Summary (Examination Guide)
- Spinal cord consists of inner gray matter, outer white matter, and central ependyma-lined central canal (Figs 26.2 and 26.3).
- Gray matter has
  - Anterior horn: It shows large multipolar anterior horn cells
  - Posterior horn: It shows small neurons
- Gray matter also has neuroglial cells.
- White matter consists of posterior, lateral, and anterior white columns. These columns have myelinated axons that are surrounded by neuroglial cells.
- Spinal cord is having deep ventral fissure and dorsal median septum.

CEREBELLUM

Q. Draw a well-labelled diagram of histology of cerebellum.

- Cerebellum (*small brain*, in Latin) is highly folded to accommodate millions of neurons in a small area.
- This folding is called *arbor vitae.*
- Cerebellum has two *cerebellar hemispheres* that are connected to each other by a median *vermis* (Figs 26.4 and 26.5).
- Cerebellum is divided into number of lobules by fissures.

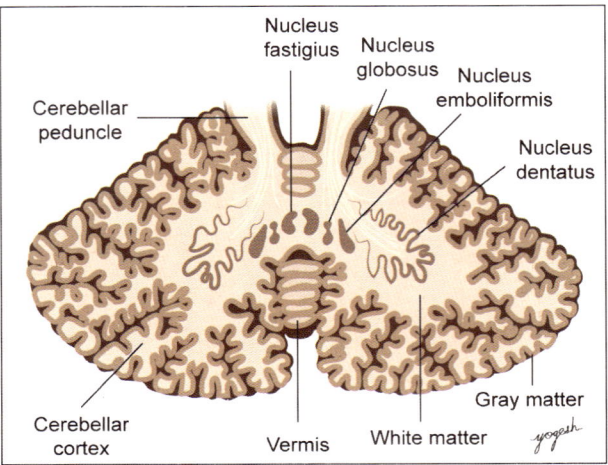

Fig. 26.4: Cerebellar nuclei.

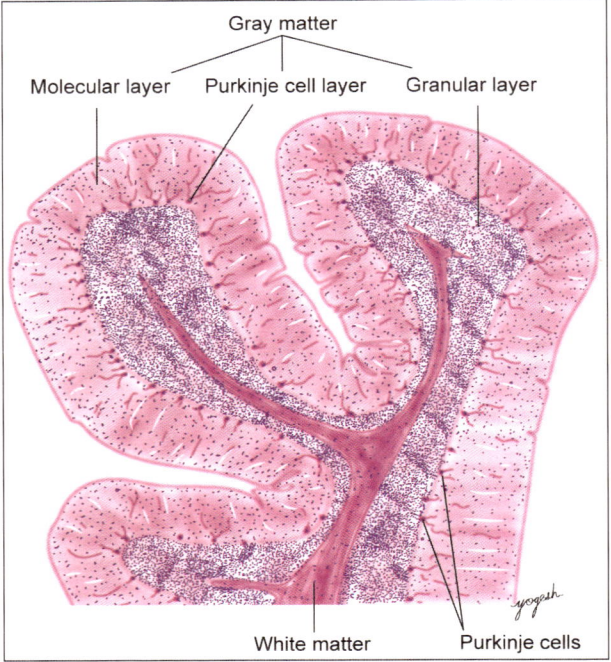

Fig. 26.5: Histology of cerebellum (practice figure).

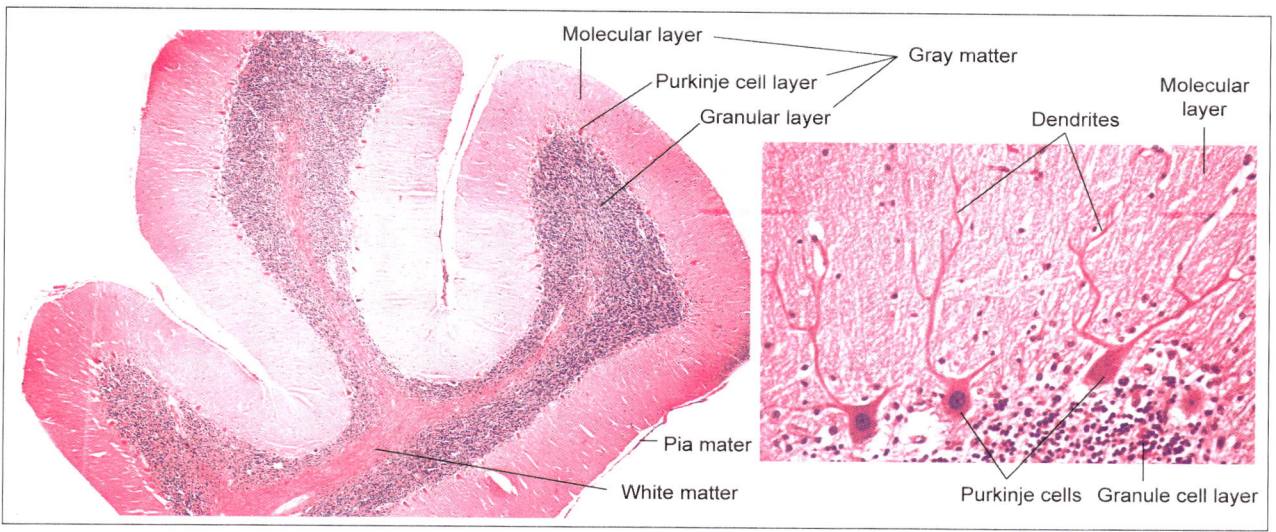

Fig. 26.6: Photomicrograph. Histology of cerebellum (low magnification on left, high magnification on right).

Histology of Cerebellum

- The structure of cerebellum is uniform throughout (homotypical).
- It has outer cortex (gray matter) and inner white matter (Figs 26.5, 26.6 and Flowchart 26.2).
- In the substance of white matter, it has four masses of gray matter as nucleus dentatus, nucleus globosus, nucleus emboliformis, and nucleus fastigius.
- Cerebellar cortex shows three layers: Outer molecular, middle Purkinje cell layer, and inner granular layer (Fig. 26.7). *Identification feature*

Molecular Layer

- Molecular layer lies just deep to the pia matter.
- It is a lightly stained layer with hematoxylin and eosin stain. *Identification feature*

Flowchart 26.2: Histology of cerebellum

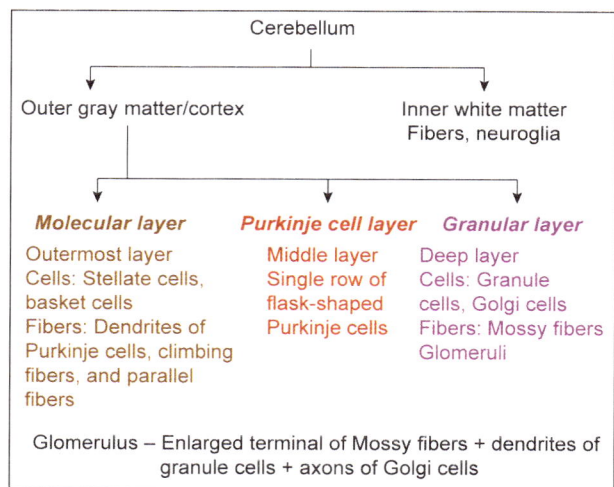

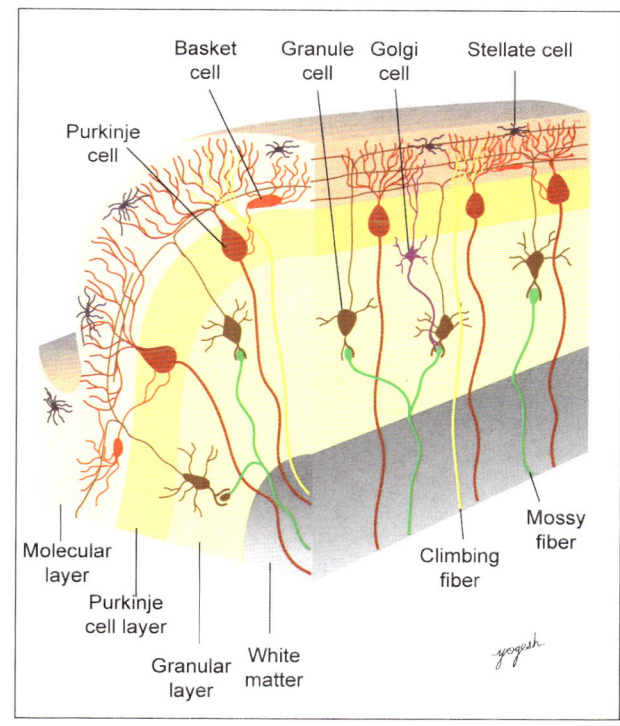

Fig. 26.7: Layers and cells of cerebellum.

- It consists of few cells and more fibers.
- Cells: Molecular layer has stellate cells in superficial part and few basket cells in deeper part.
- Fibers: Molecular layer shows numerous branching processes of Purkinje cells, axons of granule cells, and climbing fibers.

Purkinje Cell Layer

- This layer consists of a single row of Purkinje cell bodies that are arranged between molecular and

granular layer [Jan Evangelista Purkinje, 1767–1863 Czech Anatomist]. *Identification feature*
- Purkinje cells are large, flask-shaped neurons.*Viva*
- Dendrites of Purkinje cells arise from apex of flask and enter into the molecular layer.
- Single axon arises from the base that passes through the granular layer and white matter to the cerebellar nuclei.

Granular Layer
- It lies between Purkinje cell layer and white matter.
- It stains dark with hematoxylin because of closely packed, numerous, small granule cells.*Identification feature*
- Cells: Granular layer has granule cells and Golgi cells. *Granulae cells* are small neurons with round nucleus. *Golgi cell* are large, stellate cells.
- Fibers: Granule cells has *Mossy fibers* that brings information from pons to granule cells (pontocerebellar fibers). *Climbing fibers* and axons of Purkinje cells passes through the granular layer.
- *Glomeruli:* Mossy fibers end as dilated terminal. This dilated terminal is surrounded by dendrites of granule cells and axons of Golgi cells. Mossy fiber terminal with surrounding dendrites and axons form light-stained areas in granular layer. These areas are called glomeruli of cerebellum.

White Matter
- The white matter is composed of fibers and neuroglial cells.

Various cells of cerebellum are listed in Table 26.1.

Box 26.1: Afferent fibers of cerebellum
- Cerebellum receives input from Mossy fibers and climbing fibers.

Climbing fibers*Viva*
- These are olivocerebellar fibers (axons) arising from inferior olivary nucleus.
- They synapse in molecular layer with Purkinje cells. (one fiber for one cell).

Mossy fibers*Viva*
- These are other than olivocerebellar fibers.
- These include vestibulocerebellar, pontocerebellar, and spinocerebellar fibers.
- Mossy fibers have dilated terminal in granular layer.
- They synapse with dendrites of granule cells and axons of Golgi cells. This synapse forms light staining *cerebellar glomeruli* (Fig. 26.8).

Summary (Examination Guide)
- Cerebellum has outer cortex (gray matter) and inner white matter.
- Gray matter has three layers: Outer molecular, middle Purkinje cell layer, and inner granular layer.
- Molecular layer is lighter on *H&E* staining. It has numerous nerve fibers, stellate cells, basket cells, and neuroglia.
- Purkinje cell layer consists of a single row of flask shaped Purkinje cells.
- Granular layer is dark on *H&E* staining. It has numerous small granule cells and larger Golgi cells.
- White matter is composed of fibers and neuroglial cells.

Q. List the cells of cerebellar cortex.

Table 26.1: Cells of cerebellum

Cell	Location	Features	Dendrites	Axon
Stellate cells	Just beneath the surface of cerebellum in molecular layer	Small neuron	Confined to molecular layer Synapse with parallel fiber of granule cells	Confined to molecular layer Synapse with dendrites of Purkinje cells
Basket cells	Deeper part of molecular layer	Small nucleus	Few dendrites Synapse with parallel fibers bodies of granule cells, Purkinje cells, climbing and Mossy fibers	Synapse with Purkinje cell
Purkinje cells	Purkinje cell layer	Large flask-shaped cells	Arborize in molecular layer	Single axon to deep cerebellar nuclei
Granule cells	Granular layer	Small, spherical neurons	Dendrites form glomeruli with Mossy fibers	Axon runs parallel to each other and enter into molecular layer
Golgi neurons	Superficial part of granular layer	Large stellate cells GABAnergic inhibitory neurons	Dendrites enter molecular synapse with parallel fibers	Axon ends in glomeruli

Nervous System

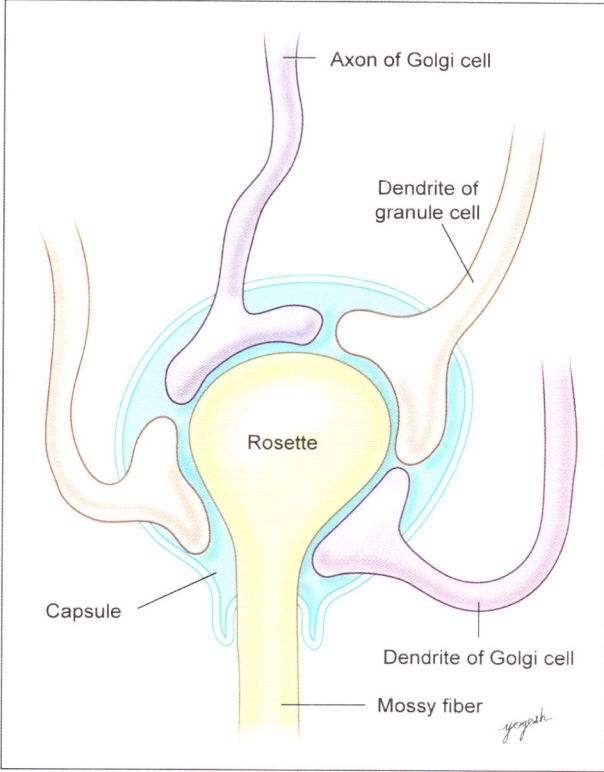

Fig. 26.8: Structure of cerebellar glomerulus.

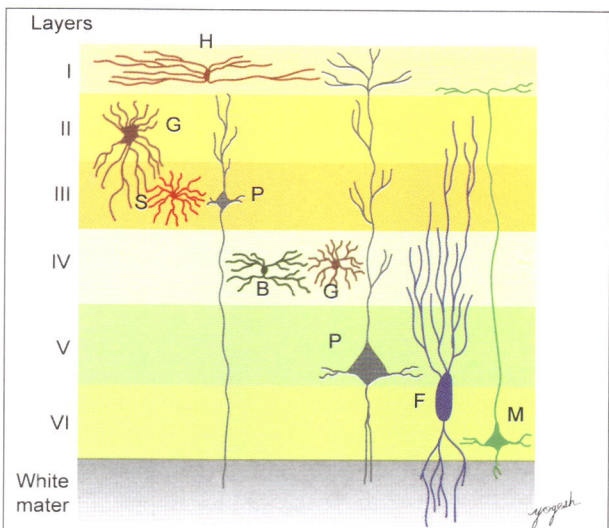

Fig. 26.9: Cells of cerebral cortex. H-horozontal cell of Cajal, G-granule cell, S-stellate cell, B-basket cell, P-pyramidal cell, F- fusiform cell, M-cells of Martinoti

CEREBRUM

Q. Draw a well-labelled diagram of histology of cerebral cortex.

- Cerebrum has outer gray matter and inner white matter.
- Gray matter of cerebrum is called cerebral cortex.
- Gray matter consists of numerous cell bodies of neurons, neuroglia, processes of neurons and neuroglia, and blood vessels.
- Gray matter has numerous synapses between neuronal processes.
- In the cerebral cortex, neurons are arranged in six layers.

Neurons of Cerebral Cortex

- Cerebral cortex consists of neurons of various size and shape, various lengths and branching pattern of neuronal processes.
- Cortex has pyramidal cells, stellate cells, fusiform cells, horizontal cells of Cajal, basket cells, cells of Martinoti, double bouquet cells, and Chadelier cells (Fig. 26.9).

Pyramidal Cells *Identification feature*

- About two-third of all cortical neurons are pyramidal cells.
- Pyramidal cells are multipolar neurons.
- These are triangular in shape. Apex of the triangle is directed toward surface of cerebral cortex.
- Pyramidal cells have the following processes:
  1. Apical dendrites arise from the apex and extend toward surface of cerebrum.
  2. Basal dendrites arise from basal angles of cell.
  3. Axon arises from base of the pyramidal cell.

Martinotti Cells

- These are small triangular or polygonal cells.
- They are present mostly in external pyramidal layer of cerebral cortex.
- Their axons travel toward the surface of cortex.

Stellate Neurons

- These are small, multipolar neurons.
- These are star-shaped neurons.
- These neurons look similar to granules; hence, also called as granular neurons.

Layer of Cerebral Cortex

- Neurons of the cerebral cortex are arranged in six layers: Molecular or plexiform layer, external granular layer, pyramidal cell layer, internal granular layer, ganglionic layer, and multiform layer (Figs 26.10, 26.11 and Flowchart 26.3). *Viva, Identification feature*

I. Molecular or Plexiform Layer

- This layer is situated just beneath the pia mater.
- It consists predominantly of fibers of neurological cells and few capillaries.
- This layer also has few horizontal cells of Cajal.

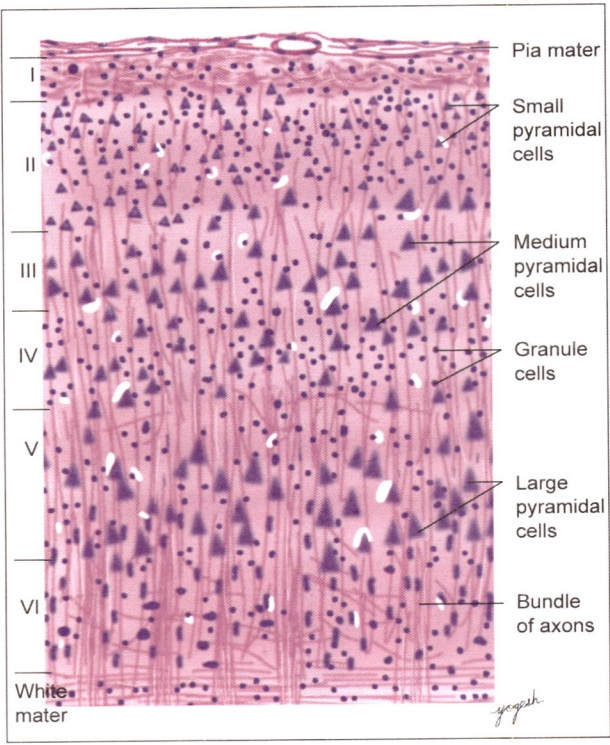

Fig. 26.10: Histology for cerebral cortex (low power, H&E stain, practice figure). I-Molecular or plexiform layer, II-external granular layer, III-external pyramidal cell layer, IV-internal granular layer, V-ganglionic layer, and VI-multiform layer.

- Only nuclei of the neurological cells can be identified; however, their cytoplasm is indistinguishable from nerve fibers.

II. External Granular Layer

- It is also called the small pyramidal cell layer.
- This layer shows two types of neurons: Small pyramidal cells and stellate/granule cells.

III. External Pyramidal Layer

- It is also called layer of medium pyramidal cells.
- It has medium pyramidal cells, few stellate cells, and cells of Martinotti.
- Axons of pyramidal cells form association and commissural fibers.

IV. Internal Granular Layer

- It consists of closely packed numerous small granular/stellate cells.
- It has horizontal fibers and called as *external band of Baillarger*. [Jules Baillarger, 1809–1890, French neurologist and psychiatrist].

V. Internal Pyramidal Layer

- This layer consists of large pyramidal cells.
- In the motor area of cerebrum, these cells are very big, and they form large *pyramidal cells of Betz* [Vladimir Alekseyevich Betz, 1834–1894, Ukrainian anatomist and histologist]. *Viva. Identification feature*
- This layer also contains horizontal fibers that form *internal band of Baillarger*.

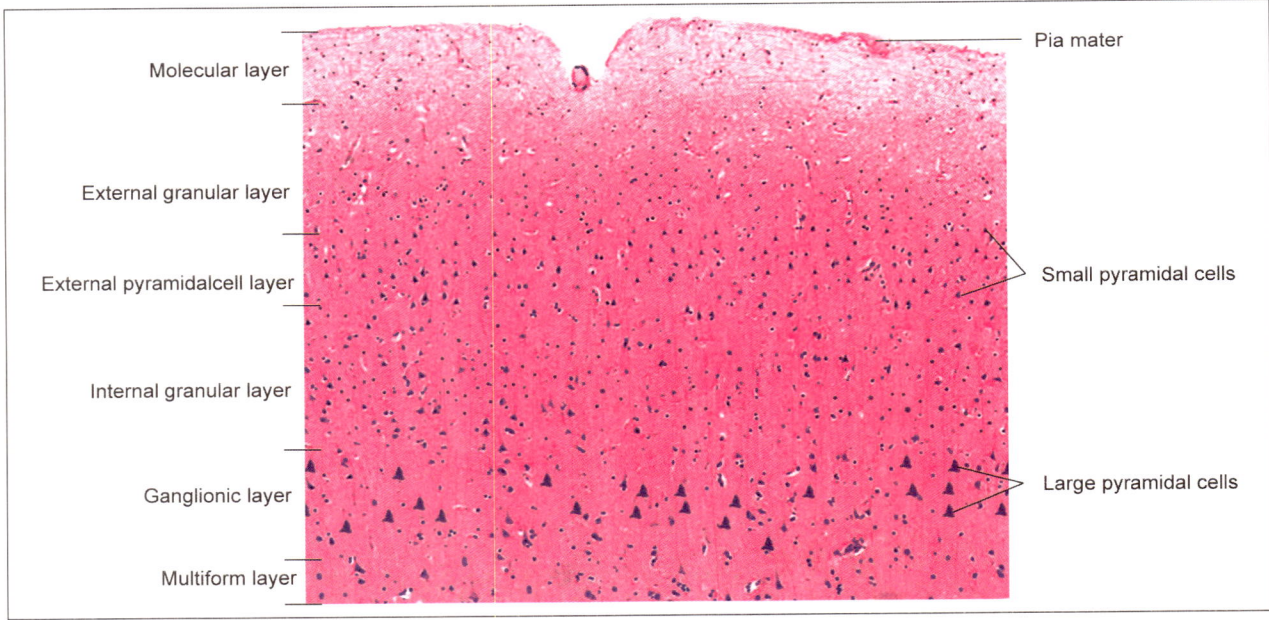

Fig. 26.11: Photomicrograph. Histology of cerebral cortex (low power, H&E stain).

Flowchart 26.3: Histology of cerebral cortex

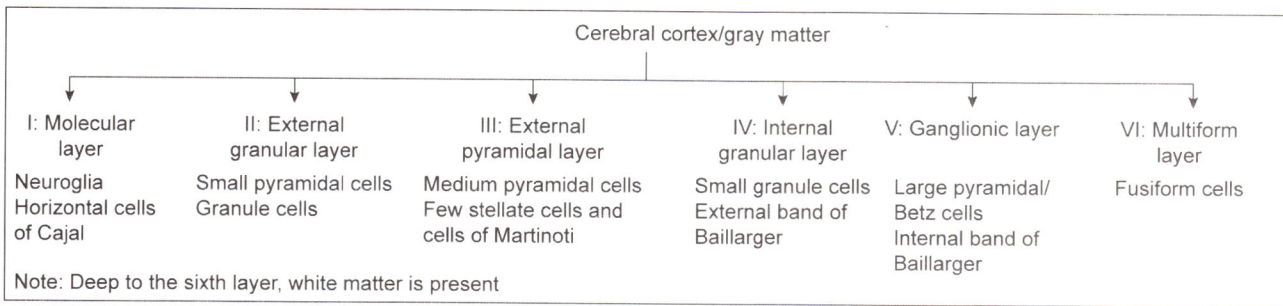

- Along with Betz cells, this layer has few cells of Martinotti, fusiform cells, and granule cells.

VI. Multiform Layer/Layer of Polymorphic/Fusiform Cells

- This layer has spindle-shaped fusiform cells, few stellate cells, and Martinotti cells.
- Fusiform cells lie perpendicular to the surface with axon coming out from center of the cell and dendrites from both ends.

White Matter

- Deep to the sixth layer, white matter of cerebral cortex is present.
- White matter consists of small round nuclei of neuroglial cells and numerous nerve cell processes.

Some Interesting Facts

- Histologically, cerebral cortex is classified as
  1. Agranular cortex: It has predominant pyramidal cells in layer III and V. It is found in motor area (precentral gyrus/area 4).
  2. Granular cortex: It has well-developed granular layer and less defined pyramidal cells. It is mainly sensory cortex.
- *Stria of Gennari* is a prominent external band of Baillarger in visual cortex (occipital lobe) that gives striate appearance to visual cortex [Francesco Gennari, 1750-1797, Italian anatomist].

Box 26.2: Connective tissue of central nervous system

- Brain and spinal cord are covered by dura, arachnoid, and pia maters.
- Dura mater has two layers: Meningeal layer that lies toward brain and endosteal layer that lies toward skull bones.
- These layers are separated to enclose dural venous sinuses.
- Arachnoid mater is a delicate layer of connective tissue.
- Trabeculae extends from arachnoid mater to pia mater. These fibers traverse subarachnoid space.
- Subarachnoid space contains cerebrospinal fluid.
- Pia mater is a delicate connective tissue layer that covers external surface of brain and spinal cord.
- Pia mater sends extensions around vessels of brain and spinal cord to form perivascular connective tissue sheaths.

CHAPTER 27

Special Senses I: Eye

Chapter Outline
- Cornea
- Sclera
- Uvea
  - Choroid
  - Ciliary body
  - Iris
- Retina
- Crystalline lens
- Vitreous body
- Structures associated with eyes
  - Optic nerve
  - Eyelid
  - Lacrimal gland

Competency achievement: The student should be able to:
AN43.2 Identify, describe and draw the microanatomy of cornea, retina

INTRODUCTION

- Eye is a peripheral organ of vision located in the bony orbit.
- Eye is spherical in shape (25 mm in diameter).
- Its movements are facilitated by six extraocular muscles and the eyeball is surrounded by adipose tissue cushion.
- Wall of eyeball consists of three structural layers (Fig. 27.1):
  1. Outer fibrous layer — sclera and cornea
  2. Middle vascular coat/uvea — choroid, ciliary body, and iris
  3. Inner nervous coat — retina
- Eyeball has three chambers as follows:
  1. Anterior chamber: Space between cornea and iris (Fig. 27.2)
  2. Posterior chamber: Space between iris and anterior surface of lens
  3. Vitreous chamber: Space between posterior surface of lens and retina
- Anterior chamber contains aqueous humor (watery fluid), whereas posterior chamber contains gel-like vitreous humor.
- Cornea, lens, aqueous humor, and vitreous humor are transparent refractive media of eyeball.*Neet*

CORNEA

- Cornea is the anterior transparent part of outermost coat of eyeball (Figs 27.1 and 27.2).
- Cornea continues with sclera at sclerocorneal junction (limbus).
- Cornea is an avascular structure.*Neet*
- Thickness: 1 mm
- Cornea is convex forward, colorless, and richly supplied with nerves.

Histology of Cornea (Figs 27.3, 27.4 and Flowchart 27.1)

- Cornea consists of five layers: Corneal epithelium, Bowman's membrane, corneal stroma, Descemet's membrane, and corneal endothelium.

Corneal Epithelium

- Outermost lining of cornea is *nonkeratinized stratified squamous epithelium*.*Neet, Viva*
- Cells of the deepest layer are low columnar with round, ovoid nuclei. Cells of superficial layer are disc-shaped (flat) with flat, pyknotic nuclei.
- Corneal epithelium regenerates rapidly (within 7 days).
- Cells of deepest layer divide and migrates superficially. During migration, these cells lose most of the cell organelles.

Special Senses I: Eye

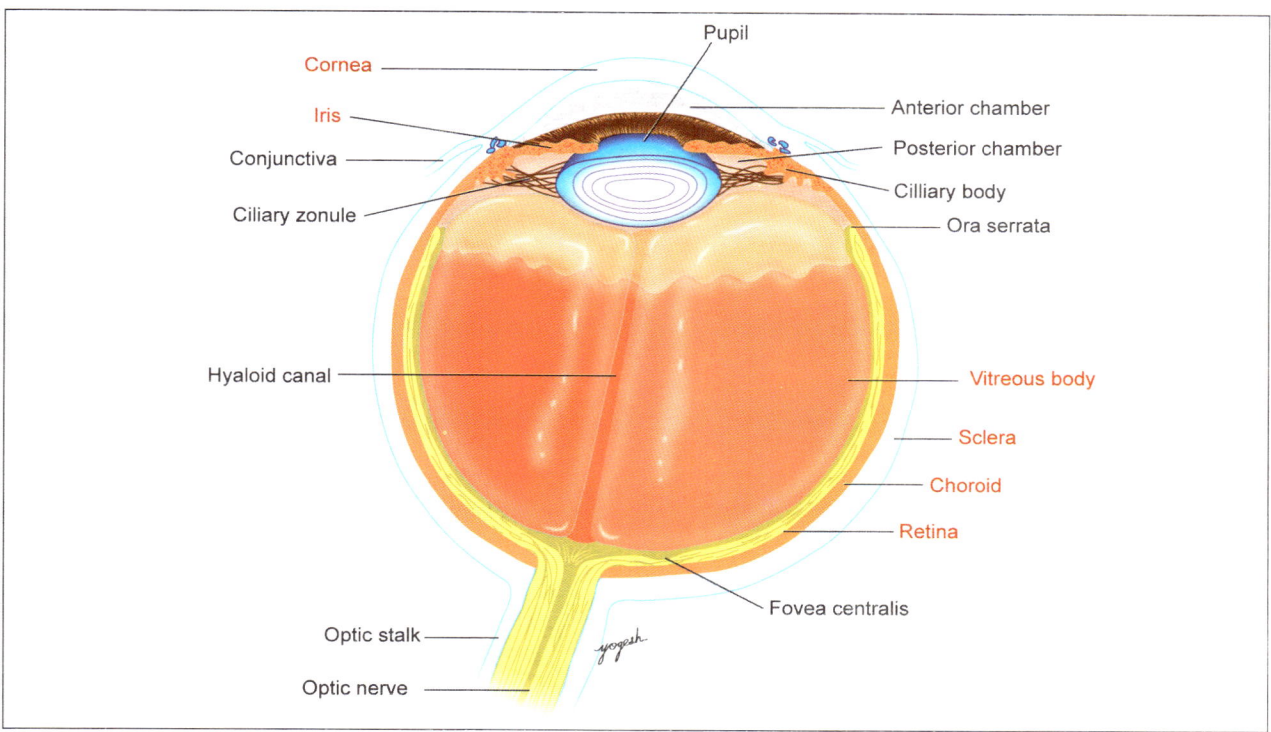

Fig. 27.1: Structure of eyeball (Source: Textbook of Human Embryology, Yogesh Sontakke, 1st edn., CBS Publishers).

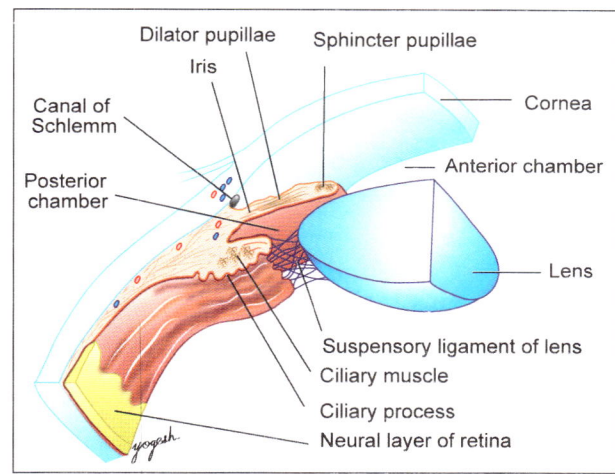

Fig. 27.2: Sclerocorneal junction, ciliary body, and suspensory ligament of lens.

- *New concept:* Stem cells for corneal epithelium are present at corneoscleral limbus.
- *Free nerve endings* in corneal epithelium make cornea extremely sensitive for touch (ophthalmic division of trigeminal nerve).
- Superficial layer of corneal epithelium shows presence of *microvilli* on external surface. These microvilli help to hold the film of tear on the cornea.

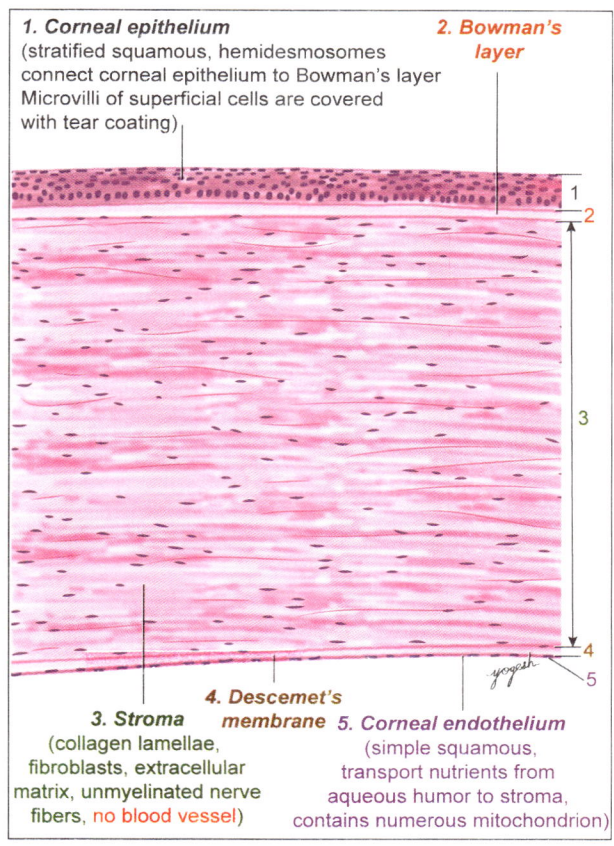

Fig. 27.3: Histology of cornea (practice figure).

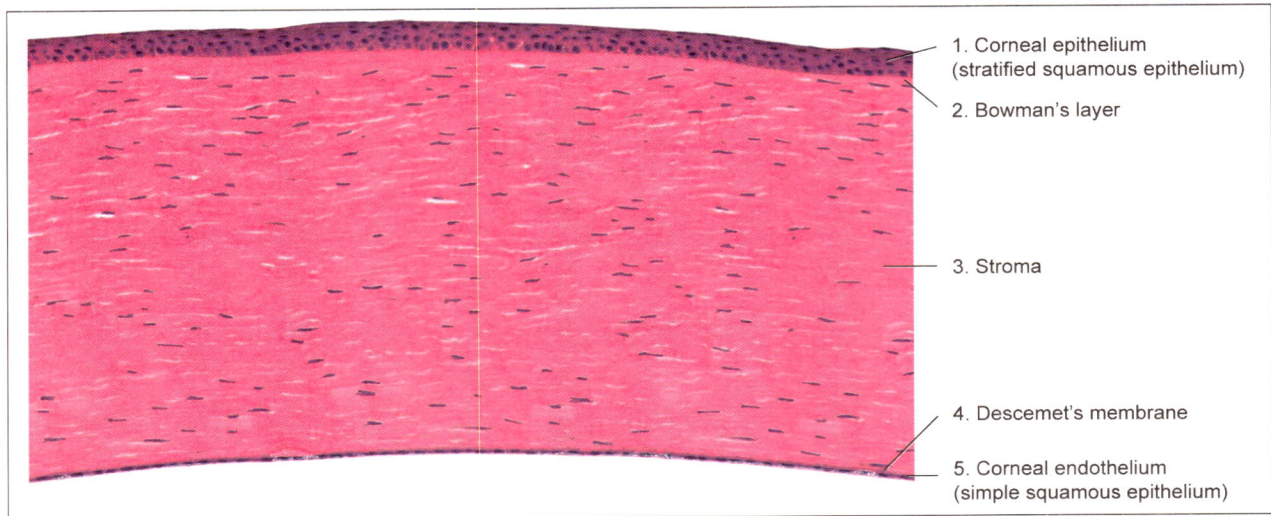

Fig. 27.4: Photomicrograph. Cornea (high magnification, *H&E* stain).

Flowchart 27.1: Histology of cornea

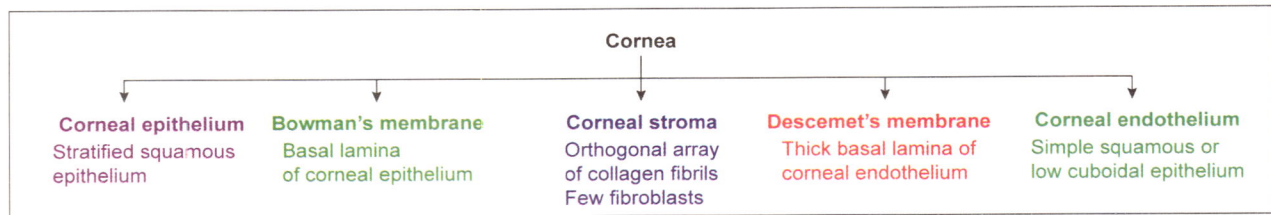

Some Interesting Facts

- *Recent concept:* Ferritin is present in corneal epithelial nuclei. This ferritin protects the nuclear DNA from the UV light exposure damage, and thus prevents cancerous changes. *Neet*
- Stem cells present at the sclerocorneal junction (limbus) are essential for corneal transparency. Any damage to these cells causes *conjunctivatization of cornea* (vascularization of cornea). It causes diminished vision. *Neet*
- Bowman's membrane does not regenerate. *Neet* Hence, damage to Bowman's membrane heals with an opaque scar that may impair vision.

Bowman's Membrane (Anterior Basement Membrane/Limiting Lamina)

- It is homogeneous lamina on which corneal epithelium rests.
- Thickness: 8–10 μm.
- It consists of randomly oriented collagen fibrils.

Functions
- It acts as a barrier that prevents the spread of infections.
- It provides support to corneal epithelium.

Corneal Stroma (Substantia Propria)

- It constitutes about 90% of corneal thickness.
- Corneal stroma has lamellae of *type I collagen* fibrils and ground substance.
- Fibers in each lamella are arranged parallel to each other, whereas the fibers are perpendicular to each other in adjacent lamellae.
- Stroma is transparent because of orderly arrangement of collagen fibrils (called orthogonal array).
- Between adjacent lamellae, ground substance and flattened fibroblasts are present.
- Ground substance contains proteoglycans (sulfated glycosaminoglycans).
- Fibroblasts are star-shaped on surface view. They are also called *keratocytes or corneal corpuscles*.

Descemet's Membrane

- It is also called *posterior basement membrane* or *posterior limiting lamina*.
- It is a thin, homogenous basal lamina of posterior endothelial cells of cornea. It is a *true basement membrane*.
- It is intensely positive to periodic acid–Schiff (PAS) and gives bright magenta color on PAS staining.

- *Pectinate ligament:* Peripheral fibers of Descemet's membrane extend beneath the sclera to form a meshwork as pectinate ligament.
- Some fibers of Descemet's membrane extend into sclera and ciliary muscle. These fibers help to maintain the curvature of cornea.

Corneal Endothelium

- Corneal endothelium lines the posterior surface of cornea.
- It is a single layer of squamous cells (some authors mentioned it as low cuboidal).
- It forms anterior endothelium of anterior chamber of eyeball and remains in contact with aqueous humor.
- Adjacent corneal endothelial cells are connected by zonulae adherens, leaky zonulae occludans, and desmosomes.
- Corneal endothelium maintains water balance in the corneal stroma. It pumps out excess water from corneal stroma and helps to maintain proper corneal transparency.

Some Interesting Facts

- After the injury, swelling of cornea causes disruption of orthogonal array of cornea. This leads to corneal opacity.
- In corneal inflammation, lymphocytes enter corneal stroma from blood vessels that lie at sclerocorneal junction.
- Bowman's membrane cannot regenerate but Descemet's membrane can regenerate.
- As cornea is avascular structure, severely damaged cornea can be easily treated with corneal transplantation.

Summary (Examination Guide)

- Cornea is a transparent, colorless, avascular structure that covers anterior one-sixth of the eyeball.
- Cornea has five layers:
  1. *Corneal epithelium* consists of nonkeratinized stratified squamous epithelium.
  2. *Bowman's membrane*/anterior limiting lamina is thickened basal lamina of corneal epithelium.
  3. *Corneal stroma* consists of layers of collagen fibrils having orthogonal array and few fibroblasts.
  4. *Descemet's membrane*/posterior limiting lamina is the thickened basal lamina of corneal endothelium.
  5. *Posterior endothelium* consists of simple squamous (low cuboidal) epithelium.

SCLERA

- External thick white opaque fibrous cover of posterior five-sixths of the eyeball is called *sclera*.
- Sclera consists of
  1. Bundles of collagen fibers
  2. Few elastic fibers
  3. Ground substance
  4. Scattered fibroblasts
- Reason for white color/opacity of sclera: Irregular arrangement of collagen fibers that make sclera white or opaque similar to other dense connective tissue.

Layers of Sclera (Ill-defined)

- Episclera/episcleral layer: It is an external covering of loose connective tissue.
- *Tenon's capsule:* It is also called *substantia propria* or sclera proper. It consists of a dense network of collagen fibers.[Neet]
- *Suprachoroid lamina:* It is also called *lamina fusca*. It is the innermost layer of sclera that consists of delicate connective tissue fibers.

Some Interesting Facts

- Extraocular muscles insert on Tenon's capsule or substantia propria of sclera.
- *Tenon's space:* It is space around the episcleral layer of sclera. This space is also called *episcleral space* and allows movement eyeball.
- Tenon's capsule is also called *fascia bulbi* or bulbar sheath.
- Sclerocorneal (corneoscleral junction)/limbus: Anteriorly, sclera continues with cornea at limbus.
- *Corneolimbal stem* cells lie along the corneoscleral limbus (junction) that help to regenerate corneal epithelium.
- *Canal of Schlemn:* These are endothelium lined-tubes or canals that lie just behind the corneoscleral junction. Canal of Schlemn drains aqueous humor from the anterior chamber into the episcleral vessels.

Previous concept: Canal of Schlemn is sclera venous channel; hence, also called *sinus venosus sclerae*.

New concept: Canal of Schlemn is a lymphatic vessel as its endothelium express many lymphatic endothelium-specific proteins (PROX1, VEGFR3, CCL21, and so on) [Friedrich Schlemn, German anatomist, 1795–1858].

- Smooth surface of sclera allows the movement of eyeball.

UVEA/VASCULAR COAT

- Deep to sclera, there is a vascular coat of eyeball. It consists of choroid, ciliary body, and iris.

Choroid (Fig. 27.1)

- Choroid is a dark brown vascular coat that lies deep to sclera and superficial to retina.
- Choroid consists of two layers: Choriocapillary layer and Bruch's membrane.

Choriocapillary Layer

- It lies superficial to Bruch's membrane.
- It consists of a network of blood vessels and supportive collagen fibers.
- It also contains many pigmented cells that give dark color to choroid.
- Outer vascular lamina of choricocapillary layer has larger vessels, whereas inner capillary lamina (choroidocapillaries) contains a network of capillaries.
- Choricapillary layer is externally supported by a nonvascular connective tissue coat called suprachoroid lamina or lamina fusca.^MCQ

Bruch's Membrane/Lamina Vitrea

- It lies between choriocapillary layer and retina.
- It is a thin amorphous refractile layer.
- It consists of layers of elastic and collagen fibers.
- Choroid extends from optic nerve to ora serrata.

Ciliary Body (Figs 27.1 and 27.2)

- Ciliary body is the thickened circular anterior portion of vascular coat of eyeball.
- It posteriorly continues with the choroid and anteriorly with iris.
- It is connected to lens by suspensory ligaments.
- Ciliary body consists of *ciliaris* muscles and vascular connective tissue.
- Ciliaris muscle consists of three functional groups of smooth muscle fiber as follows:
  - Longitudinal portion that helps to open iridocorneal angle and facilitate drainage of aqueous humor.
  - Oblique portion that causes flattening of lens during distant vision
  - Circular portion that reduces tension of lens during accommodation for near vision.
- *Ciliary processes:* These are approximately 75 thickenings of ciliary body that are covered by a double layer of columnar epithelium cells (ciliary epithelium).
- Ciliary epithelium secretes aqueous humor and maintains blood–aqueous barrier.
- Outer cells layer of epithelium is pigmented, whereas inner cell layer secretes aqueous humor.
- Zonular fibers arise from suspensory ligament of the lens.

Iris (Figs 27.1 and 27.2)

- Iris is the anterior most part of vascular coat of eyeball.
- Iris is attached peripherally to sclera, at about 2 mm posterior to corneoscleral junction.
- *Pupil:* Central aperture of the iris is called pupil.
- Iris forms a contractile diaphragm in front of lens that controls entry of light in the eyeball.
- Iris consists of two parts:
  Posterior pigment epithelium
  Anterior connective tissue stroma
- Posterior pigment epithelium consists of two layers: Posterior densely pigmented epithelium and anterior pigmented myoepithelial cells.
- Stroma of iris consists of smooth muscle fibers, fibroblasts, melanocytes, connective tissue fibers, and blood vessels.
- Smooth muscle fibers are arranged as
  - Circumferentially oriented sphincter pupillae muscle
  - Longitudinally (radially) oriented dilator pupillae muscle
- Numerous melanocytes are present in the stroma of iris. These melanocytes decide the color of iris.

RETINA

Q. List the layers of retina.

Q. Draw a well-labeled diagram showing histology of retina.

- Retina is the innermost layer of eyeball.
- Retina lines posterior three-fourth surface of eyeball.
- Embryologically, retina is derived from two layers of optic cup.
- Retina basically represents these two layers of optic cup in the form of:
  - Inner layer of neural retina or retina proper. This layer consists of photoreceptor (rods and cones), which are essential for vision.
  - Outer layer of retinal pigmented epithelium.
- *Retinal detachment:* It is a pathological condition that involves the separation of neural retina from retinal pigmented epithelium.
- Retina shows (Fig. 27.1):
  1. *Optic disc* or *optic papilla:* This is the spot where optic nerve leaves the eyeball. In the region of

optic disc, there are no photoreceptors; hence, this region is also called 'blind spot'. *Viva, MCQ*
2. Fovea centralis is the region of retina that is located 2.5 mm lateral to the optic disc. Fovea centralis is responsible for acute vision.
3. Macula is a broad area of yellow pigmentation. Macula includes (surrounds) fovea centralis.

Layers of Retina

Q. List the layers of retina.

Histologically, retina consists of ten layers as follows (Figs 27.5 to 27.7):
1. Retinal pigmented epithelium (REP)
2. Layer of rods and cones
3. Outer limiting membrane
4. Outer nuclear layer
5. Outer plexiform layer
6. Inner nuclear layer
7. Inner plexiform layer
8. Ganglion cell layer
9. Layer of optic nerve fibers
10. Inner limiting membrane

The components of retina are listed in Flowchart 27.2.

Layer 1: Retinal Pigmented Epithelium (RPE)

- It consists of a single layer of *low cuboidal cells.*
- RPE is separated from choroid (vascular coat of eyeball) by *Bruch's membrane.*
- RPE shows numerous melanin pigment. *Identification feature*
- Surface of RPE (facing toward layer of rods and cones) has apical cytoplasmic processes that extend for a short distance between rods and cones.
- Functions of RPE
  1. RPE produces melanin
  2. RPE absorbs light and prevents light reflection
  3. RPE forms a major component of blood–retinal barrier
  4. RPE removes shaded membranous discs of rods and cones by phagocytosis

Layer 2: Rod and Cones

- Photoreceptors in retina are of two types: Rod and cones. These cells convert light energy into electrical stimulus.
- Retina contains 120 million rods and 27 million cones.
- In fovea centralis, only cones are present. *MCQ* Cones are mainly responsible for color vision.
- Optic disc is devoid of photoreceptors; hence, it is called a blind spot.
- Dimensions:
  – Rods: Length – 50 μm
  – Cones: Length – 25–85 μm

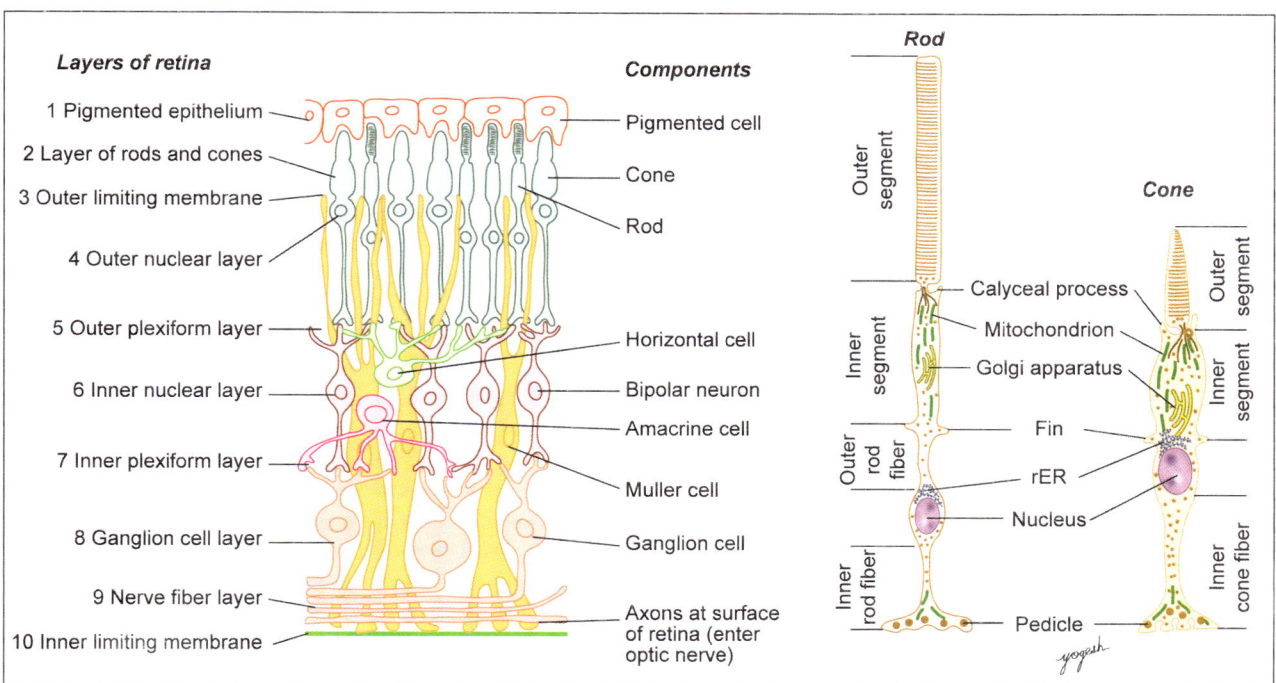

Fig. 27.5: Layers of retina and ultrastructure of rod and cone (Source: Textbook of Human Embryology, Yogesh Sontakke, 1st edn., CBS Publishers).

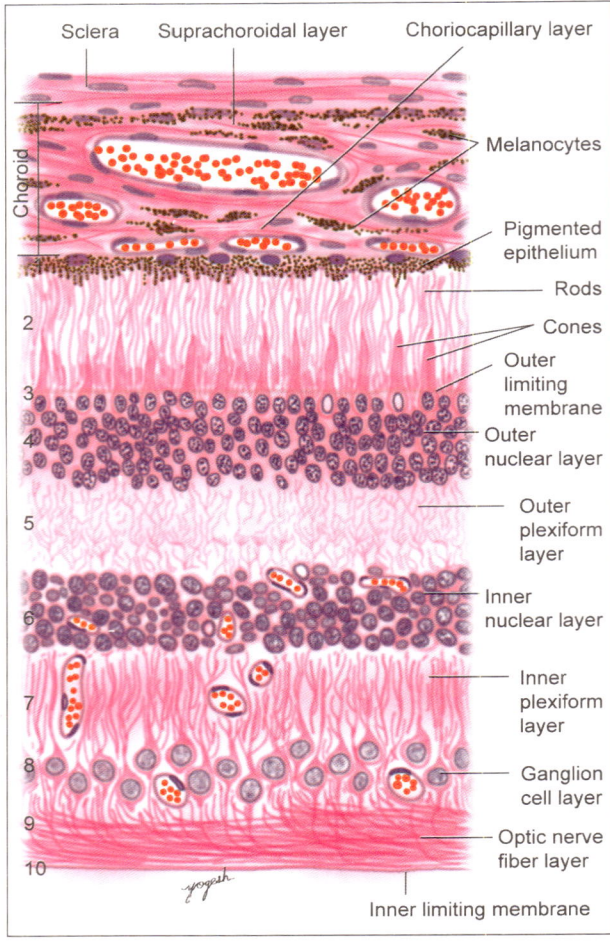

Fig. 27.6: Histology of retina (practice figure).

Structure

- Photoreceptor cell (rod and cone) has three parts as follows:
  1. Outer segment
  2. Connecting stalk
  3. Inner segment
- Outer segments of rods are cylindrical, whereas that of cones are conical in shape (outer segment is highly modified cilium).*Neet*

Flowchart 27.2: Components of retina

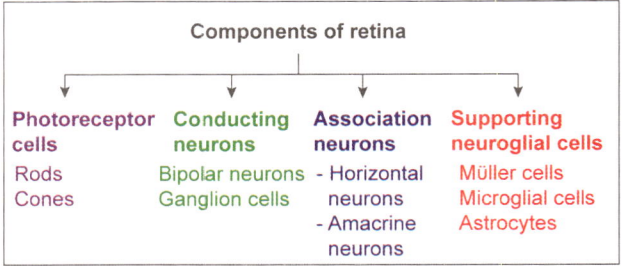

- Connecting stalk is a constricted region that connects outer and inner segment.
- Inner segment has numerous Golgi apparatus and mitochondria.
- Electron microscopy: Outer segment of photoreceptors (rods and cones) has 600–1000 horizontal discs.
- These discs are transverse infoldings of plasma membrane.
- Rods and cones shed discs. These discs are removed by pigmented epithelium by phagocytosis.
- *Visual pigment*
  - Rod contains rhodopsin (visual purple)
  - Cone contains idopsin
  - Each visual pigment (rhodopsin and idopsin) has *opsin* (membrane-bound subunits) and light-sensitive *chromophore.*
  - Rod has rhodopsin and cones has photopsin as *opsin subunit.*
  - Vitamin A is essential in the formation of chromophore.

Types of Cones

- According to the response to light, cones are of three types as follows:
  1. Long wavelength sensitive or red color (588 nm)
  2. Medium wavelength sensitive or green color (531 nm)
  3. Short wavelength sensitive or blue color (42 nm).
- Hence, cones are responsible for color vision.

Layer 3: Outer Limiting Membrane

- It is the third layer of retina.
- It consists of *zonulae adherents* between Müller's cells.
- Outer limiting membrane is not a true membrane.

Layer 4: Outer Nuclear Layer

- It consists of the nuclei of rods and cones.
- These nuclei are arranged in several layers.
- The nuclei of cone stain lightly; they are larger than rod nuclei.

Layer 5: Outer/External Plexiform Layer

- Outer plexiform layer consists of synapse between rods and cones with the dendrites of bipolar cells and amacrine and horizontal cells.
- The expanded terminal part of rod is called *spherule* and that of cone is called *pedicle.*
- Many rods synapse with single bipolar neurons, whereas a single cone synapses with single bipolar neuron.*Viva*

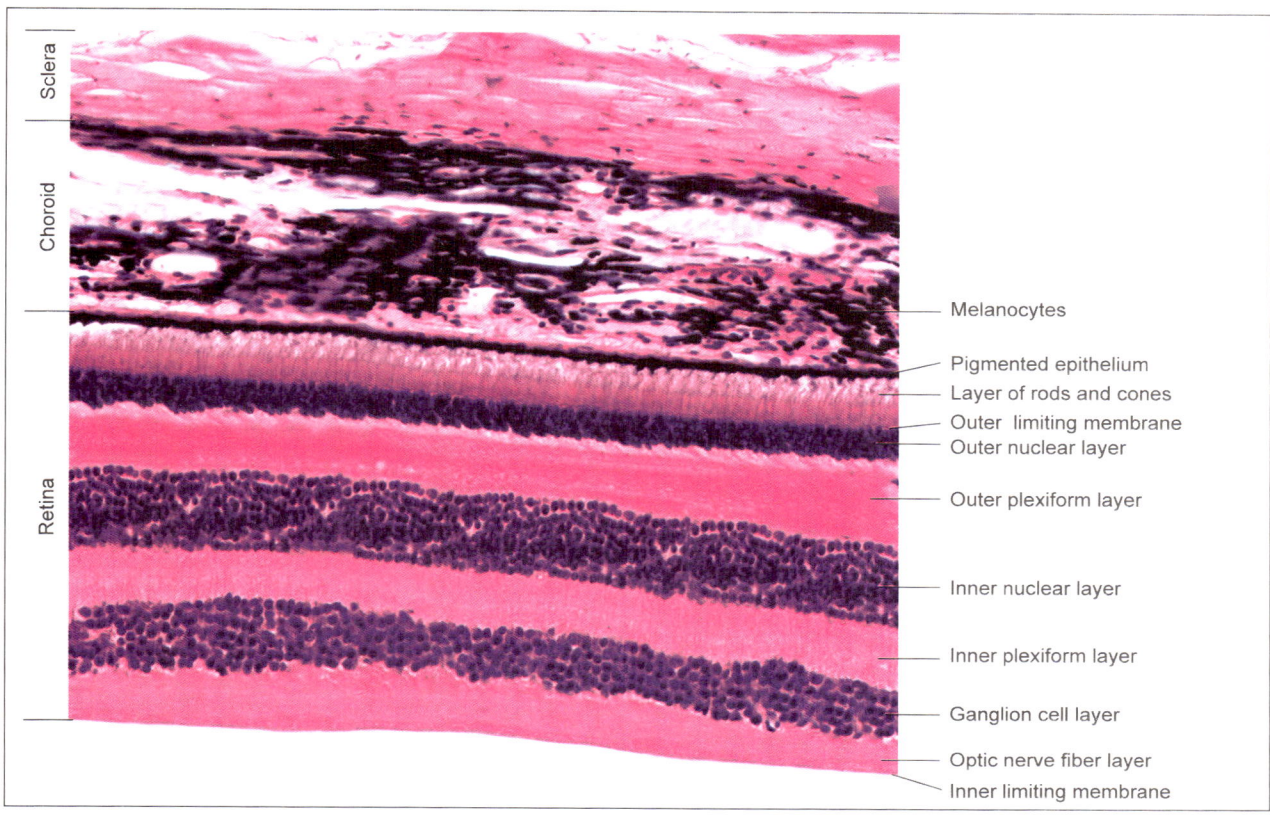

Fig. 27.7: Photomicrograph. Histology of retina (High magnification, H&E stain).

Layer 6: Inner Nuclear Layer

- Inner nuclear layer consists of nuclei of bipolar, horizontal, amacrine, and Müller cells.
- *Müller cells:* These are supporting (neuroglial) cells. These cells extend from outer to inner limiting membrane. (Heinrich Müller, German anatomist, 1820–1864).
- *Bipolar cells:* These are conducting cells that convey signal from rod and cone cells to ganglion cells.
- *Horizontal cells:* These cells synapse in outer plexiform layer with rods, cones, and bipolar cells.
- *Amacrine cells:* These cells synapse in inner plexiform layer with bipolar and ganglionic cells.
- Cells of Müller are also called retinal gliocytes. These cells nourish neurons of retina.

Layer 7: Inner Plexiform Layer

- Inner plexiform layer is a synaptic layer between bipolar neurons, cells, and ganglion cells.

Layer 8: Ganglion Cell Layer

- Ganglion cell layer consists of bodies of multipolar neurons. Nuclei of these cells are round, large, and lightly stained with prominent nucleoli. These nuclei are arranged in 2–3 layers.
- Dendrites of ganglion cells receive impulses from bipolar neurons and their axons enter optic nerve.
- In fovea, single ganglion cell synapse with single bipolar neuron, whereas in peripheral region single ganglion cell may synapse with hundreds of bipolar neurons.

Layer 9: Layer of Optic Nerve Fibers

- *Axons of ganglion cells* run toward optic disc. These axons form layer of optic nerve fibers.
- After leaving the eyeball, fibers of optic nerve become myelinated.
- Layer of optic nerve fibers also contains blood vessels of retina.

Layer 10: Inner Limiting Membrane

- Müller cells rest on the basal lamina that forms inner limiting membrane.
- This inner limiting membrane separates retina from vitreous body.

Some Interesting Facts

- **Macular pucker** or *epiretinal membrane*: In older individuals, on the inner surface of retina, a semi-translucent membrane may be formed. This membrane is called *macular pucker*. It shows macrophages, fibroblasts, and other cells. In macular pucker, there is blurring of vision and even blindness.
- Through the center of optic nerve, central artery and central vein of retina traverse. Each artery is divided into superior and inferior divisions that later give rise to nasal and temporal branches.
- Retinal vessels form capillary plexus in inner nuclear layer. Remaining outer retinal layer receives nutrition by diffusion through the vascular choriocapillary layer of choroid.
- Branches of the retinal artery are end arteries (they do not anastomose). *Neet*
- The differences between rods and cone cells are listed in Table 27.1.

CRYSTALLINE LENS

- Crystalline lens of eye is a transparent, biconvex, avascular structure (Figs 27.1 and 27.2).
- Lens is suspended from ciliary body by zonular fibers.
- Lens lies between aqueous humor and vitreous humor.
- Lens has the following three components (Fig. 27.8):
  1. Lens capsule
  2. Lens epithelium
  3. Lens substance

Lens Capsule

- Lens capsule is a transparent homogenous basal lamina of lens epithelium.
- Capsule consists of type IV collagen fibers and glycoproteins.
- Capsule is produced by lens epithelium.

Lens Epithelium

- Deep to capsule, anterior surface of lens is covered by a layer of *cuboidal epithelium*. This is also called *anterior lens epithelium* or subcapsular epithelium.

Summary (Examination Guide) (Fig. 27.6)

- Histologically retina consists of **ten layers** from outside inward as follows:
  1. *Retinal pigment epithelium*: It is the outermost layer. It has single layer of *cuboidal cells* containing *melanin*.
  2. *Layer of rods and cones*: These are photoreceptor cells.
  3. *Outer limiting membrane*: It is a sieve-like membrane formed by apical boundary of Müller cells.
  4. *Outer nuclear layer*: It consists of nuclei of rods and cones.
  5. *Outer plexiform layer*: It consists of synapses between rods, cones, bipolar neurons, and horizontal cells.
  6. *Inner nuclear layer*: It contains nuclei of Müller cells, bipolar cells, and amacrine cells.
  7. *Inner plexiform layer*: It contains synapses between bipolar cells, ganglion cells, and amacrine cells.
  8. *Ganglion cell layer*: It contains nuclei of ganglion cells.
  9. *Layer of optic nerve fibers*: It consists of *axons of ganglion cells* that later form the optic nerve.
  10. *Inner limiting membrane*: It a composed of basal lamina of Müller cells.

Table 27.1: Differences between rods and cone cells

Character	Rods	Cones
Outer segment	Rod-shaped	Cone-shaped
Number	More numerous than cones	Few in number
Distribution	Distributed evenly over retina, absent in fovea centralis	More concentrated in fovea centralis
Visual acuity	Gives less visual acuity, but sensitive to low light (night vision)	Gives more acuity, sensitive to high light intensity (day vision)
Color vision	Does not provide (achromatic/black and white)	Provide color vision
Light-sensitive pigment	Rhodopsin	Iodopsin
Physiological types	One	Three (according to types of iodopsin)

Special Senses I: Eye

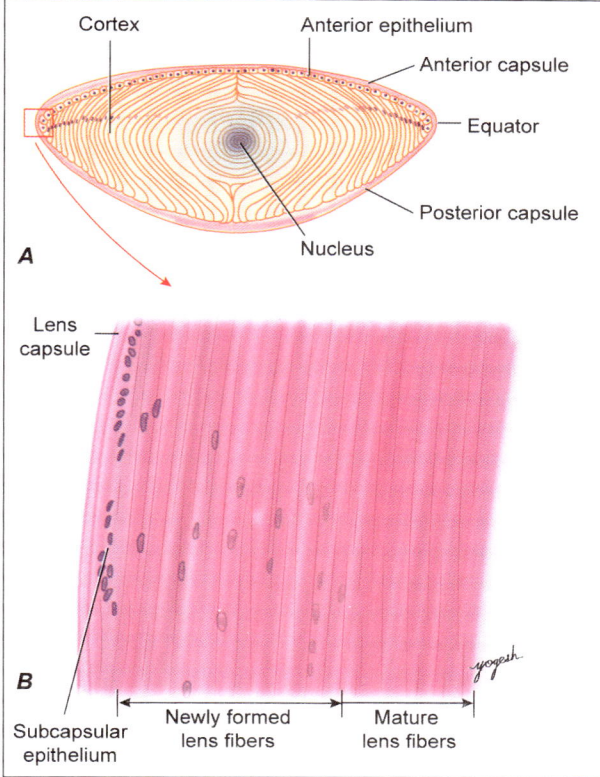

Fig. 27.8: Structure of lens. (A) Schematic drawing of the lens indicating its structural components. Basal lamina of lens fiber or capsule of lens. Germinal zone of lens lies at lens equator, where cells divide and differentiate into the lens fiber cells. Lens nucleus consists of organelle-free lens fiber cells. (B) Histological section of germinal zone of lens shows newly formed lens fiber cells from the subcapsular epithelium and old mature lens fibers that do not possess nuclei.

- Toward periphery, cells of epithelium become progressively longer and ultimately get converted into long fibers that form substance of the lens.

Lens Fibers (Lens Fiber Cells)

- Lens epithelium develops to form lens fibers. These are composed of soluble proteins called *crystallins*.

Box 27.1: Vitreous body

- Interior of the eyeball contains transparent, jelly-like substance called *vitreous body/chamber*.
- Vitreous body is loosely attached to retina.
- Composition of vitreous body
- 1. 99% water
  2. Collagen, glycosaminoglycans (hyaluronan)
  3. Hyalocytes
- Hyalocytes synthesize vitreous humor.[Neet, Viva]
- *Hyaloid or Cloquet's canal:* It is a remnant of pathway of hyaloid artery. It runs from optic disc to posterior surface of lens.[MCQ]

OPTIC NERVE

Q. Write a short note on histology of optic nerve.

- Optic nerve (cranial nerve II) transmit visual information from retina to brain. It extends from optic disc of eyeball to optic chiasma.
- Optic nerve consists of nerve fibers (axons) of ganglion cells of retina and supporting glial cells. Optic nerve is derived from optic stalk during seventh week of development.

Histology (Fig. 27.9, 27.10)

- Optic nerve is covered by three sheaths: Outermost dura mater, middle arachnoid mater, and innermost pia mater.[Identification feature]
- Optic nerve is covered by meninges because it develops as outpouching of brain (diencephalon).
- Note: There is no endoneurium, perineurium, and epineurium in optic nerve.[Identification feature]
- There are no Schwann cells in optic nerve.
- Myelin is produced by oligodendrocytes in optic nerve.[Viva]
- From pia mater, septa arise that divide optic nerve into number of fascicles.
- Each fascicle consists of *myelinated axons of ganglion cells of retina*. Each axon is surrounded by myelin produced by oligodendrocytes.[Identification feature]

Clinical Correlation

Cataract
- Normally, crystalline lens of eyeball is transparent.
- Because of various causes, it loses its transparency and it becomes opaque. The opacity of lens is called cataract.
- Causes of cataract: Old age, trauma, congenital disorders such as Down's syndrome, exposure to ultraviolet radiation, and so on.
- Treatment of cataract can be done with removal of lens and transplant with plastic lens implantation.

Presbyopia
- With increasing age, crystalline lens loses its elasticity and power of accommodation for near vision (reading). These changes are more evident by the age of 40 to 45 years and the condition is called *presbyopia*. It can be corrected with convex lens.[MCQ]

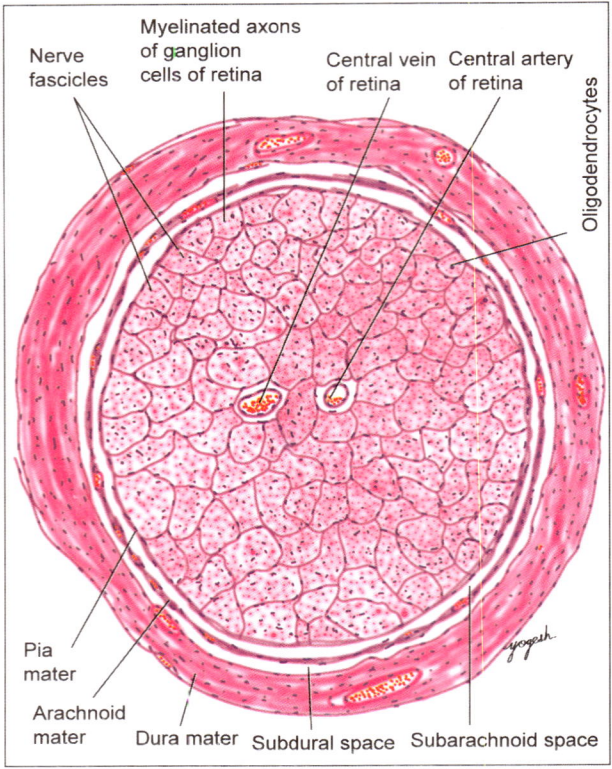

Fig. 27.9: Transverse section of optic nerve (practice figure).

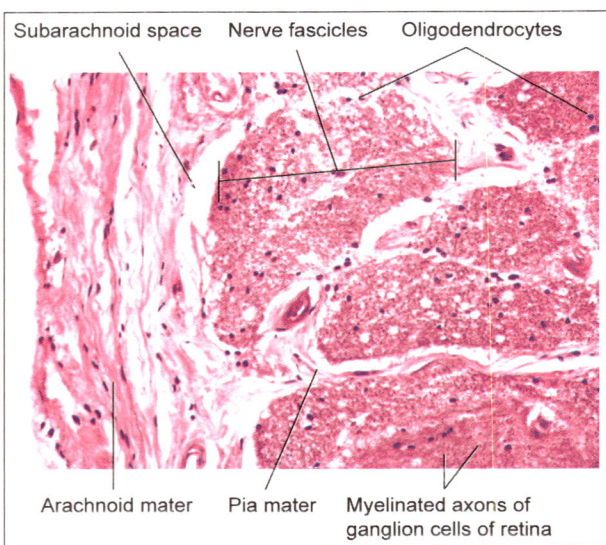

Fig. 27.10: Photomicrograph. Transverse section of optic nerve (high magnification, *H&E* stain).

- In the center of optic nerve, central artery and vein of retina are present.
- Note: As myelin is not produced in optic nerve by Schwann cells; hence, peripheral neuropathies (Guillain Barré syndrome) do not affect optic nerve.

EYELID

- An eyelid is a fold of skin that protects eyeball and helps to keep cornea moist.
- Eyelid consists of the following layers (outside inward) (Fig. 27.11)
  1. Skin
  2. Subcutaneous loose connective tissue
  3. Orbicularis oculi muscle
  4. Tarsal plate
  5. Palpebral conjunctiva
- Skin of eyelid is thin, loose, and elastic in nature.
- Subcutaneous loose connective tissue of eyelid is devoid of fat.
- Deep to subcutaneous tissue, skeletal muscle fibers of orbicularis oculi are present.
- Tarsal plate consists of dense connective tissue. It forms a thick skeleton of eyelid.
- Upper eyelid shows presence of levator palpebrae superioris muscle that opens the eyelid.
- Inner surface of eyelid is lined by *palpebral conjunctiva*. It consists of stratified squamous epithelium with goblet cells. It rests on lamina propria.

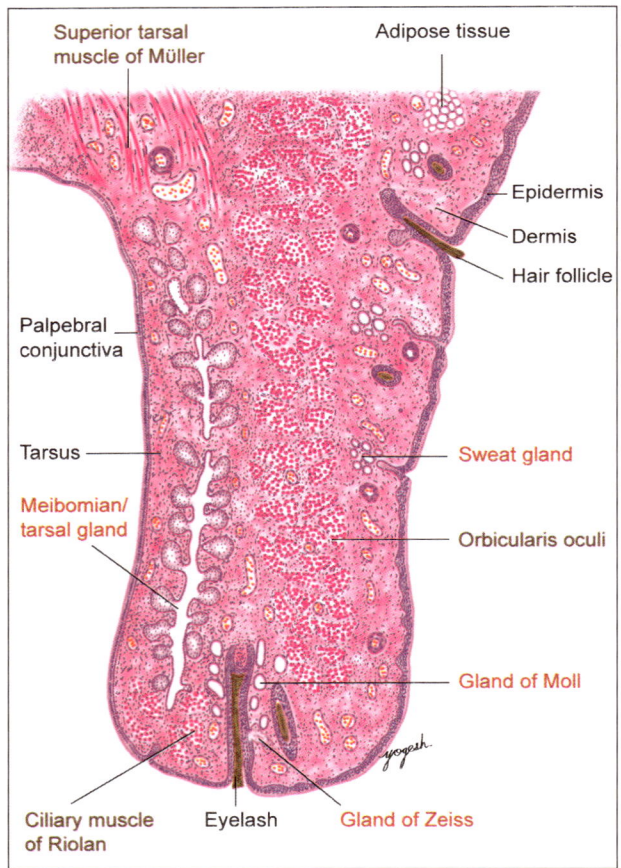

Fig. 27.11: Histology of eyelid (practice figure).

Glands of Eyelid (Fig. 27.11) *High yielding facts*

- Eyelid contains following four glands:*Neet*
  1. *Meibomian/tarsal glands:*
     These are 20–25 long *sebaceous glands* that are embedded in the tarsal plates.*Neet* These produce vertical yellow streaks in tarsal plate. Meibomian gland produces oily secretion that retards evaporation of tears.
  2. *Gland of Zeiss* (*sebaceous glands* of eyelashes): These are small, modified sebaceous glands. These glands are connected with root of eyelashes.*Neet*
  3. *Gland of Moll* (apocrine glands of eyelashes): These are *modified sweat glands* present near the free edges of eyelids. These are also called *ciliary glands.*Neet*
  4. *Glands of Wolfring* and *glands of Krause:*
     These are *accessory lacrimal glands*. Structurally, they are compound tubuloalveolar serous glands. Glands of Wolfring are located on inner surface of upper eyelid, whereas glands of Krause open into the fornix of lacrimal sac.*Neet*

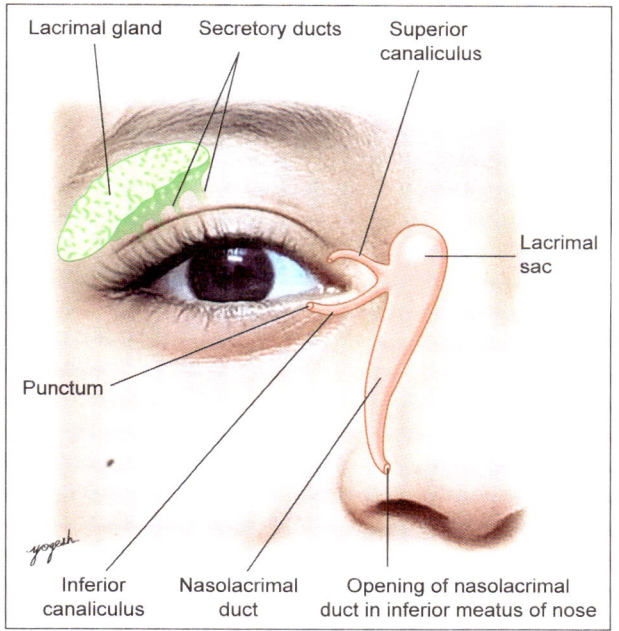

Fig. 27.12: Components of lacrimal apparatus (schematic representation).

Clinical Correlation

- *Chalazion:* It is an inflammation and blockade of tarsal gland. It appears as painless cyst, usually in upper eyelid. Usually, it does not require any treatment. It disappears in few months.
- *Style* (hordeolum): It is a bacterial infection of gland of Zeiss. It produces painful inflammation and redness of eyelid.
- *Conjunctivitis* (pink eye): Conjunctivitis is an inflammation of the conjunctiva. Most commonly it is caused by viruses. Clinical symptoms include redness, irritation, and watery discharge from eye.
  Usually, viral conjunctivitis does not need any treatment other than warm compression and artificial tears.

LACRIMAL GLAND

- Lacrimal gland is a compound tubuloalveolar gland (Fig. 27.12).
- Lacrimal gland produces tear.
- Lacrimal gland is similar to other *serous glands* of the body (Fig. 27.13).

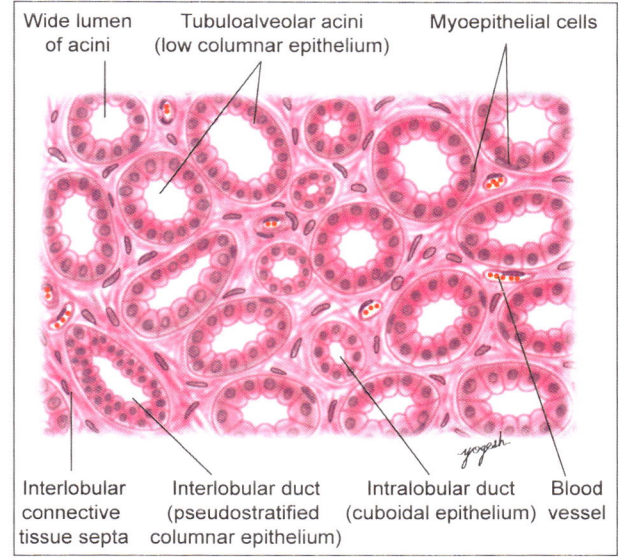

Fig. 27.13: Histology of lacrimal gland (high magnification, practice figure).

Table 27.2: Histological differences between serous salivary gland and lacrimal gland*Viva*

Lacrimal gland	Serous salivary gland
Acini are larger and have wider lumen	Acini are smaller and have narrow lumen
Cells of acini are low columnar	Cells of acini are high columnar (pyramidal)
H&E staining: Eosinophilic cells	H&E staining: Darkly stained basophilic cells (apical eosinophilia and basal basophilia)
Acini are irregular or elongated	Acini are regular or oval

- Some of the differences between lacrimal gland and other serous glands are listed in Table 25.2.
- Smaller ducts of lacrimal gland are lined by cuboidal epithelium.
- Larger ducts of lacrimal gland are lined by pseudostratified columnar or stratified columnar epithelium.
- Myoepithelial cells are located within the basal lamina of acini. These cells help in ejection of tears.
- Ducts of lacrimal gland drain into superior conjunctival fornix.
- *Glands of Krause:* These are accessory lacrimal glands present near the superior conjunctival fornix. [Karl Krause, German anatomist, 1797–1868].

CHAPTER 28

Special Senses II: Ear

Chapter Outline
- Internal ear
  - Bony labyrinth
  - Membranous labyrinth
- Organ of Corti
- Macula
- Ampullary crests

INTRODUCTION
- Ear is the sensory organ of hearing and equilibrium.
- Ear consists of three parts: External ear, middle ear, and internal ear (Fig. 28.1).
- External ear consists of auricle and external acoustic meatus.
- *Auricle* is shaped irregular because of presence of irregularly shaped *elastic cartilage*.

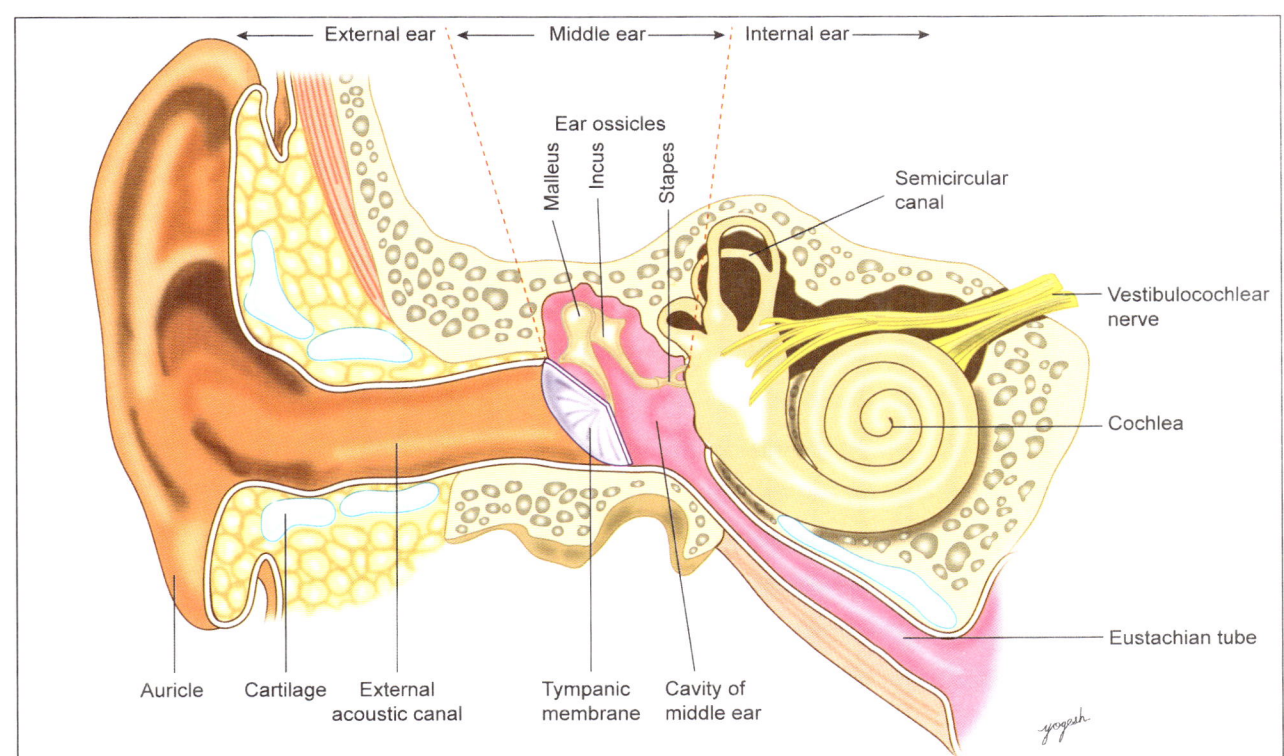

Fig. 28.1: Parts of ear.

- Auricle consists of an elastic cartilage that is covered on both side by tightly adherent layers of thin skin.
- Skin of auricle shows presence of hair follicles, sweat glands, and sebaceous glands.
- Auricle helps to gather sound waves.
- *External auditory meatus*
    - It is a tubular canal that extends from concha to the tympanic membrane.
    - It has two parts: Outer one-third (8 mm) is cartilaginous and inner two-thirds (16 mm) is bony part.
    - It is covered by thin skin.
    - It has *ceruminous glands* (modified apocrine sweat glands) that secrete cerumen or *earwax.*
    - The external ear is separated from middle ear by tympanic membrane

Middle Ear

- Middle ear is a small space in the petrous part of temporal bone
- Middle ear is lined by ciliated columnar or cuboidal epithelium.
- Middle ear contains three ossicles (incus, malleus and stapes) that are composed of compact bone.
- Middle ear contains two skeletal muscles (tensor tympani and stapedius muscles) that control movement of ear ossicles.
- Auditory tube/Eustachian tube connects middle ear cavity with nasopharynx.

Internal Ear

- Internal ear lies within the petrous part of temporal bone.
- It has *bony labyrinth* and *membranous labyrinth.*
- Bony labyrinth consists of three parts: Cochlea, vestibule, and semicircular canals.
- Within the bony labyrinth, there is a system of ducts that constitutes membranous labyrinth

> **Box 28.1: Tympanic membrane**
>
> - Tympanic membrane is a thin partition between external acoustic meatus and middle ear.
> - Shape and size: Oval and 9 mm × 10 mm.
> - It has two surfaces: Outer and inner.
> - Histologically, tympanic membrane consists of the following three layers:
> - 1. Outer cuticular layer of skin
> - 2. Middle fibrous layer
> - 3. Innermost mucous layer
> - Fibrous layer has superficial radiating fibers and deep circular collagen fibers.
> - Inner mucous layer is lined by ciliated simple columnar epithelium.

INTERNAL EAR

- Internal ear lies in the petrous part of temporal bone.
- It consists of two parts as follows:
    1. *Bony labyrinth:* It has three parts: Cochlea, vestibule, and semicircular canals.
    2. *Membranous labyrinth:* It consists of duct of cochlea, semicircular ducts, ductus reuniens, utricle, saccule, and endolymphatic duct and sac.
- Membranous labyrinth is filled with a fluid called *endolymph.*
- Membranous labyrinth is separated from the bony labyrinth by *perilymph* (fluid).

Bony Labyrinth

- Bony labyrinth consists of three parts: Cochlea anteriorly, vestibule in the middle, and semicircular canals posteriorly (Fig. 28.2).

Cochlea

- Bony cochlea resembles the shell of a common snail.
- It is cone shaped, spirally arranged bony canal.
- It has a conical central axis/*modiolus* around which cochlea makes two and three-quarter (2¾) turns.
- A spiral ridge of bone (*spiral lamina*) projects from modiolus and divide the bony cochlear canal into *scala vestibuli* above and *scala tympani* below.
- Scala vestibuli and scala tympani are filled with perilymph.
- *Basilar membrane* completes the division of bony cochlear canal.
- Scala vestibule communicates with the scala tympani at the apex of cochlea by a small opening called *helicotrema.*
- Cochlear nerve emerges from the base of cochlea.

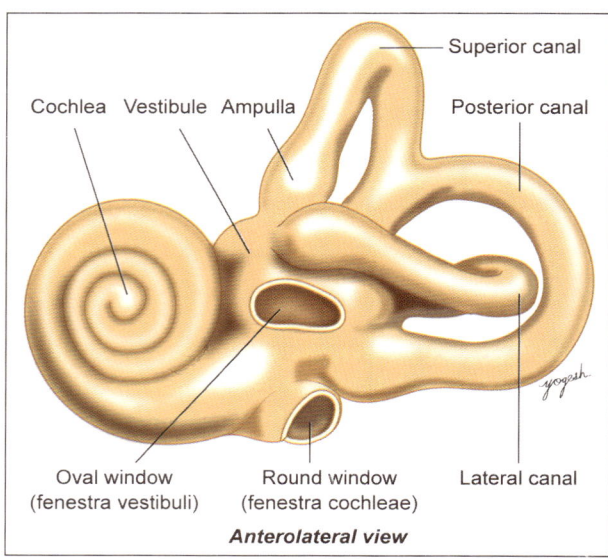

Fig. 28.2: Left bony labyrinth.

Vestibule

- This is the central part of bony labyrinth.
- It opens into the middle ear by two openings:
  1. *Fenestra vestibuli/oval window* that is closed by foot plate of stapes.
  2. *Fenestra cochleae/round window* that is closed by a membrane called *secondary tympanic membrane.*
- Three bony semicircular canals open into the vestibule through five openings.
- Vestibule has opening for *aqueduct of vestibule* and it is closed by *ductus endolymphaticus.*

Semicircular Canals

- There are three bony semicircular canals: Superior, posterior, and lateral.
- Dilated end of each canal is called *ampulla.*
- These three semicircular canals open into the vestibule by five openings.
- These canals lie perpendicular to each other.

Membranous Labyrinth

- It is a membrane-bound cavity filled with *endolymph.*
- Membranous labyrinth has three receptors—organ of Corti (for sound), maculae (for static balance), and cristae (for kinetic balance).
- Membranous labyrinth consists of following parts (Fig. 28.3):
  1. Spiral duct of cochlea or organ of Corti (lies within cochlea)
  2. Utricle and saccule with maculae (lie within vestibule)
  3. Semicircular ducts with cristae (lie within bony semicircular canals).

Duct of Cochlea/Scala Media

- The spiral duct occupies the middle part of cochlear canal between scala vestibuli and scala tympani (Figs 28.4 and 28.5).
- It is triangular in cross section.

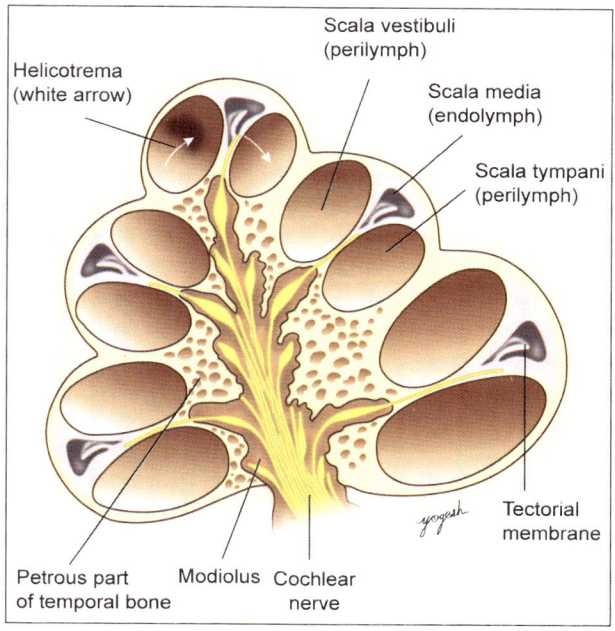

Fig. 28.4: Section of cochlea.

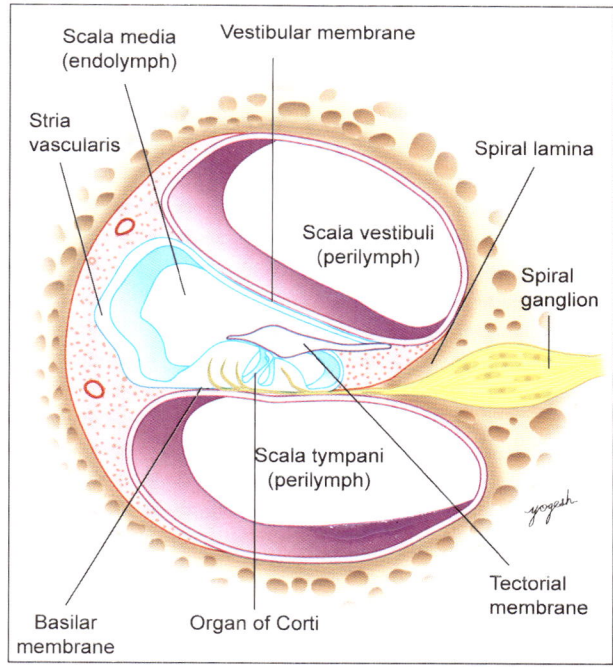

Fig. 28.5: Section of cochlea.

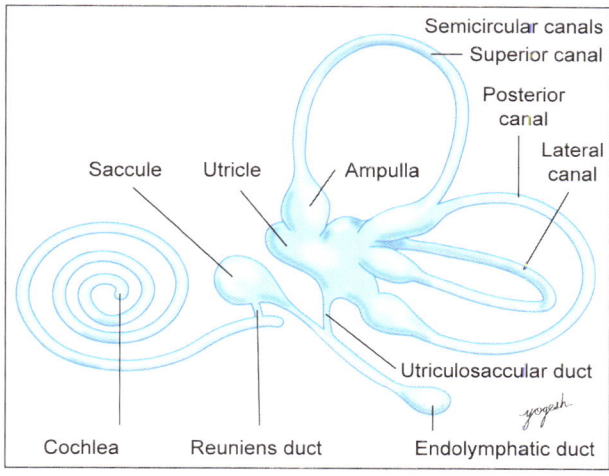

Fig. 28.3: Membranous labyrinth.

- It has three walls
  - Floor – basilar membrane
  - Roof – vestibular/Reissner's membrane
  - Outer wall – bony wall of cochlea
- Scala media contains *endolymph.*
- *Basilar membrane* supports the organ of Corti (end organ for hearing).
- Organ of Corti is innervated by peripheral processes of bipolar cells located in spiral ganglion. Central processes of bipolar cells form cochlear nerve.
- *Vestibular/Reissner's membrane* extends from spiral lamina to the lateral wall of cochlear canal. Vestibular membrane separates cochlear duct from scala vestibuli.
- *Basilar membrane* is a fibrous sheet that extends from free edge of spiral lamina to the spiral ligament.
- *Spiral ligament* is the thickened endosteum of lateral wall of cochlear canal.
- Cochlear duct is connected to saccule by narrow *ductus reuniens.*
- *Stria vascularis* is highly vascular zone in the lateral wall of cochlear duct.

Saccule and Utricle

- These are parts of membranous labyrinth. These consist of thin fibrous sheet lined with simple squamous or cuboidal epithelium.
- Saccule lies within vestibule and is connected to cochlear duct by *ductus reuniens.*
- Utricle also lies within vestibule.
- Utricle communicates ampulla of semicircular ducts through five openings.
- Duct of saccule and ducts of utricle unites with *ductus endolymphaticus.*
- Ductus endolymphaticus has terminal dilatation called *saccus endolymphaticus.*
- Medial wall of saccule and utricle are thickened to form *macula* in each chamber.
- Maculae are supplied by vestibular ganglion. Macula sense linear acceleration.

Semicircular Ducts

- Three semicircular ducts lie within the bony semicircular canals (superior, posterior, and lateral).
- Each semicircular duct has dilated terminal parts called *ampulla* that open into the utricle through five openings.
- Each ampulla has *ampullary crest/crista/cupola.*
- Ducts are arranged perpendicular to each other. Hence, they help to sense angular acceleration of head.

ORGAN OF CORTI

Q. Write a short note on organ of Corti.
Q. List the names of cells of organ of Corti.

- Organ of Corti is an end organ of hearing [Alfonso Corti, 1822–1876, Italian anatomist].
- Organ of Corti is situated on the basilar membrane and extends in a spiral manner along with turns of cochlea.
- Organ of Corti consists of supporting cells, receptor hair cells, and membrana tectoria (Figs 28.6 and 28.7).

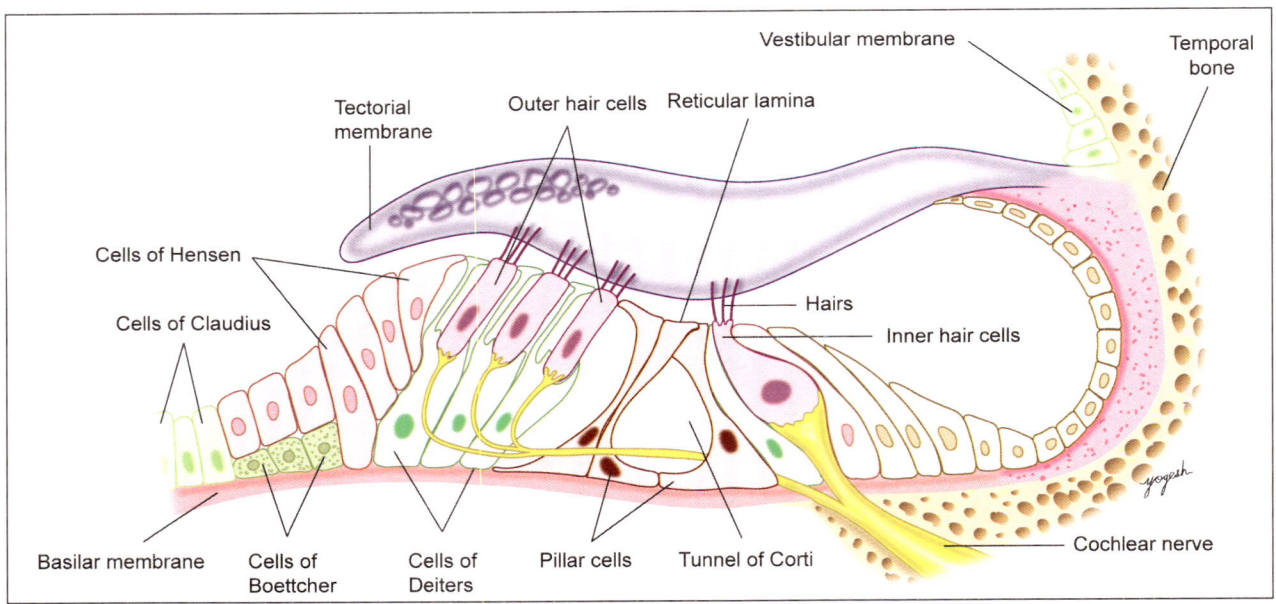

Fig. 28.6: Cells in the organ of Corti.

Special Senses II: Ear

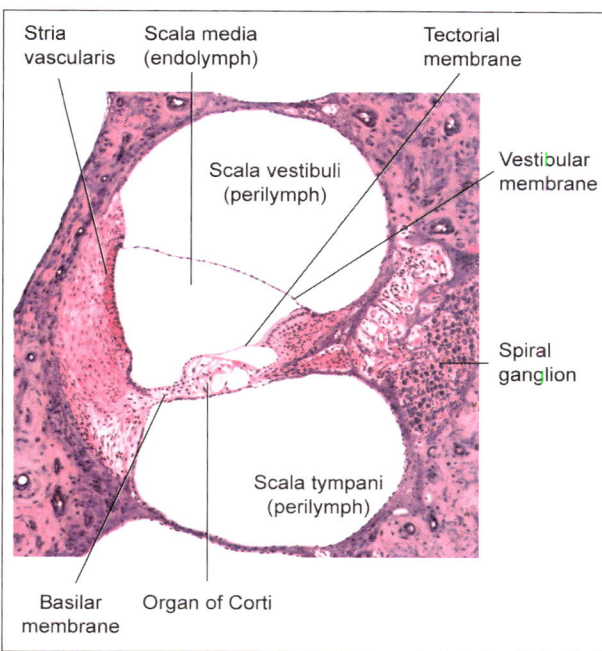

Fig. 28.7: Photomicrograph. Section of cochlea (high magnification, *H&E* stain).

- Cells of organ of Corti are covered by gelatinous membrane called *membrana tectoria.*
- Membrana tectoria is a gelatinous sheet of glycoproteins. Tips of stereocilia of hair cells are embedded in the membrana tectoria.

Supporting Cells

- Organ of Corti has supporting cells such as inner and outer rod cells, phalangeal cells of Dieters, cells of Hensen, and cells of Claudius.
- *Rod cells:* Rod cells have broad base/footplate/crus that rests on basilar membrane and elongated middle part/rod. Rod cells are arranged in two rows as inner and outer rod cells. Heads of these cells have expanded horizontal processes/pharyngeal processes. These processes join to form reticular lamina.
- *Tunnel of Corti:* Rod cells enclose a cavity called tunnel of Corti. It contains *cortilymph* fluid.
- Phalangeal cells of Deiters: These cells rest on basilar membrane and support the outer hair cells [Otto Deiters, 1834–1863, German neuroanatomist].
- *Hensen cells:* These cells support phalangeal and outer hair cells.
- *Cells of Claudius:* These are cuboidal cells that lie lateral to the Hensen cells [Friedrich Claudius, 1822–1869, German anatomist].
- *Bottcher cells:* These are polygonal cells that lie deep the cells of Claudius and rest on basilar membrane [Bottcher Jacob, 1831–1889, German pathologist and anatomist].

Hair Cells

- These are receptor cells of hearing.
- These are columnar/pyriform cells.
- They rest on phalangeal cells (do not reach basilar membrane).
- Their apical surface has thickened cuticular plate and bundle of stereocilia (hairs).
- Cuticular plates of adjacent cells are attached with each other.
- Each hair cell has 30–100 stereocilia.
- Few stereocilia are embedded within the membrana tectoria.
- Hair cells are arranged into two groups: Inner hair cells (a single row) and outer hair cells (3–4 rows).
- Peripheral processes of bipolar neurons end in hair cells.
- *Spiral limbus* bulges into the scala media from the inner angle between the points of modiolus origin of vestibular membrane and basilar membrane.
- Spiral limbus provides attachment to the tectorial membrane.

Box 28.2: Macula

- Maculae are thickened zone in the utricle and saccule (otolith organs) and are called macula utriculi and saccular macula (Fig. 28.8).
- Macula utriculi has ~33,000 hair cells, whereas saccular macula has ~18,000 hair cells.
- Striola is a narrow-curved line in the center that divides macula into two areas.

Structure

- A macula has two parts: Sensory neuroepithelium and otolithic membrane.

Sensory neuroepithelium

- It has hair cells and supporting cells.
- Supporting cells are tall columnar cells with basal nuclei. These cells produce gelatinous otolith membrane.
- Each hair cell has numerous stereocilia at its free surface and one long cilium called *kinocilium.*
- Both kinocilia and stereocilia are embeded in the otolith membrane.
- There are type I and type II hair cells.
- Type I hair cells are flask-shaped, whereas type II cells are columnar.

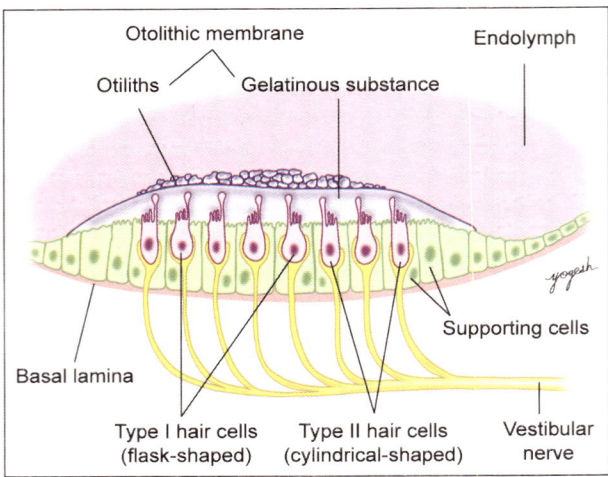

Fig. 28.8: Macula of utricle and saccule.

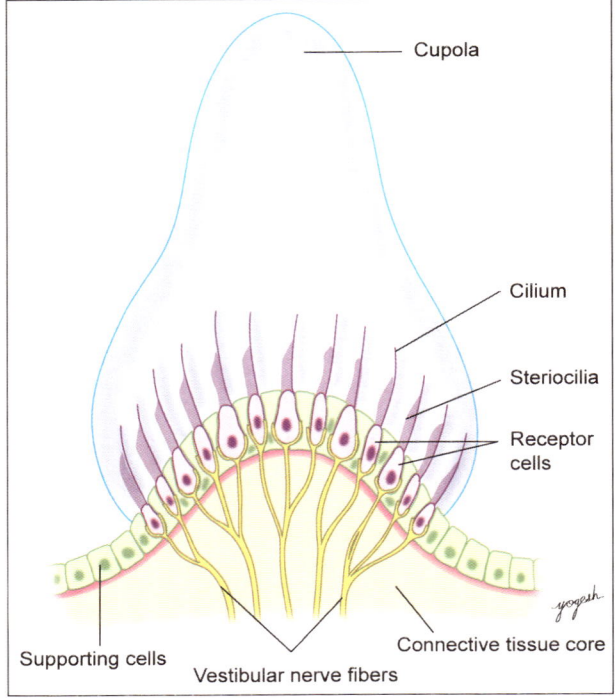

Fig. 28.9: Structure of ampullary crest.

Otolithic membrane
- It consists of a gelatinous membrane.
- It consists of gelatinous mass and otoliths.
- Otoliths (otoconia or statoconia) are crystals of calcium carbonate with organic protein matrix. They are multitude of small cylindrical and hexagonally shaped bodies with pointed ends. They lie on the top of the gelatinous mass.
- The cilia of hair cells project into the gelatinous layer.
- They also have an influence on body posture (through the vestibular nuclei).

Functions
- Macula are the organs of static balance. It appreciates position of head in response to gravity and linear acceleration.
- Macula of saccule sense low frequencies of sound.

Box 28.3: Ampullary crests

- Ampulla of each semicircular ducts has elongated projection called ampullary crest.
- Long axis of the crest lies at right angles to that of the semicircular duct.
- Crest is lined by a columnar epithelium with hair and supporting cells (Fig. 28.9).

Hair cells
- Apical surface of hair cells has two types of hairs: Single large kinocilium and numerous stereocilia (large microvilli).
- *Cupula:* It is a conical gelatinous mass that covers hair cells. Hairs extend into cupula.
- Type I hair cells (inner hair cell) are flask-shaped, whereas type II hair cells are columnar.
- Each hair cell is innervated by terminals of afferent fibers of the vestibular nerve.

Supporting/sustentacular cells
- Supporting cells are elongated and may be shaped like hour glasses (narrow in the middle and wide at each end).
- They support the hair cells and provide them with nutrition.
- They may also modify the composition of endo-lymph.

Function
- Ampullary crests are stimulated by the movements of head.
- When the head moves, a current is produced in the endolymph of the semicircular ducts by inertia.
- This movement causes deflection of the cupula to one side distorting the hair cells and generates signals.

Index

A

A band 93
Aberrations 5
Accessory pancreatic duct of santorini 232
ACE inhibitors 241
Acetyl cholinesterase 99
Achalasia cardia 201
Achondroplasia 75
Acidophils 294
Acinus/acini
    liver 225
    mixed 192
    mucous s 192
    pancreatic 232
    pulmonary 177
    secretory 191
    serous 191
Acne vulgaris 161
Acromegaly 296
Acrosomal cap 253
Acrosome 253
Actin 20, 94
Addison's disease 306
Adenohypophysis 292, 293
Adhesion spots 39
Adhesive belts 39
Adhesive strips 39
Adipocytes 62, 67, 78
Adrenal cortex 302
Adventitia 196, 198
Age pigment 18
Aggrecan 61
Agranular cortex 315
Agranulocytes 64
Albinism 156
Aldosterone 302
Alkaline phosphatase 88
Alopecia areata 160
Alpha keratin 163
Alveolar ductile 279
Alveolar septum 180
Alveoli 177, 180
Alzheimer's disease 21
Ameloblasts 185
Amnion 284
Ampulla 332
    of vater 227
Ampullary crest 332, 334
Anagen 160
Anal columns of morgagni 220
Androgens 304
Androstenol 163
Aneurysm 144
Angiotensin II receptors 240
Annulospiral nerve endings 99
Ansa nephoni 243
Anterior gray horn 309
Antibodies 108
Antrum 270
Apical eosinophilia 31, 49
Apocrine secretion 163, 281
Apoptosis 23
Appendices epiploicae 217
Appendicitis 219
APUD 305
Aqueduct of vestibule 332
Arbor vitae 310
Area cribrosa 238
Areola 279
Areole 66
Argentaffin 211
Artery/arteries 136, 139
    afferent 238
    arcuate 244
    conducting 139
    efferent 238, 244
    elastic 140, 139
    helicine 265
    medium-sized 139
    muscular 139, 142
    renal 244
    small 139
    spiral 274
    trabecular 118
    umbilical 287
Arteriole/arterioles 136, 139, 143
    afferent 244
    muscular 143
    penicillar 118
    structure of 144
    terminal 143
Arteriovenous shunts 147
Arylsulfatase B 19
Asthma 179
Astrocytes 126
Atheromatous plaque 144
Atherosclerosis 144
Atrial natriuretic factor 100
Auditory meatus external 330
Auditory tube 330
Auricle 329
Autocrine signaling 52
Autolysis 18
Autophagy 18
Autorhythmicity 100
Axial filament 254
Axon hillock 124
Axoneme 44
Axons 123
Axoplasm 124

B

Barr body 22
Barrier
    blood–air 181
    blood–aqueous 320
    blood–nerve 131
    blood–retinal 321
    blood–testis 251, 257
    blood–thymic 115
    placental 285, 287
Basal basophilia 31, 49
Basal lamina 36
Basophils 64, 294, 295
Benign prostatic hyperplasia 262
Benign prostatic hypertrophy 263
Bile 223
Bile canaliculi 224, 227
Birefringent substances 3
Bladder stones 248
Blastocyst 284
Blind spot 321
Body/bodies
    balbiani 268
    birbeck 156
    Call–Exner 270
    ciliary 316
    ciliary 320
    Herring 296
    lamellar 155, 181
    Langerhans 156
    Raynaud residual 253
    Russell 63
    tennis-racket-shaped 156
    ultimobranchial 297
    vitreous 325
    Weibel-Palade 143
Bone
    bone marrow 77
    cancellous 85
    cartilaginous 88
    compact 81, 82
    compact 82
    fibrous 82
    formation of 86
    general features of 77
    growth of long 89
    lamellar 82
    matrix 81

membranous 86
spongy 81, 85
trabecular 85, 89
uncalcified 87
woven 81
woven 82
Bony labyrinth 330, 331
Bouton terminal 129
Boutons en passant 129
BP230 39
Brain 308
Brain natriuretic factor 100
Brain sand 306
Brest cancer 282
Brittle-bone disease 56, 91
Bronchi
- intrapulmonary 175
- secondary 175
- segmental 175
- tertiary 175
Bronchial tree 175
Bronchiole 177
- respiratory 177, 179
- terminal 177
Bronchitis 181
Bulboid corpuscle 158
Bullous pemphigoid disease 39

C

C-cells 297
Cadherin 39
Calcitonin 299
Canal/canals
- anal 220
- Cloquet's 325
- Haversian 82
- hyaloid 325
- of hering 227
- of Schlemn 319
- osteonal 82
- pilosebaceous 160
- semicircular 331
- semicircular 332
- Volkmann's 83
Canaliculi 82
Capacitation 254
Capillaries 136, 139, 145
- continuous 139, 145
- discontinuous 146
- fenestrated 139
- glomerular 244
- lymph 109
- peritubular 244
- sheathed 118
- sinusoidal 139
Capsule
- Bowman's 238
- Tenon's 319
Carcinoid 219
Carcinoma
- basal cell 154

epidermoid 154
squamous cell 154
Cardiac myocytes 100
Cardiospasm 201
Cartilage 69
- canals 69
- cellular 75
- elastic 73, 172
- epiphyseal 89
- hyaline 69
  - calcification of 75
- Santorini's 232
- tracheal 174
- yellow elastic 73
- zones of epiphyseal 89
Catagen 160
Catalase 19, 227
Cataract 325
Catecholamines 174, 305
Cathelicidin 161
Cave of Retzius 232
Cavity amniotic 284
CD151 40
Celiac disease 222
Cell/cells 12
- A2 234
- alpha 234
- amacrine 323
- anterior horn 309
- antigen-presenting 62, 108
- apical domain 41
- B 108
- basket 312, 313
- beta 234
- bipolar 323
- bone-lining 81
- bottcher 333
- brush 168, 174, 181
- caveolated tuft 217
- centroacinar 232
- Chadelier 313
- chief 205, 300
- choroid epithelial 126
- chromaffin 305
- clara 178
- clear 162
- cornec'imbal stem 319
- D1 234
- dark 162, 244
- decidual 285
- delta 234
- dendritic 63
- double bouquet 313
- dust 63, 181
- endothelial 136
- enterochromaffin 28, 206, 211, 305
- epithelioreticular 115
- eukaryotic 12
- extraglomerular mesangial 241
- F 234
- fat 62

follicular 268, 297
follicular dendritic 109
fusiform 313
gitter 126
glial 306
goblet 32, 53, 210, 217, 312
granulae 312
granulosa 270
hair 333, 334
halo 256
heart failure 181
Hensen 333
hepatic stellate 226
Hofbauer 285
horizontal 323
Hortega 126
intercalated 244
Ito 146
junctions 38
juxtaglomerular 241
Kulchitsky 174, 305
Kupffer 63, 146, 226
Lacis 240, 241
langerhans 63
Langhans 62
lens fiber 325
Leydig 249, 250, 252
liver 223
M 217
Martinotti 313
mast 62
mesangial 240
mesenchymal 64
Mott's 63
mucous 50, 192
mucous neck 204
Müller 322, 323
mural 147
myoepithelial 105, 162, 192, 280, 328
myoid 105
peritubular 252
natural killer 63, 108
nests 72
of alveolar epithelium 180
of Claudius 333
of connective tissue 61
of epidermis 155
of Hensen 333
of Lymphoid System 107
of Martinoti 313
of Merkel 156
of small intestine 210
olfactory 168
organelles 15
osteoprogenitor 79
oxyntic 205
oxyphil 300
paneth 211
parafollicular 297
parietal 205
pigment 63

plasma 63, 108
PP 234
Purkinje 312
pyramidal 313
receptors 291
resident 55
reticular 109
rod 333
rouget 147
satellite 135
Schwann 127
serous 50, 191
sertoli 249, 251
small granule 168, 174
spermatogenic 251
Stave 118
stellate 312, 313
surface receptors 291
sustentacular 168, 169, 251, 334
T 108
theca interna 270
theca lutein 271
transient 55
umbrella-shaped 35
wandering 55
zymogen 211
zymogenic 204
Cementoblasts 186
Cementocytes 186
Cementum 185
Cementum 186
Central arterioles 117
Central canal 309
Central lymphoid organs 106
Centrioles 21
Centrosome 21
Cerebellar glomeruli 312
Cerebellar hemispheres 310
Cerebellum 310
    afferent fibers of 312
    histology of 311
Cerebrospinal fluid 315
Cerebrum 313
Cervical canal 277
Cervix 274
    histology of 277
Chalazion 327
Channels
    CFTR protein 163
    ligand-gated ion 15
    mechanical-gated ion 15
    voltage-gated ion 15
Cheilitis 184
Cholecystitis 230
Cholelithiasis 230
Chondrocytes 69, 70, 72, 73, 75
Chondronectin 61
Chondrosarcoma 75
Choriocapillary layer 324
Chorion 283

Chorion 284
Chorionic frondosum 284
Chorionic leave 284
Chorionic plate 285
Choroid 316, 320
Chromaffin reaction 305
Chromatic aberration 5
Chromatin 22
Chromophils 294
Chromophobes 294
Chromophore 322
Chromosomes 23
Chyle 109
Chylomicrons 109
Cilia 31, 43
    motile 44
    nodal 44
    primary nonmotile 44
Ciliaris 320
Ciliary processes 320
Circulation
Closed 118
Open 118
Splenic 118
Cis-face 16
Clasmatocytes 62
Classical liver lobule 224
Claudins 40
Clearing 9
Climacterium 267
Clinical crown 185
Cluster of differentiation 107
Cochlea 330, 331
Collagen
    synthesis of 57
    type I 56, 318
    type II 56
    type III 56
    type III 57
    type IV 56
    type XVII 40
Collecting tubules 243
Colloid 297
Colon 217
    adenocarcinoma of 221
Color vision 321
Colostrum 282
Comedo 161
Concentric lamellae 82
Conchae 168
Cones 321
Conjunctiva palpebral 326
Conjunctivitis 327
Connexons 40
Contour lines of Retzius 186
Conus medullaris 309
Copulins 163
Cord pattern 67
Cords of Billroth 118
Cornea 316

conjunctivatization of 318
histology of 316
Corneal
    corpuscles 318
    stroma 318
Corona radiata 270
Corpora amylacea 262
Corpora arenacea 306
Corpora cavernosa 264
Corpus albicans 271
Corpus luteum 271
Corpus spongiosum 264
Corpuscles
    Meissner's 157
    Pacinian 157
    Ruffini 157
Cortex cerebral 313
Cortex cerebral neurons of 313
Cortical labyrinths 238
Corticotropes 295
Cortilymph fluid 333
Cortisol 306
Cotyledons 282
Cretinism 299
Cristae 17, 332
Cryptorchidism 249, 257
Crypts of Lieberkühn 210
Crystalline lens 324
Crystallins 325
Crystals of Reinke 252
Cumulus oophorous 270
Cupola 332, 334
Cushing's disease 306
Cuticle 159, 160, 163
Cystic fibrosis 163
Cystitis 248
Cytochrome C 17
Cytocrine secretion 155
Cytoskeleton 19
Cytosol 12
Cytotrophoblasts 286

D

Decalcification 9
Decidua 283
Decidualization 284
Deep venous thrombosis 149
Dehydration 9
Dehydroepiandrosterone 304
Delta basophils 295
Demyelination 310
Dendrites 123
Dendritic cells of Langerhans 156
Dendritic trees 123
Dense bodies 104
Dental caries 186
Dentine 185, 186
Dentineal tubules 186
Dentinoenamel junction 185
Dermal papillae 154
Dermatoglyphics 154

Dermis 150, 154
Desmin 20, 95
Desmoplakin 39
Desmosine 58
Desmosomes 39, 102, 152
Desquamation 155
Detoxification 16
Detrusor muscle 248
Diabetes insipidus 296
Diabetes mellitus 234, 236
Diaphysis 77
Diastolic pump 140
Dictyotene stage 267
Diencephalon 292
Dihydrotestosterone 262
Dihydroxyphenylamine 156
Dipalmitoylphosphatidylcholine 181
Diphtheria 170
Distal convoluted tubule 243
Distal straight tubule 243
Drumstick body 22
Duchenne muscular dystrophy 21, 95
Duct/ducts
    accessory bile 227
    collecting 243
    excretory 190
    intercalated 190
    intralobular 280
    lactiferous 279
    of cochlea 332
    of Luschka 227
    of Santorini 232
    pancreatic 232
    salivary 189
    semicircular 332
    semicircular 332
    striated 190
    thyroglossal 297
Ductus deferens 257
Ductus endolymphaticus 332
Ductus reuniens 332
Duodenum 212
Dwarfism 75
Dynein 20
Dystrophin 95

E

E-face 14
Ear
    internal 330
    ossicles 330
Earwax 330
Eccentric arteriole 117
Ectocervix 277
Ectopia vesicae 248
Ectopic pregnancy 274
Edema 138
Efferent ductules 250, 254
Elastin 58
Eleidin 153
Ellipsoids 118
Embedding 9
Embryoblast 284
Emphysema 16, 181
Enamel 185
End-bulb of Krause 158
Endocardium 29
Endocervix 277
Endochondral ossification 86, 88
Endocytosis 15, 19
Endolymph 331, 332
Endometrial stroma 274
Endometrium 274
Endomysium 93
Endoneurium 130
Endoplasmic reticulum 15
Endosomes 19
Endosteum 78, 85
Endotendineum 67
Endothelin 137, 138
Endothelium 29, 136, 239
    corneal 318, 319
    functions of 137
    lymphatic 109, 319
Enkephalin 295
Entactin 61
Enterocytes 210
Eosin 9
Eosinophil 64
Ependyma 309
Ependymal cells 126
Epiblast 284
Epidermal ridges 154
Epidermis 150
Epidermolysis bullosa 40
Epididymis 255
Epiglottis 171
Epimysium 93
Epineurium 131
Epiphyses 77
Epiphysis cerebri 306
Episclera 319
Epitendineum 67
Epitheliocytes 115
Epithelium
    ciliated pseudostratified columnar 31
    classification of 28
    corneal 316
    definition 27
    features of 27
    functions of 27
    keratinized stratified squamous 32
    nonkeratinized stratified squamous 33
    parakeratinized 183
    pseudostratified 28, 31
    retinal pigmented 321
    seminiferous 250
    simple 28
    simple ciliated columnar 31
    simple columnar 29, 30
    simple cuboidal 29
    simple squamous 29
    stratified 28, 32
    stratified columnar 35
    stratified cuboidal 34
    stratified squamous 32
    transitional 35, 247
Eponychium 163
Erbin 39
Erectile function 147
Ergastoplasm 16
Erythropoietin 237
Esophagus 198
    Barrett's 201
    functions of 200
    histology of 198
Estradiol 271
Estrogens 267
Euchromatin 22
Exfoliative cytology 37
Exocytosis 15, 50
External anal sphincter 221
External band of Baillarger 315
External os 274, 277
Extracellular matrix 55, 59, 69
Extraembryonic mesoderm 284
Eye 316
Eyelashes 327
Eyelid 326
Eyepiece 4

F

F-actin chain 95
Facia adherens 102
Facilitated diffusion 15
Factor/s
    decapacitation 256
    endothelial-derived relaxing 137
    mullerian inhibiting 249
    oocyte maturation inhibitor 268
    platelet-derived growth 240
    testis-determining 249
    von Willebrand 137
Fascia
    adherens 39
    Buck's 264
    bulbi 319
Fat cells 67
Fenestra cochleae 332
Fenestra vestibule 332
Fenestrated capillaries 146
Fiber/s
    argyrophilic 57
    climbing 312
    collagen 56
    elastic 58
    fast glycolytic 98
    fast oxidative 97
    intermediate 97
    Mossy 312
    muscle 92

intrafusal 99
skeletal 97
nerve 130
    layer of optic 323
    motor 130
    sensory 130
    type I 97, 98
    type II b 98
    type IIa 97
    type IIa 98
    type IIb 98
nuclear bag 99
nuclear chain 99
of Tomes 186
pontocerebellar 312
ragged red 17
red 97
reticular 56, 57
Sharpey's 78, 186
slow oxidative 97
white 98
zonular 320
Fibrillin-1 58
Fibrinolysin 262
Fibroadenoma 282
Fibroblasts 61
Fibrocartilage 74
Fibrocyte 61
fibromuscular stroma 262
Fibronectin 61
Fibrous astrocytoma 126
Filament/s
    beaded 20
    intermediate 20
    thick 95
    thin 95
Filopodia 20
Filtration slits 239
Filum terminale 309
Fimbriae 271
Fistulas 221
Flagellum 254
Fluorophore 3
Focal length 5
Follicular atresia 271
Follicular phase 274
Foramen cecum 187
Fordyce' spots 184
Forms of chromatin 22
Fovea centralis 321
Free nerve endings 157
Freeze fracture 14
Fundus 274

G

G cells 207
G-actin 20
Galactosyl ceramidase 19
Gallbladder 229
Gametogenesis 267
Ganglion/ganglia 122,130, 132

autonomic 135
parasympathetic 135
sensory 132
sympathetic 135
Gap junctions 40, 102, 104
Gastric canals 201
Gastric pits 201, 202
Gastric ulcer 207
Gastric ulcers 201
Gastrin 207
Gastritis 207
Gastroesophageal reflux disease 201
Gastrointestinal tract 196
Gaucher disease 19
Gene 22
    AQP 2 244
    fibrillin 59
    SRY 249
Germinal center 109
Germinal epithelium 267
Gigantism 296
Gland/s 45
    accessory lacrimal 327
    accessory sex 259
    acinar 49
    adrenal 302
    alveolar 49
    apocrine 45, 51
    Bartholin 278
    Bowman's 169
    Brunner's 213
    cardiac 200
    ceruminous 330
    cervical 277
    ciliary 327
    circumanal 221
    classification of 45
    compound 48
    Cowper's 263
    eccrine 50
    endocrine 45
    exocrine 45, 46
    gastric 203
    holocrine 45, 51
    lacrimal 327
    luteal 271
    mammary 279
    Meibomian 327
    Meibomian 48
    merocrine 45, 50
    mixed 50
    modified 163, 279, 327
    mucous 49
    multicellular 45
    of eyelid 327
    of Krause 327, 328
    of Moll 327
    of Wolfring 327
    of Zeiss 327
    olfactory 169
    parathyroid 300

parathyroid 300
parotid 192
pineal 306
pituitary 292
saccular 49
salivary 189
salivary 189
sebaceous 160
serous 49
    of von Ebner 187
simple 48
sublingual 195
submandibular 192
suprarenal 302
sweat 161
    apocrine 162, 163
    eccrine 162
tarsal 327
thyroid 297
tubular 48
unicellular 45, 53
uterine 274
Glial cells 295
Glial limitans 126
Gliosis 126
Glisson's capsule 223
Glomerulonephritis 241
Glomerulus 238
Glomus 147
Glucagon 234
Glucocerebrosidase 19
Glucocorticoids 304
Glycocalyx coat 14
Glycogen 21
Glycoproteins 61
Glycosaminoglycans 60, 61
Goiter 299
Golgi apparatus 13
Golgi complex 16
Gonadotropes 295
Graafian follicle 270
Granular cortex 315
Granular layer of Tomes 186
Granules
    azurophilic 18
    keratohyalin 32
    lipofuscin 18
Granulocytes 64
Granuloma 184
Grave's disease 299
Grossing 9
Ground Substance 59, 81

H

H-band 94
Hair/s 158
    follicle 159
    papilla 159
    shaft 159

exclamation mark 160
terminal 160
vellus 160
Hashimoto's thyroiditis 299
Hassall's corpuscles 115
Haustrations 217
Haversian system of lamellae 82
HCl 206
Helicotrema 332
Hematoxylin 9
Hematoxylin and eosin staining 9
Hematuria 241
Hemidesmosomes 39
Hemorrhoidal plexuses 221
Hemorrhoids 149
    external 221
    internal 221
Hemosiderin 21
Heparin 63
Hepatic coma 228
Hepatitis 228
Hepatocytes 223
Heterochromatin 22
    constitutive 22
    facultative 22
Heterophagy 18
High endothelial venules 112
Histamine 63, 138, 207
Histaminocytes 62
Histiocytosis X 156
Histocytes 62
Holocrine secretion 161
Hordeolum 327
Horizontal cells of cajal 313
Hormone 45, 291
    adrenocorticotropic 295
    antidiuretic 296
    follicle stimulating 295
    luteinizing 295
    melanocyte stimulating 295
    parathyroid 301
    receptors 291
    thyroid stimulating 295, 299
    thyrotropin releasing 299
    β-lipotropic 295
Horn posterior gray 309
Howship's lacuna 80
Humor
    aqueous 316
    vitreous 316
Hyaline membrane diseases 181
Hyalocytes 325
Hyaloplasm 12
Hyaluronic acid 61
Hydrogen peroxide 19
Hydroxyapatite 81
Hymen 278
Hyperadrenalism 306
Hyperparathyroidism 301
Hyperpigmentation 306
Hypertension 144
Hyperthyroidism 299

Hypertrophy 102
Hypoadrenalism 306
Hypoblast 284
Hypodermis 150
Hyponychium 163
Hypoparathyroidism 301
Hypophysis cerebri 292
Hypothalamo-hypophyseal tracts 292
Hypothyroidism 299

I
I band 93
Idopsin 322
Ileum 214
Immunity 106
    acquired 106
    active 106
    cell-mediated 108
    humoral 108
    innate 106
    native 106
    passive 106
Incisura myelini 128
Inclusion bodies Charcot–Böttcher 251
Inclusions 21
Incremental lines of von Ebner 186
Incus 330
Infertility 257
Infiltration 9
Infundibulum 271, 292
Inhibin 251
Insulin 234
Interalveolar pores 180
Intercalated disc 100, 101
Intercellular space 38
Internal anal sphincter 221
Internal band of Baillarger 315
Internal ear 331
Internal os 274, 277
Internal remodeling 72
Interneurons 124
Interstitial implantation 274
Interterritorial matrix 71
Intervertebral discs 74
Intracellular receptors 291
Intrahepatic biliary tree 227
Intrinsic factor 206
Iris 316, 320
    diaphragm 4
Islets of Langerhans 234
Isodesmosine 58
Isogenous group 72
Ito cells 226

J
Jejunum 214
Junctional adhesion molecule 40
Juxtaglomerular apparatus 241

K
K-cells 174
Kallikrein–3 262
Keratan sulfate 70
Keratinization 155
Keratinocytes 155
Keratins 20
Keratocytes 318
Kidney 237
Kinesins 20
Kinocilium 334
Kniest dysplasia 56
Kohler illumination, 5
Koilonychia 164
Krabbe disease 19

L
L-iduronate sulfatase 19
Lactotrophs 294
Lacunae 70, 82
Lamellae 81
    circumferential 84
    interstitial 84
Lamellipodia 20
Lamina densa 36
Lamina fusca 319
Lamina lucida 36
Lamina vitrea 320
Laminin 61, 40, 332
Lamins 20
Langer's lines 155
Laryngitis 171
Larynx 170
Choriocapillary 320
Layer/s
    episcleral 319
    external granular 314
    external plexiform 322
    ganglion cell 323
    ganglionic 314
    granular 312
    Henle's 160
    Huxley's 160
    inner nuclear 323
    inner plexiform 323
    internal granular 314
    Malpighian 151
    multiform 315
    of cerebral cortex 313
    outer nuclear 322
    plexiform 313
    prickle cell 151
    Purkinje cell 311
    pyramidal cell 314
Lens 324, 325
Leukotriene C 63
Levator palpebrae superioris 326
Ligament 67
    elastic 67
    pectinate 319
    periodontal 185, 186

spiral 332
of Cooper 279
Limbus 316
Line/s
   cement 84
   neonatal 186
   pectinate 221
   Zwischenscheibe 94
   milk 279
   of Schreger 186
Lip 183
Lipase 236
Lipid inclusions 21
Lipid rafts 13
Lipofuscin 21, 169
Liquor folliculi 270
Liver 223
   cirrhosis of 228
   failure 228
   lobules 224
   sinusoids 226
Lochia rubra 285
Loop of Henle
   thin segment of 243
Ludwig's angina 170
Lung 175
Lung cancer 181
Lunula 163
Lymph 109
Lymph node 110
Lymphadenitis 112
Lymphatic follicle 109
Lymphatic nodule 109
Lymphatic vessels 109
Lymphocyte/s 63,107, 108
Lysosomal storage diseases 19
Lysosomes 13, 18, 19

M

M cells 211
M-line 94
Macrophages 62, 63
   alveolar 181
Macula 321, 332, 333
Macula adherens 39, 102
Macula densa 241
Macula pellucida 271
Maculae 332
Macular pucker 324
Magnification 5
Major calyces 237
Major histocompatibility complex 14, 108
Malignant melanoma 156
Malleus 330
Mallory bodies 21
Malpighian corpuscle 117, 238
Mammary ridges 279
Mamotropes 294
Mannose-6-phosphate 19
Mastocytes 62
Mater

   arachnoid 308, 315
   dura 308, 315
   pia 315
Matrix 70
Matter
   gray 308, 309
   white 308, 309, 315
Mechanism of erection 265
Mechanism of hormone action 291
Mechanoreceptor 156
Media-Golgi network 16
Mediastinum testis 250
Medullary cords 112
Medullary rays of Ferrein 238
Medullary sinuses 112
Megaesophagus 201
Melanin 155
Melanin pigments 151
Melanocytes 63, 155, 320
Melanophores 155
Melanosomes 156
Melatonin 306
Membrana tectoria 333
Membrane/s
   basement 36
      glomerular 239
   basilar 332
   Bowman's 318
   Bruch's 320, 321
   cell 12
   Descemet's 318
   epiretinal 324
   filtration slit 239
   Heuser's 284
   inner limiting 323
   internal elastic 139
   otolithic 334
   outer limiting 322
   plasma 12, 13
      abaxonal 127
      adaxonal 127
      functions of 14
      modified fluid-mosaic model 13
      transport Across 14
   postsynaptic 129
   Reissner's 332
   tympanic 330, 331
   vestibular 332
Membranous labyrinth 330, 331, 332
Menarche 267
Menisci 74
Menopause 267
Menstrual cycle 267
   endometrium in 274
Menstrual phase 274, 275
Merkel discs 158
Merocrine secretion 163, 281
Mesangium 240
Mesaxon 127
Mesenchyme 64
Mesothelium 29
Metachromasia 63

Metaphysis 89
Metaplasia 37, 181
Metarterioles 145
Metastasis 112
Method
   Cajal's gold chloride 10
   freeze-drying 59
   Gomori's silver impregnation 10
   Gordon–Sweet's 10
   hall's 10
   hexamine–silver 10
   leuco patent blue V 10
   luxol fast blue 10
   Masson-Fontana 10
   osmium tetroxide 10
   PAS 10
   Pearse's staining 10
   Periodic acid–Schiff 10
   Verhoeff–van gieson 10
   Verhoeff's 59
   von Kossa 10
   Weight's resorcin–fuchsin 10
Microfilaments 20
Microglia 126
Microglia 63
Microscope/s
   binocular 4
   bright-field 3
   compound 3
   compound light 3
   dark-field 3
   electron 3, 6
   fluorescence 3
   microscope tube 5
   monocular 4
   optical 3
   phase-contrast 3
   polarized light 3
   scanning probe 3
   simple 3
Microscopy
   confocal 6
   fluorescence 6
Microtome 9
Microtubule organizing center 20, 21
Microtubules 19, 44
Microvilli 31, 41, 210
Middle ear 330
Milk pores 279
Mineralocorticoids 302
Minor calyces 237
Mitochondria 13, 17
Mitochondrial DNA 17
Mitochondrial matrix 17
Mitochondrial porins 17
Mode of milk secretion 281
Modiolus 331
Molecular details of myofibrils 95
Moles 156
Monocytes 63, 64
Mononuclear phagocytic system 63
Motor area 315

Motor end plate 98, 99
Motor unit 98
Mounting 9
Mucinogen granules 204
Mucosa 196
    cervical mucous 277
Mucularis externa 198
Multinodular goiter 299
Multinucleated syncytium 92
Multiple sclerosis 128, 310
Muscle/s
    albinus 232
    arrector pili 160
    bulbospongiosus 278
    cardiac 92, 100
    ciliary 319
    contraction 96
    dilator pupillae 320
    extraocular 316
    involuntary 92
    orbicularis oculi 326
    Santorini's 232
    skeletal 92
        nerve supply of 98
        ultrastructure of 94
    smooth 92
    sphincter pupillae 320
    spindle 99
    striated 92
    striated involuntary 100
    trachealis 174
    visceral striated 92
    voluntary 92
Muscularis externa 196
Muscularis mucosae 197
Myasthenia gravis 99, 115
Myelin
    composition of 127
    osmium staining for 131
Myelin sheath
    formation of 127
    functions of 127
Myocardial sleeves 149
Myoclonic epilepsy 17
Myocytes 92
Myofibril 94
Myofibroblast 61, 105, 116
Myofilaments 94
Myometrium 274
Myosin II protein 94
Myotatic reflex 100
Myxedema 299

N

Nabothian cyst 277
Naevocellular naevi 156
Nail 163
    bed 163
    clubbing 164
    plate 163
    ram's horn 164

    structure of 163
Nasal cavities 167
    vestibule of 168
Nasal septum 167
Nebulin 95
Necrosis 23
Nephron/s 238
    cortical 238
    intermediate 238
    juxtamedullary 238
    types of 238
Nerve
    cochlear 332
    fascicle 131
    olfactory 169
    optic 325
    peripheral 129
    peripheral
    supply of skin 157
Nervi vasorum 139
Neurilemma 127
Neurilemmal sheath 127, 128
Neurites 123
Neurofibrils 123
Neurofilaments 20
Neuroglia 125, 313
    central 126
    peripheral 126, 127
Neurohypophysis 292, 295
Neurolemmocytes 127
Neuromuscular junction 99
Neuron/s 122, 123
    Golgi type II 125
    postganglionic 135
    preganglionic 135
    structure of 123
    bipolar 124
    classification of 124
    Golgi type I 125
    motor 124, 125
    multipolar 124
        postganglionic 135
    pseudounipolar 124, 133
    sensory 125
    unipolar 124
Neurotoxins 99
Neutrophil 64
Nexus 40
Niemann–Pick disease 19
Nipple 279
Nissl bodies 123
Nissl granules 309
Nitric oxide 137, 138
Nodal cells 102
Node of Bizzozero 153
Node of Ranvier 126, 128
Nodules
    singer 171
    teacher's 171
Nuclear envelope 22
Nuclear pores 22

Nucleolus 23
Nucleoplasm 22
Nucleosomes 22
Nucleus 21
Nucleus
    dentatus 311
    emboliformis 311
    fastigius 311
    globosus 311
    pyknotic 23
Numerical aperture 4, 5
Nurse cells 115

O

Objective lens 4, 6
    plan-apochromatic 6
    achromatic 6
    apochromatic 6
    plan 6
    semi-apochromatic 6
Occuldin 40
Odontoblasts 186
Oil red-O 10
Oligodendrocytes 126
Omental appendices 217
Onychia 164
Onychogryposis 164
Onycholysis 164
Oogenesis 267
Oogonia 267
Opsin 322
Optic disc 320, 321
Optic papilla 320
Optic stalk 325
Ora serrata 320
Orcein 59
Organ of Corti 332
Organelles
    membrane-bound 12
    nonmembrane-bound 12
Orthogonal array 67, 318
Ossification 86
Osteitis deformans 82
Osteoarthritis 72
Osteoblasts 79
Osteoclast 63, 80
Osteocyte 80
Quiescent 80
Osteogenesis imperfecta 56, 91
Osteoid 87, 88
Collagen 81
Osteolysis osteolytic 80
Osteoma osteosarcoma 91
Osteon 82
Osteonectin 61
Osteoporosis 91
Otoconia 334
Oval window 332
Ovarian Follicles 267
Ovary 267

Ovulation 271
Oxytocin 296

P

P-face 14
Pace maker 100
Paget-Schroetter disease 82
Paget's abscess 82
Paget's disease 82
Pancreas 231, 232
    endocrine 234
    exocrine 232
Pancreatic duct of Wirsung 232
Pancreatitis
    acute 236
    chronic 236
Panniculus adiposus 62
Panniculus carnosus 155
Pap smear 277
Papanicolaou smear 277
Papillae
    circumvallate 187
    filiform 187
    foliate 187
    fungiform 187
Papillary duct of Bellini 243
Paracortex 111
Paracrine signaling 52
Paraffin block making 9
Parathyroid
    III 300
    IV 300
Superior 300
Paresthesia 301
Paronychia 164
Pars distalis 292, 295
Pars intermedia 292
Pars nervosa 292, 295
Pars tuberalis 292, 295
Peg cells 273
Pemphigus vulgaris 39
Penis 264
Pepsinogen 207
Periarterial lymphatic sheaths 117
Pericellular matrix 71
Pericentriolar area 21
Perichondrium 69, 72
Pericytes 62, 145
Perikaryon 123
Perilymph 331
Perimetrium 274
Perimysium 93
Perineurium 131
Perinuclear cisternal space 22
Perionychium 163
periosteal bud 88
periosteal collar 89
Periosteum 78
Periosteum 85
Peripherin 20
Perl's prussian blue reaction 10

Pernicious anemia 207
Peroxisomes 13, 19
Peyer's patches 197, 216, 217
Phagocytosis 15, 62
Phalangeal cells of dieters 333
Pharynx 169
Pheochromocytes 305
Pheochromocytoma 305
Pheromones 163
Phospholipids 13
Physiological syncytium 41, 102
Pigment
    lipofuscin 223, 304
    visual 322
    lipochrome 259
Pinealocytes 306
Pink eye 327
Pinocytosis 15
Pituicytes 295
Pituitary gland 292
Placenta 282
    functions of 287
    mature 286
    previa 274
Placental septa 284, 285
Plasmalemma 12
Plasmatocytes 63
Plasminogen activator 251
Plasminogen-activator inhibitor 137
Plectin 39
Plexus
    Auerbach's 198
    Meissner's 198
    myenteric 198
    rete cutaneum 157
    rete subapapillare 157
Plicae circularis 197, 209
Pneumocytes
    type I 180
    type II 181
Pneumonia 181
Podocytes 239
Polydipsia 296
Polyribosome 18
Polysome 16
Polyuria 296
Pompe disease 19
Pores of Kohn 180
Porocytosis 129
Portal hypertension 228
Portal lobule 225
Portal triad 224
Portio vaginalis 277
Power houses 17
Power stroke 97
Precapillary sphincter 144
Precentral gyrus 315
Predentine 186
Premelanosomes 155
Premilk 282
Preovulatory phase 274

Presbyopia 325
presynaptic knob 129
Prickle cells 153
Primary
    areole 88
    ciliary dyskinesia 44
    follicle 268
    lymphoid organs 106
    nodules 109
    oocytes 267
    yolk sac 284
Primordial follicle 268
Principal piece 254
Prismatic rod sheath 185
Pro-opiomelanocortin 295
Progesterone 267
Progesterone 271
Prolactin 294
Proliferative phase 274
Prostacyclin 137
Prostaglandins 201, 259
Prostate 261
    adenocarcinoma of 262
    histology of 261
    transurethral resection of 262
Prostate-specific antigen 262
Prostatic acid phosphatase 262
Prostatic cancer 262
Prostatic concretions 262
Prostatic fluid 262
Prostatitis 262
Protein/s
    androgen-binding 251
    clara cell secretory 178
    fibrillin-1 59
    G-actin 95
    glial fibrillary acidic 20
    myosin II 95
    surface active 178
    actin-binding 20
    carrier 15
    channel 15
    histone 23
    ribosome docking 16
Proteinuria 241
Proteoglycans 60
Protio vaginalis 277
Protoplasm 12
Proximal convoluted tubule 242
Proximal straight tubule 243
Psoriasis 155
Pulp cavity 185
Pupil 320
Purkinje fibers 102
Pyloric glands 206
Pyramidal cells of Betz 315

R

Ramus chorii 284
Rathke's pouch 292, 295
Receptors B cell 108

Red pulp 116, 118
Reflex
    milk ejection 282
    stretch 100
Reinke crystalloids 271
Relaxation of muscle fiber 97
Renal
    columns of bertin 238
    corpuscle 238
    microvasculature 244
    pelvis 237
    pyramids 237
    tubule 242
    veins 245
Renin 237, 241
rER 13
Resolution 5
Resorption 80
Respiratory bronchiolar unit 179
Rete pegs 154
Rete ridges 154, 184
Rete testis 250, 254
Reticular lamina 37
Retina 316, 320
Retinal detachment 320
Rhodopsin 322
Ribosomes 13, 18
Rickets 91
Rima glottdis 170
Rima vestibuli 170
Rod 321
Rokitansky–Aschoff sinuses 230
Round window 332
Rugae 201

S

Saccule 332
Saccus endolymphaticus 332
Salivary corpuscles 121
Santorini 232
Santorini's concha 232
Sarcolemma 92
Sarcomere 94
Sarcoplasm 92
Sarcoplasmic reticulum 16, 92
Sarcosome 92
Satellite cells 127
Scala media 332
Scala tympani 331
Scala vestibuli 331
Scalloping of colloid 299
Schmidt–Lanterman 127
Schmidt–Lanterman clefts 126
Sclera 316, 319
Sclerocorneal junction 316, 319
Scrotum 249
Scurvy 57, 91
Seborrhea 161
Second messenger 291
Secondary areolae 88
Secondary follicle 270

Secondary lymphoid organs 107
Secondary nodules 109
Secretory phase 274, 275
Secretory vesicles 13
Seminal fluid 259
Seminal vesicles 259
Seminiferous tubules 250
Sensory cortex 315
Sensory neuroepithelium 333
sER 13
Serine proteases 63
Serosa 196, 198
Serous acini 49
Serous demilunes 50, 192
Sertoli cell barrier 257
Serum amylase 236
Sign
    Chvostek's 301
    Trousseau 301
Signet ring appearance 68
Simple diffusion 14
Sinus
    lactiferous 279
    of Morgagni 170
    renal 237
    venosus sclerae 319
Sinusoid 139, 146
    hepatic 224
Situs invertus 44
Skin 150
    appendages of 158
    blood supply of 157
    glabrous 150
    structure of 150
    thick 150
    thin 150
    types of 150
Sliding filament theory 96
Slit diaphragm
Soloplate 99
Soma 123
Somatomedin C 72
Somatostatin 234
Somatotrophs 294
Space/s
    Bowman's 238
    episcleral 319
    of disse 224, 226
    of mall 225
    perisinusoidal 226
    subarachnoid 315
    Tenon's 319
    intervillous 284
Spatial pinhole 6
Sperm Structure of Mature 253
Spermatocytosis 252
Spermatogenesis 252
    factors affecting 257
Spermatogenic cycle 251
Spermatogonia
    type A dark 252

    type A pale 252
    type B 252
Spermiation 253
Spermiogenesis 253
Spherical aberration 5
Spherule 322
Sphincter
    external urethral 248
    lower esophageal 200
    of oddi 227
    vesicae 248
Sphingomyelinase 19
Spinal cord 308
Spiral lamina 331
Spiral limbus 333
Spleen 116
Splenectomy 119
Splenic nodule 117
Splenic sinusoids 118
Splenomegaly 119
Spongiocytes 304
Spot baldness 160
Spot-welding 39
Stain
    cresyl fast violet 10
    Masson's trichrome 10
    orcein 10
    special 9
Staining 9
Stapes 330
Statoconia 334
Stellate neurons 313
Stem cells 206
Stereocilia 255
Stereocilia 42, 257
Sterile matrix 163
Stigma 271
Stomach 201
Straight tubule 250, 254
Stratum 153
Stratum basale 150, 151, 274
Stratum compactum 274
Stratum corneum 32, 150, 153
Stratum epitheliale pallidum 160
Stratum germinativum 151
Stratum granulosum 150, 153
Stratum lucidum 150
Stratum spinosum 150, 151
Stratum spongiosum 274
Stratum vascularae 274
Stria of Gennari 315
Stria vascularis 332
Striola 333
Style 327
Subcapsular sinus 111
Subcutaneous fat 62
Subendothelial cushions 288
Submucosa 196, 197
Substage condenser 4
Substantia propria 318
Suicide bags 18

Sulcus terminalis 187
Suprachoroid lamina 319
Suprarenal medulla 304
Synapse 128, 129
Synaptic cleft 129
Synaptic cleft 99
Syncytial knots 286
Syncytiotrophoblast 284
Syndecan 61
Syndecan 61
Syndrome
    acute respiratory distress 181
    Alport 57
    cerebrohepatorenal 19
    Cushing's 306
    DiGeorge 115
    Ehlers–Danlos 56, 144
    Guillain–Barré 128, 310
    Hunter 19
    immotile cilia 44, 181, 257
    Kartagener 21, 44, 181, 257
    Marfan 59, 144
    Maroteaux–Lamy 19
    mitochondrial cytopathy 17
    Peutz–Jeghers 184
    Zellweger 19
Syphilis 144
System
    central nervous 308
    endocrine 291
    hypothalamo-hypophyseal portal 293
    nervous 308
        autonomic 122
        central 122
        peripheral 122, 308
        somatic 122
    renin–angiotensin–aldosterone 302

T

T cell receptor 108
T-tubules 97
Taenia coli 217
Tanycytes 127
Tarsal plate 326
Taste buds 187
Tay–Sachs disease 19
Tears 327
Teeth 184
Telogen 160
Tenascin 61
Tendinocytes 67
Tendon 66
Terminal button of axon 99
Terminal cistern 97
Terminal web 39
Territorial matrix 71
    Schamroth's window test 164
Testis 249
Testosterone 249, 252
Tetany 301
Theca externa 270
Theca interna 270
Thermoregulation 147
Thick ascending limb 243
Third ventricle 292
Thymic corpuscles 115
Thymic involution 113
Thymoma 115
Thymus 113
Thymus-dependent cortex 111
Thyroglobulin 299
Thyrotoxicosis 299
Thyrotropes 295
Thyroxine 297
Tight junction 40
Tissue 55
    adipose 67
        brown 68
        yellow 67
    areolar 65
    connective 55
        components of 55
        dense 66
            irregular 66
            regular 66
        embryonic 64
        fibers of 56
        loose 65
        mucoid 288
        specialized 69
        subendothelial 139
    embryonic connective 55
    epithelial 55
    eixation 8
    general connective 55
    lymphatic 106
        bronchus-associated 174
        gut-associated 197
        dense 107
        diffuse 107
        mucosa-associated 107, 119
    mucous connective 64
    muscle 55
    nerve 55
    nervous 122
    processing 8
    regular fibrous 66
    sectioning 9
    specialized connective 55
    structure of erectile 264
    white fibrous 66
Titin 95
Tongue 186
    papillae of 187
Tonsil
    functions of 121
    lingual 187
    palatine 119
Tonsillar crypts 120
Tonsillectomy 121
Tonsillitis 121
Tooth
    decay 186
Toxic thyroid adenoma 299
Trabeculae 86
Tabecular sinus 111
Trachea 172
Trans-face 16
Transcytosis 146
Transport
    active 15
    axoplasmic 124
    passive 14
    transepithelial 146
    vesicular 15
Triad 97
Trigone 248
Triiodothyronine 297
Trophoblast 284
Trophoblastic shell 285
Trophoectoderm 284
Tropomodulin 95
Tropomyosin 95
Troponin 95
Truncus chorii 284
Tube
    eustachian 330
    fallopian 271
    uterine 271
Tubercles of Montgomery 279
Tubuli recti 250
Tubuli recti 254
Tubulin 19
Tunica adventitia 139, 141
Tunica albuginea 250, 264, 267
Tunica intima 138, 144
Tunica media 139
Tunica vasculosa 250
Tunnel of Corti 333
Turbinate 168
Typhoid ulcer 222
Tyrosinase 156

U

Ulcerative colitis 222
Ultra-microtome 7
Umbilical cord 287
Unguis incarnates 164
Ureters 245
Urethra 248
Urethra penile 264
Urinary bladder 246
Urothelium 35
Uterus 274
    cervix of 277
Utricle 332
Uvea 316, 320

V

Vacuoplasm 16
Vagina 278
Vaginitis 278
Valves anal 221

Valves of Kerckring 209
Varicose veins 149
Vas deferens 257
Vasa nervorum 131
Vasa recta 244
Vasa vasorum 139 139
Vascular resistance 144
Vasopressin 296
Vein/s 136, 137, 149
    central adrenomedullary 149
    Santorini's 232
    hypophyseal 293
    hypophyseal portal 293
    large 140, 148
    medium-sized 140, 147
    Santorini's plexus of 232
    small 140, 147
    umbilical 287, 288
Venules 136, 139, 147
    high endothelial 147
    muscular 147
    post-capillary 147
Vermiform appendix 219

Vermilion 184
Vermis 310
Vesicle
    olfactory 169
    synaptic 129
    afferent lymph 109
Vestibular folds 170
Vestibule 331, 332
Vibrissae 168
Villi 197, 209
Villi
    microscopy of 285
    placental 284
    primary 284
    secondary 285
    tertiary 285
Vimentin 20
Visible mucus 201
Visual cortex 315
Visual purple 322
Vitamin A 322
Vitamin D3 237
Vitiligo 156, 306

Vitreous chamber 316
Vocal folds 170

W

Waldeyer tonsillar ring 119
Wear and tear pigment 21
Wharton's jelly 65, 287, 288
White fibrocartilage 74
White line of Hilton 221
White pulp 116
Wilson disease 228

Z

Z-disc 94
Z-line 94
Zona fasciculata 302
Zona glomerulosa 302
Zona occludens 40
Zona pellucida 269
Zona reticularis 302, 304
Zonula adherens 39
Zymogen granules 232